MILADY'S STANDARD
Professional Barbering

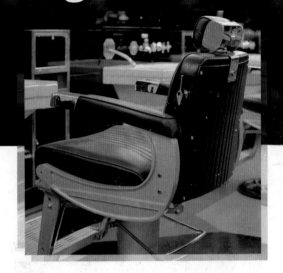

Maura Scali-Sheahan, Ed D

Endorsed by
www.barbersinternational.com

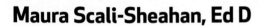
CENGAGE
Learning™

Australia • Brazil • Japan • Korea • Mexico • Singapore • Spain • United Kingdom • United States

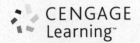
CENGAGE
Learning™

MILADY'S STANDARD Professional Barbering, Fifth edition
Maura Scali-Sheahan
Contributors: Donald Baker Sr. and Donald Baker, Jr.

President, Milady: Dawn Gerrain

Publisher: Erin O'Connor

Acquisitions Editor: Martine Edwards

Product Manager: Jessica Mahoney

Editorial Assistant: Maria Hebert

Director of Beauty Industry Relations: Sandra Bruce

Senior Marketing Manager: Gerard McAvey

Production Director: Wendy Troeger

Senior Content Project Manager: Nina Tucciarelli

Senior Art Director: Joy Kocsis

For product information and technology assistance, contact us at
Professional & Career Group Customer Support, 1-800-648-7450

For permission to use material from this text or product, submit all requests online at **cengage.com/permissions**
Further permissions questions can be e-mailed to **permissionrequest@cengage.com**

Library of Congress Control Number: 2010926975

ISBN-13: 978-1-4354-9715-3

ISBN-10: 1-4354-9715-5

Milady
5 Maxwell Drive
Clifton Park, NY 12065-2919
USA

Cengage Learning is a leading provider of customized learning solutions with office locations around the globe, including Singapore, the United Kingdom, Australia, Mexico, Brazil, and Japan. Locate your local office at: **international.cengage.com/region**

Cengage Learning products are represented in Canada by Nelson Education, Ltd.

For your lifelong learning solutions, visit **milady.cengage.com**

Visit our corporate website at **cengage.com**

Notice to the Reader
Publisher does not warrant or guarantee any of the products described herein or perform any independent analysis in connection with any of the product information contained herein. Publisher does not assume, and expressly disclaims, any obligation to obtain and include information other than that provided to it by the manufacturer. The reader is expressly warned to consider and adopt all safety precautions that might be indicated by the activities described herein and to avoid all potential hazards. By following the instructions contained herein, the reader willingly assumes all risks in connection with such instructions. The publisher makes no representations or warranties of any kind, including but not limited to, the warranties of fitness for particular purpose or merchantability, nor are any such representations implied with respect to the material set forth herein, and the publisher takes no responsibility with respect to such material. The publisher shall not be liable for any special, consequential, or exemplary damages resulting, in whole or part, from the readers' use of, or reliance upon, this material.

Printed in the United States
2 3 4 5 XX 14 13 12 11 10

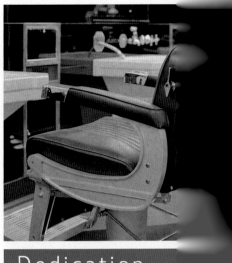

A sincere thank you to Cengage Learning, Jessica Mahoney, Product Manager, and the entire Milady staff for their commitment to maintaining a high standard of excellence of instructional materials dedicated to the barbering profession. It has been my pleasure, once again, to serve the barbering profession through the development of these materials.

Dedication

This edition is dedicated to the educators, students, barbers, state board members, and industry professionals who continue to foster the art and science of barbering. May your commitment to our time-honored profession facilitate the achievement of your goals and professional success.

Sincerely, Maura T. Scali-Sheahan Jacksonville, Florida

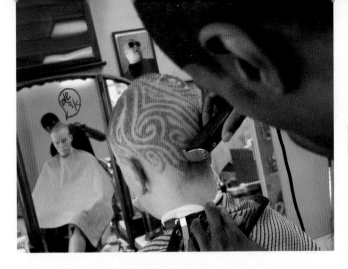

contents in brief

table of contents

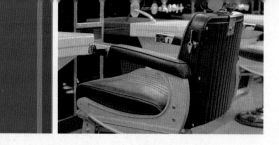

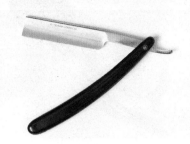

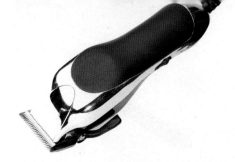

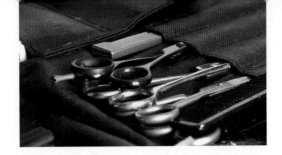

PROCEDURES, PRACTICE SESSIONS, AND TREATMENTS

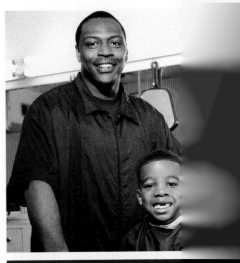

TO THE STUDENT

Congratulations! You have chosen a career filled with unlimited potential, one that can take you in many directions as you become a confident, successful professional. As a barber, you will play a vital role in the lives of your clients. They will come to rely on you to provide professional services and expertise that enables them to look and feel their best.

Milady's Standard Professional Barbering, Fifth Edition was created to provide you with the information you will need to pass the state licensure exams as well the most contemporary techniques to ensure your success in school and employment on the job. This textbook introduces you to a whole new world of technical and human relations skills that will be continually perfected as you spend time working in the profession.

You will learn from gifted instructors who will share their skills and experiences with you. You will learn the latest techniques and specific product knowledge at seminars, workshops, and conventions and you can use your participation to build a network of professionals to turn to for career advice, opportunity, and direction. Whatever direction you choose, we wish you an enjoyable and successful journey.

TO THE INSTRUCTOR

As with previous editions, Milady's *Standard Professional Barbering, Fifth Edition* was prepared with the help of industry instructors and professionals. This involved the hosting of a special focus group made up of national barber board members to review Chapter 14, "Shaving and Facial Hair Design," to make sure the techniques aligned with state board exam criteria. Additionally, a special panel of infection control experts was formed to address health and safety and decontamination guidelines. Next, we collaborated with educational experts to clarify certain portions of the content so various types of learners could understand and process it. Finally, we sent the finished manuscripts to yet more subject-matter experts to ensure the accuracy and thoroughness of the material. What you hold in your hands is the result.

Milady's Standard Professional Barbering, Fifth Edition contains updated or new information on many subjects, including microbiology, infection control, anatomy, shaving, haircutting, and hair replacement. In keeping with the previous revision, this edition provides even more full-color photos and illustrations, along with expanded procedure sections.

NEW ORGANIZATION AND CHAPTERS

The text organization helps to present the material in a logical, sequential order. To help you locate information more easily, the chapters are grouped into five main parts:

Part 1, Orientation to Barbering, consists of three chapters that cover the history of barbering and the personal skills needed to become successful. Chapter 1, "Study Skills," focuses on the kind of techniques and habits needed to get the most out of your education. Chapter 2, "The History of Barbering," outlines the origins of barbering and important facts about its evolution as a profession. Chapter 3, "Professional Image," stresses the importance of attitude, ethics, and health as well as a professional appearance.

Part 2, The Science of Barbering, includes important information to keep barbers and customers alike safe and healthy. Chapter 4, "Microbiology," contains current facts about infectious viruses and bacteria, including MRSA. Chapter 5, "Infection Control and Safe Work Practices," explains how to prevent the spread of infection in the barbershop and the decontamination procedures required by law. Chapter 6, "Implements, Tools, and Equipment," provides detailed information on the tools most used by barbers and how to care for them properly. Chapter 7, "Anatomy and Physiology," Chapter 8, "Chemistry," and Chapter 9, "Electricity and Light Therapy," provide essential scientific information that will affect how you work with clients and products. Chapters 10 and 11, "Properties and Disorders of the Skin" and "Properties and Disorders of the Hair and Scalp," provide the essential knowledge to recognize various disorders and those services that licensed barbers are qualified to offer their clients.

Part 3, Professional Barbering, which includes Chapter 12, "Treatment of the Hair and Scalp, Chapter 13, Men's Facial Massage and Treatments, Chapter 14, Saving and Facial Hair Design, Chapter 15, Men's Haircutting and Styling, and Chapter 16, "Men's Hair Replacement," offers updated material and step-by-step procedures accompanied by full-color photographs for accurate presentation of the material.

Part 4, Advanced Barbering Services, contains four chapters devoted to additional services often found in the barber shop—"Women's Haircutting and Styling," "Chemical Texture Services," "Haircoloring and Lightening," and "Nails and Manicuring"—for those states requiring proficiency in these areas.

Part 5, The Business of Barbering, opens with the newly repositioned Chapter 21, "State Board Preparation and Licensing Laws," followed by Chapter 22, "The Job Search," and Chapter 23, "Barbershop Management". In Chapter 21, students are provided with various methods to prepare for licensure examination and a general overview of barber licensing law. New content in Chapter 22 explains worker classifications important to job seekers, as does Chapter 23 as it applies to shop owners.

ELEMENTS

This edition includes the many features that were new to the previous edition with a few additions to help students master key concepts and techniques.

- *Boxed Features:* Elements such as *Focus On, Did You Know, FYI, Here's a Tip,* and *Caution* provide hints, interesting information, and targeted concepts to help sharpen skills and draw attention to special situations. New to this edition is the *Tip from the NABBA* feature that provides students with professional insights from state barber board members.
- *Key Terms:* The words students need to know in each chapter are given at the beginning in a list of key terms. The first time a word is used and defined in the text, the word appears in boldface. If the word is difficult to pronounce, a phonetic pronunciation appears after it in parentheses.
- *Chapter Glossary:* All key terms and their definitions are included in the glossary at the end of the chapter, as well as the Glossary/Index at the end of the text.
- *Learning Objectives:* Each chapter begins with a list of learning objectives that highlight important information in the chapter.
- *Review Questions:* Each chapter ends with questions designed to test student's understanding of the information. The answers appear in the Instructor's Course Management Guide.

FRESH NEW DESIGN

The changes in this edition of *Milady's Standard Professional Barbering* go far beyond the new content and features. Over 400 new four-color illustrations and photographs enhance this book, along with a totally new text design that incorporates easy-to-read type and easy-to-follow layout. Photographs using mannequins and live models are included to illustrate styles and procedures. New structure graphics are used to show lines, forms, reference points, and more, ensuring comprehension of the theory underlying general principles.

EXTENSIVE LEARNING/TEACHING PACKAGE

While *Milady's Standard: Professional Barbering, Fifth Edition* is the center of the curriculum, students and educators have a wide range of supplements from which to choose. All supplements have been revised and updated to complement the new edition of the textbook, including a new technology component, *Milady's Standard Barbering WebTutor.* Below you can find more information on the supplements offered with this edition.

STUDENT WORKBOOK

The Workbook is designed to reinforce classroom and textbook learning and contains chapter-by-chapter exercises, including fill-in-the-blank, matching, and labeling. All are coordinated with the material from the text.

EXAM REVIEW

The Exam Review contains chapter-by-chapter questions and three sample state board examinations in a multiple-choice format to help students prepare for licensure. The questions are for study purposes only and are not the exact questions students will see on the licensure exam.

STUDENT CD-ROM

The student CD-ROM is an interactive student product designed to reinforce classroom learning, stimulate the imagination, and aid in preparation for board exams. Featuring more than 20 video clips and graphic animations to demonstrate practices and procedures, this tool also contains a text test bank with 1,000 chapter-by-chapter or randomly accessed multiple-choice questions to help students study for the exam. There is also a game bank and a pronunciation glossary that pronounces and defines each term.

INSTRUCTOR'S PRINT COURSE MANAGEMENT GUIDE

The Course Management Guide contains all the materials educators need in one package. Included in this bound book are lesson plans, chapter review questions and answers, chapter tests and answer keys, supplements, and student workbook answer keys. A transition tools guide provides a synopsis of each chapter to help instructors find material that has been moved or changed in the new edition of the textbook. Also included is a lesson plan activity and supplement index for easy reference and pre-lesson planning.

INSTRUCTOR'S COURSE MANAGEMENT GUIDE ON CD-ROM

Everything found in the print version of the Course Management Guide is contained on this easy-to-use CD-ROM. The print material is formatted in easy-to-print PDF format so only select material need be printed and used at any given time. The CD-ROM also includes a computerized test bank containing multiple-choice questions that instructors can use to create random tests from a single chapter or the entire book. Answer keys are automatically created.

DVD SERIES

Milady continues to offer a two-hour DVD series that offers interactive content for classroom use. This two-disc set provides instructors with easy-search features and optional Spanish subtitles.

POWERPOINT® PRESENTATION

The new Instructor Support Slides use a PowerPoint® presentation to make lesson delivery simple yet incredibly effective. Complete with photos and art, this chapter-by-chapter CD-ROM has ready-to-use presentations that will help engage students' attention and keep their interest throughout the lesson.

ONLINE LICENSING PREPARATION

Milady's Online Licensing Preparation helps students to study for their state board licensing examinations. In the course, you can select chapter-specific questions or comprehensive 100-question exams. The program scrambles the test questions to ensure you have a new exam every time you log on!

WEBTUTOR ADVANTAGE ON WEBCT, ANGEL, AND BLACKBOARD

The WebTutor Advantage is an eHomework solution product. It is new to this addition, and contains the following elements: flashcards with audio using the text's glossary terms, quiz questions for each chapter, learning objectives and printable study notes, Hangman, labeling games, situational problems and questions for every chapter as well as short video clips from the DVD series, and links to other helpful websites.

The author and publisher wish to thank the professionals who took their valuable time to provide their insight and suggestions in the development of this book. We are indebted to them.

FOCUS GROUP PARTICIPANTS

- Charles Kirkpatrick, Arkadelphia Beauty College, Arkadelphia, AR
- David Jones, Georgia State Board of Barbers, GA
- Ed Barnes, King's Row Hairstyling, Lexington, S.C.
- Lee Roy Tucker, Tucker's Style Shop, Midwest City, OK
- Larry M. Little, AR College of Barbering & Hair Design Inc., Little Rock, AR
- Gene Record, Cold Spring, KY
- Gussie O'Connor, Coeur d'Alene, ID
- David A. Reed, Oklahoma City, OK
- Derek Davis, Washington, D.C.
- Joyce Voss, Phoenix, AZ
- Sam La Barbera, Arizona State Board of Barbers, Phoenix, AZ
- Sam Barcelona, Arizona State Board of Barbers, Phoenix, AZ
- Theresa Iliff, Northstar Center, Minneapolis, MN

REVIEWERS

- Arthur D. Knox, Universal Barber College, Phoenix, AZ
- Christopher D. Felder, The Long Island Barber Institute, Hempstead, NY
- Dale Sheffield, Roffler-Moler Hairstyling College, Marietta, GA
- Dawn N. Mango, John Paul Institute, Saratoga, NY
- Debbie Eckstine-Weidner, DeRielle Cosmetology Academy, Mechanicsburg, PA
- Deborah Beatty, former instructor at Columbus Technical College, Columbus, GA
- Derek Davis, Davis Barber and Beauty Services, Washington, DC
- Dr. Carolyn R. Kraskey, Central Beauty School. Minneapolis & Cambridge, MN
- Edwin Barnes, King's Row, Columbia, SC
- Ernestine Pledger-Peete, Tennessee Technology Center, Memphis, TN
- Frances L. Archer, Cat's Barber & Style, Columbia, SC
- Glynis Powell, A-1 Beauty & Barber College, Portsmouth, VA
- Johnnie T. Major, Master Barber and Instructor, Columbia, SC
- Joseph P. Kincheloe, Sr., Southern Arizona Barber College, Tucson, AZ
- Joyce Voss, Arizona Board of Barbers, AZ
- Ladell Walker-Chalk, Chalk Board Enterprise, Mid Cities Barber College Dallas, TX
- Larry M. Little, Arkansas College of Barbering and Hair Design, AR
- Lisa Sparhawk, Private Educator, Albany, NY
- Maria Moffre Lynch , Cosmetology Consultant, Round Lake, NY
- Mary Bryant, New Tyler Barber College, Inc., North Little Rock, AR
- Michael J. DeRiggi, DeRiggi's Hair Studio, Allison Park, PA
- Nancy Barsic, Success Schools LLC, IN
- Phyllis M. Causey, M. Ed., Instructional Designer, TX

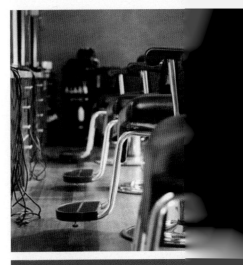

Acknowledgme

- Ray Grypp, Quad City Barber & Hairstyling College, IL
- Ronald L. Brown, Roffler School of Hair Design, Austin, TX
- Sam J. Barcelona, Arizona State Board of Barbers, Phoenix, AZ
- Sandra Peoples, Pickens Technical College, CO
- Suzi Lynch, O'Brien's Training Center, South Burlington, VT
- Thamer S. Hite & Lynell Hite , Master Barbers, Founder of The Barber School, UT
- Theodore Taylor, Flint Institute of Barbering, Inc., Flint, MI
- Tom McArthur, ABC Barber College, AR
- Walter J. Lupu, School Director, Barber/Styling College Inc., Lansing, MI
- Zane Skerry, Executive Director Massachusetts Board of Barbers, MA

Special thanks to the following contributors for their support and assistance:

- Javier Rivera, Maestro's Barbershop, Latham, New York, for use of his shop for the photo shoot and for being so accommodating to all of the staff and models.
- Deb Windus at Burmax for her help with locating mannequin and supplies for the photo shoot. Mannequins provided by Burmax.
- Gregory Zorian, III, Master Barber, Gregory's Babershop, Clifton Park, New York and Steve Vilot, Sims Barbershop, Guilderland, New York. Thank you for allowing us the use of your beautiful location for photographs and for performing haircuts as part of the shoot.
- Nelson Dauila, Master Barber, Springfield, Massachusetts, for participating as a barber and locating models. The shoot would not have been such a success without your involvement and expertise.
- Tunika "Tek-nik" Beard, Barber, Albany, NY, for assisting in haircutting and chemical texture services, as well as locating models for the photo shoot.
- Andis, Marvy Company, Wahl, and 44/20 for use of product photographs.
- The Worshipful Company of Barbers, London, England, for use of image of the Holbein painting, *King Henry VIII issuing charter to the Barber-Surgeon's company.*
- Austin Spa & Technology School, Albany, New York, for use of their excellent facility for the photo shoot. Also to their barbering instructor and students for graciously participating as models and/or barbers for the photo shoot.
- Advanced Hair Products Inc. for supplying the hair replacement systems and additional supplies for the hair replacement chapter.

GUEST BARBERS AND NAIL TECHNICIANS

The author and editors would like to thank the following for their assistance:

- Donald Baker, Sr., Master Barber, Wallace, NC
- Donald Baker, Jr., Master Barber, West Palm Beach, FL
- Gregory Zorian, III, Master Barber, Delmar, NY
- Larry M. Little, Master Barber and school owner, Little Rock, AR
- Nelson Dauila, Master Barber, Springfield, MA
- Zane Skerry, Executive Director, Massachusetts Barber Board
- Javier Rivera, Barber, Latham, NY

- Tunika Beard, Barber, Albany, NY
- Joseph Johnson, Austin Beauty School, Instructor and Barber, Albany, NY
- Juliette Vilot, Nail Technician, Sims Barbershop, MA
- Glenn Smith, Barber, Schenectady, NY
- Orlondo Hundley, Barber, Schenectady, NY

PHOTOGRAPHERS

- Yanik Chauvin, Professional Photographer, Montreal, Canada (http://www.touchphotography.com)
- Dino Petrocelli, Professional Photographer, Albany, NY (http://www.dinopetrocelli.com)
- Paul Castle, Castle Photography, Inc., Troy, NY (http://www.castlephotographyinc.com)
- Michael Dzaman Photography © Michael Dzaman/Dzaman Photography (http://www.dzamanphoto.com)

PHOTO CREDITS

Chapter 1: chapter opener, Figure 1-4 © Milady, a part of Cengage Learning. Photography by Dino Petrocelli. Figure 1-1, 1-3 © Milady, a part of Cengage Learning.

Chapter 2: chapter opener, Barber Shop Sign © Sherry Ann Elliott, 2010; used under license from Bigstock™; Figure 2-1 © Milady, a part of Cengage Learning. Photography by Paul Castle. Figure 2-3 Corbis. Figure 2-4, 2-14 © Milady, a part of Cengage Learning. Figure 2-2 courtesy of Manx National Heritage. Figures 2-5, 2-6 and 2-7 with permission of The Worshipful Company of Barbers, London, UK. Figure 2-8 (traditional barber shop pole) Peter Blazek, 2009; shutterstock.com. Figure 2-9 New York State Archives; Series 12979-79, Union label registration application files, ca. 1901-1943 (Box 2, Folder 27, No. 101). Applications (with a copy of the label) were received by the Secretary of State for registration of trade union labels, marks, names, brands or devices that graphically designate the products of the labor of associations or unions. Figure 2-10 excerpt from The Associated Master Barbers and Beauticians of America. Figure 2-11 courtesy of Kojo Kanau. Figure 2-12 courtesy of William Marvy Company.

Chapter 3: chapter opener, (barber standing outside shop); © Monkeybusiness images, 2010; used under license from Dreamstime.com. Figure 3-1, 3-2, 3-8 © Milady, a part of Cengage Learning. Photography by Paul Castle. Figure 3-3 © Milady, a part of Cengage Learning. Figure 3-4 to 3-7, 3-9, 3-10 © Milady, a part of Cengage Learning. Photography by Yanik Chauvin. Figure 3-11, Getty Images.

Chapter 4: chapter opener, (microscope); © STILLFX, 2010; used under license from Shutterstock.com. Figure 4-1 to 4-6 © Milady, a part of Cengage Learning. Figure 4-7 Courtesy of Godrey F. Mix, DPM Sacramento, CA. Figure 4-8 courtesy of Robert A. Silverman, MD, Clinical Associate Professor, Department of Pediatrics, Georgetown University. Figure 4-9 The National Pediculosis Association, Inc®.

Chapter 5: chapter opener, Figure 5-17 © Milady, a part of Cengage Learning. Photography by Yanik Chauvin. Figure 5-1 Courtesy of U.S. Department of Labor. Figure 5-2 © Milady, a part of Cengage Learning. Photography by Dino Petrocelli. Figures 5-3, 5-4, and 5-5 courtesy of William Marvy Company. Figure 5-6 to 5-16, 5-19 © Milady, a part of Cengage Learning. Photography by Paul Castle. Figure 5-18 © Milady, a part of Cengage Learning. Photography by Larry Hamill.

Chapter 6: chapter opener, Figures 6-4, 6-12, 16-14 to 16-16b, 6-33, 6-44 to 6-50, 6-52b © Milady, a part of Cengage Learning. Photography by Yanik Chauvin. Figures 6-1 to 6-3, 6-5 to 6-11, 6-16c to 6-20, 6-34a, 6-34b to 6-40, 6-42, 6-43, 6-53a, 6-54, 6-62 © Milady, a part of Cengage Learning. Photography by Paul Castle. Figure 6-13, 6-41, 6-61, 6-63 © Milady, a part of Cengage Learning. Figures 6-21 to 6-29 courtesy of the Andis Company. Figures 6-30 to 6-32b, 6-52a, 6-53b, 6-55 to 6-57 © Milady, a part of Cengage Learning. Photography by Dino Petrocelli. Figure 6-51 courtesy of Morris Flamingo, Inc./Campbell Lather King. Figures 6-58 to 6-60 © Milady, a part of Cengage Learning. Photography by Larry Hamill.

Chapter 7: chapter opener, (Xray bronze Vitruvian man); © James Steidl, 2010; used under license from Shutterstock.com. Figures 7-1 to 7-17 © Milady, a part of Cengage Learning.

Chapter 8: chapter opener, (render of molecule); © suravid, 2010; used under license from Shutterstock.com. Figures 8-1 to 8-16 © Milady, a part of Cengage Learning.

Chapter 9: chapter opener, (hot pulse); © Jodi Baglien Sparkes, 2010; used under license from Shutterstock.com. Figures 9-1 to 9-7, 9-10 to 9-12 © Milady, a part of Cengage Learning. Figure 9-8, 9-9 © Milady, a part of Cengage Learning. Photography by Larry Hamill.

Chapter 10: chapter opener, (side view of young man); © Robert Kneschke, 2010; used under license from Shutterstock.com. Figures 10-1 to 10-5, 10-9 © Milady, a part of Cengage Learning. Figures 10-6, 10-7, 10-10, 10-13, 10-16, 10-17c and d, 10-18, 10-19, 10-21, 10-23, 10-24, and 10-25 Reproduced with permission from the American Academy of Dermatology, Copyright © 2010. All rights reserved. Figure 10-8 courtesy of Timothy Berger, MD, Associate Clinical Professor, University of California San Franciso. Figure 10-14 and 10-15 courtesy of the Centers for Disease Control and Prevention (CDC). Figures 10-11, 10-12 and 10-22 T. Fitzgerald, *Color Atlas and Synopsis of Clinical Dermatology*, 3E, 1996. Reprinted with permission of The McGraw-Hill Companies. Figures 10-17a and b courtesy of Mark Lees Skin Care. Figure 10-20 courtesy of National Rosacea Society.

Chapter 11: chapter opener, (high angle view of hairdresser); © Diego Cervo, 2010; used under license from Shutterstock.com. Figures 11-1, 11-4 to 11-8, 11-11, 11-15, 11-23 © Milady, a part of Cengage Learning. Figures 11-2, 11-9, and 11-24 to 11-26 courtesy of P&G Beauty and Grooming, The World of Hair, by Dr. John Gray. Figure 11-3 Reproduced from Clairol, Inc. Figures 11-12, 11-13 © Milady, a part of Cengage Learning. Photography by Paul Castle. Figures 11-18 and 11-21 courtesy of Robert A. Silverman, MD, Clinical Associate Professor, Department of Pediatrics, Georgetown University. Figures 11-10, 11-14, and 11-16 courtesy of Pharmacia and Upjohn Company. Figures 11-17a and b photography courtesy of P & G Beauty. Figure 11-19 The National Pediculosis Association, Inc®. Figure 11-20 courtesy of Hogil Pharmaceutical Corporation. Figure 11-22 Reproduced with permission from the American Academy of Dermatology, Copyright 2010. All rights reserved.

Chapter 12: chapter opener, Figures 12-1, 12-8 to 12-25 © Milady, a part of Cengage **Learning.** Photography by Paul Castle. Figures 12-2 © Milady, a part of Cengage Learning. Figures 12-3a to 12-7 © Milady, a part of Cengage Learning. Photography by Dino Petrocelli. All procedure photos, © Milady, a part of Cengage **Learning.** Photography by Paul Castle. Illustrations in procedures, © Milady, a part of Cengage Learning.

Chapter 13: chapter opener, (adult male getting a facial); © 2010; used under license from Fotosearch.com. Figure 13-1a-b to 13-4, 13-19, 13-21, 13-22 © Milady, a part of Cengage Learning. Figures 13-5 to 13-11 © Milady, a part of Cengage Learning. Photography by Paul Castle. Figures 13-12 to 13-18, 13-20, 13-23 to 13-25 © Milady, a part of Cengage Learning. Photography by Larry Hamill. Illustrations in procedures, © Milady, a part of Cengage Learning. All procedure photos, © Milady, a part of Cengage Learning. Photography by Paul Castle.

Chapter 14: chapter opener, Figures 14-2 a-d, 14-4, 14-5, 14-9 to 14-12, 14-15 to 14-36 © Milady, a part of Cengage Learning. Photography by Yanik Chauvin. Figure 14-1, 14-3, 14-6 to 14-8, © Milady, a part of Cengage Learning. Procedure 14-1, steps B1a and B1b, 14-13a to 14-14i, 14-37 to 14-52 © Milady, a part of Cengage Learning. Photography by Paul Castle. All other Procedure photos © Milady, a part of Cengage Learning. Photography by Yanik Chauvin.

Chapter 15: chapter opener, Figures 15-36 to 15-38a, 15-39 to 15-41, 15-52 to 15-58, 15-61, 15-64, 15-102, 15-103, 15-113 to 128, 15-132, 15-133, 15-137 to 15-150 © Milady, a part of Cengage Learning. Photography by Paul Castle. Figures 15-1 to 15-33b, 15-35, 15-74 to 15-98, 15-104 to 112, Procedure 15-1 illustrations © Milady, a part of Cengage Learning. Figure 15-34a photos used with permission of the authors, Martin Gannon and Richard Thompson, as featured in their book, *Mahogany: Steps to Colouring and Finishing Hair.* Copyright Martin Gannon and Richard Thompson. 1997. Figures 15-34b and 15-72a provided by Anetta Nadolna. Figure 15-38b, 15-42 to 15-51, 15-59a to 15-60, 15-62 to 15-63b, 15-65 to 15-70c, 15-72b, 15-73, 15-99 to 15-101, 15-129a to 131b, 134a to 136b © Milady, a part of Cengage Learning. Photography by Yanik Chauvin. Figure 15-71, courtesy of William Marvy Company. Figure 15-151 Preston Phillips. Procedures 15-1, 15-2, 15-3, 15-6, 15-7 to 15-9 © Milady, a part of Cengage Learning. Photography by Paul Castle. Procedure 15-4, 15-5 © Milady, a part of Cengage Learning. Photography by Yanik Chauvin.

Chapter 16: chapter opener, Figures 16-3, 16-13a to 16-16b, Procedures 16-2 to 16-4, Procedure 16-6 © Milady, a part of Cengage Learning. Photography by Yanik Chauvin. Figures 16-1, 16-2, 16-4, 16-5, Procedure 16-1, 16-6 to 16-12 © Milady, a part of Cengage Learning. Photography by Paul Castle. Illustration in Procedure 16-1 © Milady, a part of Cengage Learning.

Chapter 17: chapter opener, Figures 17-35 to 17-39, Procedure 17-10 © Milady, a part of Cengage Learning. Photography by Yanik Chauvin. Figures 17-1, 17-4 to 17-7, 17-10, 17-12, 17-14, 17-16, 17-20 17-23, 17-28 17-32 to 17-34, 17-40a, 17-41, 17-45 to 17-48 © Milady, a part of Cengage Learning. Figure 17-3, 17-29, 17-40b, 17-44 to 17-43, Procedures 17-1 to 17-8 © Milady, a part of Cengage Learning. Photography by Paul Castle. Figures 17-2, 17-13, 17-19, 17-25, and 17-30 photos used with permission of the authors, Martin Gannon and Richard Thompson, as featured in their book, *Mahogany: Steps to Colouring and Finishing Hair.* Copyright Martin Gannon and Richard Thompson. 1997. Figure 17-8, hair by Geri Mataya, makeup by Mary Klimek, photo by Jack Cutler. Figure 17-9, Getty Images. Figure 17-11 courtesy of Gebhart International, hair by Dennis and Syliva Gebhart, makeup by Rose Marie, production by Purely Visual, photo by Winterhalter. Figure 17-15, John Paul Mitchell Systems, hair by Jeanne Braa, photo by Albert Tolot. Figure 17-22, John Paul Mitchell Systems, The Relaxer Workshop, photo by Sean Cokes. Figure 17-24, Mario Tricoci Hair Salons & Day Spas, hair by Tricoci, makeup by Shawn Miselli. Figure 17-27, John Paul Mitchell Systems, hair by People and Schumacher, photo by Andreas Elsner. Figures 17-17 hair by Brian & Sandra Smith, makeup by Rose Marie, wardrobe by Victor Paul, photo by Taggart/Winterhalter, production by Purely Visual. Figures 17-26, 17-31 Preston Phillips. Figures 17-18, 17-21 © Milady, a part of Cengage Learning.

Chapter 18: chapter opener, © Milady, a part of Cengage Learning. Photography by Paul Castle. Procedure 18-2 and 18-3 © Milady, a part of Cengage Learning. Photography by Yanik Chauvin. Figures 18-1a to 18-4, 18-7 to 18-9, 18-16 to 18-30,18-35, 18-36, 18-38, 18-39 © Milady, a part of Cengage Learning. Figure 18-5, 18-6, 18-11 to 18-15, 18-31 to 18-34, 18-37, 18-40 to 49, Procedure 18-1 © Milady, a part of Cengage Learning. Photography by Paul Castle. Figure 18-10 © Milady, a part of Cengage Learning.

Chapter 19: chapter opener, Figures 19-1a-b, 19-17b © Milady, a part of Cengage Learning. Photography by Yanik Chauvin. Figure 19-2 to 19-16 © Milady, a part of Cengage Learning. Figures 19-17a, Procedure 19-1 to 19-7 © Milady, a part of Cengage Learning. Photography by Paul Castle. Figure 19-18, 19-19 © Milady, a part of Cengage Learning.

Chapter 20: chapter opener, Procedures 20-1, 20-3 and 20-4 © Milady, a part of Cengage Learning. Photography by Yanik Chauvin. Figure 20-1, 20-2, 20-5, 20-6, 20-12, 20-13, 20-16, 20-19 to 20-21 © Milady, a part of Cengage Learning. Figures 20-4, 20-15, 20-22 courtesy of Robert Baran, MD (France). Figures 20-7, 20-9, 20-10, 20-11, 20-14 courtesy of Godfrey Mix, DPM, Sacramento, CA. Figure 20-8 © Milady, a part of Cengage Learning. Photography by Paul Castle. Figure 20-17 courtesy of Orville J. Stone, MD, Dermatology Medical Group, Huntington Beach, CA. Figure 20-23 Collins Manufacturing Company. Figure 20-24, 20-35 © Milady, a part of Cengage Learning. Photography by Michael Dzaman. Figure 20-27, 20-31 to 20-33, Procedure 20-2 © Milady, a part of Cengage Learning. Photography by Dino Petrocelli. Figure 20-30 © Milady, a part of Cengage Learning. Photography by Trevor Ehmann. Figures 20-3, 20-18, 20-25, 20-26, 28, 29, 34

Chapter 21: chapter opener, Figure 21-1© Milady, a part of Cengage Learning. Photography by Dino Petrocelli. Figure 21-2, 21-4 © Milady, a part of Cengage Learning. Figure 21-3 provided by Anetta Nadolna.

Chapter 22: chapter opener, (employment form on clipboard with pen); © Sideways Design, 2010; used under license from Shutterstock.com. Figures 22-1© Milady, a part of Cengage Learning. Photography by Yanik Chauvin. Figures 22-2 to 22-6 © Milady, a part of Cengage Learning.

Chapter 23: chapter opener, (barber standing proud outside barbershop), Jupiterimages, 2010. Figure 23-1, Getty Images. Table 23-2: IRS, Sample Form 4070A from Publication 1244. Figure 23-2 © Milady, a part of Cengage Learning. Photography by Paul Castle. Figure 23-3, 23-4, 23-5, 23-8 © Milady, a part of Cengage Learning. Figures 23-6, 23-9 © Milady, a part of Cengage Learning. Photography by Yanik Chauvin. Figures 23-7 © Milady, a part of Cengage Learning. Photography by Dino Petrocelli.

FILLER PHOTOS CREDITS

Chapter 1

33153607 (book with colorful 3D characters): © panco, 2010; used under license from Shutterstock.com. 13237186 (Vector illustration of a creative thinking mind background with alphabet letters coming from the head and gearwork moving inside. Knowledge concept): © DCD, 2010; used under license from Shutterstock.com. 45474337 (TIP- theory into practice concept, colorful reminder notes and white chalk handwriting on blackboard): © marekuliasz, 2010; used under license from Shutterstock.com. 15590923 (Male college student reaching for a library book): © Monkey Business Images, 2010; used under license from Shutterstock.com. 15906880 (A shot of an Asian student working on his laptop at the campus): © Supri Suharjoto, 2010; used under license from Shutterstock.com. 41577490 (laptop): © jimmi, 2010; used under license from Shutterstock.com. 24425842 (vector illustration of notebook with pencil): © Sonia.eps, 2010; used under license from Shutterstock.com. 625524 (Young man studies): © Yuri Arcurs, 2010; used under license from Shutterstock.com. 44840959 (A diverse group of young adult students): © Christopher Futcher, 2010; used under license from Shutterstock.com.

Chapter 2

8212888 (Antique Barber Chair isolated on white): © Classic Visions, 2010; used under license from Shutterstock.com. 9839160 (Giulio Cesare portrait): © PaoloGaetano, 2010; used under license from iStockphoto.com 19880236 (Monk in stained glass): © Panaspics, 2010; used under license from Shutterstock.com. 38809156 (Bust of Alexander the Great in white marble isolated on white): © kmiragaya, 2010; used under license from Shutterstock.com. 8928580 (Barber Shop image showing chairs in a row): © Jorge R. Gonzalez, 2010; used under license from Shutterstock.com. 95979189(Barber Shop sign): © Lori Slater, 2010; used under license from iStockphoto.com.

Chapter 3

11798566 (golden way to success): © pdesign, 2010; used under license from Shutterstock.com. 11416451 (ten positive emotions): © marekuliasz, 2010; used under license from iStockphoto.com. 9550268 (personal development concept on blackboard): © marekuliasz, 2010; used under license from iStockphoto.com. 8732859 (After Workout): © LattaPictures, 2010; used under license from iStockphoto.com. 8861577 (body, mind, soul, spirit and you on blackboard): © marekuliasz, 2010; used under license from iStockphoto.com. 10518557 (Young Professional Checking the Time): © Camrocker, 2010; used under license from iStockphoto.com. 46196227 (The worker at office with a notebook and the handle): © Vira, 2010; used under license from Shutterstock.com 11416453 (creativity word cloud on blackboard): © marekuliasz, 2010; used under license from iStockphoto.com. 9346157 (mind map for setting personal life goals): © marekuliasz, 2010; used under license from iStockphoto.com. 42357388 (organizer): © S.P., 2010; used under license from Shutterstock.com.17673187 (Barber cutting hair): © Josh Resnick, 2010; used under license from Shutterstock.com.

Chapter 4

5269969 (Petri dish): © Bertrand Collet, 2010; used under license from Shutterstock.com. 8815489 (bacteria): © Sebastian Kaulitzki, 2010; used under license from Shutterstock.com. 3427368 (Microbial fractal): © herrumbroso, 2010; used under license from iStockphoto.com. 19044466 (MRSA bacteria): © Michael Taylor, 2010; used under license from Shutterstock.com. 29354905 (Finger prick): © Sean Gladwell, 2010; used under license from Shutterstock.com. 8539633 (viruses): © Sebastian Kaulitzki, 2010; used under license from Shutterstock.com. 42546331 (High detailed hepatitis virus view isolated with clipping path): © WOODOO, 2010; used under license from Shutterstock.com. 8881042 (HIV virus): © Sebastian Kaulitzki, 2010; used under license from Shutterstock.com. 12052901 (hi virus infecting cell): © Eraxion, 2010; used under license from iStockphoto.com. 4605866 (Model of HIV Protease): © theasis, 2010; used under license from iStockphoto.com. 15472690 (A person washing their hands in the bathroom sink): © ARENA Creative, 2010; used under license from Shutterstock.com. 9461736 (Human immune system and bacteria): © Henrik5000, 2010; used under license from iStockphoto.com.

Chapter 5

29376910 (Close-up of barber hair trimmer on white): © Bochkarev Photography, 2010; used under license from Shutterstock.com. 19486594 (gold medal with a green approved tick on it): © argus, 2010; used under license from Shutterstock.com. 3449330 (Biohazard label on a bottle in a research lab): © Olivier Le Queinec, 2010; used under license from Shutterstock.com. 476926 (Hazard Icons and Symbols): © highhorse, 2010; used under license from iStockphoto.com. 4033449 (Set of major Hazardous Signs): © Christophe Testi, 2010; used under license from Shutterstock.com. 644836 (MSDS Binder): © Travis Klein, 2010; used under license from Shutterstock.com. 8928580 (Barber shop image showing chairs in a row): © Jorge R. Gonzalez, 2010; used under license from Shutterstock.com. 15753481 (A bucket of cleaning supplies isolated on white): © Joe Belanger, 2010; used under license from Shutterstock.com. 29377666 (Cleaning Supplies): © Jocicalek, 2010; used under license from Shutterstock.com. 433883 (Biohazard Label): © Andrei Orlov, 2010; used under license from Shutterstock.com. 25630579 (Set of men's cosmetics on white background): © vnlit, 2010; used under license from Shutterstock.com. 6430570 (Barber supplies): © Gaby Kooijman, 2010; used under license from Shutterstock.com. 1486676 (Chair in salon): © Georgethefourth, 2010; used under license from iStockphoto.com. 1790318 (Barber Salon Chairs): © rafal, 2010; used under license from iStockphoto.com. 10146676 (Little boy getting haircut): © Christophe Testi, 2010; used under license from Shutterstock.com. 1532143 (Barber's Chair): © CraigPJ, 2010; used under license from iStockphoto.com.

Chapter 6

1212459(barber pole): © EyeMark, 2010; used under license from Bigstockphoto.com. 530328 (razor-blade): © Mats, 2010; used under license from Shutterstock.com. 4544636 (Old Time Razor and Strop): © Chuckee, 2010; used under license from iStockphoto.com. 503308 (Old time barber shop c. 1915 when the pace of life was slower): © Robert Kyllo, 2010; used under license from Shutterstock.com. 2610819 (shaving kit): © Evgeny Burgasov, 2010; used under license from Shutterstock.com. 2090727 (Hair Dryer): © Andyd, 2010; used under license from iStockphoto.com.

Chapter 7

5066220 (Vitruvian man): © mpabild, 2010; used under license from iStockphoto.com. 3252606 (Portrait of a young businessman standing comfortably): © Yuri Arcurs, 2010; used under license from Shutterstock.com. 2427966 (man getting a massage facial from therapist): © Yanik Chauvin, 2010; used under license from Shutterstock.com. 8613763 (skin cross section showing the sweat glands and the surrounding tissue): © Jubal Harshaw, 2010; used under license from Shutterstock.com. 7292219 (Cells dividing): © Henrik5000, 2010;

used under license from iStockphoto.com. 6827829 (x-ray human body of a man with skeleton running): © angelhell, 2010; used under license from iStockphoto.com. 6847593 (Human body of a man with transparent muscles and skeleton): © angelhell, 2010; used under license from iStockphoto.com. 6708409 (Anatomical Overlays): © Linda Bucklin, 2010; used under license from Shutterstock.com. 8566343 (Synapse and Neurons): © Animean, 2010; used under license from iStockphoto.com. 6025392 (Circulatory system): © mpabild, 2010; used under license from iStockphoto.com. 6388713 (human heart): © Eraxion, 2010; used under license from iStockphoto.com. 10819113 (Blood Cells): © raulov, 2010; used under license from iStockphoto.com. 5444616 (Antique Medical Illustration Carotid Artery): © mstroz, 2010; used under license from iStockphoto.com. 6204934 (Antique Medical Illustrations Neck Arteries): © mstroz, 2010; used under license from iStockphoto.com. 2371227 (lymphatic system): © Eraxion, 2010; used under license from iStockphoto.com. 9047417 (Digestive system): © mpabild, 2010; used under license from iStockphoto.com. 11662148 (Stratified Squamous Epithelium): © BeholdingEye, 2010; used under license from iStockphoto.com.

Chapter 8

1438064 (Element Table): © davidf, 2010; used under license from iStockphoto.com. 4029376 (Atom): © lenm, 2010; used under license from iStockphoto.com. 143857 (PlasmaLights CircleFlow): © Capsule, 2010; used under license from iStockphoto.com. 9450965 (molecule): © _arh0n, 2010; used under license from iStockphoto.com. 877085 (Blue water world 13): © Grafissimo, 2010; used under license from iStockphoto.com. 2623327 (pH-Paper): © Sudo2, 2010; used under license from iStockphoto.com. 9211138 (Match): © SusanneB, 2010; used under license from iStockphoto.com. 44089690 (makeup powder isolated): © Jakub Pavlinec, 2010; used under license from Shutterstock.com. 3062074 (Mixing blue and yellow solutions in a flask to make green): © Katrina Leigh, 2010; used under license from Shutterstock.com. 20960776 (close up of syrup, spoon and bottle on white background): © Picsfive, 2010; used under license from Shutterstock.com. 8829859 (Beauty Lotions and Creams): © PhotoNotebook, 2010; used under license from iStockphoto.com. 47208202 (tube with ointment or cream coming out): © Kesu, 2010; used under license from Shutterstock.com. 4879996 (Plastic tube of hair conditioner ready for use): © Brett Mulcahy, 2010; used under license from Shutterstock.com. 37972012 (beauty cream box on white): © Graphic design, 2010; used under license from Shutterstock.com. 25108477 (Spray Bottle isolated on a white background): © Michele Cozzolino, 2010; used under license from Shutterstock.com. 31233724 (Miniature shampoo bottles isolated against a white background): © Kitch Bain, 2010; used under license from Shutterstock.com. 23063947 (Hand and finger pushing spray can): © Paul Matthew Photography, 2010; used under license from Shutterstock.com. 5839732 (Closeup of container of moisturizing face cream and white chrysanthemum on green toned background with ice cubes): © Bochkarev Photography, 2010; used under license from Shutterstock.com. 25126105 (Hair mousse): © M.antonis, 2010; used under license from Shutterstock.com. 11559404 (Medical Items): © tammykayphoto, 2010; used under license from iStockphoto.com.

Chapter 9

143532 (prism and rainbow): © Lexy Sinnott, 2010; used under license from Shutterstock.com. 26692675 (A seamless blue electric lightning storm art): © Kentoh, 2010; used under license from Shutterstock.com. 640866 (Gold Dimmer Switch on isolated background): © Dainis Derics, 2010; used under license from Shutterstock.com. 32921773 (Electricity, power and energy icons): © stoyanh, 2010; used under license from Shutterstock.com. 17093869 (electrical plug isolated on white): © david n madden, 2010; used under license from Shutterstock.com. 28488043 (Electric plug isolated on the white background): © Elnur, 2010; used under license from Shutterstock.com. High frequency machine, courtesy of Jellen Products, Inc. (www.jellenproducts. com) 25837522 (solarium): © Karkas, 2010; used under license from Shutterstock.com. 18937960 (viewable colours frequencies): © italianestro, 2010; used under license from Shutterstock.com.

Chapter 10

11662181 (Hair Bearing Skin): © BeholdingEye, 2010; used under license from iStockphoto.com. 25788133 (Skin-labeled): © Blamb, 2010; used under license from Shutterstock.com. 31162276 (The center portion of a hair follicle showing a sebaceous gland): © Jubal Harshaw, 2010; used under license from Shutterstock.com. 4422514 (Neurons): © ktsimage, 2010; used under license from iStockphoto.com. 3266121 (casual smiling man portrait isolated over a white background): © Andresr, 2010; used under license from Shutterstock.com. 329487

(Big Pimple): © pjjones, 2010; used under license from iStockphoto.com. 39000460 (basal cell carcinoma cancer skin being treated with 5 percent fluorouracil. Upper arm of a 58 year old woman): © R. Michael Ballard, 2010; used under license from Shutterstock.com. 11373840 (Skin Mole): © zlisjak, 2010; used under license from iStockphoto.com. 10615958 (Skin Wart): © zlisjak, 2010; used under license from iStockphoto.com. 9596357 (Hand's man affected by vitiligo): © piccerella, 2010; used under license from iStockphoto.com.

Chapter 11

48759364 (Human hair macro): © Kletr, 2010; used under license from Shutterstock.com. 31460794 (3D Cross section of skin): © Blamb, 2010; used under license from Shutterstock.com. 6258316 (Image of amino acid cysteine): © stanislaff, 2010; used under license from Shutterstock.com. 37655029 (beautiful shiny healthy style hair): © Raia, 2010; used under license from Shutterstock.com. 21976129 (beautiful blond long hair and wood comb): © Bairachnyi Dmitry, 2010; used under license from Shutterstock.com. 65938 (Hair): © jfegan, 2010; used under license from iStockphoto. com. 13169032 (male head with hair loss): © Anastasios Kandris, 2010; used under license from Shutterstock. com.13169035 (male balding head): © Anastasios Kandris, 2010; used under license from Shutterstock. com. 34765969 (Dandruff issue on man's shoulder): © Zurijeta, 2010; used under license from Shutterstock. com.

Chapter 12

15008269 (Hair Salon – a hair washing sink and chair): © ARENA Creative, 2010; used under license from Shutterstock.com. 8069955 (Shampoo and conditioner, in bottles): © WEKWEK, 2010; used under license from iStockphoto.com. 16429456 (Hand being washed with soap under tap): © Brian A. Jackson, 2010; used under license from Shutterstock.com. 2612300 (beauty products): © gvictoria, 2010; used under license from iStockphoto.com. 1136746 (Young man getting a shampoo at beauty salon): © Alfred Wekelo, 2010; used under license from Shutterstock.com.

Chapter 13

1361493 (A man receives a facial treatment in the spa): © Mag. Alban Egger, 2010; used under license from Shutterstock.com. 45176902 (Mans irritated skin): © val lawless, 2010; used under license from Shutterstock. com. 78481577 (Woman steaming her face): © Comstock, 2010; used under license from Thinkstock.com.29023825 (uv lamp on table. Blue): © Andrey Sukhachev, 2010; used under license from Shutterstock.com. 11547615 (Infrared fomentation): © eROMAZe, 2010; used under license from iStockphoto.com. 12362632 (Isolated close up on the face of an elder man): © Mehmet Dilsiz, 2010; used under license from Shutterstock.com. 16087669 (Close-up shot of a part of man's face. Isolated on white background): © Andrejs Pidjass, 2010; used under license from Shutterstock.com. 25417900 (portrait of man): © photobank.ch, 2010; used under license from Shutterstock.com. 4122493 (three quarter view close up of a African American male's eyes): © 4736202690, 2010; used under license from Shutterstock.com. 18051880 (Middle-aged man face fragment): © Andrejs Pidjass, 2010; used under license from Shutterstock.com. 48232420 (Plastic grey cosmetics tube isolated on white): © Coprid, 2010; used under license from Shutterstock. com. 7271134 (vial with lotion): © Galushko Sergey, 2010; used under license from Shutterstock.com. 41483857 (Cosmetics cream. Isolated on the white background): © NatUlrich, 2010; used under license from Shutterstock. com. 159043 (Close up of exfoliating cream): © Johanna Goodyear, 2010; used under license from Shutterstock. com. 25630576 (set of men's cosmetics): © vnlit, 2010; used under license from Shutterstock.com.

Chapter 14

14738776 (Isolated razor): © ethylalkohol, 2010; used under license from Shutterstock.com. 20986732 (A shaving razor and a sharpening leather on white): © Milos Luzanin, 2010; used under license from Shutterstock.com. 11709745 (Close up of African American Male in suite): © dapoopta, 2010; used under license from iStockphoto.com. 1852868 (At the Barber Shop 2): © Martine Oger, 2010; used under license from Shutterstock.com. 1547172 (young male lips): © LesByerley, 2010; used under license from iStockphoto.com. 29278465 (Beard): © echo3005, 2010; used under license from Shutterstock.com. 27590707 (Beard and facial hair styles in vector silhouette): © LHF Graphics, 2010; used under license from Shutterstock.com.

Chapter 15

24459115 (Barber cutting a pattern into a man's hair): © Ronald Sumners, 2010; used under license from Shutterstock.com. 14142592 (Young casual man posing, isolated in white background): © Hugo Silveirinha Felix, 2010; used under license from Shutterstock.com. 33617269 (Male portrait and abstract geometric pattern. 3d digitally created

illustration): © dimitris_K, 2010; used under license from Shutterstock.com. 11344012 (Cheerful young businessman against white background): © Yuri Arcurs, 2010; used under license from Shutterstock.com. 29222536 (Good looking young man with modern HairStyle over a grunge wall background): © IKO, 2010; used under license from Shutterstock.com. 26676598 (Portrait of a young happy teenager): © Ghaint, 2010; used under license from Shutterstock.com. 3100684 (Portrait young serious businessman, looks in chamber, close up): © Andriy Solovyov, 2010; used under license from Shutterstock.com. 1546039 (At the hair salon): © Susan_Stewart, 2010; used under license from iStockphoto.com. 10592697 (Caucasian Handsome Young Male Fashion Model Portrait, Copy Space): © quavondo, 2010; used under license from iStockphoto.com. 13153000 (A portrait about a trendy cute guy who is smiling and he has an attractive look. He is wearing sunglasses, a stylish black suit and a scarf): © Henri Schmit, 2010; used under license from Shutterstock.com. 41385193 (Fashion Shot of a Young Man A trendy European man dressed in contemporary cloth): © Aleksandar Todorovic, 2010; used under license from Shutterstock.com. 8319034 (A black man with dreadlock hair isolated on a white background): © martin garnham, 2010; used under license from Shutterstock.com.

Chapter 16

9371111 (Bald): © fatihhoca, 2010; used under license from iStockphoto.com. 15818959 (beautiful hair, brown, thick): © Dolly, 2010; used under license from Shutterstock.com. 22342207 (Blond and auburn red hair): © Anne Kitzman, 2010; used under license from Shutterstock.com. 2179646 (tape measure): © milosluz, 2010; used under license from iStockphoto.com. Page 502, before and after bonding © Milady, photography by Yanik Chauvin. 426844 (wigs): © martyw, 2010; used under license from iStockphoto.com. 43927894 (Brown glass bottle of organic solvent isolated on white): © Coprid, 2010; used under license from Shutterstock. com. 1582763 (products for dying hair): © Graca Victoria, 2010; used under license from Shutterstock. com. Page 516, before and after tattooing photos, courtesy of Cheryl Rosenblum, Hair Simulation.

Chapter 17

11620280 (Serious Young Woman With Bare Shoulders): © chrisgramly, 2010; used under license from iStockphoto.com. 9545116 (Cutting hair): © Casarsa, 2010; used under license from iStockphoto.

com. 4892492 (Blonde fashion): © kaleenakatt, 2010; used under license from iStockphoto.com. 7981875 (Close-up of Woman's Face with Red Hair): © chrisgramly, 2010; used under license from iStockphoto.com. 8937354 (Lovely Latin Woman): © jhorrocks, 2010; used under license from iStockphoto.com. 8745108 (African American Young Woman Beauty Shot): © quavondo, 2010; used under license from iStockphoto.com. 8061088 (Beauty hairstyle): © DomenicoGelermo, 2010; used under license from iStockphoto.com. 4765546 (Young Woman Curly Blond Hair, Portrait): © hammondovi, 2010; used under license from iStockphoto.com 9281018 (Attractive Woman in a Striped Top): © chrisgramly, 2010; used under license from iStockphoto.com. 1151551 (Portrait of Young Woman Wrapped in Red Shawl): © aldra, 2010; used under license from iStockphoto.com.

Chapter 18

973296 (redhead hair): © zinchik, 2010; used under license from iStockphoto.com. 8925584 (rays of light and chemical formulas): © Vladimir, 2010; used under license from iStockphoto.com. 2978060 (3d rendering illustration emulating nanophotography): © Yannis Ntousiopoulos, 2010; used under license from Shutterstock.com. 28089517 (high angle view of hairdresser using comb): © Diego Cervo, 2010; used under license from Shutterstock.com. 5078355 (colourful curlers on a dummy head): © pidjoe, 2010; used under license from iStockphoto.com. 10490214 (Curlers): © nesharm, 2010; used under license from iStockphoto.com. 31162276 (The center portion of a hair follicle showing a sebaceous gland. Enhanced. Magnification 100x): © Jubal harshaw, 2010; used under license from Shutterstock.com. 11231809 (Beauty Treatment): © herkisi, 2010; used under license from iStockphoto.com. 10185654 (Handle rake and hair rollers): © TimArbaev, 2010; used under license from iStockphoto.com. 41095363 (An old barbers comb running through black hair): © Ronald Sumners, 2010; used under license from Shutterstock.com.

Chapter 19

38190790 (Palette of hair color sample and hairdresser's tools): © Ivanova Inga, 2010; used under license from Shutterstock.com. 66540 (Vintage portrait of a man with a big mustache): © Elena Ray, 2010; used under license from Shutterstock.com. 30297307 (beautiful shiny healthy hair texture): © Raia, 2010; used under license from Shutterstock.com. 21693952 (Vector color wheel): © Romanova Ekaterina, 2010; used under license from Shutterstock.com. 826233 (Close up of raw Henna powder used for natural color dyeing): © Steve Lovegrove, 2010; used under license from Shutterstock.com. 6430573 (barber supplies): © Gaby Kooijman, 2010; used under license from Shutterstock.com. 7055731 (bleaching hair with bleach upclose): © Andi Berger, 2010; used under license from Shutterstock.com. 2159605 (women having hair foiled): © Lorraine Kourafas, 2010; used under license from Shutterstock.com. 9949654 (hair in the process of being colored): © Lorraine Kourafas, 2010; used under license from Shutterstock.com. 37266403 (hair coloring): © Vladislav Gajic, 2010; used under license from Shutterstock.com. 9949657 (hair coloring being applied): © Lorraine Kourafas, 2010; used under license from Shutterstock.com. 18401239 (close-up of wavy blond hair): © originalpunkt, 2010; used under license from Shutterstock.com. 21187921 (Senior African man with beard and sad expression isolated on white): © Four Oaks, 2010; used under license from Shutterstock.com.

Chapter 20

10885969 (Manicure treatment-soaking off the old nail set): © Christopher Elwell, 2010; used under license from Shutterstock.com. 24129097 (Anatomy of the fingernail): © Blamb, 2010; used under license from Shutterstock.com. 11670772 (small finger on the white background, wound and bruise): © Tramper, 2010; used under license from Shutterstock.com. 1872593 (Care of nails and manicure): © Andrey Chmelyov, 2010; used under license from Shutterstock.com. 3056905 (Band-aid at thumb): © Schaefer Elvira, 2010; used under license from Shutterstock.com.

Chapter 21

37830070 (Classic Barber Pole): © TerryM, 2010; used under license from Shutterstock.com. 1651377 (Young student reading and taking notes): © Yuri Arcurs, 2010; used under license from Shutterstock.com. 16647424 (Exam): © Carla Donofrio, 2010; used under license from Shutterstock.com. 6148949 (Haircutting): © TimMcClean, 2010; used under license from iStockphoto.com. 9646167 (Salon Hair Styling): © tomeng, 2010; used under license from iStockphoto.com. 1580662 (Young man doing work at home. Contemporary looking guy doing an assignment.); © Yuri Arcurs, 2010; used under license from Shutterstock.com. 502067 (Hairdresser): © the huhu, 2010; used under license from iStockphoto.com. 1647823 (government regulations, magnifier, pencil); © James Steidl, 2010; used under license from Shutterstock.com.

Chapter 22

9103786 (Careers (job search)): © zorani, 2010; used under license from iStockphoto, com. 300415 (barber chair); © Jorge Figueiredo, 2010; used under license from Shutterstock.com. 8941303 (Mens Haircut): © powerofforever, 2010; used under license from iStockphoto.com. 10414230 (man in black hides behind money): © PhotonStock, 2010; used under license from iStockphoto.com. 9121836 (Isolated Clipboard with Job Application Form): © sidewaysdesign, 2010; used under license from iStockphoto.com. 15769243 (designer portfolio bag); © yienkeat, 2010; used under license from Shutterstock.com. 3707309 (Waiting for the interview): © oddrose, 2010; used under license from iStockphoto.com.

Chapter 23

Page 739, © Milady, photography by Yanik Chauvin. 86520998 (Boy getting haircut at barbershop); © Jupiterimages, 2010; used under license from Getty Images. 200342127-001(Two male barbers standing by doorway of shop, portrait); © Michael Blann, 2010; used under license from Thinkstock.com. 200342131-001(Male barber sweeping floor); © Michael Blann, 2010; used under license from Thinkstock.com. 8928580 (barber shop image showing chairs in a row); © Jorge R. Gonzalez, 2010; used under license from Shutterstock.com. 49423750 (empty-strip-mall-with-pastel-stucco-and-stone-accents); © L Barnwell, 2010; used under license from Shutterstock.com. 35164939 (rental-contract-form-with-pen); © OfiPlus, 2010; used under license from Shutterstock.com. 5478976 (business-man-drawing-a-business-plan-on-screen-over-a-white-background); © Andresr, 2010; used under license from Shutterstock.com. 32336302 (taxi-billboard-close-up-at-night); © Jorge Salcedo, 2010; used under license from Shutterstock.com. 51732460 (word-of-mouth-advertising-is-the-best-way-to-capture-new-customers-without-paying-for-it-it); © Vlue, 2010; used under license from Shutterstock.com. 1194588 (Customer service feedback): © guyerwood, 2010; used under license from iStockphoto.com. 49854274 (man-is-confused-on-the-phone); © doglikehorse, 2010; used under license from Shutterstock.com. 56473517 (close-up of bottles in a hair salon); © George Doyle, 2010; used under license from Thinkstock.com. ist2_3959279 (Cosmetics in cabinet): © peepo, 2010; used under license from iStockphoto.com.

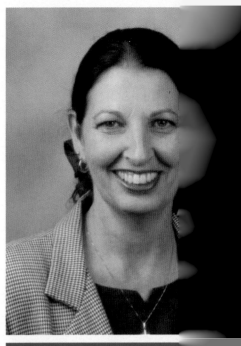

MAURA SCALI-SHEAHAN, ED.D.

Master Barber, Educator, and Consultant
In addition to holding a Master Barber license since the 1970s, Maura earned a doctorate in education and a master's degree in workforce education training and development. She is the Education Director for Barbers International and has served on a variety of college councils, advisory boards, the Illinois and Florida State Barber Boards, and the former AMBBA Executive Board. She was inducted into the NABBA Barbering Hall of Fame in 2008.

Dr. Scali-Sheahan has been a Career Institute educator since 2001 and an instructor since 1991. In addition to teaching and freelance writing for the industry, she is also an adjunct instructor for Southern Illinois University's Workforce Education Development programs. She is dedicated to promoting the longevity of the barbering profession through enhanced barbering education and provides professional development and enrichment venues for barbering programs, instructors, and students. Her services include all aspects of program design and development to help prepare the next generation of barbers and educators for the profession.

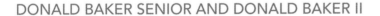

DONALD BAKER SENIOR AND DONALD BAKER II

Contributors to Chapter 16, Men's Hair Replacement
Donald Ray Baker, Sr. and Donald Ray Baker II are a father and son team who have taken the hair replacement industry to a new level. Donald Ray Baker, Sr. started a small barbershop in Wallace, North Carolina in 1973, which grew into a successful family business.

In 1989, Donald Ray Baker II started helping his father in the barbershop and also learned the trades of a master barber and cosmetologist. The Bakers decided to open a studio focusing only on hair replacement in Wilmington, North Carolina. The shop and practice of hair replacement had such a large demand that in 2001 they opened their third location in Greenville, North Carolina.

Donald Ray Baker II went on to pursue a career with the country's largest hair replacement manufacturer, in West Palm Beach, Florida, while his father still runs the hair replacement studios today.

The combined knowledge and experience of the two Don's has led them to many awards and recognitions as leaders of the hair replacement world. They greatly appreciate the opportunity to share with you their knowledge of this ever-growing business.

PART1

ORIENTATION TO BARBERING

1 Study Skills

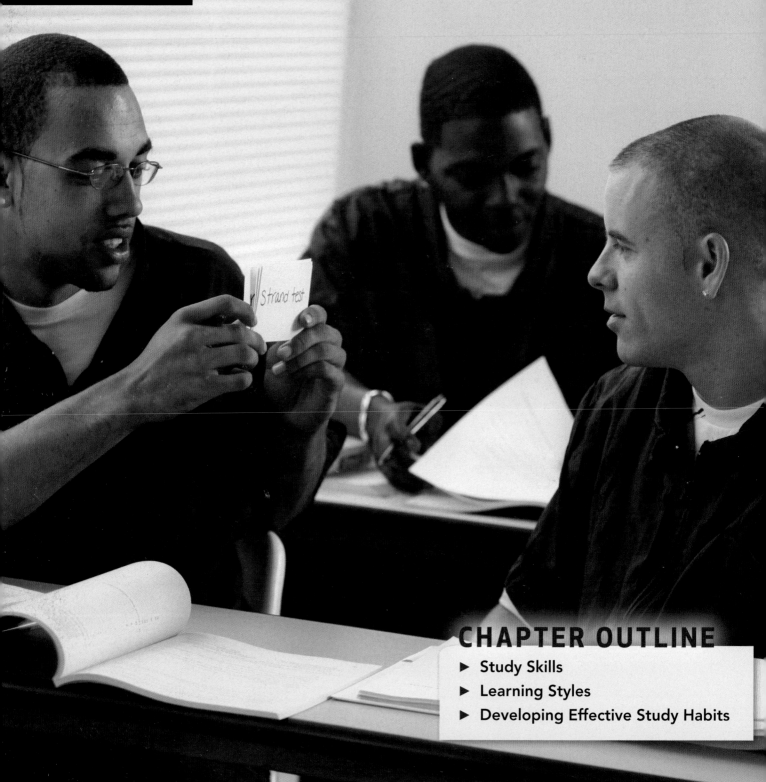

☑ Learning Objectives

AFTER COMPLETING THIS CHAPTER, YOU SHOULD BE ABLE TO:

1 Discuss study skills that can enhance your understanding of new information.

2 Discuss methods for mind-mapping a topic.

3 Identify the four steps of the writing process.

4 Identify your preferred learning style.

5 Discuss effective study habits.

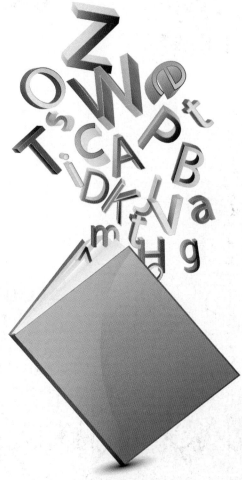

Key Terms

PAGE NUMBER INDICATES WHERE IN THE CHAPTER THE TERM IS USED.

drafting / 7	mind-mapping / 5	planning / 7
editing / 7	mnemonics / 5	repetition / 4
learning styles / 8	organization / 4	revising / 7

Your orientation to the study of barbering begins with a review of the study skills you may have developed or forgotten over the years since your last school experience. For some of you, the program you have begun may be your first postsecondary educational experience. For others, it might signal the preparation for a second or even third career after military service or years spent in other professions. Still others may be returning to barbering after an extended absence from the industry. Regardless of prior experience, your barbering career begins now and good study skills will help you achieve your educational and professional goals within it.

One of the most important keys to your success as a student is your ability to learn and master new information. Some of you learned effective study skills early on and should have a relatively smooth time understanding and applying new information. Others may not have developed these skills and may struggle with new information or learning situations. In either case, this chapter should help you develop new ways of receiving and processing information for the purpose of optimizing your educational experiences. As you develop your personal study skills, bear in mind that practice and a sense of discipline toward your studies will help you *understand* and *apply* what is taught.

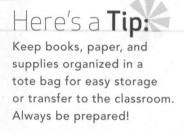

Here's a **Tip:**

Keep books, paper, and supplies organized in a tote bag for easy storage or transfer to the classroom. Always be prepared!

Study Skills

Your personal study skills are highly individualized methods or tools that help you absorb and retain new information. As such, they should help you organize, store, and recall information. The following information-processing methods can be used to optimize the effort you put toward your studies:

- *Repetition:* **Repetition** improves your short-term memory. Whether you repeat information in your head, say it out loud, write it down, or practice it hands-on, repetition helps your short-term memory secure a firmer grasp on the information. This makes the information easier to retrieve when you need it.

- *Organization:* You can use **organization** to process new information for both short-term and long-term memory use. To enhance your short-term memory, try categorizing the information into smaller segments. For example: The skin consists of two primary divisions with three distinct layers. These are the epidermis, dermis, and subcutaneous tissue layers. Contained within these divisions are eight layers of skin structures. Rather than trying to remember all eight layers, use the categories of the skin divisions to break the information down into three sections. Begin with the epidermis. The epidermis consists of five layers or strata: the stratum corneum, stratum lucidum, stratum granulosum and stratum spinosum (not always listed separately), and the stratum germinativum. Once you have mastered this information and the characteristics of these

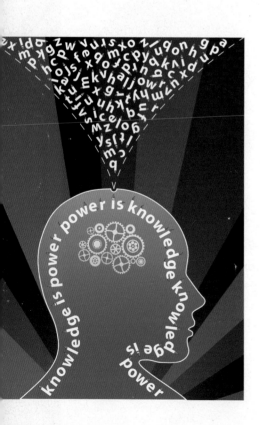

layers, you can move on to learning about the features of the dermis and subcutaneous tissue layers. To promote better long-term memory, try to associate new information with prior knowledge through word association techniques. For example, based on what you will learn about the epidermis, use word association techniques to remember the names and characteristics of the layers as demonstrated in the following:

> ▶ Outermost layer: stratum corneum—a.k.a. horny layer; continually being shed; *corn* rhymes with *horn*.

> ▶ Second layer: stratum lucidum—a.k.a. clear layer; light penetrates through; *lucid* means *clear*; *lucid* is the root word of *lucidum*.

A.K.A. means "also known as."

- Similar word associations can be developed for the remaining layers of the epidermis as well. Create word associations that mean something to you so that you truly learn the material and are not just memorizing it for the short term.

- *Mnemonics:* Yet another way to trigger your memory is through the use of mnemonics. **Mnemonics** can be acronyms, songs, rhymes, sentences, or any other device that helps you recall information.

> ▶ Using the first letters in a series of words creates acronyms. For example, remember the functions of the skin using the word SHAPES—sensation, heat regulation, absorption, protection, excretion, and secretion. This is a particularly good acronym because skin also gives *shape* to the body.

> ▶ Songs or rhymes don't have to be complicated. Something as simple as "keep the *air* and the *hair* moving when blow-drying" to prevent burning the client's scalp or "rock 'n' roll rodding creates a spiral perm" to illustrate a permanent wave rodding technique can be effective reminders during application procedures.

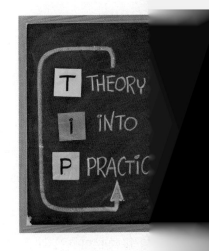

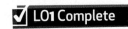
☑ LO1 Complete

- *Mind-mapping:* **Mind-mapping** is a fun and creative way to take notes or solve a problem. Write the main topic or problem in the center of a piece of paper. Jot down key words or ideas that come to mind and connect them to the main topic. Then, using the key words or ideas, create subconnections to other thoughts or information. Use color or symbols to highlight important information. For example, the skin structure topic used previously to organize information for understanding and memory is mind-mapped with accompanying notes in **Figure 1-1**.

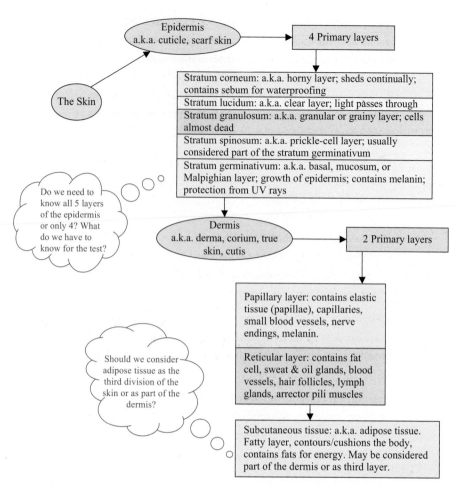

▲ FIGURE 1-1

Mind-mapping skin divisions and layers.

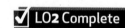

I. First main idea

   A. subtopic

      1. detail

      2. detail

   B. subtopic

      1. detail

      2. detail

   C. subtopic

      1. detail

      2. detail

      3. detail

II. Second main topic

   A. subtopic

   B. subtopic

III. Third main topic, etc.

▲ FIGURE 1-2

Topic outline for note taking.

- *Note taking:* One of the most useful ways of taking notes is to write them down in outline form. An outline typically begins with the "big picture" of an idea or topic and provides a format with which to record important information in manageable components. Begin by titling your outline with the topic or concept to be covered. Next, use the Roman numeral I to identify the first main topic or idea, and then use a capital letter A for the first subtopic. Under subtopic A, list any details using 1, 2, 3, and so forth, as necessary to cover the material. If the situation arises where the details require further notes for understanding, use lowercase letters followed by a period. The letter B and subsequent detail numbers will identify the next subtopic introduced, and so on (**Figure 1-2**).

- *Report writing:* Now, what happens if your instructor assigns a research paper on a particular topic? Where do you start? First of all, don't panic; the process is not as daunting as it might seem. The writing process has four distinct steps that can help you develop an informative presentation or well-written paper. These steps are planning, drafting, revising, and editing.

Planning, or prewriting, involves anything you do prior to writing the first draft of your paper. This includes brainstorming, researching, taking notes, and so forth, and helps you organize the writing process.

Drafting includes formal outlining and putting? thoughts and information into cohesive sentences and paragraphs. This is where you should bring the information together.

Revising requires the writer to look at the content from the reader's or listener's perspective. This step includes rewriting or reorganizing the material as necessary.

Editing involves proofreading and correcting your work. Check the punctuation, spelling, grammar, and appearance of the paper. Practice an oral presentation to make sure the delivery flows within the allotted time.

Now, let's put these steps into action. You might begin with the mind-mapping exercise to get your thoughts, questions, and ideas into a loosely organized model. Identify criteria associated with the project such as length, due dates, and so forth. Then jot down some topic ideas and possible research sources. Next, decide what the topic is going to be and narrow it down to a manageable concept or category. For example, the topic of Egyptian hairstyles is a very broad category that would require in-depth research and a lot of time to cover in any detail. Conversely, a report that summarizes the use of wigs by ancient Egyptians narrows the focus of the study to a more manageable topic (planning).

Once the topic has been selected, create an outline that includes an introduction, body paragraphs, and a conclusion. You can write the topic in either a note-taking outline form (Figure 1-2) or in a report outline form (**Figure 1-3**). The introduction should inform the reader what your report is about. Body paragraphs should contain specific topic sentences that introduce what is discussed in each particular paragraph, and the conclusion should summarize and make relevant to the reader the information delivered (drafting).

Now that you know what you want to say, revisit your draft to determine how you're going to say it and the order in which it will be presented. Group related information or concepts and provide supporting evidence or material when needed. Check your transitions from one paragraph to the next so that the information flows smoothly (revising).

The final step requires a thorough review of your paper to check sentence structure, clarity, word usage, and punctuation. Don't depend exclusively on your computer spell-checker to find spelling errors, as it does not know whether you mean to say *hair* or *hare,* for example (editing).

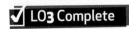 LO3 Complete

TOPIC

I. Introduction

  A. Main points or ideas

    1. category one

    2. category two

II. Body paragraphs

  A. Category one

    1. details

    2. details

  B. Category two

    1. details

    2. details

III. Conclusion

  A. summarize

  B. relevance

▲ **FIGURE 1-3**

Topic outline for report writing.

Learning Styles

One way to hone your study skills is to recognize that we all have different **learning styles** and that it helps to know what kind of learner you are. Knowing your particular learning style often makes it easier to organize new information because the methods used for retrieval and application are made more relevant and meaningful to you personally **(Figure 1-4)**.

Learning styles are classifications that are used to identify the different ways in which people learn. Learning takes place through our individual *perceptions* of reality and the way in which we *process* information and experiences. Some individuals *feel* their way through new information or situations, while others *think* their way through. Therefore, perceptions of reality tend to be either more emotionally centered or more analytically based. When processing new information or experiences, some people watch and absorb while others act and do. When the two different ways of perceiving are combined with the two different ways of processing, four distinct learning styles emerge. Review the following learning style descriptions to determine the learning style that you think—or feel—is most like you.

1. *Interactive learners:* Interactive learners (also known as imaginative or innovative learners) learn best by watching, listening, and sharing ideas. These are "idea people" who function best through social interaction and the opportunity to ask "why?" or "why not?" They tend to appreciate a learning environment that is interactive, supportive, sympathetic, and friendly. Interactive learners like to engage in classroom discussions and usually study well with a group of people.

2. *Reader/listener learners:* These individuals (also called analytic learners) are interested in facts and details. They learn best by

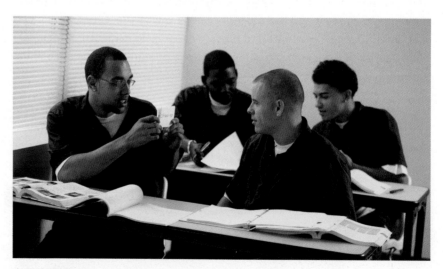

▲ **FIGURE 1-4**
An interactive learning environment.

thinking through the ideas or concepts they have read or heard. Since the analytic learner's favorite question is "what?" they tend to work well in structured environments with instructors who answer their questions freely and keep them focused on the subject matter.

3. *Systematic learners:* The systematic learner (also known as the common-sense learner) benefits more from new information when he or she can connect it to real-life situations. These learners need to know how things work, enjoy practical applications, and tend to concentrate best when studying alone. The systematic learner's favorite question is "how?" and they favor a learning environment that challenges them to "check things out."

4. *Intuitive learners:* Intuitive learners (also called dynamic learners) like to learn through trial and error and self-discovery. They are open to possibilities and to new ways of doing things, and tend to ask "what if?" Intuitive learners want to try out what they read about and actually experience what they study. Since they like variety, intuitive learners usually respond best to learning environments that facilitate the stimulation of ideas and the exploration of different ways to achieve the desired outcome.

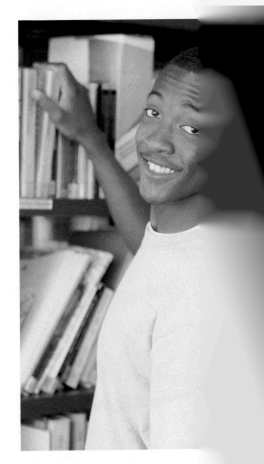

Once you recognize your particular learning style, think about the ways in which these characteristics might be applied to your study habits to maximize your effectiveness as a student. Here are a few tips for classroom note taking that have been designed around the four learning styles.

1. *Interactive learners:* Apply personal meaning to the topic. For example, ask yourself "Why is the topic important and how does it relate to me and my future?" Picture yourself in that future. Ask for clarification or examples when needed to fully understand concepts or procedures.

2. *Reader/listener learners:* List key words and facts. Analyze the concepts (*what* the topic consists of) during study time for greater clarity and understanding as to *why* the facts are what they are. This should allow you to think things through so you can move more easily and logically from point A to point B during practical applications.

3. *Systematic learners:* List key information—especially procedures—in an orderly fashion. You won't want to miss a step! In theory class, make notations along the margins that remind you to experiment with concepts that can be transitioned into practical applications. Ask questions or experiment until you understand how concepts are related or how a procedure works.

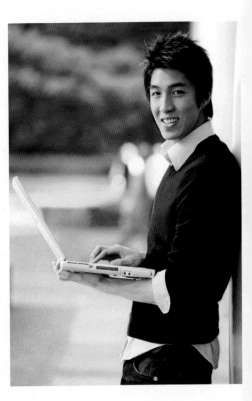

4. *Intuitive learners:* Be open to accepting what is already known since doing so can eliminate some of the frustration associated with learning exclusively through the trial-and-error method. Pay attention to key concepts and list procedural steps when taking notes. When an idea comes to mind, note it in the margins for later exploration; if a topic triggers interest in another area, mark it for some independent study or experimentation. Experiment with incorporating your own "what if" ideas when questioning concepts that require more examples for understanding or exploring other ways of performing procedures.

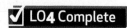

Developing Effective Study Habits

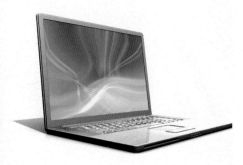

An important part of developing effective study habits is to know what, when, where, and how to study. Here are some pointers to keep in mind.

What

- Review textbook chapter headings and subheading to identify key topics.

- Use notes from class discussions or demonstrations to focus on key points.

- Question instructors about what you don't understand or need clarification to understand.

- Outline, mind-map, or diagram key points or procedures to show their interrelationships in a visual way.

When

- Estimate how many hours of study you need.

- Plan your study time around the times of day when you are most energetic and motivated.

- Use "down" times, such as riding on a bus, to study.

Where

- Select a quiet location where you will not be disturbed or interrupted.

- Study sitting in a chair or standing instead of lying down.

- Maintain a routine by studying in the same place whenever possible.

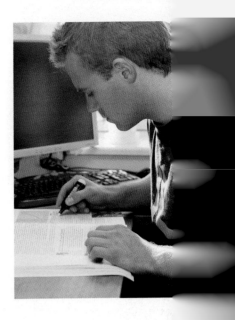

How

- Stay focused on your reason for studying by keeping your goals in mind.

- Stay motivated by declaring your intentions aloud or on paper and make a promise to yourself to follow though.

- Resist distractions during study time.

- Be persistent, disciplined, and determined.

- Think about tackling the tougher chapters or topics first.

- Pace yourself with breaks, healthy snacks, and physical movement.

The development of good study habits is a skill that can be used beyond your barbering training or the classroom environment. It is a transferable skill that will be utilized throughout your lifetime as you grow to achieve your full personal and professional potential. For example, consider the ways in which effective study habits might help you begin the research needed to open a barbershop or to participate at a state board meeting. Each new life experience, information set, or professional challenge involves learning that will require study in some form. Effective study skills will help you create your own good luck in your present and future endeavors.

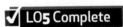

✓ **LO5 Complete**

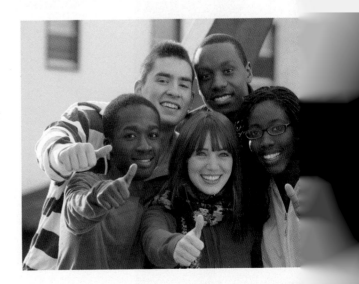

Review
Questions

1. What ability is one of the most important keys to your success as a student?

2. Identify an information-processing method that can be used to enhance short-term memory.

3. Identify an information-processing method that can be used to enhance long-term memory.

4. Create a mind-map for this chapter.

5. What are the four steps of the writing process?

6. What is your preferred learning style?

7. Design a form or template for note taking based on your preferred learning style.

Chapter Glossary

drafting putting thoughts and information into cohesive sentences and paragraphs

editing the task of proofreading and correcting a paper in terms of punctuation, spelling, grammar, and so forth.

learning styles classifications that are used to identify the different ways in which people learn

mind-mapping a graphic representation of an idea or problem that helps to organize one's thoughts

mnemonics any memorization device that helps a person to recall information

organization a method used to store new information for short-term and long-term memory

planning any action taken prior to the draft writing process when preparing a report or presentation

repetition repeatedly saying, writing, or otherwise reviewing new information until it is learned

revising the task in which a writer rewrites or reorganizes a writing project

2 THE HISTORY OF Barbering

CHAPTER OUTLINE

☑ Learning Objectives

AFTER COMPLETING THIS CHAPTER, YOU SHOULD BE ABLE TO:

1 Define the origin of the word *barber*.

2 Discuss the evolution of barbering.

3 Describe the barber-surgeons and their practices.

4 Explain the origin of the barber pole.

5 Identify some organizations responsible for upgrading the barbering profession.

6 Explain the importance and function of state barber boards.

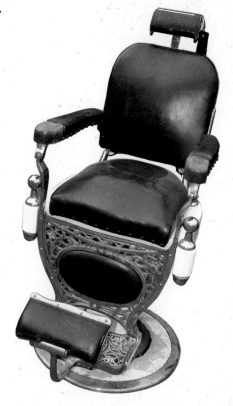

Key Terms

PAGE NUMBER INDICATES WHERE IN THE CHAPTER THE TERM IS USED.

A.B. Moler / 23

AMBBA / 23

Ambroise Pare / 21

barba / 16

barber pole / 22

barber-surgeons / 20

journeymen barber groups / 22

master barber groups / 22

Meryma'at / 17

National Association of Barber Boards of America / 25

Ticinius Mena / 17

tonsorial / 16

tonsure / 18

Barbering is one of the oldest professions in the world. With the advance of civilization, barbering and hairstyling developed from its early cultural and tribal beginnings into a recognized profession.

The study of this progression leads to an appreciation of the accomplishments, evolution, and position of high esteem attained by early practitioners. The cultural, esthetic, and technical heritage they developed provides the basis for the prestige and respect accorded to the profession and its services today.

Origin of the Barber

The word *barber* is derived from the Latin word **barba,** meaning *beard* (Figure 2-1). Another word derived from Latin, **tonsorial,** means the cutting, clipping, or trimming of hair with shears or a razor; it is often used in conjunction with barbering. Hence, barbers are sometimes referred to as tonsorial artists.

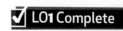 **LO1 Complete**

Archaeological studies reveal that haircutting and hairstyling were practiced in some form as early as the glacial age. The simple but effective implements used then were shaped from sharpened flints, oyster shells, or bone. Animal sinew or strips of hide were used to tie the hair back or as adornment, and braiding techniques were employed in some cultures.

Many primitive cultures believed in a connection between the body, mind, and spirit. This belief translated into superstitions and beliefs that merged religious ritual, spirituality, and medical practices together into an integrated relationship. For example, some tribes believed that both good and bad spirits entered the individual through the hairs on the head and that the only way to exorcise bad spirits was to cut the hair.

Similar belief systems were found in other regions, and tribal barbers were elevated to positions of importance to become medicine men, shamans, or priests. In one religious ceremony, long hair was worn loose to allow the evil spirits to exit the individual. Then, after ritual dancing, the barber cut the hair, combed it back tightly against the scalp, and tied it off to keep the good spirits in and the evil spirits out.

Given the archaeological evidence found in painted pottery, early sculptures, and burial mounds, it can be assumed that early cultures practiced some form of beautification and adornment, whether from esthetic sense or religious conviction. From a historical perspective, the division between what archaeological evidence leads us to *believe,* and what can be claimed as absolute *fact,* occurs with the rise of the Egyptian civilization.

The Egyptian culture is credited with being the first to cultivate beauty in an extravagant fashion. Excavations from tombs have revealed such relics as combs, brushes, mirrors, cosmetics, scissors, and razors made of tempered copper and bronze (Figure 2-2).

Coloring agents made from berries, bark, minerals, and other natural materials were used on the hair, skin, and nails. Eye paint was the most popular of

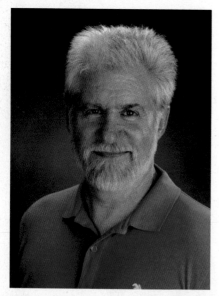

▲ **FIGURE 2-1**

The Latin word *barba,* for "beard," gives us our modern English word *beard.*

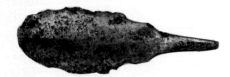

▲ **FIGURE 2-2**

Double-edged razor, early Bronze Age (2000–1400 BC)

Courtesy Manx National Heritage.

all cosmetics, and the use of henna as a coloring agent was first recorded in 1500 BC (**Figure 2-3**).

The use of barbers by Egyptian noblemen and priests 6,000 years ago is substantiated within Egypt's written records, art, and sculpture. The barber **Meryma'at** is one historical figure whose work was apparently held in such high esteem that his image was sculpted for posterity. Every third day, Meryma'at would shave the priests' entire bodies to ensure their purity before entering the temple. High-ranking men and women of Egypt had their heads shaved for comfort when wearing wigs and for the prevention of parasitic infestations.

In Africa, hair was groomed with intricately carved combs and ornamented with beads, clay, and colored bands (**Figure 2-4**). The Masai warriors wove their front hair into three sections of tiny braids and the rest of the hair into a queue down the back. Braiding was used extensively, with the intricate patterns frequently denoting status within the tribe.

Many Biblical passages refer to the barber profession. According to Leviticus, Moses (b.1391 BC) was told by God to command those who had recovered from leprosy to shave all their body hair as part of a ritual cleansing. Ezekiel referred to an ancient custom when he said, "Take thou a barber's razor and cause it to pass upon thy head and upon thy beard." Based on these and other Biblical references, it has been accepted that barbering was available to the general population during the lifetime of Moses.

Although Greek-Sicilian barbers from Sicily introduced shears to Rome sometime between 700 and 800 BC, it was in Greece during its Golden Age (500–300 BC) that barbering became a highly developed art. Well-trimmed beards became status symbols, and Greek men had them trimmed, curled, and scented on a regular basis. Barbershops became the gathering place for sporting, social, and political news, and barbers rose in prominence to become leading citizens within the social structure. Barbers were virtually unknown in Rome until 296 BC.

In the third century BC, the Macedonian troops of Alexander the Great lost several battles to the Persians as a result of the warriors' beards. The Persians would grab the Macedonian warriors by their beards and drag them to the ground, where they were either speared or beheaded. Alexander issued a decree that all soldiers were to be clean-shaven from that point on. Eventually, the general populace adopted the trend and, although the trimming of beards declined, barbers were kept busy performing shaves and haircuts.

Ticinius Mena of Sicily is credited with bringing shaving and barbering services to Rome in 296 BC. The men of Rome enjoyed tonsorial services such as shaves, haircutting and dressing, massage, and manicuring on a daily basis, with a good portion of their day spent at the barber's. While the average citizen patronized the barbers' places of business, rich noblemen engaged private *tonsors* to take care of their hairdressing and shaving needs. The Romans expanded the concept of these personal services to include communal bathing and what became known as the Roman baths.

Clean-shaven faces were the trend until Hadrian came into power in 117 AD. Emperor Hadrian became a trendsetter when he grew his beard to hide scars on his chin. This resulted in the populace following his lead, and the beard was again in fashion.

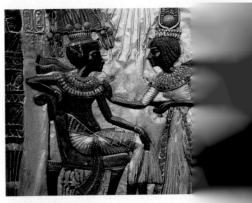

▲ **FIGURE 2-3**
The Egyptians wore elaborate hairdos and makeup.

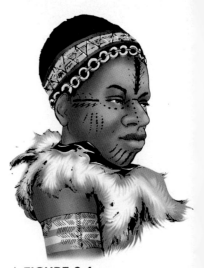

▲ **FIGURE 2-4**
Africans groomed their hair with intricately carved combs and ornamental beads, clay, and colored bands.

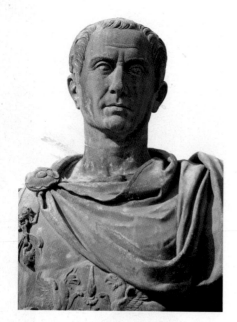

CUSTOMS AND TRADITIONS

In almost every early culture hairstyles indicated social status. Noblemen of ancient Gaul indicated their rank by wearing their hair long; this continued until Caesar made them cut it when he conquered them, as a sign of submission. In ancient Greece, boys would cut their hair upon reaching adolescence, while their Hindu counterparts would shave their heads. Following the invasion of China by the Manchu, Chinese men adopted the queue as a mark of dignity and manhood.

The ancient Britons were extremely proud of their long hair. Blond hair was brightened with washes composed of tallow, lime, and the extracts of certain vegetables. Darker hair was treated with dyes extracted and processed from plants, trees, and various soils. The Danes, Angles, and Normans dressed their hair for beautification, adornment, and ornamentation before battles with the Britons.

In ancient Rome, the color of a woman's hair indicated her class or rank. Noblewomen tinted their hair red; those of the middle class colored their hair blond; and poor women were compelled to dye their hair black. At various times in Roman history, slaves would be allowed or disallowed to wear beards, depending on the dictates of the ruler.

In later centuries, religion, occupation, and politics also influenced the length and style of hair and the wearing of beards. Clergymen of the Middle Ages were distinguished by the **tonsure** (derived from the Latin *tondere*, "to shear"), a shaved patch on the crown of the head. During the seventh century, Celtic and Roman church leaders disagreed on the exact shape the tonsure should take. The circular tonsure, called the tonsure of St. Peter, left only a slight fringe of hair around the head and was preferred in Germany, Italy, and Spain. The Picts and Scots preferred a semicircular design, known as the tonsure of St. John. After much argument, the Pope eventually decreed that priests were to shave their beards and mustaches and adopt the tonsure of St. Peter.

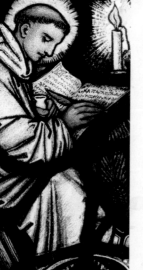

Although the edicts of the church maintained some influence over priests and the general populace for several centuries, the wearing of beards and longer hairstyles had returned by the eleventh century. Priests curled or braided their hair and beards until Pope Gregory issued another Papal decree requiring shaved faces and short hair. In 1972, the Roman Catholic Church finally abolished the practice of tonsure.

By the seventeenth century in England, political affiliation and religion could be indicated by the long, curling locks of the royalist, Anglican cavaliers and the cropped hair of the parliamentarian, Puritan roundheads. British barristers wore gray wigs, while the various branches of the law and the military wore specific styles according to their position or military corps.

Most rulers and monarchs became trendsetters by virtue of their position and power in society. Personal whim, taste, and even physical limitations could become the basis for changes in hairstyles and fashion. For example, when Francis I of France (in the sixteenth century) accidentally burned his hair with a torch, his loyal subjects had their hair, beards, and mustaches cut short.

During the reign of Louis XIV in the seventeenth century, noblemen wore wigs because the king, who was balding, did so. During the nineteenth century in France, men and women showed appreciation for antiquity by wearing variations of the "Caesar cut," the style of the early Roman emperors.

The beliefs, rituals, and superstitions of early civilizations varied from one ethnic group to another, depending on the region and social interactions with other groups. There was a general belief among many groups that hair clippings could bewitch an individual. Hence, the privilege of haircutting was reserved for the priest, medicine man, or other spiritual leader of the tribe. According to the Greek philosopher and mathematician Pythagoras, the hair was the source of the brain's inspiration, and cutting it decreased an individual's intellectual capacity. The Irish peasantry believed that if hair cuttings were burned or buried with the dead, no evil spirits would haunt the individual. Among some Native American tribes it was believed that the hair and the body were so linked that anyone possessing a lock of hair of another might work his will on that individual.

THE BEARD AND SHAVING

The importance of the beard for reasons other than personal preference or adornment lies more in the past than the present. Nonetheless, it is interesting to note the various customs associated with wearing or shaving the beard. Since the practice of shaving predates the written word, it is difficult to determine just when this form of hair removal began.

The excavation of early stone razors or scrapers from the Upper Paleolithic period (40,000–10,000 BC) indicates that early man may have used these tools for hair removal as well as for the skinning of animals. By the time of the Neolithic period (8000–5000 BC) early man had created settlements and begun to farm and raise animals. Artwork of this period shows examples of clean-shaven men, but it is unknown how the hair was removed. However, Egyptian pyramids from around 7000 BC have yielded flint-bladed razors that were used by the ruling classes to shave their heads as well as their faces, and by 4000 BC a form of tweezers was also used.

It stands to reason that the nomadic nature of many early groups would help to spread the practice of shaving throughout the rest of the world. Mesopotamians of 3000 BC were shaving with obsidian blades and by 2800 BC the Sumerians were also clean-shaven. Artwork also shows us that Greek men of 1000 BC were visiting the local barber for shaving services.

In early times, most groups considered the beard to be a sign of wisdom, strength, or manhood. In some cultures, the beard was a sacred symbol. For example, among Orthodox Jews today, the beard is a sign of religious

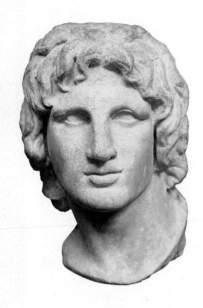

devotion and to cut off one's beard is contrary to Mosaic law. In Rome, a young man's first shave on his 22nd birthday constituted a rite of passage from boyhood to manhood and was celebrated with great festivity.

Certain rulers required that beards be removed. As previously mentioned, Alexander the Great ordered his soldiers to shave so their beards could not be seized in battle. Peter the Great encouraged shaving by imposing a tax on beards. In 1096, the Archbishop of Rouen in France prohibited the wearing of a beard, which resulted in the formation of the first known barber organization.

During the spread of Christianity, long hair came to be considered sinful and the clergy were directed to shave their beards. Although the shaving of the beard was still forbidden among Orthodox Jews, the use of scissors to trim or shape excess growth was permitted. The Muslims took great care in trimming their mustaches and beards after prayer. The hair that was removed was preserved so that it could be buried with its owner.

During the Middle Ages (400 to 1500 AD), three hairs from the English king's beard were imbedded in the wax of the royal seal on a charter written in 1121. Later, it became fashionable to dye the beard and cut it into a variety of shapes during the reign of Queen Elizabeth in England.

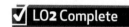

The Rise of the Barber-Surgeons

By the Middle Ages, barbers not only provided tonsorial services but also entered the world of medicine, where they figured prominently in the development of surgery as a recognized branch of medical practice. This was the result of the barbers' interaction with the religious clerics of the day. As the most learned and educated people of the Middle Ages, monks and priests had become the physicians of the period. One of the most common treatments for curing a variety of illnesses was the practice of bloodletting, and barbers often assisted the clergy in this practice. But in 1163 at the Council of Tours, Pope Alexander III forbade the clergy to "draw blood or to act as physicians and surgeons" because it was contrary to Christian doctrine "for ministers of God to draw blood from the human body" (Moler, 1927). It was at this point in history that the barbers took over the duties previously performed by the clergy. They continued the practices of bloodletting, minor surgery, herbal remedies, and tooth pulling. For centuries, dentistry was performed only by barbers, and for more than a thousand years they were known as **barber-surgeons**.

The barber-surgeons formed their first organization in France in 1096 AD and by the 1100s had formed a guild of surgeons that specialized in the study of medicine. By the middle of the thirteenth century, these barber companies had also founded the School of St. Cosmos and St. Domain in Paris to instruct barbers in the practice of surgery.

The Worshipful Company of Barbers guild was formed in London, England in 1308 with the objective of regulating and overseeing the profession. The Barbers' Company was ruled by a master and consisted of two classes of barbers: those who practiced barbering and those who specialized in surgery. By 1368, the surgeons formed their own guild with oversight by the Barber's Guild that lasted until 1462 (**Figure 2-5**). Although there is reason to believe that competition and antagonism existed between the two organizations, a parliamentary act united the two groups in 1450, but separated the practices of each profession. Barbers were limited to the practices of bloodletting, cauterization, tooth pulling, and tonsorial services, and the surgeons were forbidden to act as barbers. The merged guilds became the Company of Barber-Surgeons (**Figure 2-6**).

In 1540, Henry VIII reunited the barbers and surgeons of London through an Act of Parliament by granting a charter to the Company of Barber-Surgeons. The Company commissioned Hans Holbein the Younger, a noted artist of the time, to commemorate the event (**Figure 2-7**).

With the advancement of medicine, the practice of bloodletting became all but obsolete. Although the barber-surgeons' medical practice dwindled in importance, they were still relied upon for dispensing medicinal herbs and pulling teeth. Finally, in 1745, a law was passed in England to separate the barbers from the surgeons and the alliance was completely dissolved.

Barber-surgeons had also flourished in France and Germany. As previously mentioned, the first barber-surgeons' corporation was formed in France in 1096. Later, French barber-surgeons who were under the rule of the king's barber formed another guild in 1371, which lasted until about the time of the French Revolution (1789). It is interesting to note that **Ambroise Pare** (1510–1590), who began his work as a barber-surgeon, is considered the greatest surgeon of the Renaissance period and the father of modern surgery.

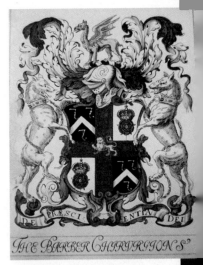

▲ **FIGURE 2-5**

The Worshipful Company of Barbers Coat of Arms.
With permission of The Worshipful Company of Barbers, London, UK.

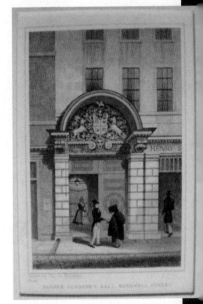

▲ **FIGURE 2-6**

19th Century engraving depicting the first Barber-Surgeon's Hall in London, built in the 1440s.
With permission of The Worshipful Company of Barbers, London, UK.

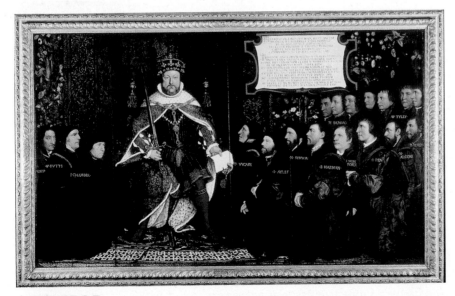

▲ **FIGURE 2-7**

Hans Holbein painting. Henry VIII issuing a charter to the Company of Barber Surgeons.
With permission of The Worshipful Company of Barbers, London, UK.

During the eighteenth and early nineteenth centuries (1700–1800s), wigs became so elaborate and fashionable that a separate corporation of barber-wigmakers was founded in France. Not until 1779 was a similar corporation formed in Prussia, but this was disbanded in 1809 when new unions were started.

Many Europeans had become so dependent upon the services of the barber-surgeons that Dutch and Swedish settlers brought barber-surgeons with them to America to look after the well being of the colonists.

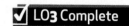

THE BARBER POLE

The symbol of the **barber pole** evolved from the technical procedures of bloodletting performed by the barber-surgeons. The pole is thought to represent the staff that the patient would hold tightly in order for the veins in the arm to stand out during bloodletting. The bottom end-cap of modern barber poles represents the basin that was used as a vessel to either catch the blood during bloodletting or to lather the face for shaving. The white stripes on the pole represent the bandages that were used to stop the bleeding and were hung on the staff to dry. The stained bandages would then twist around the pole in the breeze, forming a red-and-white pattern. One interpretation of the colors of the barber pole is that red represented the blood, blue the veins, and white the bandages. Later, when the Barber Surgeon's Company was formed in England, barbers were required to use blue-and-white poles and surgeons red-and-white poles. It is also thought that that the red, white, and blue poles displayed in the United States originated in deference to the nation's flag. Modern barbers have retained the barber pole as the foremost symbol of the business and profession of barbering. In fact, it is prohibited in some states to display a barber pole at any establishment that is not a licensed barbershop with licensed barbers employed (**Figure 2-8**).

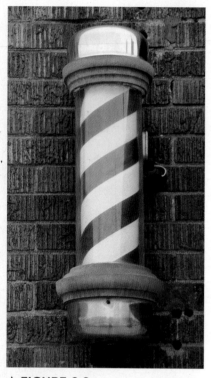

▲ **FIGURE 2-8**
An example of the barber pole.

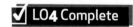

Modern Barbers and Barbering

By the end of the nineteenth century, barbering had completely separated from religion and medicine and began to emerge as an independent profession. During the late 1800s, the profession's structure changed and it began to follow new directions. The formation of employer organizations known as **master barber groups** and employee organizations known as **journeymen barber groups** were the first steps toward upgrading and regulating the profession. During this era the emergence and growth of these organizations helped to establish precedents and standards that are part of today's barbering profession.

The Barbers' Protective Association was organized in 1886. In 1887, it became the Journeymen Barbers' International Union of America at its first convention in Buffalo, New York, and affiliated with the American Federation

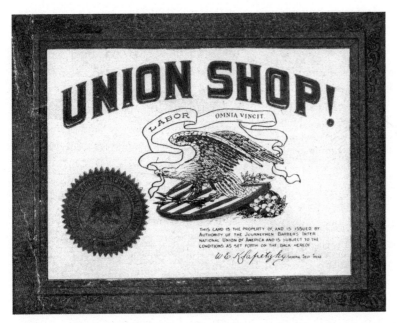

◄ **FIGURE 2-9**
Union label of the Journeymen Barber's
International Union of America.

of Labor. By 1963 the name had changed again to the Journeymen Barbers,
Hairdressers, Cosmetologists, and Proprietors International Union of America
(**Figure 2-9**).

In 1893, **A. B. Moler** established America's first barber school in Chicago,
Illinois. In the same year, he published the first barbering textbook, *The Moler
Manual of Barbering*.

Minnesota was the first state to pass a barber-licensing law. This legislation,
passed in 1897, set standards for sanitation and minimum education and
licensing requirements for barbers and barbershops in that state. The setting
of standards was important because at the time it was common for towels,
shaving brushes, and other barbering tools to be used on more than one
customer without the benefit of being disinfected inbetween. These practices
provided ample opportunity for bacteria or parasites like ringworm, herpes,
or head lice to be spread from one person to another, casting a bad light on
barbers and barbershops overall. Similar laws that included hand washing,
powdered (rather than stick) astringents, regular floor sweeping, and the disinfection of tools were soon passed in other states as result of the need
to protect the public from infectious conditions.

Awareness of the importance of cleaning practices in preventing disease
became so prevalent that the Terminal Methods system was enacted in
1916 in New York City. At that time, it was common to see barbershops,
beauty shops, and other small business enterprises at the main railway
terminals in larger cities. The Terminal Methods system included strict
disinfection and cleaning practices, such as boiling tools in view of
customers and the airtight storage of disinfected implements. The system
soon spread to other shops throughout New York, providing customers
with sanitary and superior service.

In 1924, the Associated Master Barbers of America was organized in Chicago,
Illinois. The name was changed in 1941 to the Associated Master Barbers and
Beauticians of America (**AMBBA**) and represented barbershop and beauty
salon owners and managers.

Code of Ethics

A statement of the responsibility of this shop to its patrons.

We recognize the fact that you are entitled to every possible protection against infection and contagion while in this establishment, and we endeavor to discharge this responsibility by scrupulous adherence to all sanitary precautions.

We believe that you are entitled to the same courteous, careful and conscientious treatment from every practitioner in this establishment, whether you wish all of the services we have to offer or only one, and we sincerely try to carry out this principle.

The preparations dispensed in this establishment and sold for home use are all standard merchandise of the highest quality, bearing the original manufacturer's label.

We consider it our professional duty to suggest and explain to our patrons such services and applications as we think may be needed in any particular case. However, we do not mean to be offensive, overbearing or insistent, and will at all times respect the wishes of our patrons.

We regard the cosmetics for sale in our shop as legitimate aids to the preservation and beautification of hair and the proper care of the skin and scalp.

We feel that we owe the responsibilities enumerated above to every patron of this establishment, regardless of the frequency of his, or her, visits, and the owner would appreciate having called to his attention any lapse on his or her part or on the part of any of our co-workers.

▲ FIGURE 2-10
Barber Code of Ethics.

By 1925, the AMBBA established the National Educational Council with the goal of standardizing and upgrading barber training. The council was successful in standardizing the requirements of barber schools and barber instructor training, establishing a curriculum, and promulgating the passage of state licensing laws.

The National Association of Barber Schools was formed in 1927. Working in cooperation with the Associated Master Barbers and Beauticians of America, the association developed a program that standardized the operation of barber schools.

By 1929, the National Association of State Board of Barber Examiners was organized in St. Paul, Minnesota. Its purpose was to standardize the qualifications required for barber examination applicants and the methods of evaluation to be used. The Associated Master Barbers and Beauticians of America adopted a Barber Code of Ethics to promote professional responsibility in the trade (**Figure 2-10**) and later published a barbering textbook.

Did **You** Know...

Elijah Pierce began woodcarving as a young boy. As an adult, he became a minister and barber, working in both fields for the rest of his life. Elijah would carve during the down times between customers in his barbershop and eventually started displaying his work there. His work became nationally known during the 1970s and, after numerous exhibitions and awards, he is known as one of America's most prominent folk artists. The National Association of Barber Boards of America inducted Elijah Pierce into the Barbering Hall of Fame in 1991 (**Figure 2-11**).

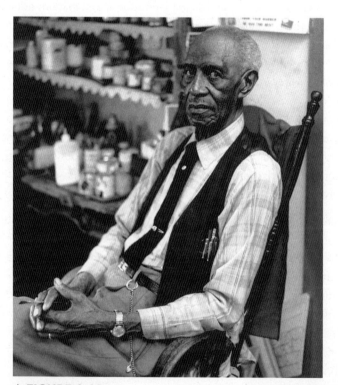

▲ FIGURE 2-11
Elijah Pierce in 1971.

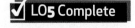

State Barber Boards

Since 1929, all states, with the exception of several counties in Alabama, have passed laws regulating the practice of barbering and hairstyling. The state boards are primarily concerned with the protection of the health, safety, and welfare of the public. They do this through the maintenance of high educational standards to assure competent and skilled service, the licensing of individuals and shops, and the enforcement of infection control laws. Today's state barber boards meet up to twice a year as members of the **National Association of Barber Boards of America** (NABBA). The NABBA established the month of September as National Barber Month "in recognition of the contributions of the barbers to the fabric of our society." The mission and objectives of the NABBA, as posted at http://www.nationalbarberboards.com, are as follows:

- The National Association of Barber Boards of America represents over 300,000 and the icon of the independent businessperson.
- The tonsorial arts have been a tradition in the United States of America since its inception.
- The time-honored tradition of the neighbor barbershop continues to grow and prosper.

Objectives:

1. To promote the exchange of information between state barber boards and state agencies examining, licensing, and regulating the barber industry.

2. To develop standards and procedures for examining barbers.

3. To develop standards for licensing and policing the barber industry.

4. To develop curriculum for educating barbers.

5. To promote continuous education in the barber industry.

6. To develop and promote procedures for insuring that the consumer is informed and protected.

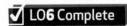 **LO6 Complete**

In this chapter we have seen the progression of barbering from early man to today's regulatory agencies. As a profession, barbering has risen from tribal beginnings to carry the practice of haircutting, styling, and shaving to all parts of the world. Barbers have served as surgeons, dentists, and wig-makers. They have adapted to the eras into which they were born by using the tools at hand **(Figure 2-12)**, from the earliest scissors to the hand clippers of the 1890s or the high-quality electrical tools available today. Barbers have had to adapt to trends, politics, and technological advances to maintain their profession and their livelihoods. Some of these changes were challenging, such as the change brought about by kings who mandated the wearing of wigs, while other

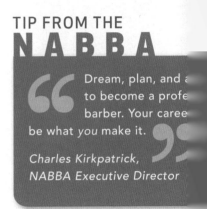

TIP FROM THE
NABBA

"Dream, plan, and ̲ to become a profe̲ barber. Your caree̲ be what *you* make it."

Charles Kirkpatrick,
NABBA Executive Director

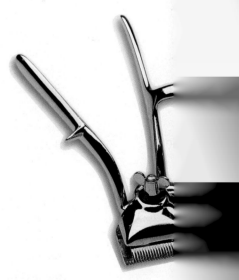

▲ **FIGURE 2-12**
Barbers have adapted to the eras into which they were born using the tools at hand.

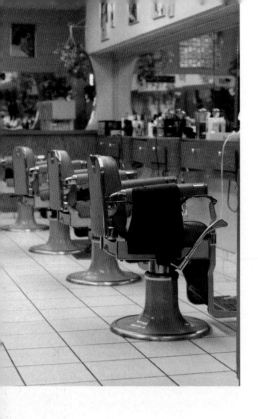

changes have served the profession in a beneficial way. Some of the changes that improved the practice of barbering during the twentieth century include:

1. The implementation of regulatory and educational standards.

2. Improved cleaning practices in the barbershop.

3. The availability and use of better implements and tools.

4. The availability and use of electrical appliances in the shop.

5. The study of anatomy dealing with those parts of the head, face, and neck serviced by the barber.

6. The study of products and preparations used in facial, scalp, and hair treatments.

The enforcement of state barber laws, the advancement of the industry, and the protection of the health, safety, and welfare of the public in the performance of barbering services must rest with today's barbers and their schools, shops, associations, and state boards. As a student of barbering, you are now a member of this profession with its long and established history (**Figure 2-13**). Along with that membership comes a responsibility to maintain and enhance standards, continue the quest for knowledge, and to perfect the technical and social skills so necessary to this profession.

HISTORY OF BARBERING TIMELINE

2.5 million years ago	Stone Age; refers to man's technological history predating the use of metal, which varies in different parts of the world up to 5000 BC; early cutting tools of bone, flint, antler, and shell are produced 600,000 to 700,000 years ago.	1300–900 BC	Iron Age: Smelting processes and metallurgy are refined.
		700–800 BC	Greek-Sicilian barbers from Messina introduce shears to Rome for cutting hair.
		595 BC	The Biblical prophet Ezekiel writes of a "barber's razor."
BC or BCE	*Before the Christian Era*	500 BC	Barbers are prominent and well-trimmed beards fashionable in Greece.
9000–6000 BC	Middle East Neolithic communities develop (late Stone Age).		
5000 BC	Barbering services performed in Egypt.	500–300 BC	The Golden Age of Greece.
3000–1200 BC	Bronze Age: The process of smelting is developed.	334 BC	Alexander the Great prohibits the wearing of beards in battle.
2000–3000 BC	Earliest known scissors appear in Middle East.	325 BC	Shaving is a common practice in Macedonia.
1391–1271 BC	Barbering becomes available to general populace of the Middle East by Moses' time.	296 BC	According to Pliny, barbering and shaving were introduced to Rome by Ticinius Mena.
		100 BC–AD 100	Being clean-shaven is a rule in Rome.

▲ **FIGURE 2-13**

History of Barbering Timeline

AD	*Anno Domini* (Latin: "In the year of our Lord"); the era following the birth of Jesus Christ.	1450	English surgeon and barber guilds merge and become the Company of Barber-Surgeons until 1745; barbers restricted to bloodletting, tooth drawing, cauterization, and tonsorial services.
30–325	Early Christian era; barbers practice shaving throughout Europe and assist physician-clergy until the twelfth century (AD 1100–1199).	1500–1599	Europeans colonize America.
1–100	Galen writes of medical practices, hair treatments, and cosmetic customs in Greece. Cross-bladed shears developed in Rome.	1540	Henry VIII of England reunites the barbers and surgeons through an Act of Parliament to set up the Company of Barbers and Surgeons of London.
117–138	Hadrian grows his beard to hide scarring and sets a new fashion trend.	1541	Painting by Hans Holbein the Younger depicts Henry VIII granting charter to the Company of Barber-Surgeons.
400–1500	Considered to be the millennium of the Middle Ages.		
400–500	Cross-bladed shears developed with center pivot in Rome.	1600–1699	Dutch and Swedish settlers bring barber-surgeons to America.
700–800	Charlemagne sets the trend for long, flowing hair.	1700–1799	Indentured servants and black barbers perform tonsorial services.
1096	William, Archbishop of Rouen (France), prohibits wearing of beards, resulting in formation of the first known barber organization; barber-surgeons travel and practice throughout Europe.	1745	Surgeons again separate from the barbers and form the Company of Surgeons (becomes Royal College of Surgeons in 1800); complete separation of barbers from surgeons enacted by law; barbers keep the barber pole as the sign of their profession.
1163	Council of Tours prohibits clergy to draw blood or act as physicians; barber-surgeons assume medical duties of the clergy, including dentistry.	1750–1850	Wigs in vogue in Europe and worn in the American colonies by the upper classes; barbers add wig-making and maintenance to tonsorial services.
1200–1290	School of St. Cosmos and St. Domain established by barber-surgeons in Paris to instruct barbers in surgery.	1861–1899	American Civil War (1861–1865); beards become popular; barbershops established in towns by English, French, German, and Italian immigrants.
1308	Worshipful Company of Barbers guild founded in London, England; two groups formed: barbers who practiced barbering and those who practiced surgery.	1886	Barbers' Protective Union represented at AFL founding convention in Columbus, Ohio.
1371	French barber-surgeons form a guild under the rule of the king's barber.	1887	Journeymen Barbers' International Union formed at convention in Buffalo, New York (later renamed the Barbers, Beauticians, and Allied Industries International Association).
1368	Surgeon group of Worshipful Company of Barbers form separate guild with oversight by Barber's Guild until 1462.		

▲ **FIGURE 2-13**

(Continued)

1888	Official AFL charter issued to Journeymen Barbers' International Union.	1943	Barbers and Beauty Culturists Union holds first convention in New York City.
1893	A. B. Moler opens first barber school in Chicago and publishes first barbering textbook.	1948	International Barber Schools Association formed in Indianapolis, Indiana.
1897	Minnesota passes the first barber licensing laws.	1950	William Marvy begins manufacture of barber poles.
1916	The Terminal Methods system is established in New York City.	1958	National Barber Show held in New York City.
1921	Matthew Andis, Sr. develops working model of an electric clipper and sells it door-to-door to barbershops; opens Andis Company in 1922.	1959	Edmond ("Pop") O. Roffler develops the Roffler Sculptur-Kut based on European razor-cutting techniques.
		1960s	Social and cultural influences set the stage for the "long hair revolution."
1924	Associated Master Barbers of America (AMBA) organized in Chicago, Illinois; John Oster invents motor-driven hand clipper.	1975	Over 6,000 barbers have been trained in the Roffler Method; still used today.
1925	Associated Master Barbers of America establishes the National Education Council to improve and standardize barbering education.	1980	Barbers, Beauticians, and Allied Industries International Association (formerly the Journeymen Barber International Union) merges with the United Food and Commercial Workers International Union (UFCW).
1927	National Association of Barber Schools organized in Cleveland, Ohio.	1985	Over 50 percent of barber students reported to be female.
1929	National Association of Barber Examiners organized in St. Paul, Minnesota.	1988	Ed Jeffers establishes Barber Museum in Canal Winchester, Ohio.
1931	AMBA publishes textbook of barbering.	1995	Over 50 percent of barber students reported to be African American.
1935	John Oster invents Stim-U-Lax massager, and Oster Lather machine in 1937.	2000–	Resurgence in barbering taking place; new schools opening in many states; new barbershops, both independent and franchised, feature traditional skills and an atmosphere geared to the male consumer.
1940–1949	Flat top, butch cut, crew cut, and Princeton cut become popular hairstyles.		
1941	Associated Master Barbers of America changes name to Associated Master Barbers and Beauticians of America.		

▲ **FIGURE 2-13**

(Continued)

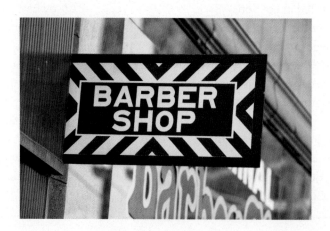

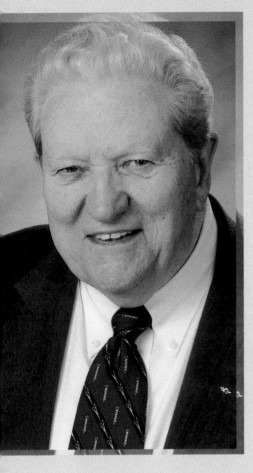

THE ED JEFFERS BARBER MUSEUM

The Ed Jeffers Barber Museum is located in Canal Winchester, Ohio, and is open to the public by appointment. A virtual tour is available at http://www.edjeffersbarbermuseum.com.

Entering the Ed Jeffers Barber Museum is like taking a step back in time. The first thing that catches the eye is the number and variety of barber poles, including a one-of-a-kind antique red-and-white barber pole that must stand over 6 feet tall. Beautiful oak barber stations with red plush–upholstered seats invite one to sit down and relax while having a good old-fashioned "shave and a haircut."

The Ed Jeffers Barber Museum was started in Canal Winchester in 1988 with fewer than a dozen pieces. Today it has grown to several thousand individual artifacts from as early as the 1700s. Housed in over 3,500 square feet, the museum was created to preserve the roots and document the progression of the barbering profession. "It's important to know where we've come from and how we've progressed, in order to know where we're going," said museum founder Ed Jeffers in a brief interview.

Since its beginning, the museum has welcomed visitors from more than 44 states and 10 countries. It has been featured on television shows on the Discovery Channel and the Family Channel, as well as on television in Japan. The museum has also been featured in journals such as *Smithsonian* magazine and on the front page of the *Wall Street Journal* (July 30, 1999).

Jeffers was able to collect rare items from all over the country due to the positions he held during his lifetime. A barber for over 48 years, he was a member of the Ohio State Barber Board for over 36 years and an officer with the National Association of Barber Boards of America for over 33 years. Edwin C. Jeffers passed away on July 5, 2006, but many remember him with affection and respect for his dedication and contributions to the barbering industry.

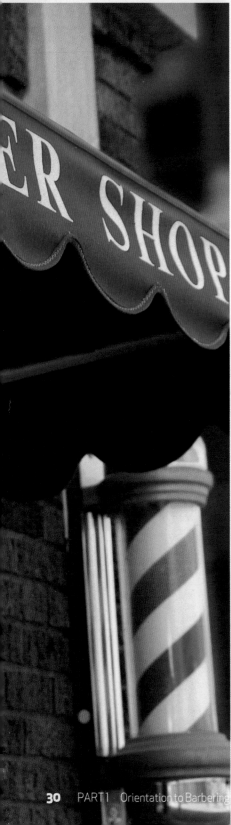

2 Review Questions

1. What is the origin of the word *barber?*

2. What is the name of the Egyptian barber commemorated with a sculpture?

3. Which country is credited with being the first to cultivate beauty in an extravagant fashion?

4. Name the person credited with bringing barbering and shaving to Rome.

5. Explain the duties of Egyptian barbers associated with the priests of that culture.

6. List the human characteristics sometimes associated with the wearing of a beard.

7. Explain the duties of the barber-surgeons.

8. Explain the origin of the modern barber pole.

9. Which ethnic groups brought barber-surgeons to America?

10. Identify the name of the early barber employer organizations.

11. Identify the name of the early barber employee organizations.

12. In what year did A. B. Moler open the first barber school in America?

13. Who was the author of the first barbering textbook?

14. Name the first state to pass a barber licensing law and the year in which it was passed.

15. Explain the primary function of state barber boards.

16. What does NABBA stand for?

Chapter
Glossary

A. B. Moler wrote the first barbering textbook; opened the first barber school in Chicago in 1893

AMBBA Associated Master Barbers and Beauticians of America

Ambroise Pare French barber-surgeon who became known as the father of surgery

barba Latin for beard

barber pole most often a red, white, and blue striped pole that is the iconic symbol of the barbering profession

barber-surgeons early practitioners who cut hair, shaved, and performed bloodletting and dentistry

journeymen barber groups barber employee unions

master barber groups barber employer unions

Meryma'at Egyptian barber commemorated with a statue

National Association of Barber Boards of America the association of the state barber boards

Ticinius Mena Sicilian credited with bringing barbering and shaving to Rome in 296 BC

tonsorial related to the cutting, clipping, or trimming of hair with shears or a razor

tonsure a shaved patch on the head

3 Professional Image

☑ Learning Objectives

AFTER COMPLETING THIS CHAPTER, YOU SHOULD BE ABLE TO:

1 Define *professional image.*

2 Discuss the ways in which life skills, values, and beliefs influence your professional image.

3 Explain the relationship between personality and attitudes and the demonstration of professional behavior.

4 List the guidelines to maintaining personal and professional health.

5 Demonstrate an understanding of effective human relations and communication skills.

6 List the rules of professional ethics.

7 Discuss the basic principles of personal and professional success.

8 Explain the concepts of motivation and self-management.

9 Create short-term and long-term goals.

10 Discuss time-management skills.

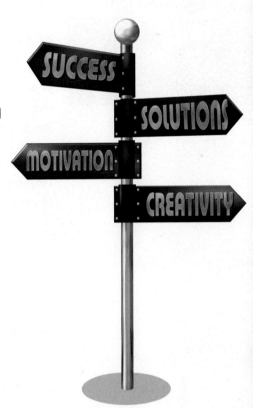

Key Terms

PAGE NUMBER INDICATES WHERE IN THE CHAPTER THE TERM IS USED.

attitude / 36	goal setting / 48	rapport / 41
beliefs / 35	life skills / 34	receptivity / 36
compartmentalization / 46	motivation / 47	self-management / 47
diplomacy / 36	personal hygiene / 37	values / 35
ergonomics / 40	personality / 36	
ethics / 44	professional image / 34	

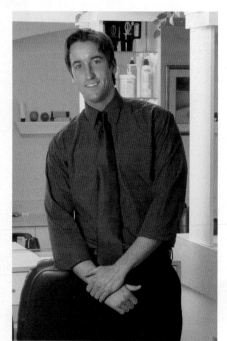

▲ FIGURE 3-1

Project a professional image.

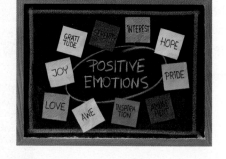

Do you know that you are a unique and complex individual? Indeed, we are all unique and complex due to both the many similarities and the many differences each of us has with regard to others. In this chapter, you will explore a variety of factors that originate from your innermost self—factors that have the ability to influence your professional image.

Your Professional Image

The image you project to others is a reflection of you as an individual. Your personality, attitude, abilities, appearance, and moral character all help to create emotional and mental pictures in the hearts and minds of every person you interact with in daily life. This image is the *impression* you make on others in your personal and professional lives. And although your personal image may differ somewhat from your professional image, the values and beliefs that guide you in both capacities stem from the inner source of the real and authentic you.

In this chapter, we define your **professional image** as the impression that you project as a person engaged in the profession of barbering. Your professional image consists of the outward appearance, attitude, and conduct that you exhibit in the workplace. In addition, it reflects your prior learning and the life experiences or life skills that continually add to your total professional development. Ultimately, the professional image you project to coworkers and clients will impact your present and future success (**Figure 3-1**).

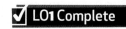

LIFE SKILLS

We begin our discussion of your professional image with some insights into what are known as life skills. **Life skills** are an important basis from which to begin because they are the tools and guidelines that prepare you for living as a mature adult in a challenging and often complicated world. Life skills provide the foundation that will help you face life's difficulties, successfully manage situations you find challenging, and empower you to reach your full personal and professional potential.

Life skills are developed through learning and experience. As such, many life skills are learned through our parents and families. Being considerate of others' feelings or valuing honesty are life skills that many of us have been taught from an early age. Other life skills, such as patience or adaptability, may have been learned from actual experiences or situations that required the application of these particular skills in order to benefit from the experience or handle the situation. In either scenario, once a life skill has been learned and practiced, it can become part of your personal foundation so that you are better prepared to successfully manage future life experiences.

While there are many life skills that can provide you with a solid foundation from which to support your personal and professional journey through life, some of the most important are:

- Genuine concern and caring for other people
- The ability to adapt to different situations

- The development and achievement of goals

- Persistence and a "can-do" attitude

- Follow-through in the completion of jobs, tasks, and commitments

- The development and use of common sense

- The establishment of positive and healthy relationships

- Approaching everything with a strong sense of responsibility and a positive attitude

- Feeling good about yourself

- Being cooperative

- Being organized

- Maintaining a sense of humor

- Being patient with yourself and others

- Being honest and trustworthy

- Striving for excellence

You are now at the beginning of your barbering education and training. Each student embarks upon this training with a set of life skills based on prior learning environments and opportunities that should grow and expand with new experiences. New experiences can be used as stepping stones toward the development and enhancement of your personal and professional life skills. The attitude with which each individual meets and learns from each new experience originates from his or her personal values and beliefs.

- *Values:* The deepest feelings and thoughts we have about ourselves and about life are called values. **Values** consist of what we think, how we feel, and how we act based on what we think and feel. For example, let's say you value loyalty. You *think* it is important in a friendship and expect it in your relationships. One day you overhear a friend sharing with someone else something you've said to him or her in confidence and you *feel* hurt and betrayed. The way in which you react to the situation is an *action* that is taken in response to what you are *thinking* and *feeling*.

- *Beliefs:* Specific attitudes that occur as a result of our values and that have a strong influence on how we act or behave in situations are called **beliefs.** For example, if you value responsibility, you probably take on more than your share of commitments to your family, school, workplace, or community. This example shows us the link between a positive belief and a resulting positive behavior; however, beliefs can be negative in nature as well.

When you tell yourself or others that you can't do something, you are setting yourself up for a negative self-fulfilling prophecy that comes true simply because you *think* it will come true. Conversely, you can initiate a positive self-fulfilling prophecy to inspire change, action, or a commitment to your goals by substituting "I can" for "I can't." Changing your beliefs will change your behavior, and focusing on *what is* rather than *what is not* is a much more positive approach to attaining your goals.

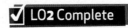 ✔ **LO2 Complete**

PERSONALITY

Your **personality** plays an important role in both your personal and professional life. Personality can be defined as the outward reflection of inner feelings, thoughts, attitudes, and values. It is expressed through your voice, speech, and choice of words, as well as through your facial expressions, gestures, actions, posture, clothing, grooming, and environment. Your personality defines who you are and distinguishes you from others, making you the unique individual that you are. In the people-oriented profession of barbering, your personality becomes one of the most important demonstrations of your particular style of professionalism. In this section we will explore the many personal characteristics that are expressed through one's personality.

ATTITUDE

There is an old adage that says, "The only difference between a good day and a bad day is your **attitude**." This is an effective reminder that we are in control of our attitudes and the outlook we have on life at any given point. Although one's attitude stems from innate values and beliefs, the adage also reminds us that an attitude does not have to be stagnant or "written in stone." Rather, attitudes can be altered or changed if we remain open minded to new insights. This ongoing process is called *attitude development* and it can expand with each new life experience.

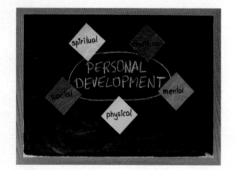

Although there are times when our attitudes may be influenced by friends, family, or circumstances, the extent to which we allow others or situations to *change* our attitude is really up to us. We can assume positive, negative, or neutral attitudes, but we also have to live with the consequences of our reactions. We also need to remember that attitude is one of the most obvious and apparent aspects of personality. It is there for all to see in both personal and professional life. Review the following aspects of a well-developed attitude to determine how you might enhance your own attitude development.

- *Diplomacy:* **Diplomacy** is the art of being tactful, and being tactful means having the perception and skill to say or do the right thing without offending or being critical.

- *Emotional stability:* Learn to control your emotions. Do not reveal negative emotions such as anger, envy, and dislike. An even-tempered person is usually treated with respect.

- *Sensitivity:* Your personality shines the most when you show concern for the feelings of others. Sensitivity is a combination of understanding, empathy, and acceptance that leads to being compassionate and responsive to other people.

- *Receptivity:* **Receptivity** means being interested in and responsive to the ideas, feelings, and opinions of others.

- *Courtesy:* Courtesy and good manners reflect your thoughtfulness toward others. Good manners are expressed by treating other people with respect, exercising care of their property, being tolerant and understanding of their shortcomings and efforts, and being considerate of those with whom you work. Courtesy is one of the most important keys to a successful career.

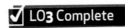 **LO3 Complete**

PERSONAL AND PROFESSIONAL HEALTH

In accordance with the general concept of a profession that helps others to look their best, barbers should strive to reflect their own best image. An important aspect of this representation is the barber's personal health and physical appearance. To achieve success in this area, it is helpful to follow a set of guidelines that help to maintain both a healthy body and a healthy mind.

- *Hygiene:* Hygiene is the branch of applied science concerned with healthful living; its main purpose is to preserve health. **Personal hygiene** is the daily maintenance of cleanliness and healthfulness through certain sanitary practices. These include daily bathing or showering, shaving, using deodorant or antiperspirant, brushing and flossing teeth, using mouthwash, and maintaining clean, well-groomed hair and nails **(Figure 3-2)**.

- *Personal grooming and appearance:* Personal grooming is an extension of personal hygiene that includes your hairstyle, facial hair or makeup design, and choice of apparel. A well-groomed barber is one of the best advertisements for the barbershop or salon. If you present a poised and attractive image, your clients will have confidence in you as a professional. Many shop owners consider appearance, personality, and poise to be as important as technical knowledge and manual skills.

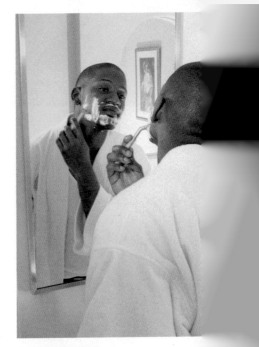

▲ FIGURE 3-2
Practice personal hygiene every day.

- Although many shop owners do not require their barbers to wear standard uniforms, they may have a specific dress code for the shop. For example, some may require the wearing of a barber's jacket, a smock, or even a tie! Select your outfits so that you reflect the image of the shop and dress for success. Clothes should be clean, pressed, and fit well; avoid excessively baggy clothing that can get in the way of your work. Shoes should be supportive, polished, and kept in good repair. Jewelry should be chosen with care; avoid long chains that can dangle in a client's face or get caught on equipment. Wristwatches should be waterproof and will help you maintain your schedule on the job.

- *Rest and relaxation:* Adequate sleep is essential for good health because without it you cannot function efficiently. The body needs to be allowed to recover from the fatigue of the day's activities and should be replenished with a good night's sleep. Body tissues and organs are rebuilt and renewed during the sleeping process. The amount of sleep needed to feel refreshed varies from person to person. Some people function well with 6 hours of sleep while others need 8 hours. An average of 7 or 8 hours of sleep each night is recommended by medical professionals. Relaxation is also important as a change of pace from day-today routines. Going to

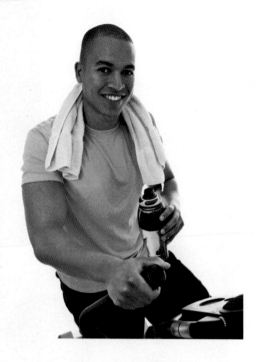

a movie or a museum, reading a book, watching television, playing sports, or dancing are just some ways to "get away from it all." When you return to work, you should feel refreshed and eager to attend to your duties.

- *Nutrition:* What you eat affects your health, appearance, personality, and performance on the job. The nutrients in food supply the body with energy and ensure that the body functions properly. A balanced diet should include foods containing a variety of important vitamins and minerals. Drink plenty of water daily. Try to avoid sugar, salt, caffeine, and fatty or highly refined and processed foods.

- *Exercise:* Exercise and recreation in the form of walking, dancing, sports, and gym activities tend to develop the muscles and help to keep the body fit. Regular physical activity benefits the body by improving blood circulation, oxygen supply, and proper organ function.

- *Stress management and a healthy lifestyle:* Stress is defined as the inability to cope with a real or imagined threat that results in a series of mental and physical responses or adaptations. The way in which individuals perform under stressful situations depends on their personality type, temperament, physical health, and coping skills. Practice stress management through a combination of rest, relaxation, exercise, and daily routines that provide you with time to calm the body and its systems. To maintain a healthy lifestyle, avoid substances that can have a negative effect on health, such as tobacco, alcohol, and drugs. Live a life of moderation in which work and other activities are balanced so that you can achieve a sense of harmony in your life.

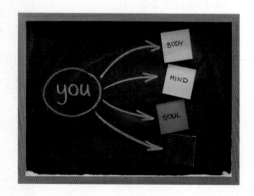

- *Healthy thoughts:* The body and mind operate as a unit; therefore thoughts and emotions can influence the body's activities. A thought may either stimulate or depress the way the body functions. Strong emotions such as worry and fear have a harmful effect on the heart, arteries, and glands. Depression weakens the functioning of the body's organs, thereby lowering resistance to disease.

- *Posture:* Your posture is an aspect of your physical presentation that is important to your professional image. Good posture presents your personal appearance to its best advantage, helps to create an image of confidence, lessens fatigue, and reduces the opportunity for other physical problems to occur.

Working as a barber, you will spend most of your time in a standing position. Raising your arms to work at the top of the client's head or bending over at the shampoo bowl are repetitive motions that can create physical stress in the hand, wrist, arm, shoulder, and lower back areas. When such stresses occur, physical or movement therapies may be required to maintain proper body alignment **(Figure 3-3)**.

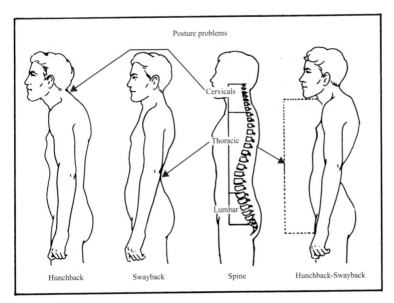

Posture problems

Cervicals

Thoracic

Lumbar

Hunchback   Swayback   Spine   Hunchback-Swayback

◀ **FIGURE 3-3**

Posture problems.

Compare the barber's posture in **Figures 3-4** and **3-5**; then practice the following guidelines for maintaining a more stress-free standing posture behind the chair.

▶ Keep your head up and chin parallel to the floor.

▶ Keep the neck elongated and balanced above the shoulders.

▶ Lift your upper body so that your chest is up and out—do not slouch.

▶ Hold your shoulders level and relaxed.

▶ Stand with your spine straight.

▶ Pull in your abdomen so it is flat.

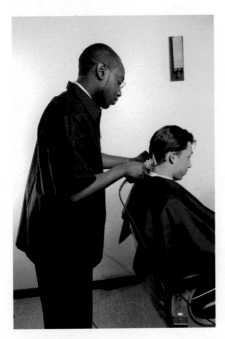

▲ **FIGURE 3-4**

Poor standing posture.

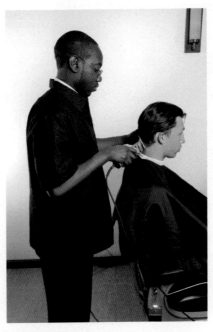

▲ **FIGURE 3-5**

Good standing posture.

Just as there is a mechanically correct posture for standing, there is also a correct sitting posture. Compare the barber's sitting posture in **Figures 3-6** and **3-7**; then use the following guidelines to learn to sit correctly in a balanced position.

▶ Keep your hips level and horizontal, not tilted forward or backward.

▶ Flex your knees slightly and position them over your feet.

▶ Lower your body smoothly into a chair, keeping your back straight.

▶ Keep the soles of your feet on the floor directly under your knees.

▶ Have the seat of the chair even with your knees. This will allow the upper and lower legs to form a 90-degree angle at the knees.

▶ Rest the weight of your torso on the thighbones, not on the end of the spine.

▶ Keep your torso erect.

▶ When sitting at a desk, make sure it is at the correct height so that the upper and lower parts of your arm form a right angle when you are writing.

• *Ergonomics:* **Ergonomics** is the study of human characteristics for a specific work environment that attempts to fit the tasks, equipment, and environment to the worker, rather than the worker to the job. As previously mentioned, barbers are particularly susceptible to problems of the hands, wrists, arms, shoulders, neck, back, feet, and legs.

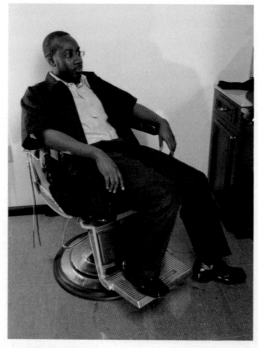

▲ **FIGURE 3-6**
Poor sitting posture.

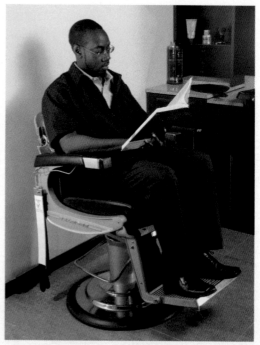

▲ **FIGURE 3-7**
Good sitting posture.

Prevention is the key to avoiding these problems by fitting your work to your body and not your body to your work **(Figure 3-8)**. Practice some of the following suggestions to work more comfortably and effectively.

► Do not grip or squeeze tools and implements too tightly.

► Do not bend the wrist up or down constantly when cutting hair or using a blow-dryer.

► Try to position your arms at less than a 60-degree angle when holding your arms away from your body while working.

► Avoid bending or twisting your body.

► Wear appropriate and supportive shoes or footwear.

► Adjust the height of the chair so that the client's head is at a comfortable working level.

► Tilt the client's head as necessary for better access during hair services.

► Keep your wrists in a straight or neutral position as much as possible.

► Keep tools and implements sharpened and well lubricated.

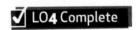 **LO4 Complete**

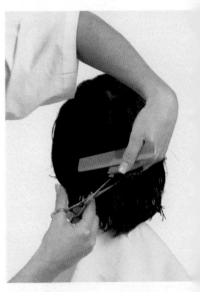

▲ **FIGURE 3-8**
Improper positioning of body, arms, hands, wrists, and shears.

Human Relations

Human relations is the psychology of getting along well with others. Effective human relations skills help you build rapport with clients and coworkers. **Rapport** may be defined as a close and empathetic relationship that establishes agreement and harmony between individuals. Your professional attitude is expressed by your self-esteem, confidence, and the respect you show others. Good habits and practices acquired during your education lay the foundation for a successful career in barbering. The following guidelines for good human relations will help you gain confidence, deal courteously with others, and become a successful professional.

• Always greet clients by name, using a pleasant tone of voice. Address clients by their last name, as in "Mr. Jones" or "Mrs. Smith," unless the client prefers first names or it is customary to use first names in the barbershop.

• Be alert to the client's mood. Some clients prefer quiet and relaxation; others like to talk. Be a good listener and confine the conversation to the client's needs. Never gossip or tell off-color stories.

• Topics of conversation should be carefully chosen. Friendly relations are achieved through pleasant conversations. Let the client guide the topic of conversation. In a business setting it is best to avoid such controversial topics as religion and politics, personal problems, or issues relating to other people. Never discuss other clients or coworkers, and always maintain an ethical standard of confidentiality. Never discuss personal wages, tips, rent, or tax information.

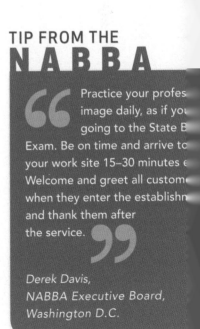

TIP FROM THE
NABBA

" Practice your profes image daily, as if yo going to the State E Exam. Be on time and arrive to your work site 15–30 minutes e Welcome and greet all custom when they enter the establishm and thank them after the service. "

Derek Davis,
NABBA Executive Board,
Washington D.C.

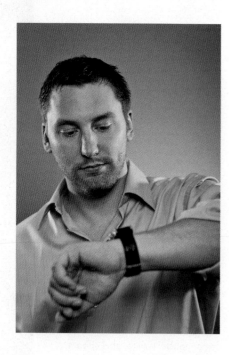

- Make a good impression by looking the part of the successful barber and by speaking and acting in a professional manner at all times.

- Cultivate self-confidence and project a pleasing personality.

- Show interest in the client's personal preferences and give the client undivided attention.

- Use tact and diplomacy when dealing with problems you may encounter.

- Deal with all disputes and differences in private. Take care of all problems promptly and to the client's satisfaction.

- Be capable and efficient.

- Be punctual. Arrive at work on time and keep appointments on schedule. Plan each day's schedule so that you manage your time effectively.

In addition to basic human relations skills, barbering students need to cultivate other aspects of a professional image that can impact their success in the profession. Some desirable qualities for effective client relations are:

- *Talking less, listening more:* There is an old saying that we were given two ears and one mouth for a reason. When you practice good listening skills, you are fully attentive to what the other person is saying. If there is something that you don't understand, ask questions to gain understanding **(Figure 3-9)**.

- *Emotional control:* Learn to control your emotions. Try to respond rather than to react. Do not reveal negative emotions such as anger, envy, and dislike through gestures, facial expressions, or conversation. An even-tempered person is usually treated with respect.

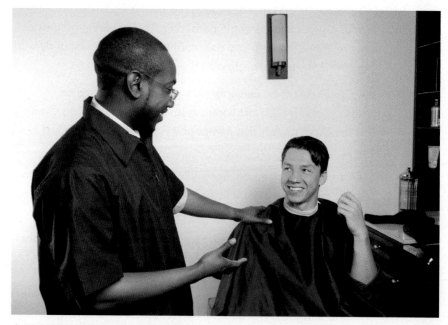

▲ **FIGURE 3-9**

Ask questions to gain understanding.

- *Positive approach:* Be pleasant and gracious. Be ready with a smile of greeting and a word of welcome for each client and coworker. A good sense of humor is also important in maintaining a positive attitude. A sense of humor enriches your life and cushions the disappointments. When you are able to laugh at yourself, you will have gained the ability to accept and deal positively with difficult situations.

- *Good manners:* Good manners reflect your thoughtfulness toward others. Treating others with respect, exercising care of other people's property, being tolerant and understanding of their shortcomings and efforts, and being considerate of those with whom you work all express good manners. As previously mentioned, courtesy is one of the most important keys to a successful career.

- *Mannerisms:* Gum chewing and nervous habits such as tapping your foot or playing with your hair detract from the effectiveness of your image. Yawning, coughing, and sneezing should be concealed with your hand in front of your mouth. Control negative body language—sarcastic or disapproving facial grimaces, for example. Exhibiting pleasant mannerisms and attractive gestures and actions should be your goal at all times.

EFFECTIVE COMMUNICATION SKILLS

Effective communication is one of the barber's most important human relations skills. Communication includes listening skills, voice, speech, and conversational ability—all of which are necessary to forming satisfying relationships with customers and coworkers.

Communication is the act of transmitting information in the form of symbols, gestures, or behaviors to express an idea or concept so that it is clearly understood **(Figure 3-10)**. This requires sending and receiving

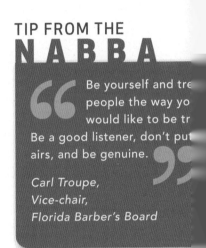

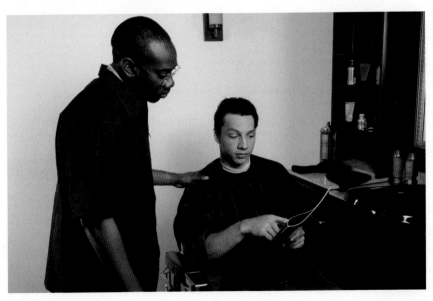

▲ **FIGURE 3-10**
Communication is the act of transmitting information.

messages in order to establish a relationship, or rapport, with the client. The following steps can be used to help you determine your clients' service expectations.

- *Organize your thoughts:* What question or information do you want your client to understand? For example, a client with medium-length hair that covers the top part of the ears says he wants a trim. You will need to determine just what the client's definition of a trim is and may ask if he wants the tops of his ears covered or not.

- *Clarify:* The next step is to clarify what the client is telling you. In the preceding scenario, let's say the client's response to the question is that he wants his hair "over the ears." This answer still does not provide you with the information you need to proceed with the haircut. Why? Because you now have to clarify what the client means by "over the ears." Does it mean covering the tops of the ears, or does it mean above and/or around the ears?

- *Repeat:* Once you have an understanding of the client's definition of "over the ears" or any other description used, repeat to the client your interpretation of what you think he told you. This communication step will provide you with further clarification and the opportunity to make other changes and to reach an understanding of the client's expectations.

There are many ways in which effective communication skills can impact your professional success. Review the following barbershop or salon activities that benefit from effective communication skills.

- Making contacts and networking

- Meeting and greeting clients

- Understanding a client's service needs, likes, dislikes, desires, and expectations

- Self-promotion and building a clientele

- Selling services and products

- Telephone conversations and appointment bookings

- Conversation and interaction with the shop or salon staff, clients, and vendors

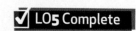 **LO5 Complete**

PROFESSIONAL ETHICS

Ethics are the principles and standards of good character, proper conduct, and moral judgment. The governing board or commission of a particular occupation often creates a code of ethics, which specifically relates to the characteristics of that profession. For example, state barber boards set the ethical standards that all barbers must follow while working in each state.

Ethics, however, goes beyond a set of rules and regulations. In barbering, ethics is also a code of conduct that is expressed through your personality, human relations skills, and professional image.

Ethical conduct helps build the client's confidence in you. Having clients speak well of you is the best form of advertising and helps build a successful business. All professional barbers should practice the following rules of ethics:

- Give courteous and friendly service to all clients. Treat everyone honestly and fairly; do not show favoritism.

- Be courteous and show respect for the feelings, beliefs, and rights of others.

- Keep your word. Be responsible and fulfill your obligations.

- Build your reputation by setting an example of good conduct and behavior.

- Be loyal to your employer, managers, and associates.

- Obey all the barber board laws and rules in your state.

- Practice the highest standards of sanitation and decontamination to protect your health and the health of your coworkers and clients.

- Believe in your chosen profession. Practice it faithfully and sincerely.

- Do not try to sell clients a product or service they do not need or want.

- As a student, be loyal and cooperative with school personnel and fellow students. Comply with all school policies and procedures.

Questionable practices, extravagant claims, and unfulfilled promises violate the rules of ethical conduct and cast an unfavorable light on barbers. Unethical practices affect the student, practicing barbers, schools, barbershops or salons, and the entire industry.

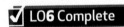
✔ **LO6 Complete**

The Psychology of Success

Defining *success* is a highly individualized and personal matter. For some, money is the measure of their success; for others, career satisfaction or helping others makes them feel successful and fulfilled. Regardless of your personal definition of success, there are some basic principles that form the foundation of personal and professional success.

- *Build self-esteem:* Self-esteem is based on inner strength and begins with trusting in your ability to reach your goals. It is a form of self-belief that helps you feel good about yourself and what you can accomplish.

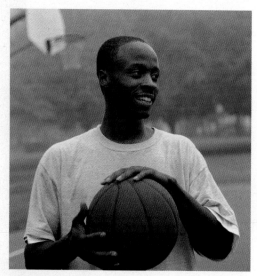

▲ FIGURE 3-11

Recreational activities help you build on strengths and maintain a positive self-image.

Getty Images.

- *Visualize:* Visualize yourself in whatever scenario is relevant to the situation or environment that requires your attention. Picture yourself as a confident and competent person who earns the trust and respect of the others involved in the scenario. The more you practice visualization techniques, the more easily you can turn possibilities and dreams into realities.

- *Build on your strengths:* Spend time doing whatever it is that helps you maintain a positive self-image. Use areas of personal interest to provide incremental challenges that help you build on strengths and expand your success-building options **(Figure 3-11)**.

- *Be kind to yourself:* Put a stop to self-critical and negative thoughts that can work against you. If you make a mistake, think about what you could have done differently, forgive yourself, and plan to do your best next time.

- *Define success for yourself:* Be a success in your own eyes and do not depend on other person's definition of success. What is right for others may not be right for you.

- *Practice new behaviors:* Practicing new behaviors that are not a part of your regular lifestyle can help you develop personally and professionally. For example, if you are nervous about speaking in front of your classmates, practice! Take advantage of every opportunity to hone your speaking skills and create a stepping-stone path to success that will make it easier for you each time you engage in the activity. Remember that creating success is a skill that can be learned, so don't be afraid to try new things.

- *Keep your personal life separate from your work or school life:* Another aspect of success psychology is the ability to keep your personal and professional lives separate. While we all have responsibilities and concerns that impact our multidimensional lives, it is important to know when, where, and to what extent it is permissible to talk about personal issues. In the work and school environments, the answer is almost never. People who talk about themselves (or others) at work or school can negatively impact and undermine the professional atmosphere that is an important aspect of work and learning environments. In the barbershop or salon, clients should not be subjected to comments about coworkers, personal opinions, or complaints. Clients patronize a barbershop to receive personal services and should be treated with utmost professionalism. If you find it difficult to keep your personal life out of these environments, try an exercise known as **compartmentalization.** Imagine that you have two filing cabinets; one is labeled Personal and the other, Professional. Visualize yourself locking the Personal file cabinet before leaving for work or school and opening the Professional cabinet when you arrive at your destination. This exercise helps you store things away in the different compartments of the mind—and it works.

- *Keep your energy up:* Successful people know how to pace themselves. Get enough rest, exercise, eat a nutritious diet, and spend time with family and friends. Successful people know that having a clear head, a fit body, and the ability to refuel and recharge are important conditions for maintaining a successful lifestyle.

- *Respect others:* Make a point of relating to everyone you know with a conscious feeling of respect. This includes basic principles such as using good manners; using words like *please, thank you,* or *excuse me* are common courtesies that should be practiced at all times. Avoid interrupting or speaking when someone else is talking. Be respectful of others and they will be respectful of you.

- *Stay productive:* The three habits that can keep you from maintaining peak performance are procrastination, perfectionism, and the lack of a game plan. Work on eliminating these troublesome habits and you will see an almost instant improvement in your ability to achieve your goals.

- *Remind yourself:* Success is a choice—and it is your choice.

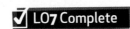 **LO7 Complete**

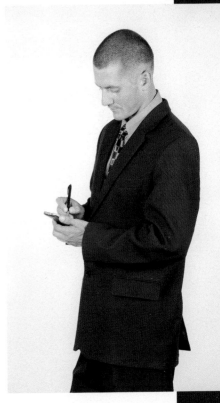

MOTIVATION AND SELF-MANAGEMENT

Motivation originates from a desire for change and serves as the ignition for success. **Self-management** is the fuel that will keep you going on the long ride to your destination. It is important to feel motivated, especially when you are a student. The best motivation for learning comes from an inner (intrinsic) desire to know more about a particular interest or subject matter. If you have always been interested in the profession of barbering, then you are likely to be interested in the material you will be studying in barbering school. If your motivation stems from some external (extrinsic) source such as parents or friends, you may not complete your studies because you will need more than a push from others to make a career for yourself. You need to feel a sense of excitement and have a good reason that begins *within yourself* for staying the course. No one should have to motivate you to study other than yourself. *You are in charge of managing your own life and learning!*

While motivation propels you to do something and may originate from within you instinctually, self-management is a well-thought-out process for the long term. For example, since you want to be a licensed barber, you are motivated to the extent that you enrolled in a barbering program to reach that goal. But that is just the beginning, isn't it? You've probably already used some self-management skills to arrange your schedule, financing, transportation, or the like to begin this program. Now you will have to use other self-management skills to apply yourself to your studies and to complete the program.

☑ **LO8 Complete**

ACCESS YOUR CREATIVE CAPABILITIES

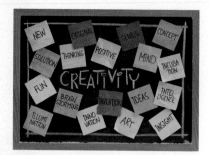

In most conversations, when we use the word *creative* we think of particular talents or abilities in the arts such as painting, singing, acting, or even hairstyling. But being creative or having a sense of creativity is not limited to these artistic expressions. Creativity also functions as an unlimited inner resource of ideas and solutions for the many challenges you face in your lives and it can be accessed to find new ways of thinking and problem solving. To enhance your creative skills, keep the following guidelines in mind:

- *Stop criticizing yourself:* Criticism blocks the creative mind from exploring ideas and discovering solutions to challenges.

- *Refrain from asking others what to do:* In one sense, this can be a way of hoping that others will motivate you instead of you finding the motivation from within. This does not rule out the importance of mentors or of what can be learned from others, but being able to tap into your own creativity is the best way to manage your own success.

- *Change your vocabulary:* Build a positive vocabulary of active problem-solving words such as *explore, analyze, determine, judge, assess,* and so on.

- *Ask for help when you need it:* Being creative does not mean doing everything by yourself. The best self-managers ask for help, utilizing family, friends, peers, coaches, and mentors to stimulate their creativity. Sometimes creativity is best stimulated in an environment in which people work together, brainstorm, and pool their ideas.

GOAL SETTING

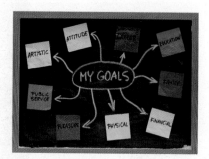

What are you working toward at this time in your life? What do you dream about doing? Turning dreams into reality is what **goal setting** is all about. Picture a goal in your mind. Is it working in a barbershop or salon, or do you see yourself owning your own business? Do you think you have the drive and desire to make your dreams happen? If so, do you also have a realistic plan for reaching your goals? Goal setting helps you decide what you want out of life, and when you know what your goal is, you can map the best route for getting to your destination. Setting goals is like bringing a map along on a road trip to somewhere you've never been before.

There are two types of goals: short term and long term. *Short-term goals* usually refer to those goals you wish to accomplish within a year or less.

Long-term goals are measured in longer segments of time such as 5 years, 10 years, or even longer. Both require careful thought and planning.

Goal setting is a process. The first step is to identify both your short-term and long-term goals. Then write them down! Seeing your goals in written form will help you focus on them so that you can develop a plan for achieving them. As you develop your plan, keep the following guidelines in mind:

- Express your goals in a positive way and be specific.

- Make your goals measurable and set deadlines for accomplishing each one.

- Plan for your goals and make a list of the tasks that need to be completed.

- Check off each item on the list as it is accomplished.

Remember, the important elements of goal setting are having a plan, reexamining it often so that you can make sure you are on track, and being flexible to changes that may have to be made along the way.

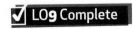 **LO9 Complete**

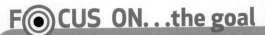

F◉CUS ON...the goal

Try this visualization exercise: Visualize a pathway of stepping stones. Your ultimate goal is at the far end of the pathway, and each stone represents the successful completion of a step that you will have to take toward attaining your goal. Map out realistic short- and long-term goals. Visua[lize] checkpoint signs along the way so that yo[u] know when you are close to achieving a g[oal] and when you have arrived. Then celebrat[e] the accomplishment!

TIME MANAGEMENT

One way to reach your goals more effectively is to manage your time as efficiently as you can. According to time management experts, everyone has an "inner organizer" and can learn to manage their time efficiently. Here are some tips from the experts:

- Learn to prioritize by listing tasks in the order of most to least important.

- Schedule in blocks of unstructured time for flexibility.

- Stress is counterproductive, so pace yourself and don't take on more than you can handle.

- Learn problem-solving techniques to save time when seeking solutions.

- Take time out when you need to reenergize.

- Carry a notepad with you to record great ideas or reminders.

- Make daily, weekly, and monthly schedules.

- Identify your peak-energy and low-energy times of the day and plan accordingly.

- Utilize to-do lists.

- Make time management a habit.

- Reward yourself for work well done.

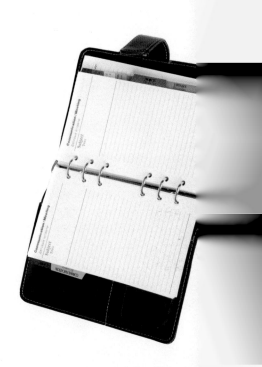

Guidelines for Student Success

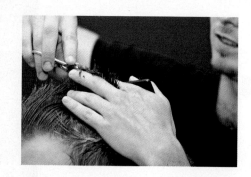

- Participate in the classroom in a courteous manner.

- School regulations are important—obey them all.

- Turn off pagers, cell phones, iPods, and other electronic devices. Personal calls interfere with teaching and learning.

- Be careful with all school equipment and supplies.

- Be clean and well groomed at all times.

- Cooperate with teachers and school personnel.

- Use notebooks and workbooks as important review aids.

- Avoid loafing as it makes a poor impression on others and wastes valuable learning time.

- Be courteous and considerate at all times.

- Be tactful and polite to faculty, fellow students, staff, and clients.

- Observe safety rules and prevent accidents.

- Develop a pleasing personality.

- Think and act positively.

- Attend trade shows and conventions to increase knowledge.

- Stay on task and carefully complete all homework assignments.

- Keep clothes and uniforms spotlessly clean.

- Follow teachers' instructions and techniques.

- Demonstrate interest and sincerity.

- Maintain good attendance.

- Ask for clarification of anything you do not understand.

- Bathe daily and use a deodorant.

- Develop and exhibit good manners at all times.

- Be respectful to teachers and supervisors.

- Develop good work habits essential to success.

- Comply with state board laws, rules, and regulations that govern the profession. These regulations are designed to contribute to the health, safety, and welfare of the public and your community.

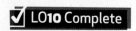

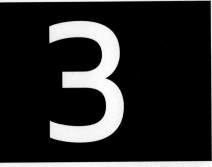

Review
Questions

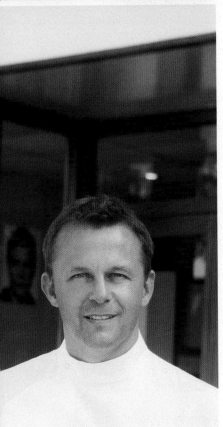

1. Define *professional image*. What personal elements does a professional image consist of?

2. Define *life skills*. List five life skills that you would like to enhance for your own professional growth.

3. Identify and list five values that are the most important to you personally.

4. Explain one way in which attitudes can be altered or changed.

5. List nine basic requirements for personal and professional health.

6. Define *ergonomics*.

7. Define *human relations* and list five desirable qualities for effective client relations.

8. Define rapport.

9. List three communication steps that will help determine a client's service expectations.

10. Define *professional ethics*. Identify three actions that violate the rules of ethical conduct and cast an unfavorable light on barbers.

11. Explain the vision of professional success you have for yourself.

12. Where does the best motivation for learning originate?

13. List a minimum of three short-term goals and three long-term goals that you have developed for yourself.

14. What are state board laws, rules, and regulations designed to do?

Chapter
Glossary

attitude a manner of acting, posturing, feeling, or thinking that shows a person's mood, disposition, mindset, or opinion

beliefs specific attitudes that occur as a result of our values

compartmentalization the capacity to keep different aspects of your mental activity separate so you can achieve greater self-control

diplomacy the art of being tactful

ergonomics the study of human characteristics related to the specific work environment

ethics principles of good character, proper conduct, and moral judgment, expressed through personality, human relations skills, and professional image

goal setting the identification of short- and long-term goals

life skills tools and guidelines that prepare you for living as an adult in a challenging world

motivation a desire for change

personal hygiene the daily maintenance of cleanliness and healthfulness through certain sanitary practices

personality the outward expression of inner feelings, thoughts, attitudes, and values reflected through voice, gestures, posture, clothing, grooming, and environment

professional image the impression projected by a person in any profession, consisting of outward appearance and conduct exhibited in the workplace

rapport a close and empathetic relationship that establishes agreement and harmony between individuals

receptivity the extent to which one is interested in and responsive to others' ideas, feelings, and opinions

self-management the ongoing process of planning, organizing, and managing one's life

values the deepest feelings and thoughts we have about ourselves and about life

PART 2

THE SCIENCE OF BARBERING

4 Microbiology

Learning Objectives

AFTER COMPLETING THIS CHAPTER, YOU SHOULD BE ABLE TO:

1. Identify the two types of bacteria.
2. Identify the classifications of pathogenic bacteria.
3. Describe the growth and reproduction of bacteria.
4. Explain how bloodborne pathogens can be transmitted.
5. Understand the differences between bacterial and viral infections.
6. Discuss hepatitis transmission and prevention.
7. Discuss HIV/AIDS transmission and prevention.
8. Discuss plant and animal parasites.
9. Understand immunity and related terms.

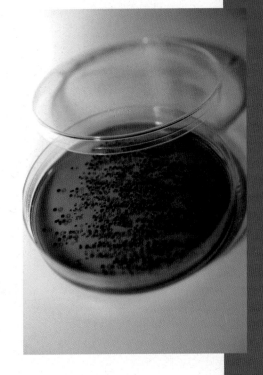

Key Terms

PAGE NUMBER INDICATES WHERE IN THE CHAPTER THE TERM IS USED.

acquired immunodeficiency syndrome (AIDS) / 62

acquired immunity / 68

active (vegetative) stage / 58

aseptic / 60

bacilli / 57

bacteria / 56

bloodborne pathogens / 60

cocci / 57

contagious (communicable) / 59

diplococci / 58

flagella / 58

fungi / 67

general infection / 59

hepatitis / 61

human disease carrier / 68

human immunodeficiency virus (HIV) / 62

immunity / 68

inactive stage / 58

infection / 59

local infection / 59

mitosis / 58

MRSA / 59

natural immunity / 68

nonpathogenic / 57

objective symptoms / 60

parasites / 67

pathogenic / 57

pediculosis / 67

pus / 59

scabies / 67

sepsis / 60

spirilla / 57

spore-forming bacteria / 59

staphylococci / 57

streptococci / 57

subjective symptoms / 60

virus / 61

Each year, the barbering industry services hundreds of thousands of clients. That means that barbers and their clients are exposed to billions of micro-organisms that can cause illness and infection. To limit the exposure and spread of disease, state barber boards, health departments, and other agencies require barbering professionals to apply infection control measures while serving the public.

As a professional barber, it is your responsibility to ensure that your clients receive their services in a safe and sanitary environment. In this chapter, you will learn the nature of various microorganisms, their relationship to disease, and how you can limit their spread in the school or barbershop. It is important to realize that contagious diseases such as skin infections and blood poisoning are just a few of the many conditions that can be caused by the transmission of infectious materials from one individual to another or through the use of contaminated tools and implements. Therefore, it is imperative that you learn how to best safeguard your health and the health of your clients through safe and sanitary work practices in your daily routine. To prepare for our discussion of infection control in Chapter 5, we need to begin with an overview of microbiology and its related studies.

Microbiology

Microbiology is the branch of science that studies living organisms, known as microbes or microorganisms, that are too small to be seen with the naked eye. Microorganisms exist everywhere and are generally classified as bacteria, viruses, fungi, protozoa, or algae. They exist in a variety of shapes and sizes, serve different functions, and require magnification to be seen. Microorganisms that are capable of causing infectious diseases in plants or animals are called *pathogens*. This text focuses on the more common microbial forms that will be of interest to you and your work in the barbershop.

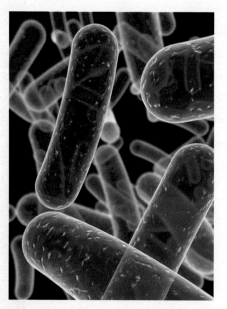

Bacteriology

Bacteriology (bac-ter-i-OL-o-gy) is the science that deals with the study of the microorganisms (my-kroh-OR-gan-iz-ums) called bacteria.

Bacteria (bac-TER-i-a), are one-celled (unicellular) microorganisms that exist almost everywhere: on the skin; in water, air, and decayed matter; and in bodily secretions. Although bacteria are commonly known as germs or microbes because of their association with disease, most bacteria actually perform helpful or harmless functions that are necessary to life.

Some bacteria perform useful functions such as decomposing dead matter, recycling nutrients through soils, or aiding human digestion, while others are disease-producing organisms. Like other microorganisms, bacteria can only be seen with the aid of a microscope and are so small that 1,500 rod-shaped bacteria barely reach across the head of a pin.

TYPES OF BACTERIA

All of the many different kinds of bacteria are classified into two general types—nonpathogenic and pathogenic bacteria.

1. **Nonpathogenic** (non-path-uh-JEN-ik) bacteria make up the majority of bacteria. These are beneficial, symbiotic, or harmless microorganisms that perform useful functions such as improving the fertility of the soil. Saprophytes (SAH-pruh-fyts) are a type of nonpathogenic bacteria that live on dead matter and do not produce disease. In the human body, nonpathogenic bacteria help to digest food, fight infectious microorganisms, and stimulate the immune response. For example, acidophilus (*acido* = acid, *philus* = loving) is a lactobacteria (*lacto* = milk) found in yogurt and yogurt-type products that helps neutralize harmful substances such as nitrates and nitrites in the human digestive tract.

2. **Pathogenic** (path-uh-JEN-ik) bacteria (germs), although in the minority, are harmful and can cause considerable damage by invading plant or human tissues. Pathogenic bacteria produce disease and infection, and maintaining sanitary standards in the barbershop is vital to prevent the spread of these organisms. Parasites also belong to the pathogenic bacteria group because they require living matter for their growth and survival.

✓ **LO1 Complete**

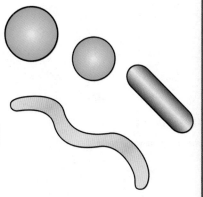

▲ **FIGURE 4-1**
Shapes of pathogenic bacteria.

CLASSIFICATIONS OF PATHOGENIC BACTERIA

Pathogenic bacteria have distinct shapes that help to identify them and are classified as cocci, bacilli, or spirilla **(Figure 4-1)**. Table 4-1 provides the pronunciation of words relating to pathogenic bacteria.

- **Cocci** are round-shaped organisms that appear singly or in the following groups **(Figure 4-2)**:

  ▶ **Staphylococci** bacteria are pus-forming organisms that grow in bunches or clusters. They cause abscesses, pustules, pimples, boils, and staph infections such as MRSA (methicillin-resistant *Staphylococcus aureus*).

  ▶ **Streptococci** bacteria are pus-forming organisms that grow in chains and cause infections such as strep throat, tonsillitis, other lung and throat diseases, and blood poisoning.

  ▶ **Diplococci** bacteria grow in pairs and cause pneumonia and gonorrhea.

- **Bacilli** are short, rod-shaped organisms. They are the most common bacteria and produce diseases such as tetanus (lockjaw), typhoid fever, tuberculosis, and diphtheria **(Figure 4-3)**. Many bacilli bacteria, such as those associated with anthrax, are endospore–producers (discussed later in this chapter).

- **Spirilla** are curved or corkscrew-shaped organisms. They are subdivided into several groups, and include pathogenic bacteria such as *Treponema pallidum*, a sexually transmitted organism that causes syphilis, or *Borrelia burgdorferi*, which causes Lyme disease **(Figure 4-4)**.

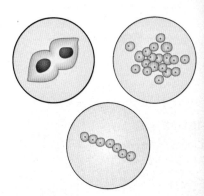

▲ **FIGURE 4-2**
Forms of cocci (round).

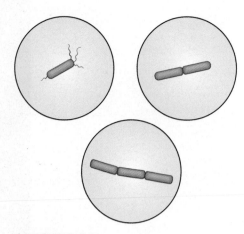

▲ FIGURE 4-3

Forms of bacilli bacteria.

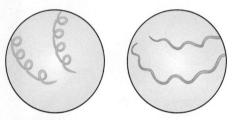

▲ FIGURE 4-4

Forms of spirilla bacteria.

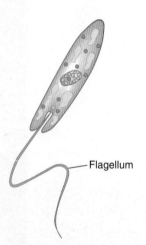

Flagellum

▲ FIGURE 4-5

Bacteria with flagellum.

> **TABLE 4-1** Pronunciation of Terms Relating to Pathogenic Bacteria

SINGULAR	PLURAL
coccus (KOK-us)	cocci (KOK-sy)
staphylococcus (staf-uh-loh-KOK-us)	staphylococci (staf-uh-loh-KOK-sy)
streptococcus (strep-toh-KOK-us)	streptococci (strep-toh-KOK-eye)
diplococcus (dip-loh-KOK-us)	diplococci (dip-loh-KOK-sy)
bacillus (bah-SIL-us)	bacilli (bah-SIL-ee)
spirillum (spy-RIL-um)	spirilla (spy-RIL-ah)

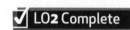

☑ **LO2 Complete**

MOVEMENT OF BACTERIA

Different bacteria move in different ways. Cocci rarely show active motility (self-movement). They may be transmitted in the air, in dust, or within the substance in which they settle. Bacilli and spirilla are both motile and use hair-like projections, known as **flagella** (fla-GEL-la) or cilia (CIL-i-a), to move about. A whip-like motion of these hairs propels the bacteria through liquids (**Figure 4-5**).

BACTERIAL GROWTH AND REPRODUCTION

Bacteria generally consist of an outer cell wall and internal cytoplasm (see Chapter 7). They receive nutrients from the surrounding environment, give off waste products, and grow and reproduce. Bacteria often have two distinct phases in their life cycle: the **active** or **vegetative stage,** and the **inactive stage.**

- *Active or vegetative stage:* During the active or vegetative stage, bacteria grow and reproduce. Generally, microorganisms multiply best in warm, dark, damp, dirty places where sufficient food is present. As food is absorbed, bacterial cells grow until their maximum growth is reached. The cells then divide through a method called *binary fission* into two new cells. This process is called **mitosis** (mi-TO-sis) and the cells that are formed are called daughter cells. As mitosis occurs, one bacterium can create as many as 16 million microbes in a 12-hour period. When favorable conditions cease to exist, bacteria either become inactive or die.

- *Inactive stage:* During the inactive stage, bacteria do not grow or reproduce. Some bacteria may become stationary or lie dormant while others simply die off. Certain bacteria, such as the anthrax and tetanus bacilli, are **spore-forming bacteria** and may survive the inactive stage by forming spherical (round) spores that have tough outer coverings to withstand periods of famine, dryness, or unsuitable temperatures. In this stage, spores can be blown about in the dust and are not harmed by most disinfectants, heat, or cold. When favorable conditions are restored, these spores may be reactivated and start to grow and reproduce.

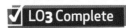

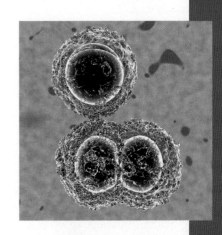

BACTERIAL INFECTIONS

Pathogenic bacteria become a menace to health when they invade the body. An **infection** occurs if the body is unable to cope with the bacteria and their harmful toxins. There can be no disease without the presence of pathogenic bacteria.

The presence of pus is a sign of infection. **Pus** is a fluid that contains white blood cells, dead and living bacteria, waste matter, tissue elements, and body cells. A **local infection** is indicated by a lesion containing pus and usually appears in a particular area of the body. Infected scrapes or cuts, pimples, and boils are examples of local infections. A **general infection** results when the bloodstream carries the bacteria and their toxins to all parts of the body, as in blood poisoning or syphilis.

Staphylococci (commonly called staph) are among the most common pus-forming human bacteria and are carried by approximately one-third of the population. Staph can be picked up from surfaces such as floors, doorknobs, or countertops but are more frequently transferred through contaminated objects or skin-to-skin contact. Antibiotics once controlled these bacteria, but certain strains of staph have become highly resistant to the drugs, making it difficult to cure infections. For example, methicillin-resistant *Staphylococcus aureus* (**MRSA**) is a type of staph infection that is resistant to antibiotics such as methicillin, oxacillin, amoxicillin, and penicillin. While these staph infections most often afflict people with weakened immune systems in hospitals or healthcare facilities, MRSA infections are also seen in athletes, military personnel, children, prisoners, and other community-associated groups. Some preventive measures that can help limit the spread of MRSA include thorough hand washing, covering scrapes and cuts, and avoiding contact with other people's wounds, bandages, or personal items. Barbers can help to limit the spread of staph and other infectious bacteria by practicing effective sanitation and decontamination procedures in the barbershop.

When a disease spreads from one person to another by contact, it is considered to be **contagious,** or **communicable.** If a disease simultaneously attacks a large number of people living in a particular area or locality, it is called an epidemic.

Some of the more contagious diseases or disorders that will prevent a barber from servicing clients are tuberculosis, the common cold, ringworm, scabies, head lice, and viral infections. The chief sources of contagion are unclean hands or implements, open sores, pus, oral or nasal discharges, and the shared use of drinking cups and towels. Uncovered coughing, sneezing, and spitting in public also spread germs. The spread of infection can be controlled through conscientious personal hygiene, effective sanitation procedures, and public sanitation.

Bloodborne Pathogens

Disease-producing bacteria or viruses that are carried through the body in blood or body fluids, such as hepatitis and HIV, are called **bloodborne pathogens.** Blood-to-blood contact might occur if you accidentally cut a client who is HIV-positive or infected with hepatitis, continue to use the implement without disinfecting it, and then puncture your skin or cut another client with the contaminated tool. Similarly, if you are shaving a client's face or neck with a razor or clipper blades, body fluids can be picked up from a blemish or open sore, making transmission possible.

HOW PATHOGENS ENTER THE BODY

Pathogenic bacteria or viruses may enter the body through:

- A break in the skin, such as a cut, pimple, or scratch.
- The mouth (contaminated food or water).
- The nose (breathing).
- The eyes or ears.
- Unprotected sex.

The body fights infection by means of its defensive forces, which include:

- The unbroken skin, the body's first line of defense.
- Body secretions such as perspiration and digestive juices.
- White blood cells, which destroy bacteria.
- Antitoxins, which counteract the toxins produced by bacteria and viruses.

Infections created by pathogenic bacteria or viruses can be prevented through personal hygiene and public sanitation.

Sepsis is the poisoned state caused by the absorption of pathogenic microorganisms and their products into the bloodstream. It is because of the possibility of poisoning due to pathogenic bacteria that barber schools and shops must maintain high standards of cleanliness and sanitation in order to achieve an environment that is as **aseptic** (free of disease germs) as possible.

Symptoms are the signs of disease. **Subjective symptoms,** such as itching, burning, or pain, can be felt only by the person with the disease. **Objective symptoms,** such as pimples, boils, swelling, or inflammation, can be observed by anyone.

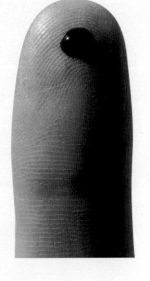

✓ **LO4 Complete**

Viruses

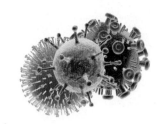

A **virus** is a submicroscopic structure so small that it can pass through a porcelain filter. Viruses are capable of infecting almost all plants and animals, including bacteria, and cause common colds, respiratory and gastrointestinal infections, influenza, measles, mumps, chicken pox, smallpox, rabies, yellow fever, hepatitis, polio, and AIDS.

Viruses live only by penetrating cells and becoming a part of them. Bacteria are organisms that can live on their own. It is for this reason that bacterial infections can usually be treated with specific antibiotics. Conversely, viruses are resistant to antibiotics and are hard to kill without harming the body in the process. Although vaccinations can prevent certain viruses from penetrating cells, vaccinations are not available for all types of viruses.

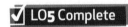
☑ LO5 Complete

Hepatitis

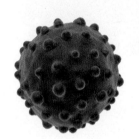

Hepatitis is a disease marked by inflammation of the liver. Although it is a bloodborne virus similar to HIV in transmission, it is more easily contracted than HIV because it is present in all body fluids. The Centers for Disease Control and Prevention list five types of viral hepatitis infections:

1. *Hepatitis A virus (HAV):* This flu-like illness usually lasts about three weeks with symptoms that include jaundice (yellowing of the skin or eyes), fatigue, nausea, fever, abdominal pain, and loss of appetite. The disease is spread through close household contact involving poor sanitation, poor personal hygiene, common bathroom use, contaminated foods and liquids, and sexual contact. Although a person who has recovered from HAV will not get it again, a vaccine is also available to prevent contraction of the disease.

2. *Hepatitis B virus (HBV):* This form of hepatitis is a serious disease that accumulates in the blood and can cause lifelong hepatitis infection, cirrhosis of the liver, liver failure, liver cancer, and death. Although the disease can mirror flu-like symptoms, about half the people infected with the disease may not show symptoms. The disease can be transmitted through saliva, sexual contact, or *parenteral exposure* to blood or blood products exposure that pierces mucous membranes or the skin barrier. A vaccine is available.

3. *Hepatitis C virus (HCV):* Hepatitis C can progress slowly and may include symptoms of fatigue and abdominal pain. The disease is transferred through parenteral contact, sexual activity with infected partners, blood transfusions with HCV-contaminated blood, and illegal drug injections. No vaccine is available.

4. *Hepatitis D virus (HDV):* Hepatitis D is a serious liver disease that is uncommon in the United States. It is transmitted through contact with infected blood and there is no vaccine available at this time.

5. *Hepatitis E virus (HEV):* Hepatitis E is another serious liver disease that is uncommon in the United States. It is usually found in countries with poor sanitation and a contaminated water supply. There is no approved vaccine available.

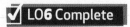

HIV/AIDS

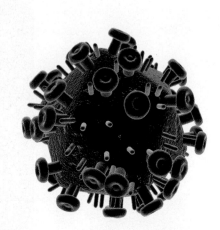

A discussion of HIV/AIDS should begin with an understanding of the terms associated with the subject. The most common terms used in conjunction with this topic include:

- **Human immunodeficiency virus (HIV)**
- **Acquired immunodeficiency syndrome (AIDS)**
- AIDS-related complex (ARC)
- Sexually transmitted disease (STD)

HIV is the virus that causes AIDS. AIDS is the onset of life-threatening illnesses that compromise the immune system as a result of HIV infection and disease.

HIV is passed from person to person through body fluids such as blood, breast milk, semen, and vaginal secretions. The most common methods of transferring the virus are through sexual contact with an infected person, the use of or sharing of dirty hypodermic needles for intravenous drug use, the transfusion of infected blood, and from mother to child during pregnancy and birth.

A person can be infected with HIV for up to 11 years without having symptoms and, if not tested, may not realize that they are infecting other people. Unlike most other viruses, HIV is not transferred through casual contact with an infected person, sneezing, or coughing, because it is not an airborne virus; nor is it transmitted by holding hands, hugging, or sharing household items like telephones or toilet seats. It can, however, enter the bloodstream though cuts and sores and may be transmitted in the barbershop by improperly disinfected sharp implements. For example, if you were to cut a client infected with HIV you might transfer blood to a haircutting implement, razor, or manicuring implement. Then, if you cut another client and transfer the infected blood to the second client through the wound, that client also risks being infected.

Although the human immunodeficiency virus may lie dormant in an infected person's system for 11 years or more, it can also mature into a fatal disease in 2 to 10 years. Testing for the virus may be performed on an anonymous basis and should be sought if an individual has engaged in any behavior that puts him or herself at risk of being infected.

The immune system works to defend the body against infection. Especially important in this process are the following body parts and systems:

- Bone marrow, where lymphocytes (white blood cells that play critical roles in the immune system) are manufactured

- The thymus gland, where lymphocytes called T cells mature

- The lymphoreticular system, which provides storage sites for mature lymphocytes

- The bloodstream, which contains cellular elements of the immune system

REMINDER

>>> HIV is not an airborne virus. It is not transmitted through casual contact with an infected person or by sharing household items.

Remember that a virus is the smallest disease-producing microorganism. Consisting of genes surrounded by a protein layer, a virus is able to reproduce within the body by utilizing specific body cells. One of the most difficult aspects of treating HIV infection is that HIV is a retrovirus. This means that the virus uses the reproductive processes of the host cell (to which it becomes attached) to duplicate itself.

When HIV enters the bloodstream, it searches for a special molecule to which it can attach itself. These molecules are present on lymphocytes called T-helper cells (among others), and often the virus attaches itself to these cells. Once attached, these cells are considered target cells. The virus then sheds its outer covering of protein and enters the target cell. Once inside, HIV begins to pass its own genes into the nucleus of the target cell, where duplication begins. The target cell then produces large numbers of new viruses, which eventually burst out of the cell. The viral process begins again, leaving the destroyed T cell in its wake. This lowers the strength of the immune system, with the result that the body becomes susceptible to opportunistic diseases, which can eventually cause death (Figure 4-6).

HIV is considered to be a weak virus when compared to other viruses such as polio. However, unlike polio, which responds to treatment, HIV is difficult to destroy once it locks into T cells in the bloodstream. HIV is not thought to survive in open environments, especially when subjected to cold surfaces, drying, or ultraviolet light, and can be killed through the use of household bleach or hospital-grade disinfectants. The virus cannot live in food or drink. There should be no risk from handling the linens of HIV-infected persons as long as universal precautions are followed and there is no direct contact with the blood or bodily fluids.

THE STAGES OF HIV/AIDS

Once HIV has entered the bloodstream and the immune response begins, antibodies will normally be produced within a range of two weeks to six months. At this point, HIV can be passed along to others.

The symptom stages are as follows:

- *Stage 1—HIV infection:* No physical indications of illness; antibodies to the virus may be present.

- *Stage 2—ARC:* Chronic fatigue; unexplained chills, fever, or night sweats; 10 percent or greater weight loss without dieting; skin disorders; enlarged liver and/or spleen; swollen lymph glands; chronic diarrhea.

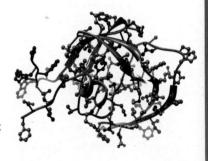

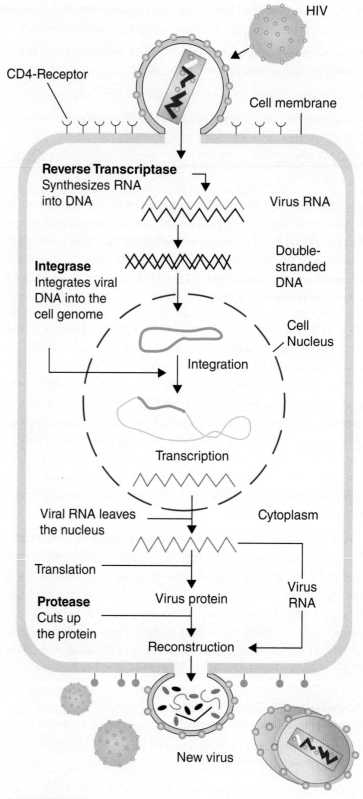

▲ FIGURE 4-6

HIV Replication Cycle.

- *Stage 3—AIDS:* All of the above symptoms, as well as hair loss; skin and other cancers; pneumonia and other infections; and nerve and brain damage. Individuals in the final stage of HIV infection (full-blown AIDS) usually exhibit the most severe characteristics of the disease.

PREVENTING HIV/AIDS

To date, there is no vaccine to prevent HIV infection, nor is there a cure for AIDS. Early intervention is the key to obtaining whatever treatments are available that may be beneficial in improving the immune response and delaying progression of the disease.

Those individuals who are at risk of contracting HIV/AIDS may be helped by eliminating all known causes of immune system suppression and by utilizing any and all therapies that stimulate immune system function. The correct diet, including vitamin, mineral, and herbal supplements; exercise; a healthy environment; and a proper mental attitude all contribute to the well being of the immune system.

In many states, professionals are currently required to attend an HIV/AIDS education course prior to licensure and license renewal. In some cases, HIV/AIDS instruction has been added to barber school curriculum requirements. Strict adherence to precautionary and sanitary measures in the workplace assists in the protection of the health, safety, and welfare of professionals and their clients. Universal precautions will be discussed in Chapter 5 and should be followed at all times when blood or bodily fluids are present.

The following suggestions may also serve as helpful reminders to student barbers:

- Avoid accidents and practice all safety precautions applicable to the shop or school.
- Wash hands with an antibacterial soap before and after servicing each client.
- Always sanitize tools and implements before and after each client.
- Sanitize equipment, such as headrests; chair backs; arm rests; and facial, massage, and manicure tables, before and after client services.
- Use disposable gloves whenever possible.
- If you cut, nick, or scrape yourself, treat the wound immediately and cover it.
- If you cut, nick, or scrape a client, apply gloves and treat the wound to the extent of your state board allowances and limitations.
- Avoid exposure and contact with another person's bodily fluids, especially blood.
- Attend available seminars and classes that provide updates on HIV/AIDS research.
- If you feel there is any chance that you have contracted HIV, or if you simply wish to ease your mind, have an HIV antibody test performed. Keep in mind your responsibility to others and to yourself to minimize the risk of spreading this disease.

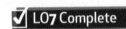 ✓ **LO7 Complete**

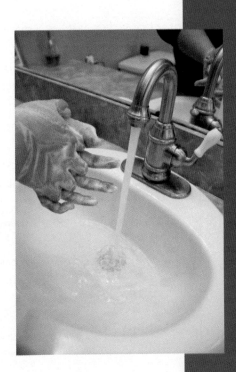

Table 4-2 lists general terms and definitions associated with diseases and disorders.

TERM	DEFINITION
acute disease	disease having a rapid onset, severe symptoms, and a short course or duration
allergy	reaction due to extreme sensitivity to certain foods, chemicals, or other normally harmless substances
aseptic	freedom from disease germs
chronic disease	disease of long duration, usually mild but recurring
congenital disease	disease that exists at birth
contagious disease	disease that is communicable or transmittable by contact
contraindication	any condition or disease that makes an indicated treatment or medication inadvisable
diagnosis	determination of the nature of a disease from its symptoms
disease	abnormal condition of all or part of the body, organ, or mind that makes it incapable of carrying on normal function
epidemic	appearance of a disease that simultaneously attacks a large number of persons living in a particular locality
etiology	study of the causes of disease and their mode of operation
infectious disease	disease caused by pathogenic microorganisms or viruses that are easily spread
inflammation	condition of some part of the body as a protective response to injury, irritation, or infection, characterized by redness, heat, pain, and swelling
objective symptoms	symptoms that are visible, such as pimples, pustules, or inflammation
occupational disease	illness resulting from conditions associated with employment, such as coming in contact with certain chemicals or tints
parasitic disease	disease caused by vegetable or animal parasites, such as pediculosis and ringworm
pathogenic disease	disease produced by disease-causing bacteria, such as staphylococcus and streptococcus (pus-forming bacteria), or viruses
pathology	science that investigates modifications of the functions and changes in structure caused by disease

TERM	DEFINITION
prognosis	foretelling of probable course of a disease
seasonal disease	disease influenced by the weather
sepsis	the poisoned state caused by the absorption of pathogenic microorganisms and their products into the bloodstream
subjective symptoms	symptoms that can be felt, such as itching, burning, or pain
systemic disease	disease that affects the body generally, often due to under- or overfunctioning of the internal glands
venereal disease	contagious disease commonly acquired by contact with an infected person during sexual intercourse, characterized by sores and rashes on the skin

Parasites

Parasites are plant or animal organisms that live on another living organism, drawing their nourishment from the host organism without giving anything in return.

Plant parasites or **fungi** (FUN-jy), such as molds, mildews, rusts, and yeasts, can produce contagious skin diseases such as ringworm or favus (FAY-vus). Nail fungus can be contracted through improperly disinfected implements or through moisture trapped under nail enhancements. Nail fungus is chronic and usually localized but can be spread to other nails and from client to client if implements are not disinfected before and after each use. Generally, treatment is applied directly to the affected area; however, serious cases require a physician's care (Figure 4-7).

Animal parasites are also responsible for contagious diseases and conditions. Itch mites can burrow under the skin causing itching and inflammation. This contagious disorder is known as **scabies** (SKAY-beez) and is pictured in Figure 4-8. **Pediculosis** (puh-dik-yuh-LOH-sis) is the technical term for an infestation caused by the head or body louse (Figure 4-9). Neither of these

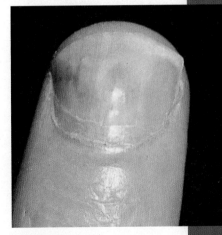

▲ **FIGURE 4-7**

Nail fungus.

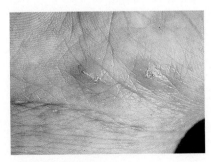

▲ **FIGURE 4-8**

Scabies.

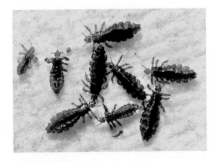

▲ **FIGURE 4-9**

Head lice.

disorders should be treated in the barbershop or school. Clients should be referred to a physician and any tools, equipment, or seating that may have come into contact with these clients should be thoroughly decontaminated with disinfectants and pesticides.

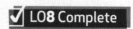

Immunity

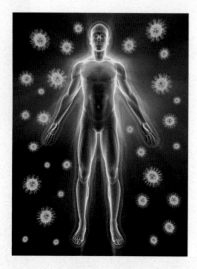

Immunity is the ability of the body to resist invasion by bacteria and to destroy bacteria once they have entered the body. Immunity against disease may be natural or acquired and is a sign of good health. **Natural immunity** is the natural resistance to disease that is partially inherited and partially developed through hygienic living. **Acquired immunity** is developed after the body has overcome a disease or through inoculations such as vaccinations.

A **human disease carrier** is a person who is immune to a disease, but harbors germs that can infect other people. Typhoid (TY-phoid) fever and diphtheria (diph-THER-i-a) are two diseases that may be transmitted in this manner.

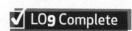

As you will learn in Chapter 5, bacteria may be destroyed through the use of chemical disinfectants; intense heat such as boiling, steaming, baking, or burning; and ultraviolet light.

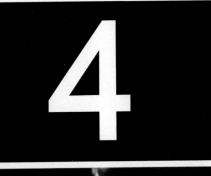

Review
Questions

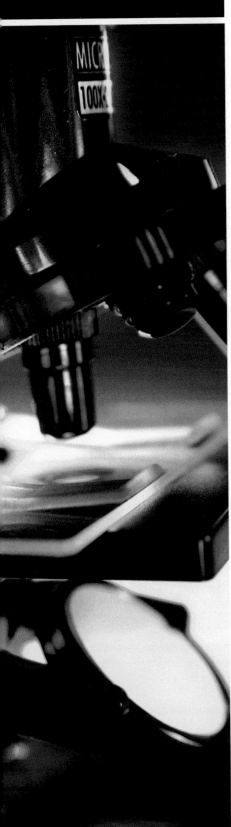

1. What are bacteria?

2. Name and describe the two main types of bacteria.

3. Name and describe three forms of pathogenic bacteria.

4. How do bacteria move about?

5. How do bacteria multiply?

6. Describe the active and inactive stages of bacteria.

7. Identify a type of pathogenic bacteria that is capable of forming protective spores.

8. Name the most common pus-forming human bacteria.

9. Identify the type of bacteria that causes MRSA.

10. Why might an MRSA infection be difficult to cure?

11. What is the difference between a local infection and a general infection?

12. What is a contagious or communicable disease?

13. How might bloodborne pathogens be transmitted during barbering services?

14. Why is hepatitis more easily contracted than HIV?

15. Identify the virus that causes AIDS. Define AIDS.

16. Name two types of parasites and the conditions they cause.

17. What is the definition of natural immunity? Acquired immunity?

18. List the methods that can be used to destroy bacteria.

Chapter
Glossary

acquired immunodeficiency syndrome (AIDS) the onset of life-threatening illnesses that compromise the immune system as a result of HIV infection and disease

acquired immunity an immunity that the body develops after it overcomes a disease or through inoculation

active (vegetative) stage the stage in which bacteria grow and reproduce.

aseptic free of disease germs

bacilli rod-shaped bacteria that produce diseases such as tetanus, typhoid fever, tuberculosis, and diphtheria

bacteria one-celled microorganisms, also known as germs or microbes

bloodborne pathogens disease-causing bacteria or viruses that are carried through the body in the blood or body fluids

cocci round-shaped bacteria that appear singly or in groups

contagious (communicable) a disease that may be transmitted by contact

diplococci round-shaped bacteria that cause diseases such as pneumonia

flagella hair-like extensions that propel bacteria through liquid

fungi plant parasites such as molds, mildew, yeasts, and rusts that can cause ringworm and favus

general infection an infection that results when the bloodstream carries bacteria or viruses to all parts of the body

hepatitis a bloodborne disease marked by inflammation of the liver

human disease carrier a person who is immune to a disease, but harbors germs that can infect other people

human immunodeficiency virus (HIV) the virus that causes AIDS

immunity the ability of the body to resist invasion by bacteria and to destroy bacteria once they have entered the body

inactive stage the stage in which bacteria do not grow or reproduce

infection the result when the body is unable to cope with the invasion of bacteria and their harmful toxins

local infection an infection that is limited to a specific area of the body

mitosis the division of cells during reproduction

MRSA acronym for methicillin-resistant *Staphylococcus aureus*; a type of staph infection resistant to certain antibiotics

natural immunity natural resistance to disease that is partially inherited and partially developed

nonpathogenic beneficial or harmless bacteria that perform many useful functions

objective symptoms symptoms that can be seen by anyone

parasites plant or animal organisms that live on other living organisms without giving anything in return

pathogenic harmful, disease-producing bacteria

pediculosis a contagious infestation caused by the head or body louse

pus a fluid that contains white blood cells, dead and living bacteria, waste matter, tissue elements, and body cells; a sign of infection

scabies a contagious disorder caused by the itch mite

sepsis a poisoned state caused by the absorption of pathogenic microorganisms into the bloodstream

spirilla curved or corkscrew-shaped bacteria that can cause syphilis and Lyme disease

spore-forming bacteria certain bacteria that have the ability to form protective spores to survive an inactive stage

staphylococci pus-forming bacteria that cause abscesses, pustules, pimples, and boils

streptococci pus-forming bacteria that cause infections such as strep throat, tonsillitis, other lung and throat diseases, and blood poisoning

subjective symptoms symptoms that can be felt or experienced only by the person affected

virus an infectious agent that lives only by penetrating cells and becoming a part of them

5 Infection Control

AND SAFE WORK PRACTICES

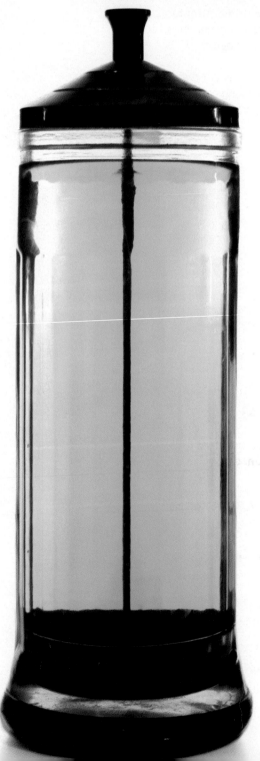

☑ Learning Objectives

AFTER COMPLETING THIS CHAPTER, YOU SHOULD BE ABLE TO:

1 Discuss the ways in which infectious materials may be transmitted in the barbershop.

2 Understand the reasons for maintaining an MSDS notebook.

3 Discuss federal and state agencies associated with infection control and safe work practices.

4 Define *decontamination* and list three levels used for the prevention and control of pathogen transmission.

5 Identify the chemical decontamination agents most commonly used in barbershops.

6 Demonstrate proper decontamination procedures for tools, equipment, and surfaces.

7 Discuss standard precautions and blood-spill disinfection.

8 Discuss disinfecting rules, decontamination safety precautions, and rules of sanitation.

9 Define safe work practices.

10 Recognize potential safety hazards in the barbershop.

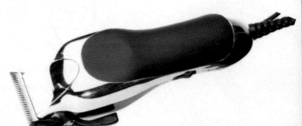

Key Terms

PAGE NUMBER INDICATES WHERE IN THE CHAPTER THE TERM IS USED.

State barber boards, health departments, and other regulatory agencies require that infection control measures and safe work practices be applied while serving the public. The implementation of infection control measures helps minimize the spread of contagious diseases, skin infections, and blood poisoning that can be caused by the transmission of infectious material from one individual to another. This transmission can also occur through the use of contaminated combs, clippers, razors, shears, or other tools and implements. Safe work practices require an awareness of the potential hazards that exist in the barbershop and the strategies that help minimize the associated risks. It is your responsibility as a professional barber to employ proper and effective decontamination methods that help safeguard your health and the health of your clients. You are also responsible for employing safe work practices that help prevent accidents and injuries from occurring in the workplace.

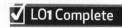

✓ **LO1 Complete**

Regulation

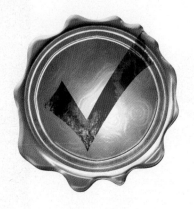

Many different federal, state, and local agencies regulate the practice of barbering. Federal agencies set guidelines for the protection of human health, the environment, and safe work practices for most occupational and manufacturing sectors. State and local agencies regulate and enforce licensing, minimum standards, workplace conduct, and a variety of other oversight responsibilities that help ensure public health and safety. For example, most states follow federal regulations to set the minimal performance standards for disinfectant and sanitizing agents approved for use in barbershops and require that the products are registered for sale within the state. As a professional barber, you should be aware of the primary agencies that regulate the health and safety practices of your profession.

ENVIRONMENTAL PROTECTION AGENCY (EPA)

The EPA develops and enforces the regulations of environmental law in an effort to protect human health and the environment. One result of environmental law is that the EPA and each individual state must approve all disinfectants. Product labels must provide the manufacturer's claims for the effectiveness of the product in killing specific organisms and display an EPA registration number.

FOOD AND DRUG ADMINISTRATION (FDA)

The **Food and Drug Administration** is responsible for enforcing rules and regulations associated with food, drug, and cosmetic products purchased and used by the public. Although the FDA does some testing of products and can take legal action against a manufacturer, the responsibility for documenting the quality and safety of their products rests with the manufacturers. Occasionally, a product or product batch is found to be defective or harmful in some way and in most cases it is the manufacturer who will issue the recall. If complaints of adverse reactions to a product reach the FDA, they will follow up with investigations and inspections.

Cosmetic preparations used in the barbershop include hair tonics, shampoos, shaving creams, conditioners, permanent wave solutions, haircolor tints, chemical processors, hair sprays, gels, and many others. Consumer products are those described as over-the-counter preparations, meaning that they can be purchased by the general public at a retail store or outlet. Professional products are those that are sold only to licensed barbers or other industry professionals. Because manufacturers do not have to adhere to the same FDA labeling regulations for professional products as they do for retail products, you may discover that some professional products do not contain a list of ingredients on the label. If in doubt about a product's ingredients, refer to the Material Safety Data Sheet (MSDS), discussed later in this chapter, or contact the manufacturer to ask specific questions.

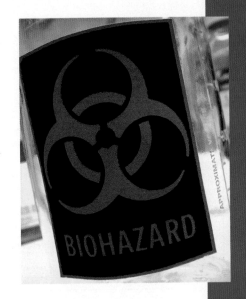

OCCUPATIONAL SAFETY AND HEALTH ADMINISTRATION (OSHA)

Created as a result of the federal **Occupational Safety and Health Act** of 1970, the primary purpose of **Occupational Safety and Health Administration (OSHA)** is to assure, regulate, and enforce safe and healthful working conditions in the workplace. Two key functions of the act include:

1. The requirement of employers to furnish their employees with a working environment that is free from recognizable hazards

2. The requirement of compliance with occupational safety and health standards as set forth by the act

Many of the OSHA regulations and standards for general industry are applicable to barbers and barbershops. For example, the OSHA Bloodborne Pathogens Standard helps protect employees from being at risk from cross-infection.

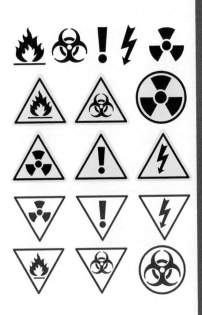

The **Hazard Communication Rule** requires that chemical manufacturers and importers evaluate and identify possible health hazards associated with their products. Some chemicals used in the barbershop may be combustible, caustic, or otherwise potentially harmful to the human body, and this rule requires the proper mixing, storage, and disposal of all chemicals in the workplace. Material Safety Data Sheets and required labeling are two important results of this rule. Additionally, the Hazard Communication Rule requires that this information be made available to workers through the Right-to-Know Law.

NOTE: Although the requirements for mixing and storing chemical products are identified on the Material Safety Data Sheets, the disposal of waste, hazardous, or outdated products requires more specific information. These procedures may be obtained from your local hazardous waste agency or office.

MATERIAL SAFETY DATA SHEETS (MSDSs)

A **Material Safety Data Sheet** provides vital information about each product, ranging from ingredient content and associated hazards to combustion levels and storage requirements. Barbershops and schools are required by law to maintain an MSDS for every product used on the premises (**Figure 5-1**).

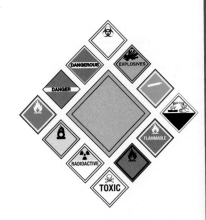

MSDSs may be obtained from the product distributor or manufacturer when an order is placed, but you must request it. Once received, the MSDS

Material Safety Data Sheet

May be used to comply with
OSHA s Hazard Communication Standard,
29 CFR 1910.1200. Standard must be
consulted for specific requirements.

U.S. Department of Labor

Occupational Safety and Health Administration
(Non-Mandatory Form)
Form Approved
OMB No. 1218-0072

IDENTITY (As Used on Label and List)	Note: Blank spaces are not permitted. If any item is not applicable, or no information is available, the space must be marked to indicate that.

Section I

Manufacturer s Name	Emergency Telephone Number
Address (Number, Street, City, State, and ZIP Code)	Telephone Number for information
	Date Prepared
	Signature of Preparer (optional)

Section II — Hazardous Ingredients/Identity Information

Hazardous Components (Specific Chemical Identity; Common Names(s))	OSHA PEL	ACGIH TLV	Other Limits Recommended	% (optional)

Section III — Physical/Chemical Characteristics

Boiling Point		Specific Gravity (H_2O - 1)	
Vapor Pressure (mm Hg.)		Melting Point	
Vapor Density (Air - 1))		Evaporation Rate (Butyl Acetate - 1)	
Solubility in Water			
Appearance and Odor			

Section IV — Fire and Explosion Hazard Data

Flash Point (Method Used)	Flammable Limits	LEL	UEL
Extinguishing Media			
Special Fire Fighting Procedures			
Unusual Fire and Explosion Hazards			

(Reproduce locally)

OSHA 174, Sept. 1985

▲ **FIGURE 5-1a**

A Sample MSDS.

Material Safety Data Sheet (MSDS)

Section V — Reactivity Data

Stability	Unstable		Conditions to Avoid
	Stable		

Incompatibility (Materials to Avoid)

Hazardous Decomposition or Byproducts

Hazardous Polymerization	May Occur		Conditions to Avoid
	Will Not Occur		

Section VI — Health Hazard Data

Route(s) of Entry:	Inhalation?	Skin?	Ingestion?

Health Hazards (Acute and Chronic)

Carcenogenicity:	NTP?	IARC Monographs	OSHA Regulated?

Signs and Symptoms of Exposure

Medical Conditions
Generally Aggravated by Exposure

Emergency and First Aid Program

Section VII — Precautions for Safe Handling and Use

Steps to Be Taken in Case Material is Released or Spilled

Waste Disposal Method

Precautions to Be Taken in Handling and Storing

Other Precautions

Section VIII — Control Measures

Respiratory Protection (Specify Type)

Ventilation	Local Exhaust	Special
	Mechanical (General)	Other

Protective Gloves	Eye Protection

Other Protective Clothing or Equipment

Work/Hygienic Practices

Page 2

▲ **FIGURE 5-1b**

A Sample MSDS.

should be kept in a notebook or file in an organized format for easy access. There are official guidelines for setting up an MSDS notebook that may be obtained from your state's department of labor.

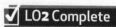

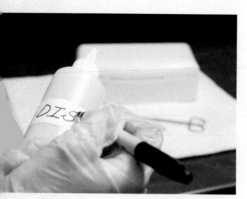

▲ **FIGURE 5-2**
All products and containers are required to be labeled.

Labeling refers to the listing of ingredients on the packaging of a product with the appropriate hazard warning. When you think about the range of products used in the barbershop or styling salon, the importance of complying with this standard becomes obvious. Disinfectants, glass and surface cleaners, alcohols, and antiseptic solutions are just a few of the chemicals that can be found in the shop or salon environment. All products and containers are required to be labeled, even spray bottles that are filled with water (Figure 5-2). Through the efforts of OSHA, the law requires that chemical product labels contain the identity of the hazardous chemical(s) and the appropriate hazard warning. This information is required in order to provide the consumer with product knowledge, the criteria for making an informed decision, and warnings about possible risks. These are the main reasons for *always* reading and following the directions provided by product manufacturers.

Federal law has provided employers and employees certain guidelines for the promotion of safe work practices. The following general information has been provided to give you a basic understanding of some of these federal mandates.

RIGHT-TO-KNOW LAW

The **Right-to-Know Law** requires that a right-to-know notice be posted in the work environment where toxic substances are present. (The notice is obtainable through your state department of labor.) This notice advises the worker of specific rights under the Right-to-Know Law. The basic guidelines of federal legislation should define the employer's responsibilities and the worker's rights as follows:

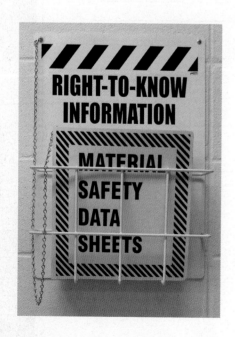

Employer's Responsibilities

• Inform the worker of toxic substances in the workplace.

• Maintain Material Safety Data Sheets and have them available upon request.

• Provide education to the worker about the proper use of the substances and emergency procedures.

• Notify the appropriate local agencies, such as the fire department and hazardous waste department, about the identity, characteristics, and location of the toxic substance(s).

Worker's Rights

• Know the characteristics and location of toxic substances in the workplace.

• Have access to relevant Material Safety Data Sheets.

- May refuse to work with a listed toxic substance if not supplied with a copy of the MSDS.

- Education and instruction (within first 30 days of employment) on the potentially adverse health effects of each toxic substance in the work environment and the appropriate emergency procedures.

- Additional information from the Toxic Substances Information Center.

- Protection from discharge, discrimination, or discipline for exercising rights.

STATE REGULATORY AGENCIES

It is the responsibility of state regulatory agencies to protect consumers' health, safety, and welfare while receiving services in the barbershop. These agencies include occupational licensing bureaus, state barber boards, health departments, building inspectors, and many others. The agencies fulfill their responsibilities to the public by enforcing the rules through inspections, investigations, and the issuance of penalties when warranted. Penalties can range from warnings to fines, probation, and suspension or revocation of licenses and can affect both the shop owner and barber employees. Ignorance of the law is no excuse for health or safety violations that might occur in the barbershop, so it is vital that you understand and follow the laws and rules governing the barbering profession in your state.

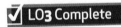

Principles of Prevention and Control

As discussed in Chapter 4, microorganisms exist almost everywhere and can be transmitted from environmental sources through the air and via human or direct contact. Consequently, the key to effective infection control is the *prevention* of the transmission of these organisms, which is primarily the responsibility of barbershop personnel.

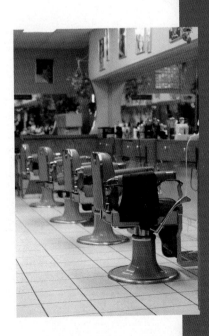

Effective infection control in the barbershop also influences the professional image of the establishment. A client's first impression of the shop begins the moment they open the door, so a clean environment should extend beyond each barber's immediate work area. All of the sights, sounds, smells, and general ambience of the barbershop meld together to form this impression regardless of how many times a client has visited the shop. In essence, this "first" impression happens over and over again because clients do not see you or the shop daily. A clean and orderly barbershop helps build client confidence and trust that continuous care is being taken to provide a safe and sanitary environment in which to receive their personal services.

CONTAMINATION

No matter how clean a surface looks, it is probably contaminated. Bacteria, viruses, and fungi act as contaminants and can be found almost anywhere. In the barbershop, these microorganisms can live on tools, implements, styling chairs, countertops, and even in the air; therefore, it is the barber's responsibility to control the spread of infection and disease through the use of effective cleaning and disinfecting products and methods.

DECONTAMINATION

It is virtually impossible to keep the barbershop free from all contamination; however, there are methods available that will ensure an optimum level of cleanliness. The removal of pathogens and other substances from tools or surfaces is called **decontamination.**

Decontamination involves the use of physical or chemical processes to remove, inactivate, or destroy pathogens to make an object safe for handling, use, or disposal. The three *levels* of decontamination are sanitation, disinfection, and sterilization. The three *steps* to decontamination are cleansing (sanitizing), disinfecting, and sterilizing.

Health departments and state barber boards recognize that it is virtually impossible to completely sterilize barbering tools and implements; therefore it is generally recognized that this equipment will be cleansed and disinfected rather than sterilized. Throughout the text, the terms *sanitize* or *sanitizing* are used to denote the act of thoroughly cleaning an item or surface with soap or detergents and water, or, as a required first step in the disinfection process. The terms *disinfect* or *disinfection* are used to indicate the process of thorough cleaning (sanitizing) followed by the application of a disinfectant to achieve an optimum level of decontamination.

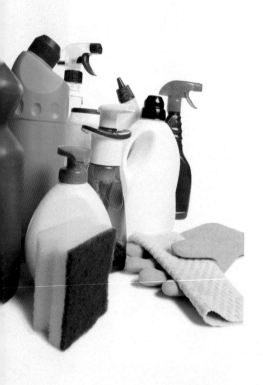

Levels of Prevention and Control

Sanitation is the first and lowest level of decontamination and means to significantly *reduce* the number of pathogens found on a surface. Barbering tools, implements, and other surfaces are *cleansed* (sanitized) by washing with soaps or detergents and are then *disinfected* through the application of chemical disinfectants. Hand washing is a frequently used form of cleansing.

Disinfection is a higher level of decontamination than sanitation and is second only to sterilization. Disinfection is the process of killing specific microorganisms by physical or chemical means on non-porous surfaces such as shampoo bowls, counter tops, clipper blades, shears, combs, or other fixtures and implements. **Disinfectants** are prepared chemical substances used to destroy harmful microorganisms such as bacteria, fungi, and some viruses on contaminated implements and surfaces, although some products may not be effective on bacterial spores.

Sterilization is the process of rendering an object germ-free by destroying all living organisms on a surface. Although it is the highest level of effective decontamination, it is not a practical option in the barbershop because the sterilization of metal implements would require either steaming in an autoclave or the application of dry heat (in the form of baking) to be rendered truly sterile. These methods are time consuming and require expensive equipment.

Public sanitation is the application of measures to promote public health and prevent the spread of infectious diseases. This is accomplished through wastewater management, water treatment facilities, ensuring food safety, and pollution control, to name but a few of the ways in which public health is protected by local, state, and federal agencies.

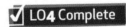 ✓ **LO4** Complete

Prevention and Control Agents

The agents or methods used to decontaminate barbering tools and shop surfaces are either physical or chemical in nature. As will be seen, chemical agents are usually the more efficient and effective choice of professional barbers and regulatory agencies.

PHYSICAL AGENTS

Physical agents such as moist heat (boiling water), steaming (in an autoclave), and dry heat are rarely used in today's barbershops. As previously mentioned, these methods are impractical, inefficient, and expensive in terms of time, convenience, and cost. The only physical methods still used routinely in barbershop sanitation procedures are the ultraviolet rays housed within an electric UV sanitizer. An **ultraviolet-ray sanitizer** will keep disinfected tools and implements sanitary until they are removed for use.

CHEMICAL AGENTS

Chemical agents are the most effective sanitizing and disinfecting methods used in barbershops to destroy or check the spread of pathogenic bacteria. Within the chemical agents group are antiseptics and disinfectants. See **Table 5-1** for a listing of these products.

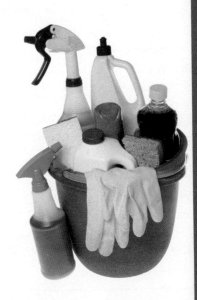

Antiseptics are substances that may kill, retard, or prevent the growth of bacteria and can generally be used safely on the skin. Because they are weaker than disinfectants, antiseptics are not effective for use on implements and surfaces. Hydrogen peroxide (3 percent solution) and tincture of iodine are good examples of antiseptics.

Disinfectants are the chemical agents used to destroy most bacteria and some viruses. They are used to disinfect and control microorganisms on hard, non-porous surfaces such as clipper blades, shears, and razors, but should *never* be used on the skin, hair, or nails. Any chemical agent or substance that is powerful enough to destroy pathogens can also damage skin.

ANTISEPTICS

NAME	FORM	SOLUTION STRENGTH	USE (FOLLOW MANUFACTURER'S DIRECTIONS)
Boric acid	Crystals	2–5%	Cleanse eyes and skin.
Hydrogen peroxide	Liquid	3%	Cleanse skin and minor cuts.
Isopropyl alcohol (Rubbing alcohol)	Liquid	50–60%	Cleanse skin and cuts; not to be used if irritation is present.
Sodium hypochlorite	Crystals	5%	Rinse the hands.
Styptic (alum)	Stick, powder, or liquid (stick styptics are impractical in the shop because they cannot be disinfected)		Stops bleeding of nicks or slight cuts in the skin. Use powder or liquid form only. Apply with cotton swab and discard.
Tincture of iodine	Liquid	2%	Cleanse cuts and wounds.

DISINFECTANTS

CATEGORY	FORM	SOLUTION STRENGTH	USE (FOLLOW MANUFACTURER'S DIRECTIONS)
Phenols (Lysol®, Pine Sol®, etc)	Liquid	Per manufacturer's directions	Cleanse surfaces, floors, sinks, etc.
Quaternary ammonium compounds (Quats) (Barbicide, H-42 Disinfectant Cleaner®, Sani-Wipe®,	Powder, tablet, liquid, or wipe	Per manufacturer's directions	Immerse for 5–20 minutes. Check state barber board law and manufacturer's directions for required disinfection time
Sodium hypochlorite (Bleach)	Liquid	10%	Immerse sharp cutting edges or glass electrodes for a minimum of 10 minutes. Used to clean non-porous surfaces.
Petroleum distillates (may be a cleaner and/or disinfection formula; H-42 Clipper Cleaner, Oster Blade Wash, etc.)	Liquids	Per manufacturer's directions	Run clipper blades through or immerse metal tools in product for recommended time

TYPES OF CHEMICAL DISINFECTANTS

All disinfectants must be approved by the EPA and each individual state. Product labels must provide the manufacturer's claims for the effectiveness of the product in killing specific organisms and have an EPA registration number.

There are four levels of disinfection **efficacy** (effectiveness) among the many **EPA-registered disinfectants** available for use in the barbershop:

1. *Limited* disinfection products have a very low efficacy level and will kill either the staphylococcus or salmonella organisms, but not both.

2. *General* disinfection products rate a low efficacy level because, although they will kill the staphylococcus and salmonella organisms, they are not effective on the organisms that cause pseudomonas or tuberculosis.

3. *Hospital-grade* disinfectants will kill staphylococcus, salmonella, and *Pseudomonas aeruginosa*, but not the more resistant tuberculosis bacillus.

4. **Hospital-grade tuberculocidal disinfectants** are effective against bacteria, fungi, viruses, tuberculosis, pseudomonas, HIV-1, and Hepatitis B. The ability to combat all of these organisms provides the optimum level of disinfection of tools, implements, and surfaces.

Consult your barber board or health department for a list of approved disinfectants in your state and consider the following requirements of a good disinfectant:

- Convenient to prepare
- Quick acting
- Preferably odorless
- Non-corrosive
- Economical
- Nonirritating to the skin (**Caution:** Most disinfectants will cause skin irritation at some point. Avoid prolonged contact.)

In addition to hospital-grade tuberculocidal disinfectants, other chemical decontamination agents commonly used in the barbershop include sodium hypochlorite, quaternary ammonium compounds, phenol- or pine-based products, alcohols, and petroleum distillate products.

- *Sodium hypochlorite:* Sodium hypochlorite (common household bleach) compounds are frequently used to provide the disinfecting agent chlorine. Although one of the key advantages of chlorine is its ability to destroy viruses, surfaces or items must be pre-cleaned with a cleaning agent and rinsed prior to application of the bleach solution. A 10 percent solution is recommended with an application or immersion time of 10 minutes. (See formulation directions in Table 5-1.)

  CAUTION: Bleach can damage certain tools and implements and will soften nylon combs.

- *Quaternary ammonium compounds (quats):* Quaternary ammonium compounds are chloride-based disinfecting agents effective for

Disinfectants must be approved by the EPA and by each individual state. When choosing a disinfectant product, look for the EPA registration number on the label. This assures you that the product is safe and effective. It should be noted that although disinfectants may be safe to use, they are still too harsh for human skin or eye contact. Always wear gloves and safety glasses to prevent accidental exposure.

sanitizing tools and cleaning countertops, but are not effective against the more resistant organisms such as tuberculosis and some viruses. Quats are odorless, nontoxic, and fast acting, requiring a short disinfection time. Most quat solutions disinfect implements in 10–15 minutes, but the time will vary depending on the strength of the solution. Check the product label to make sure that it contains a rust inhibitor and avoid long-term immersion of implements. Leaving some tools in the solution too long may damage them. Traditionally, a 1:1000 solution has been used to sanitize implements with an immersion time of 1 to 5 minutes. Refer to your state barber board rules and regulations for their specific requirements and always follow the manufacturer's directions when preparing the solution.

- *Phenols:* Phenols, like quats, have been used to disinfect implements for many years. Although caustic and toxic, phenols are relatively safe and extremely effective in their germ-killing capabilities, including effectiveness against the tuberculosis bacillus, when used according to the directions. Care should be taken with rubber and plastic materials as they may become softened or discolored with continued phenol use. In addition, phenolic disinfectants can cause skin irritation, so avoid skin contact and wear protective gear. Concentrated phenols can seriously burn the skin and eyes and are poisonous if ingested.

  Pine oil has natural antibacterial properties and is categorized as a phenol disinfectant. Products typically contain pine oil and surfactants (cleaning agents) and may irritate the skin or mucous membranes.

- *Alcohol:* Alcohol is an organic compound. While there are many types of alcohols used in science and manufacturing, the two most common forms utilized by barbers are ethyl alcohol and isopropyl alcohol, or combinations thereof. These alcohols act as limited disinfectants because although they are effective against most bacteria, fungi, and viruses, they are not as effective as the higher-grade disinfectants in eliminating bacterial spores. In some states, it may be permissible to use 70 to 90 percent ethyl or isopropyl alcohol products to disinfect implements such as shears, razors, or the glass electrodes of facial and scalp treatment appliances. A 50 to 60 percent isopropyl alcohol (also available at 91 percent and 99 percent) may be used on the skin as an antiseptic, and alcohol-based hand sanitizing gels may be used when water is not readily available.

- *Petroleum distillates:* Products containing petroleum distillates are preferred for the cleaning or disinfection of metal tools to eliminate or minimize rust formation. Oils or other chemicals may be included in the mixture, so always check the label for the manufacturer's intended use for the product.

- *Prepared commercial products:* A variety of prepared commercial products containing one or more of the chemical agents just discussed are available through barber supply and retail stores. Products such as Barbicide® and H-42® Disinfectant are multi-purpose formulations that can be used on surfaces and implements depending on the strength used. Lysol®, Pine-Sol®, and similar products are sufficient for decontaminating countertops, doorknobs, floors, and so forth. These products are generally effective against bacteria, fungi, and viruses, and some new *plus* formulas are also effective against tuberculosis, MRSA, and other resistant microbial strains. Most are available in liquid, concentrate, spray, or wipe formulas.

- Other products, like Clippercide®, H-42®, or Marvicide® sprays, are designed for the cleaning or disinfection of clippers, trimmers, and other electrical tools. As a cautionary note, commercially prepared products designed for use on these tools usually perform at least one of four functions: cleaning, disinfection, lubrication, or cooling. While there are products that may accomplish all four tasks, others may perform only one, so read labels carefully before purchasing, and know the intended function of the product.

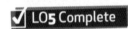 LO5 Complete

 For more information about the disinfectant properties of hypochlorites, phenols, and quats, refer to *Guideline for Disinfection and Sterilization in Healthcare Facilities, 2008* by W. A. Rutala and D. J. Weber, at http://www.cdc.gov/.

Solutions and Strengths

As a barber, your work will require the use of a variety of solutions for different purposes. As you have learned, disinfectants are essential for the decontamination of fixtures, surfaces, tools, and implements. Antiseptics are used for cleansing the hands and for treating minor cuts and abrasions.

In many cases, a premixed commercial preparation such as a blade wash will be used; however, other formulations, such as quats and phenols, are less costly when purchased in concentrated form. Concentrates must be diluted with water to achieve the required strength; they also cost less than premixed solutions.

Since the purchase of disinfectant products in concentrate form requires the formulation of a solution, it is important to become familiar with the terms associated with solution preparation.

A **solution** is the product resulting from the combining and dissolving of a solute in a solvent. The **solute** is the substance that is dissolved and the **solvent** is the liquid in which it is dissolved. For example, in a solution of sugar water, the sugar is the solute and water is the solvent.

In the preparation of a solution, the amount of *solute* indicates the strength of the solution. For example, a 10 percent solution (or strength) of sodium hypochlorite means that 10 percent, or $^1/_{10}$, of the solution is sodium hypochlorite and the remaining 90 percent, or $^9/_{10}$, is water.

 Mixing chemicals stronger than recommended by the manufacturer may counteract the effectiveness of the product. Always read manufacturers' directions.

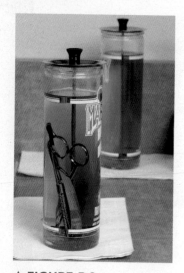

▲ FIGURE 5-3

Wet sanitizer.

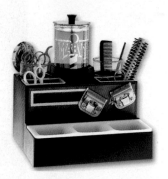

▲ FIGURE 5-4

Wet sanitizer.

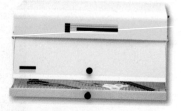

▲ FIGURE 5-5

Ultraviolet-ray sanitizer.

🏛️ STATE

The procedures for the immersion of implements into a chemical solution must conform to the state barber board, EPA, and/or OSHA regulations in your state.

The strength of a solution is identified by the percentage of solute. The percent figure indicates one of two measurements, either the percentage of solute by *weight* or the percentage of solute by *volume.*

- *Example by weight:* A container holds a total solution of 100 grams. If it is labeled as a 5% solution, it means that there are 5 grams of solute in the solution.

- *Example by volume:* A 1-gallon container contains a 20 percent by volume solution. This means that 20 percent of the solution is solute. Let's say you want to duplicate the formula. You would have to know the number of ounces of solute and solvent needed to mix the formula. There are 128 ounces in a gallon, therefore 20 percent, or 25.6 ounces of solute, and 80 percent, or 102.4 ounces of solvent, would be needed to duplicate the solution.

Because the percent figure measures either weight or volume, you need to pay attention when reading labels. Simply remember that, like strength, the percentage tells you how much solute there is in the solution.

Sanitizers

A **wet sanitizer** is a covered receptacle large enough to hold a disinfectant solution into which objects can be completely immersed. Wet sanitizers are available in a variety of shapes and sizes, so select the size most appropriate for the tools or implements that you will be disinfecting (**Figures 5-3** and **5-4**).

Ultraviolet-ray sanitizers are usually metal cabinets with ultraviolet lamps or bulbs that are used to store disinfected tools and implements. They are effective for keeping clean brushes, combs, and implements sanitary until ready for use, but they are not capable of sanitizing or decontaminating an object. Items must be thoroughly cleansed and disinfected before being placed in the sanitizer. Follow the manufacturer's directions for proper use and check your state barber board regulations concerning the use of ultraviolet-ray cabinets (**Figure 5-5**).

A **dry,** or **cabinet, sanitizer** is an airtight cabinet containing an active fumigant such as formalin. This fumigant produces a formaldehyde vapor that destroys bacteria on tools and implements. Although dry sanitizers used to be a standard barbershop fixture for the disinfection and storage of tools, modern methods and products have replaced them. Today, barbers may store their disinfected implements in closed plastic containers, plastic wrap, or zip-lock plastic bags to help prevent contamination.

Disinfection Procedures

Always disinfect tools and implements according to the manufacturer's directions. The EPA guidelines for wet disinfectants require complete immersion of the item for the required amount of time.

Procedure for Quats Solution Disinfection of Implements

1 Read the manufacturer's directions for quats, phenol, or other disinfectant solution. Mix accordingly (**Figures 5-6** and **5-7**). Note: Add the concentrate *after* filling the container with water to eliminate excessive suds formation.

2 Remove hair from combs, brushes, and other implements (**Figure 5-8**).

3 Wash item(s) thoroughly with hot water and soap.

4 Rinse item(s) thoroughly and pat dry.

5 Place item(s) in the wet sanitizer containing the disinfectant solution, immersing completely. Disinfect for the recommended time (**Figure 5-9**).

6 Remove item(s) from the disinfectant and rinse thoroughly (**Figure 5-10**).

7 Dry item(s) with a clean towel.

Store item(s) in a dry cabinet sanitizer, UV sanitizer, or other clean, covered container until needed.

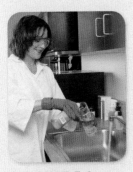

▲ **FIGURE 5-6**
Read manufacturer's directions and mix accordingly.

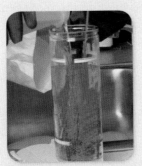

▲ **FIGURE 5-7**
Carefully pour disinfectant into the water when preparing disinfectant solution.

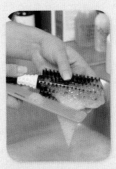

▲ **FIGURE 5-8**
Remove hair from brushes and combs before disinfecting.

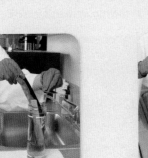

▲ **FIGURE 5-9**
Immerse combs and brushes in disinfectant solution.

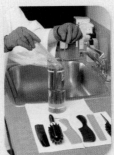

▲ **FIGURE 5-10**
Remove implements, rinse, and dry thoroughly.

CAUTION

In the past, fumigants in the form of formaldehyde vapors were used in dry cabinet sanitizers to keep sanitized implements sanitary. Tablet or liquid formalin releases formaldehyde gas, which has since proven to be irritating to the eyes, nose, throat, and lungs. Formaldehyde can cause skin allergies and has long been suspected of being a cancer-causing agent. Although formalin is an effective disinfectant, it is not safe for shop or salon disinfection. Many states have prohibited the use of formalin; refer to your state board rules and regulations for specific or updated information.

FYI Tools and implements must be cleaned prior to disinfectant immersion to comply with decontamination rules and to avoid solution contamination.

FYI Some regulatory boards require a 1:1000 quat disinfectant solution. To mix this solution, add $1\frac{1}{4}$ ounce quat solute to 1 gallon of water. Add the quats concentrate *after* filling the container with water to eliminate excessive suds formation.

DISINFECTING CLIPPERS AND OUTLINERS

The decontamination of electrical tools such as clippers and outliners requires a different approach than for non-electric tools and implements. Hair particles and bacteria become trapped between and behind clipper blades, so thorough cleaning and disinfection of these tools is very important. Since they cannot be completely immersed in water-based disinfectants, and since most spray disinfectants alone are not sufficient for thorough disinfection, products containing a petroleum distillate, such as liquid blade washes, are the usual choice for the decontamination procedure.

mini PROCEDURE

Procedure for Disinfecting Clippers and Outliners

1 Arrange all supplies, products, and tools on a clean surface (**Figure 5-11**).

2 Pour blade wash into a glass, plastic, or disposable container wide enough to accommodate the width of the clipper blades to a depth of approximately ½ inch (**Figure 5-12**).

3 Remove hair particles from clipper blades with a stiff brush (**Figure 5-13**).

4 Submerge only the cutting teeth of the clipper blades into the blade wash and turn the unit on. Run the blades in the solution until no hair particles are seen being dislodged from between the blades (**Figure 5-14**).

5 Remove the clippers and wipe the blades with a clean, dry towel (**Figure 5-15**).

6 Spray with a blade lubricant and/or spray clipper disinfectant. Grease or oil clipper parts as necessary (**Figure 5-16**).

7 Sanitize the conductor cord and store in a clean, closed container until needed for use.

8 Follow these procedures *before and after* servicing each client.

NOTE: Detachable clipper blades may be removed from the clipper, brushed clean, and immersed in blade wash for the recommended soaking time.

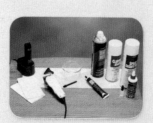

▲ **FIGURE 5-11**
Arrange products, supplies, and tools on a clean surface.

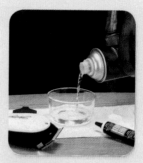

▲ **FIGURE 5-12**
Pour blade wash into container.

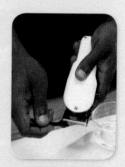

▲ **FIGURE 5-13**
Remove hair particles from clipper blades.

(Continued)

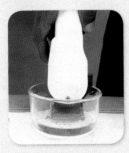

▲ **FIGURE 5-14**
Submerge only the teeth of the clipper blades into blade wash.

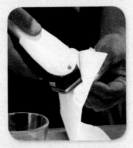

▲ **FIGURE 5-15**
Wipe clipper blades with a clean, dry towel.

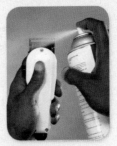

▲ **FIGURE 5-16**
Spray clipper blades with a lubricant.

DECONTAMINATING TOWELS, LINENS, AND CAPES

Clean towels and linens must be used for each client. All towels, linens, and capes that come into contact with a client's skin should be laundered with detergent and bleach according to label directions. It is advisable to maintain a sufficient supply of these items for use in the barbershop to avoid the spread of infectious agents and particles. Disposable towels or neck strips should be used to keep capes from touching the client's skin. If the neckline of a cape comes in contact with the client's skin, do not use it again until it has been laundered.

DISINFECTING WORK SURFACES

Before and after each client, an EPA-registered, hospital-grade tuberculocidal disinfectant should be used on all work surfaces and equipment that come into contact with the client or the barber's tools. This includes station countertops, barber chairs, armrests, headrests, shampoo bowls, and other surfaces.

HAND WASHING

Hand washing is one the most important and easiest ways to prevent the spread of germs from one person to another. Thorough hand washing requires rubbing the hands and under the nails with warm, soapy water for at least 20 seconds and drying with a clean paper towel. Moisturizing lotions can help prevent dry skin that may otherwise occur as a result of repeated hand washing (Figure 5-17).

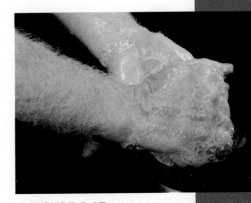

▲ **FIGURE 5-17**
Thorough hand washing helps prevent the spread of germs.

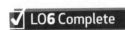
✓ **LO6 Complete**

Standard Precautions

As mentioned, there are standards that must be used when dealing with blood and the possibility of bloodborne pathogens. *Universal precautions* were established in the 1980s to reduce the spread of infection from bloodborne pathogens specifically. Since then, the Centers for Disease Control and Prevention (CDC) have required expanded precautions that cover more bodily fluids and body sites, such as broken skin, mucous membranes, secretions, and excretions. The result is a set of **standard precautions** that workers in any profession where sharp implements are used should be aware of. Precautions include hand washing; proper disinfection and decontamination of tools; use of protective equipment such as gloves and goggles; injury prevention; and the proper handling and disposal of sharp implements (such as razor blades) or contaminated dressings. Table 5-2 provides a decontamination guide for certain situations that may arise in the school or barbershop.

TABLE 5-2 Decontamination Guide

ITEM/SITUATION	LEVEL OF DECONTAMINATION	PROCEDURE/PRODUCTS
Any implement used to puncture or break the skin, or that comes into contact with pus or other bodily fluids	Sterilization	Steam autoclave and dry heat. Dispose of all sharps in a sharps container.
Non-porous tools and implements (brushes, combs, razors, clipper guards) that *have not* come into contact with bodily fluids or blood	Disinfection	Completely immerse in an EPA-registered, hospital-grade bactericidal, pseudomonacidal, fungicidal, and virucidal disinfectant for amount of time specified by the manufacturer.
Non-porous tools and implements (brushes, combs, razors, clipper guards) that *have* come into contact with bodily fluids or blood	Disinfection	Completely immerse in an EPA-registered disinfectant with demonstrated efficacy against HIV-1/HBV or tuberculosis for amount of time specified by the manufacturer.
Non-porous tools and implements (brushes, combs, razors, clipper guards) that have come into contact with parasites such as head lice	Disinfection	Completely immerse in Lysol solution (2 tablespoons in 1 quart water) for one hour.
Electrotherapy tools	Disinfection	Spray or wipe with an EPA-registered, hospital-grade disinfectant specifically made for electrical equipment.
Countertops, shampoo bowls, sinks, floors, toilets, doorknobs, mirrors, etc.	Sanitation	Use an EPA-registered cleaning product designed for surfaces.
Towels, linens, chair cloths, capes, etc.	Sanitation	Launder in hot water with detergent and bleach.
Barber's hands prior to and after each service	Sanitation	Wash with liquid antibacterial soap and warm water.

EXPOSURE INCIDENTS

Formerly known as a blood spill, an **exposure incident** is the contact with non-intact skin, blood, body fluid, or other potentially infectious materials that may occur during the performance of an individual's work duties. Accidents happen and exposure incidents occur when the barber or client sustains a cut during a service. Such incidences require **blood-spill disinfection** procedures to protect the health and safety of both individuals.

mini PROCEDURE

Cut Sustained by Client

1 Stop the service immediately and inform the client of the incident.

2 Wash your hands and apply gloves.

3 Clean the injured area.

4 Apply antiseptic or styptic using a cotton swab. Do not contaminate the container.

5 Cover the injury with an appropriate dressing.

6 Discard all disposable contaminated objects such as cotton, tissues, and so forth by double-bagging. Use the appropriate biohazard sticker (red or orange) on a container for contaminated waste. Deposit sharp disposables in a sharps box (Figure 5-18).

7 Disinfect tools and workstation using an EPA-registered disinfectant or 10 percent bleach solution. Refer to Table 5-2 for disinfection guidelines.

8 Remove gloves by peeling one glove off from the wrist, allowing it to turn inside out. Hold it in the gloved hand. Use the exposed hand to grasp a section of the inside of the second glove. When peeling off the second glove, stretch it over and around the first glove. Promptly dispose of the gloves in the appropriate biohazard container.

9 Wash your hands with soap and warm water before returning to the service.

10 Recommend that the client see a physician if signs of redness, pain, swelling, or irritation develop.

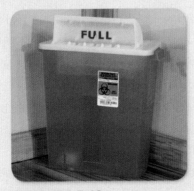

▲ **FIGURE 5-18**

A sharps box.

(Continued)

mini PROCEDURE (Continued)

Cut Sustained by Barber

1 Stop the service and check the client for possible transmission of blood.

2 Wash your hands.

3 Apply antiseptic or styptic using a cotton swab. Do not contaminate the container.

4 Cover the injury with an appropriate dressing (bandage, finger guard, or gloves as necessary).

5 Discard all disposable contaminated objects such as cotton, tissues, and so forth by double-bagging. Use the appropriate biohazard sticker on a container for contaminated waste. Deposit sharp disposables in a sharps box (Figure 5-18).

6 Disinfect tools and workstation using an EPA-registered disinfectant or 10 percent bleach solution. Refer to Table 5-2 for disinfection guidelines.

7 Wash your hands before returning to the service.

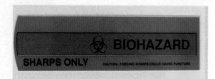

DISINFECTING RULES

- Chemical solutions in sanitizers should be changed regularly. Change the solution when it becomes dirty, contaminated, or cloudy.

- All metal implements should be disinfected, lubricated, and stored in airtight containers.

- All items must be clean and free from hair and debris before being sanitized.

- All cups, finger bowls, or similar objects must be disinfected prior to being used for another client. Do not forget to disinfect such surfaces as headrests, shampoo bowl neck rests, and other equipment.

DECONTAMINATION SAFETY PRECAUTIONS

- Purchase chemicals in small quantities and store them in a cool, dry place as they can deteriorate when exposed to air, light, and heat.

- Wear protective gloves, goggles, and aprons when mixing chemicals.

- Carefully weigh, measure, and pour chemicals.

- Keep all containers labeled, covered, and under lock and key.

- Do not smell chemicals or solutions. Some have pungent odors and can irritate the nasal membranes.

- Avoid spilling chemicals when diluting them.

- Prevent burns by using forceps to insert or remove objects from heat sources.

- Keep a complete first-aid kit on hand.
- Maintain a complete MSDS record of all chemicals and products used in the barbershop.

Public Sanitation and Rules of Sanitation

As previously discussed, public sanitation is the application of measures to promote public health and prevent the spread of infectious diseases. The importance of cleaning cannot be overemphasized. The barbering profession requires direct contact with clients' skin, scalp, and hair. Understanding sanitation and decontamination measures ensures the protection of the clients' health as well as your own.

Various government agencies protect community health by ensuring that food is wholesome, the water supply is untainted, and refuse is disposed of properly. Barber boards and boards of health in each state have formulated sanitation regulations that all barbers must follow in the pursuit of their profession. The most basic sanitation regulations apply to air quality, water quality, and infectious diseases.

The air within a barbershop should be moist and fresh. Room temperature should be about 70 degrees Fahrenheit. The shop should be equipped with an exhaust fan or an air-conditioning unit. Air-conditioning is an advantage since it permits changes in the quality and quantity of air in the shop.

Water in the barbershop should be pure. Be aware that crystal-clear water still may be unsanitary if it contains pathogenic bacteria, which cannot be seen with the naked eye. Many municipal governments require water coolers in establishments that serve the general public.

A person ill with an infectious disease puts other people's health at risk. A barber with a cold or any other contagious disease should not serve clients. Likewise, clients suffering from infectious diseases should be tactfully encouraged to postpone their appointment until after they are well. This protects you and other clients being serviced.

RULES OF SANITATION

- Barbershops must be well lit, heated, and ventilated, in order to keep them clean.
- Walls, floors, and windows in the shop must be kept clean.
- All barbering establishments must have hot and cold running water.
- All plumbing fixtures should be properly installed.
- The premises should be kept free of rodents and flies or other insects.
- Dogs (with the exception of guide dogs), cats, birds, and other pets must not be permitted in the shop.
- The barbershop should not be used for eating or sleeping or as living quarters. If square footage allows, staff may use a small room

TIP FROM THE
NABBA

"Put yourself in the client's position when it comes to sanitation. Let your clients see you disinfect your tools and implements before starting the service and be sure to drape the client so the cape does not touch his skin."

Carl Troupe,
Vice-Chair,
Florida Barber's Board

at the back of the shop during their breaks. State boards and local building inspectors can provide mandatory standards and codes.

- Clean and disinfect all implements as they are used and return them to their proper places.

- Clean work areas, chairs, and mirrors.

- Remove all hair and waste materials from the floor.

- Rest rooms must be kept in a clean condition.

- Each barber must be appropriately attired to work on clients.

- Barbers must cleanse their hands thoroughly before and after serving a client.

- Barbers must wash their hands after using the bathroom.

- A freshly laundered towel or fresh paper towel must be used for each client. Towels ready for use should be stored in a clean, closed cabinet. All soiled linen towels and used paper towels must be disposed of properly. Keep dirty towels separate from clean towels.

- Headrest coverings and neck strips or towels must be changed for each client.

- Use a neckstrip to prevent the cape from coming in contact with the client's skin.

- The common use of tools and implements is prohibited unless they are disinfected after each client.

- The common use of drinking cups, styptic pencils, or shaving mugs is prohibited.

- Lotions, ointments, creams, and powders must be kept in clean, closed containers. Use a disinfected spatula to remove creams or ointments from jars. Use sterile cotton pledgets to apply lotions and powders. Re-cover containers after each use.

- Combs and other implements must not be carried in the pockets of uniforms.

- Combs, shears, and razors must be disinfected after each use.

- All used instruments and articles must be disinfected before placing them in a dustproof or airtight container or a cabinet sanitizer.

- Objects dropped on the floor may not be used until they are disinfected.

- Maintain client record cards with emergency contact information.

The public is increasingly aware of the possibility of cross-contamination and cross-infection that can occur in barbershops and salons. Adherence to the rules of sanitation will result in cleaner and better service to the public. The manager or owner must provide the necessities for school or shop sanitation, and every student or barber should take responsibility for implementing decontamination procedures in these environments.

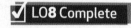

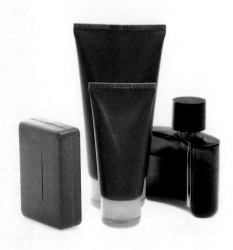

Safe Work Practices

The previous sections discussed decontamination and infection control procedures relevant to maintaining necessary sanitary conditions in the barbershop in order to prevent the spread of disease and contamination. Yet another important responsibility of barbers and stylists is to follow safety precautions and procedures for the benefit of shop personnel and patrons.

Safe work practices include the maintenance of sanitation and decontamination standards and the application of safety precautions in the workplace environment. Although the overall responsibility for maintaining safety standards in the barbershop rests with the owner or manager, it is the responsibility of each employee to comply with those standards. Be observant and recognize safety hazards, especially in areas where electricity and water are in close proximity to one another or where chemicals are stored. Learn to handle tools and implements with care and thus avoid unnecessary injuries. Try to prevent accidents before they happen. Assist clients who need help. In general, if you are conscientious, use common sense, and stay alert, many accidents can be avoided.

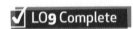

DISCLOSURE

In cases of injury to a client—minor or otherwise—always inform the client of the situation. Some implements are so sharp that the client may not immediately feel the nick of a trimmer, razor, or shears. Redness, irritation, or swelling of the skin due to a reaction to certain chemicals may also go unnoticed at first, but can intensify over time, resulting in a more severe reaction, if not rinsed and cared for immediately. Remember that honesty will help protect you, your reputation, and the client's health.

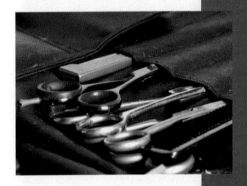

SAFETY PRECAUTIONS

Most potentially harmful situations in the barbershop can be avoided by being observant and using common sense. Learn to recognize safety hazards to minimize the occurrence of accidents.

Water

- At the shampoo bowl, be careful how you handle the spray hose. Position the client's head for comfort and access, being conscious of your own body position as well. Do not bend or twist from the waist unnecessarily. Wipe up any water spills or leaks immediately.

- If the water temperature reaches a scalding level while in the hot position, turn the thermostat on the hot-water tank down to a more acceptable temperature for application to the skin, scalp, and hair.

- As a precaution, always test the water temperature on the inside of your wrist before applying to a client's hair or scalp. The same procedure may be used to test steam towels for facials and shaves.

Electricity

- Electricity and water do not mix! Make sure that all electrical appliances and tools are stored safely, and preferably unplugged, when in close proximity to water.

- Have shop wiring checked periodically to ensure a safe, fire-free environment.

- Schedule annual safety and operational check-ups for wiring, hot-water tanks, air-conditioners, and ventilation systems.

Tools and Appliances

- Tools and equipment should be strategically placed so that the items are safely stored when not in use, yet are accessible when needed. Smaller tools, such as clippers, trimmers, blow-dryers, or curling irons, may be placed in countertop receptacles designed for that purpose. Don't forget to disinfect before and after each use. Larger equipment such as UV-ray cabinet sanitizers may be mounted under the cabinet, attached to a wall, or set on a shelf. Wet sanitizers and electric latherizers are usually placed on the station countertop, but should be set back toward a wall or partition so as not to interfere with other tools. This also limits the risk of accidental burns from a hot latherizer or the spillage of disinfectant solutions.

- All tools and implements should be in good working condition. Replace damaged electrical cords, chipped clipper blades, cracked housings, broken shears, and other tools immediately. Never subject yourself or your client to the risks of faulty or broken equipment.

- Barbering tools and implements are designed for specific purposes, so use the right tool for the job. Do not expect a trimmer to do the work of a clipper!

- Electrical cords deserve specific mention because they often become a safety hazard in the shop. Cords to clippers, trimmers, curling irons, and blow-dryers tend to become twisted and tangled during use. If the cord is too long, it can get caught on the foot or arm rests of a hydraulic chair or even on the foot of a client! Some barbers replace the factory cord with a retractable cord device or purchase cordless trimmers, which eliminate the problem altogether. A well-planned workstation with sufficient and conveniently placed outlets can also help minimize the "tangled cord syndrome."

- Do not overload electrical outlets.

Equipment and Fixtures

- Keep all hydraulic chairs, headrests, shampoo chairs, heat lamps, and lighting fixtures in good working order. Tighten screws and bolts, grease or oil hinges, and service equipment mechanisms as needed.

- Dust and clean regularly to avoid soil buildup and to maintain clean conditions.

- Maintain lighting fixtures. Change bulbs when necessary to keep workstations well lit.

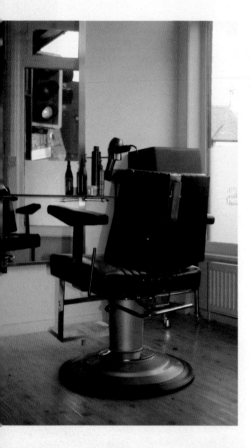

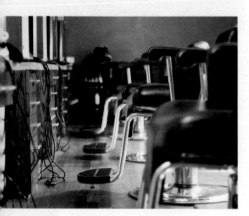

Ventilation

- Proper ventilation and air circulation are extremely important in today's shop or salon. Particles from products such as talc, hair sprays, and disinfectants can be inhaled and may cause allergies or other health problems. Heating and air-conditioning vents should be located to perform their optimum functions without inferring with client services. Fumes from chemical applications and nail care products require sophisticated filtration units that cleanse and detoxify the air. Once installed, air filters should be changed or cleaned regularly.

Attire

- Clothing should be comfortable and professional in appearance. Excessively baggy clothes can get in the way of your performance just as *easily as tight clothing can restrict it.*
- Long hair worn in a loose style has been known to get caught in blow-dryer motor vents and other appliances. Keep hair pulled back or short enough to avoid entanglements.
- Necklaces should be of an appropriate length so as not to get caught on equipment or dangle in a client's face at the shampoo bowl or during a shave. Rings should not be worn on the index and middle fingers as they might interfere with haircutting accuracy. Watches should be waterproof and shock absorbent.
- Shoes should have nonskid rubber soles with good support.

Children

- Children can cause serious risk of injury to themselves in the shop environment. Being aware of their inquisitive natures and the speed with which they can move can help prevent accidents from happening.
- Post notices in the reception area that advises patrons that children are not to be left unattended.
- Do not allow children to play, climb, or spin on hydraulic chairs.
- Do not allow children to wander freely around the shop with access to workstations, storage areas, and so forth.

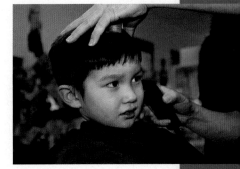

- When cutting a child's hair, try to anticipate their sudden moves. Never trust a young child to hold their head still while you approach their head area with shears or other tools. Instead, hold the child's head gently but firmly with one hand while cutting with the other. This technique is especially helpful when cutting around ears and at the nape. When trimming bangs or front hairlines, hold the hair between your fingers at a low elevation, cutting the hair on the inside of your palm, thereby putting the barrier of your fingers between the tool and the child's face.

Adult Clients

- As barbers, many of the things we do to assure client comfort also fall under the category of safety precautions. In the following chapters you will learn the proper draping procedures and chemical

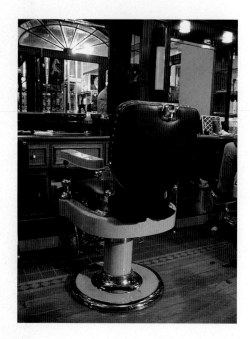

application methods to ensure client safety and comfort from the standpoint of avoiding skin irritations, burns, wet or soiled clothing, and so forth; however, there are also several common-sense services that should be performed. Using good manners and performing common courtesies will help you gain the reputation of being a safety conscious and courteous barber.

- Assist clients (especially the elderly) in and out of hydraulic and shampoo chairs.
- Always lower the hydraulic chair to its lowest level and lock it in position so that it does not spin before inviting the client to be seated or leave the chair.
- Hold doors open for clients.
- Assist clients in walking whenever necessary.
- Always support the back of the chair, and thus the client, when reclining or raising a chair back.
- Cushion the client's neck with a folded towel in the neck rest at the shampoo bowl. This is especially beneficial for clients with neck injuries such as whiplash.
- Support the client's head whenever appropriate at the shampoo bowl. Do not ask them to hold their head up for shampooing or rinsing. Instead, gently turn their head to the side for easier access to the back and nape areas.

Exits

- Exits should be well marked and identifiable. (Check with your local building inspection office for codes and requirements.)
- Employees should know where exits are located and how to evacuate the building quickly in case of fire or other emergencies. Implement fire drills to practice for this contingency.

Fire Extinguishers

- Fire extinguishers should be placed where they are readily accessible.
- All employees should be instructed in fire extinguisher use.
- It is a law that fire extinguishers be checked periodically. Be guided by the manufacturer's recommendations and state and local ordinances.

Chemicals

- Request an MSDS from your supplier(s) for each product purchased for use or sale in the shop, and maintain an MSDS notebook. Add to the notebook as new products are brought into the workplace.
- Take the time to study the MSDS from the manufacturer so that you will know how and where to store products and what procedures to follow in an emergency.
- There is a correct way to dispose of chemicals such as haircolor tints, chemical relaxers, bleach, and so forth. Contact your local hazardous-waste department or agency for disposal guidelines.

- Never mix cleaning products together—especially bleach and ammonia.

- Never mix leftover chemicals together!

- Do not allow leftover chemicals to stockpile. Dispose of products as often as necessary to maintain a safe environment.

- Check the inventory stock occasionally for plastic bottles with dents or bulges. This swelling of the container indicates that the contents are under pressure and could possibly explode.

- Wear goggles when pouring or mixing products. Add a lab apron and gloves when handling any caustic or skin-irritating material.

- Chemical spills require an absorbent material, such as sawdust, to clean up properly. Be guided by your local hazardous-waste agency.

- Every solution, liquid, cream, powder, paste, gel, and other substance should be properly labeled. This requirement goes beyond labeled products purchased from a supplier and includes spray bottles of water or setting lotions, sanitizing jars of alcohol, containers of blade wash, and any other substance used in the shop that is not contained within its original packaging (Figure 5-19).

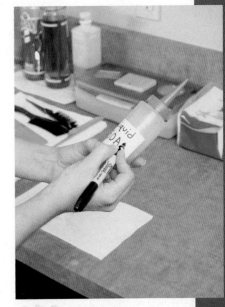

▲ FIGURE 5-19
All containers should be labeled.

Professional Responsibility

After studying this chapter, it should be clear that your responsibilities as a professional barber far exceed the requirement to perform a good haircut. This responsibility includes a certain awareness that can be developed and demonstrated through a sincere sense of caring when working with the public. It is this awareness or observation of the environment that helps you notice the little things that will make the barbershop safe for you and your clients. Responsible awareness also encourages you to do things the right way, rather than trying to take shortcuts.

Being prepared for emergencies is also a part of your professional responsibility. Every shop should have employee and clientele emergency information available near the telephone. An emergency phone number checklist should include the contact numbers for fire, police, and medical rescue departments; the nearest hospital emergency room; and taxis. Utility service companies, such as electricity, water, heat, air-conditioning, and so forth, and landlord or custodial numbers are also helpful in an emergency or if something breaks down in the shop. Update this information on an annual basis and you will always be prepared.

As your sense of awareness increases and you begin to feel more comfortable and confident working with clients, the quality of your communication and human relations skills will increase as well. Subsequently, you will reap the benefits of a loyal clientele base. Behavior that stems from a knowledgeable and caring manner is what separates a true professional from a nonprofessional, and being a *professional* is something you can take pride in.

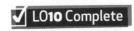

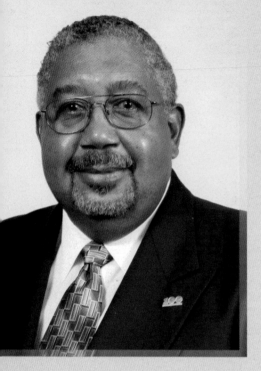

RONALD S. HAMPTON, SR.

Ronald S. Hampton Sr. is the President and CEO of Hampton Manufacturing Inc. in Fayetteville, Georgia. While studying chemistry in college, Ron was drafted into the U.S. military and later attended barber college. For the past 30 years, he has developed industrial chemical cleaners for Fortune 500 companies and the barbering industry at large. His most recent research and development has led to the formulation of a clipper disinfectant that should prove effective against the Hepatitis B and C viruses.

At the age of 10 I worked as a shopkeeper, shining shoes and keeping the Collegiate Barber Shop clean until the age of 15. After college and the military I graduated from the Capital Barber College. My college background in chemistry afforded me a career in the development, formulation, and marketing of industrial chemicals.

Then one day in 1986, I was next in line for a haircut by the barber who had cut my hair for years. I noticed that the gentlemen in the chair ahead of me had a personal hygiene issue in that his hair was extremely dirty and he appeared to have a serious scalp condition. After the gentlemen had exited the barbershop, I quietly asked my barber to clean his tools before cutting my hair. His response was that he did not like using bleach (recommended for cleaning clipper blades at the time) and after a long conversation I decided to try another shop. I also planned to do some research for him and get back later with the information. It was inevitable that this experience and my chemistry background would lead to the development of safe and effective chemical products for barbershops.

It was my technical work with companies, such as the Georgia Power Company and Norfolk Southern Rail Road, in the development of cleaners that were safe and economical alternatives to what they were using, that gave me the idea of a clipper blade cleaner that barbers would love. I decided to develop a petroleum hydrocarbon–type cleaner that could be used to clean electric hair clipper blades and eliminate the risk of electrical shock. My wife and I decided to name it H-42 Clean Clipper. It would work the same as blade wash, but unlike blade wash, it would be very pleasant to use. But this was not enough. In a visit with the Georgia State Barber Board, I was asked by one of the board members to explain some of the merits of the cleaner. After a brief introduction it was explained to me that we were entering a new era wherein barbers needed a product that would protect their clients from bacteria and viruses. This brought back to mind the scenario that had triggered my original idea for a blade cleaner—recognizing certain health threats as they existed then and the barbers' need for a germ-killing product that was safe on electric clippers.

Our research and development lead us to a process of introducing an antimicrobial without the use of water, the results of which were presented to a EPA-approved lab for testing against salmonella, pseudomonas, and staphylococcus, a community of organisms associated with MRSA. Our research and development continued as cross-contamination of Human Immunodeficiency Virus type 1 (HIV-1) was beginning to be a very serious problem. In the end, Anti-Bacterial H-42 Clean Clipper was tested under federal regulations and was found to kill HIV-1 on metal cutting blades in 60 seconds, earning our product the right to be called Virucidal Anti-Bacterial H-42 Clean Clipper. Since then, additional research and development has provided insight on testing against the hepatitis B and C viruses. These results are being prepared and will be presented to EPA for approval in the near future.

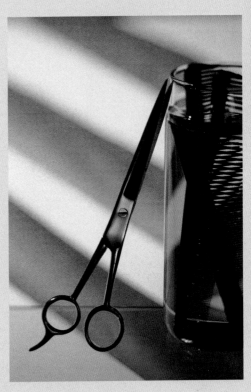

We are proud of the inroads made in formulating the only EPA-approved, patented, water-free clipper blade cleaner for the benefit of the barbering industry and its clients. Virucidal Anti-Bacterial H-42 Clean Clipper is quick and easy to use, cleanse, and disinfect without removing the clipper blades. All of our products adhere to similar safety, economy, and efficacy standards.

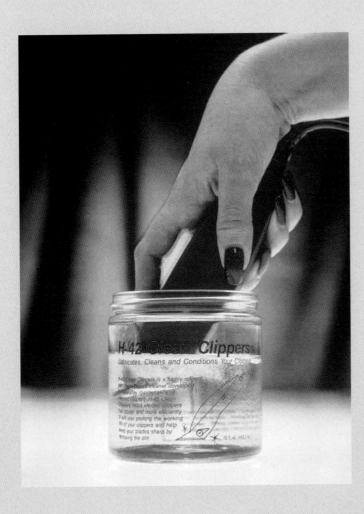

5 Review
Questions

1. Identify two ways in which infectious materials may be transmitted in the barbershop.

2. Why is it important to maintain an MSDS notebook in the school or barbershop?

3. List three federal agencies that help regulate infection control and safe work practices in the barbershop.

4. Define *decontamination.* List and explain the three levels of decontamination. List the three steps of decontamination and identify the two steps most often used in barbering.

5. List the chemical decontamination agents commonly used in barbershops.

6. Explain the differences between solutes, solvents, and solutions.

7. What two types of sanitizing units are most commonly used in barbershops?

8. List the steps used to disinfect (a) combs and brushes, (b) shears and razors, and (c) clippers, trimmers, or outliners.

9. Define *standard precautions.*

10. What blood-spill disinfection procedures should be performed when a client sustains a cut during an exposure incident?

11. What is the definition of *safe work practices*?

12. List 11 safety-precaution areas or topics barbers should be aware of in the barbershop.

Chapter
Glossary

antiseptics chemical agents that may kill, retard, or prevent the growth of bacteria; not classified as disinfectants

blood-spill disinfection the procedures to follow when the barber or client sustains an injury that results in bleeding

clean (cleaning) to remove all visible dirt and debris from tools, implements, and equipment by washing with soap and water.

decontamination the removal of pathogens from tools, equipment, and surfaces

disinfectants chemical agents used to destroy most bacteria and some viruses and to disinfect tools, implements, and surfaces

disinfection the second-highest level of decontamination; used on hard, non-porous materials

dry (cabinet) sanitizer an airtight cabinet containing an active fumigant used to store sanitized tools and implements

efficacy the effectiveness of a disinfectant solution in killing germs when used according to the label

Environmental Protection Agency also referred to as EPA; develops and enforces the regulations of environmental law in an effort to protect human health and the environment

EPA-registered disinfectant a product that has been approved by the Environmental Protection Agency as an effective disinfectant against certain disease-producing organisms

exposure incident contact with non-intact skin, blood, body fluid, or other potentially infectious materials that may occur during the performance of an individual's work duties

Food and Drug Administration also referred to as FDA; enforces rules and regulations associated with food, drug, and cosmetic products purchased and used by the public

Hazard Communication Rule requires that chemical manufacturers and importers evaluate and identify possible health hazards associated with their products

hospital-grade tuberculocidal disinfectant disinfectants that are effective against bacteria, fungi, viruses, tuberculosis, pseudomonas HIV-1, and hepatitis B and are registered with the EPA

Material Safety Data Sheet also referred to as MSDS; provides product information as compiled by the manufacturer

Occupational Safety and Health Act an act that led to the creation of OSHA

Occupational Safety and Health Administration also referred to as OSHA, whose primary purpose is to assure, regulate, and enforce safe and healthful working conditions in the workplace.

public sanitation the application of measures used to promote public health and prevent the spread of infectious diseases

Right-to-Know Law requires employers to post notices where toxic substances are present in the workplace

safe work practices the maintenance of sanitation standards and the application of safety precautions in the workplace environment

sanitation also referred to as cleaning; the lowest level of decontamination; significantly reduces the number of pathogens found on a surface

solute the substance that is dissolved in a solvent

solution the product created from combining and dissolving a solute in a solvent

solvent the liquid in which a solute is dissolved

standard precautions CDC guidelines and controls that require employers and employees to assume that all human blood and specified human body fluids are infectious for HIV, HBV, and other bloodborne pathogens

sterilization the process of rendering an object germ-free by destroying all living organisms on its surface

ultraviolet-ray sanitizer metal cabinets with ultraviolet lamps or bulbs used to store sanitized tools and implements

wet sanitizer any covered receptacle large enough to permit the immersion of tools and implements into a disinfectant solution

6 Implements, Tools, and Equipment

✓ Learning Objectives

AFTER COMPLETING THIS CHAPTER, YOU SHOULD BE ABLE TO:

1 Identify the principal tools and implements used in the practice of barbering.

2 Identify the parts of shears, clippers, and razors.

3 Demonstrate the correct techniques for holding combs, shears, clippers, and razors.

4 Demonstrate honing and stropping techniques.

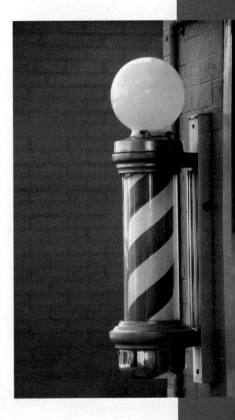

Key Terms

PAGE NUMBER INDICATES WHERE IN THE CHAPTER THE TERM IS USED.

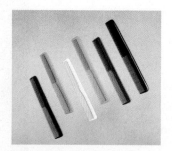

▲ **FIGURE 6-1**

Assorted all-purpose combs.

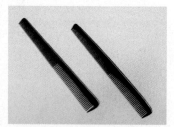

▲ **FIGURE 6-2**

Taper combs.

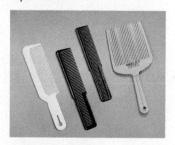

▲ **FIGURE 6-3**

Flat-top combs.

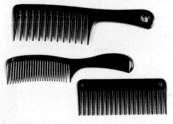

▲ **FIGURE 6-4**

Wide-toothed combs.

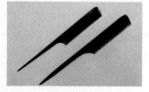

▲ **FIGURE 6-5**

Tail combs.

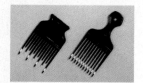

▲ **FIGURE 6-6**

Pick or Afro combs.

All of the instruments and accessories used in the practice of barbering are categorized as the implements, tools, or equipment of the profession. In this chapter, non-motorized items (combs, shears, etc.) are referred to as implements; electrically powered items (clippers, trimmers, etc.) as tools; and anything from barber chairs to steam towel cabinets are considered to be equipment.

Barbers should always use high-quality implements, tools, and equipment. When taken care of properly, well-tempered metal implements and electric tools will provide years of dependable service. Since a myriad of choices is available and can be confusing, ask your instructor or a licensed barber to assist you in making appropriate selections.

Although you will probably use all of the implements and tools associated with barbering at some time or another, the principal "tools of the trade" are combs, brushes, shears, clippers, trimmers, and razors.

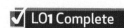 ✓ **LO1 Complete**

Combs

Combs are available in a variety of styles and sizes. The correct comb to use depends on the type of service to be performed and the individual preference of the barber. Combs are usually made of bone, plastic, or hard rubber. Since bone combs can be costly and plastic combs are not as durable as bone or rubber, most barbers prefer combs made of hard rubber.

The teeth of a comb may be fine (close together) or coarse (far apart). Fine-toothed combs may be used for general combing purposes, while wide-toothed combs are preferable for detangling or chemical processing. In either case, it is important that the teeth have rounded ends to avoid scratching or irritating a client's scalp. Some available comb styles are:

- The all-purpose comb, which may be used for general haircutting and styling. A popular size is $7\frac{3}{4}$ inches long (**Figure 6-1**).

- An all-purpose comb with a curved interior assists in lifting subsections and partings of hair while cutting. The usual size is $7\frac{1}{2}$ inches long.

- A **taper comb** is used for cutting or trimming hair in those areas where a gradual blending of the hair is required. The tapered end is especially useful for trimming mustaches, tapering necklines, and blending around the ear areas. Taper combs are available with curved or straight interior sections, as shown in **Figure 6-2**.

- A flat handle comb with evenly spaced teeth works best to achieve a flat-top style (**Figure 6-3**).

- Wide-toothed combs can be used in hairstyle finishing or to spread relaxer creams, detangle the hair, or comb through curly hair textures. They are also available with a curved interior (**Figure 6-4**).

- The tail comb is the best choice for sectioning long hair or when making partings to wrap on perm rods or rollers (**Figure 6-5**).

- The pick or Afro comb is usually the most efficient comb for combing through tight curl patterns or permanent waved hair (**Figure 6-6**).

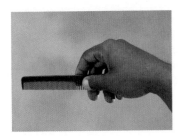

▲ FIGURE 6-7
Proper comb-holding position.

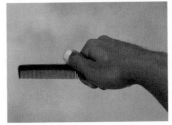

▲ FIGURE 6-8
Improper comb-holding position.

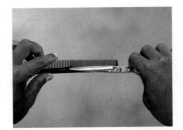

▲ FIGURE 6-9
Proper holding position for shear-over-comb cutting.

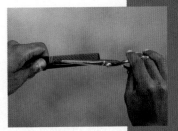

▲ FIGURE 6-10
Improper holding position for shear-over-comb cutting.

HOLDING THE COMB

The correct manner in which to hold the comb will be dictated by the type of comb used, the service being performed, and the dexterity and comfort of the barber. **Figures 6-7** through **6-10** show correct and incorrect holding positions that are often used with an all-purpose comb. Be guided by your instructor and practice, practice, practice!

CARE OF COMBS

To keep combs in good condition, avoid exposing them to excessive or prolonged heat. Combs must be disinfected before and after each client has been served, using the following procedure:

1. Remove loose hairs from the comb.

2. Wash comb thoroughly with hot water and soap or detergent.

3. Rinse thoroughly and pat dry.

4. Place in a wet sanitizer with disinfectant for the recommended disinfection time.

5. Rinse comb, wipe dry, and place in a clean, closed container, dry sanitizer, or an UV-ray electrical sanitizer until needed.

STYLING BRUSHES

Styling brushes are used to smooth, wave, or add fullness to hair or to stimulate the scalp. The choice of bristle texture, spacing, and material will depend on the hairstyle to be achieved. Most hairbrushes are manufactured with plastic, wood, or metal bases and contain either natural or artificial bristles. Some brush styles combine plastic or hard rubber handles with a cushioned rubber base into which either nylon or metal bristles are set. Boar bristle brushes clean the hair by trapping particles and polish the hair by dispersing collected sebum throughout the hair strands. These are excellent brushes for finish work, but should be purchased with a handle material that will stand up to the repeated disinfection procedures required in the barbershop. Brushes are cleaned and disinfected in the same manner as combs. As with other barbering tools and implements, the styling brushes a barber chooses to use are a matter of personal preference (Figure 6-11).

Did **You** Know...

Barbers can simplify their work when cutting hair by using light-colored combs on dark hair and dark-colored combs on light hair. This technique provides greater contrast between the comb and the hair, especially when employing shear-over-comb or clipper-over-comb cutting methods.

▥▥▥STATE

Check your state board regulations concerning the use of fumigants in dry cabinet sanitizers.

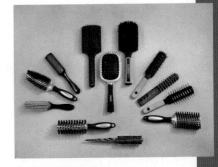

▲ FIGURE 6-11
Assorted styling brushes.

Haircutting Shears

There are two types of shears generally used by barbers: the French style, which has a brace (finger rest) for the little finger, and the German type, which does not include the finger rest. Barbers typically choose the French-style shear with either a cast or screw-in finger rest, and both are now available in ergonomically designed styles (**Figure 6-12**). Haircutting shears with detachable blades have also become very popular because the old or dull blades can be removed and replaced with new ones, thereby eliminating the need to send shears out for sharpening.

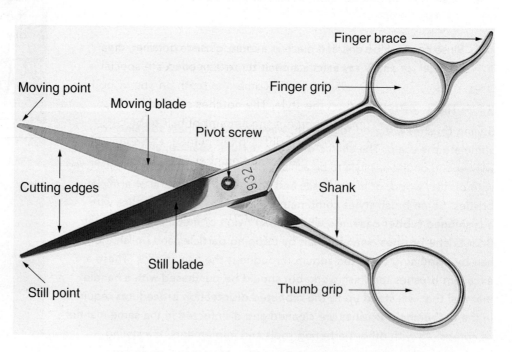

▲ **FIGURE 6-12**

Haircutting shears.

SHEAR CHARACTERISTICS

Haircutting shears are composed of two blades: one movable and the other a stationary or still blade. These blades are fastened with a tension screw that acts as a pivot. The other main parts of the shears are the points, cutting edges, shanks, finger grip, finger rest (tang), and thumb grip (**Figure 6-13**). Most shears are made from tempered stainless steel to ensure hardness and durability.

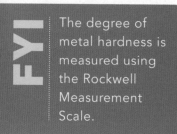

- *Size:* Shears are available in a variety of lengths, measured in inches and half inches. There are two common methods used to measure the size of shears: from the tip (points) to the end of the longest finger grip (Japanese method) or from the tip to the end of the finger rest (German method). It should be noted that a shear measuring 6.5″ using the Japanese method will measure 7″ when the German method of measurement is used. Most barbers prefer the $6\frac{1}{2}$″ to $7\frac{1}{2}$″ shears.

- *Grinds:* The grind refers to the inside construction of the blade and the way it is cut in preparation for sharpening and polishing. The flat grind is traditionally associated with German-style shears, while hollow-ground blades are typically seen in convex shear styles.

▶ **FIGURE 6-13**

Parts of haircutting shears.

Moving point • Moving blade • Pivot screw • Finger brace • Finger grip • Cutting edges • Shank • Still blade • Still point • Thumb grip

- *Blade edges:* The cutting edges of the shears may be beveled, convex, or hybrid in design. A *beveled* edge means there is an angle on the cutting surface (edge) of the blade. Beveled edges can be plain-ground with smooth, polished, or razor-edged surfaces. Beveled shears usually have one plain and one corrugated (serrated) blade (Figure 6-14). The design of the corrugations help to hold the hair in place and prevent it from sliding on the blade while it is being cut. Beveled shears work well for blunt, shear point, and shear-over-comb cutting.

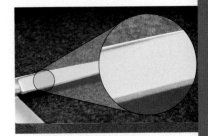

▲ FIGURE 6-14
Corrugated (serrated) shear edge.

The outside of a *convex* blade edge has a clamshell or half-moon shape. This shape is created using hollow grinding and a hone line on the inside of the blade that allows the blade to be rolled over at a rounded, graduated angle to produce extremely sharp edges. Convex blades with sharp angled edges help to facilitate a variety of cutting methods including sliding, slicing, or carving techniques.

Shears that consist of a combination of edges are called *hybrids*. For example, a convex shear may have a beveled edge put on it. Although doing so creates a shear that is no longer truly convex and the benefit of the edge work may be lost, some barbers prefer to utilize this option in blade edge design.

FYI Tempering is the process of heating and cooling metal to ensure hardness and durability.

- *Set:* The **set of the shears** refers to the angle of the blade from its tip to back (ride) and the alignment of the blades in relation to each other. This alignment is just as important as the grind or edges of the blades because even shears with the finest cutting edges will be inferior cutting tools if the blades are not set properly. Tension also affects the set and alignment of the blades and can be adjusted by turning the pivot screw.

THINNING SHEARS

Thinning shears, also called blending, tapering, or texturizing shears, are used to taper hair ends, reduce hair thickness, or create special texturizing effects. These shears have comb-like teeth on one or both shear blades, depending on the style. The notches created by these teeth help to control and portion out the amount of hair to be cut (Figure 6-15). Thinning shears also differ in the number and shape of the teeth along the blade. The greater the number of teeth, the more finely the hair strands can be cut without leaving noticeable cut marks. Recent designs include a wider tooth pattern, with slightly recessed indentations in the notching teeth, to perform alternative texturizing techniques. Thinning shears are also available in a variety of lengths and in detachable blade styles.

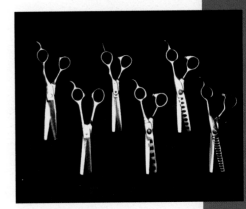

▲ FIGURE 6-15
Thinning or texturizing shears.

HOW TO HOLD HAIRCUTTING SHEARS

When picking up your shears in preparation for use, you will probably complete the following steps simultaneously.

1 Insert the ring finger into the finger grip of the still blade with the little finger resting on the finger brace. To ensure proper balance, brace the index finger on the shank of the still blade, approximately $\frac{1}{2}''$ from the pivot screw.

2 Place the tip of your thumb into the thumb grip of the moving blade. The thumb grip should be positioned halfway between the end of your thumb and the first knuckle. Do not allow the thumb grip to slide below the first knuckle or you will lose control of the cutting blade. See **Figures 6-16a** and **6-16b** for the correct finger placement and holding position of the shears. Incorrect finger placement is shown in **Figure 6-16c**.

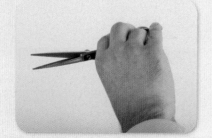

▲ **FIGURE 6-16a**

Barber's view: Correct finger placement and holding position of shears.

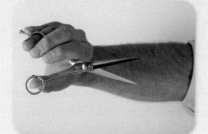

▲ **FIGURE 6-16b**

Front view: Correct finger placement and holding position of shears.

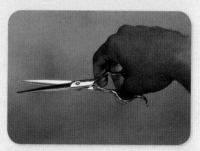

▲ **FIGURE 6-16c**

Incorrect finger placement and holding position of shears.

Palming the Shears and Comb

The shears and comb should be held at all times during a haircut that requires these tools. For safety, shears need to be closed and resting in the palm while combing the hair. This is called "**palming the shears**" and is achieved by slipping the thumb out of the thumb grip and simply pivoting the shear into the palm of the hand (**Figure 6-17**). With practice, palming will become a very natural motion. Thinning or texturizing shears should be held in the same manner as regular haircutting shears.

Once the shears are palmed, the process of combing through the hair is performed with the comb in the same hand as the shears (**Figure 6-18**). After the section of hair has been combed into position for cutting, the comb is

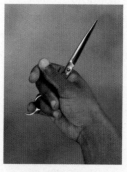

▲ **FIGURE 6-17**

Palming the shears.

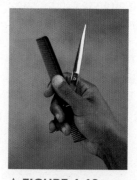

▲ **FIGURE 6-18**

Holding the comb and shears.

transferred to the opposite hand and palmed (Figure 6-19). This allows the first two fingers of that hand to be free to maintain control of the hair and the shear hand free to cut the hair section (Figure 6-20).

CARE OF HAIRCUTTING AND THINNING SHEARS

1. Avoid dropping shears! Even one drop on a hard surface can ruin the set of the shears.

2. Protect shears in a leather sheath or holder when carrying them in a kit, bag, or case.

3. Never cut anything but hair with haircutting shears.

NOTE: Use a less expensive shear on mannequin hair and save your finest tools for models and clients.

4. Do not force shear blades through a section of hair. If there is resistance, section off a thinner parting for cutting.

5. Avoid contact or prolonged immersion with corrosive chemicals, including permanent waving lotions, oxidizers, and certain disinfectants.

6. Check the tension of the shears. Hold the shears horizontally by the thumb grip (moving blade) with the thumb and index finger of the left hand. Raise the finger grip (still blade) to an open position with the thumb and index finger of the right hand. Release the still blade. The still blade should drop $\frac{1}{4}$ to $\frac{1}{2}$ of the way closed before stopping, depending on the quality of the shears. If the blades do not drop at all, the tension is too tight; if they close completely, they are too loose. Adjust a slotted tension screw as follows:

    1. Hold closed shears securely, placing the blades flat on a hard surface.
    2. Use the appropriate size of screwdriver to turn the screw in $\frac{1}{4}$-turn increments, checking the tension after each adjustment.

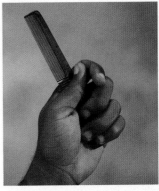

▲ FIGURE 6-19
Palming the comb.

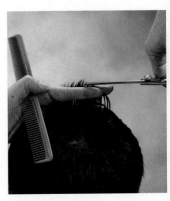

▲ FIGURE 6-20
Correct palming of comb while cutting.

CLEANING HAIRCUTTING AND THINNING SHEARS

Use the following steps to clean shears after each use:

1. Wipe hair from under the tension screw and along the blades with a clean, soft cloth.

2. Wash shears in warm, soapy water and dry thoroughly.

3. Wipe blades with an appropriate disinfectant (follow the manufacturer's cleaning directions and your state barber board regulations).

4. Lubricate according to the manufacturer's recommendations. In most cases, applying shear lubricant or light clipper oil to the pivot screw and the juncture of the blades will maintain smooth blade action. Wipe off excess product along the length of the blades.

5. Store shears in a clean, closed container or ultraviolet sanitizer until needed for use.

> ⟩Did **You** Know...
>
> The term *shears* is used to describe a cutting tool that is longer than 6″ with double-ground edges and two different-sized finger holes. The term *scissors* is used when describing a cutting tool measuring less than 6″.

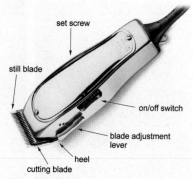

▲ FIGURE 6-21

Visible parts of an electric clipper.

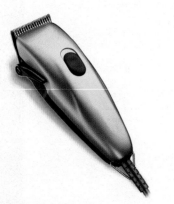

▲ FIGURE 6-22

Rotary (universal) motor clippers.

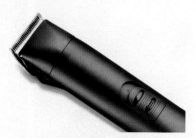

▲ FIGURE 6-23

Pivot motor clippers.

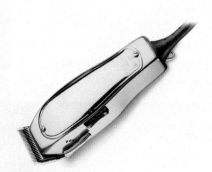

▲ FIGURE 6-24

Magnetic motor clippers.

Clippers and Trimmers

Clippers and trimmers are two of the most important tools used in barbering. **Clippers** can be used for a variety of cutting techniques, from blending to texturizing. Trimmers, also referred to as edgers or outliners, are essential for finish and detail work.

Today's barber has a vast array of clipper styles from which to choose. Function, style, weight, contour, and speed are just some of the factors that should be considered when purchasing a clipper. For example, most clipper models are single speed but there are also two-speed models available. Some clippers utilize a detachable blade system, while others have a single adjustable blade. Clippers with a single cutting head usually have a blade adjustment lever on the side of the unit and rely on clipper guards to vary the length of the hair being cut. Check with your local supplier for different models and styles.

Electric clippers are driven by one of three basic motor types: rotary motors, pivot motors, and magnetic (vibratory) motors. The visible parts of an electric clipper are the cutting blade, still blade, heel, switch, set or power screw, and conducting cord (**Figure 6-21**).

ROTARY MOTOR CLIPPERS

The *rotary motor clipper*, also called the universal motor clipper, is capable of producing a powerful cutting action and is designed for the heavy-duty, continual use that is required in barbershops. These clippers have fewer moving parts and run more quietly than pivot or magnetic motor clippers, and tend to require little maintenance. They can be used for wet or dry haircutting and have detachable cutting heads (clipper blades) that must be changed to achieve various hair lengths. If properly taken care of, these clippers can be used for many years with little or no repair (**Figure 6-22**).

PIVOT MOTOR CLIPPERS

Although the *pivot motor clipper* is not as powerful as the rotary motor clipper, it is twice as powerful as magnetic motor clippers. Pivot motor clippers produce twice the number of blade strokes because the blades are pulled both ways as opposed to the magnetic clipper, which pulls the blade in one direction only. Like rotary motor clippers, pivot motor clippers tend to require little maintenance and can be used for wet or dry haircutting. These clippers have an adjustable blade that is controlled by a lever on the side of the clipper and are usually packaged with an assortment of attachable clipper guards or combs (**Figure 6-23**).

MAGNETIC CLIPPERS

Vibratory or *magnetic clippers* operate by means of an alternating spring and magnet mechanism (**Figure 6-24**). The magnetic motor pulls the blade in one direction and then retracts, using the spring to return the blade. These clippers run faster than the rotary motor type and usually have a single cutting head, which is adjustable for cutting a variety of hair lengths. New balding clipper models are now available with fine-toothed surgical blades for extra-close cutting. Comb attachments (guards) that leave the hair longer than the original cutting head (blades) snap or slide on for easy haircutting versatility.

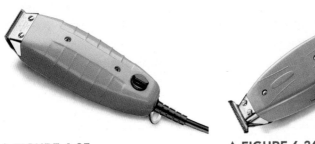

▲ **FIGURE 6-25**

Straight-blade trimmer.

▲ **FIGURE 6-26**

T-shaped blade trimmer.

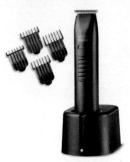

FYI
The position of the clipper blades relative to the skin, and the hair's density and texture, will determine the length of the hair that is left after cutting. Remember that angling the clipper blades toward the scalp or out toward the hair ends will produce different results.

TRIMMERS

A trimmer, also known as an outliner or edger, may utilize a magnetic or pivot motor. **Trimmers** have a very fine cutting head for outlining, arching, and design work. The cutting blade is usually available in two styles: a straight trimmer blade (**Figure 6-25**) and a T-shaped blade (**Figure 6-26**). The versatility and utility of the T-blade when trimming rounded or difficult areas makes it the first choice of many barbers and stylists. The outliner is a very valuable implement for detail, precision design, and fine finish work on haircuts and facial hair trims.

CORDLESS CLIPPERS

A number of manufacturers have produced clippers and outliners that do not require an electric cord. These tools are designed to rest in a special unit that recharges their power. Cordless clippers are a very important innovation for barbers because they are easily maneuverable and portable (**Figure 6-27**).

BLADES AND GUARDS

Clipper **blades** are usually made of high-quality carbon steel and are available in a variety of styles and sizes. Some styles are intended for use with detachable-blade clippers and others serve as replacement blades for certain clipper models. Blade sizes can also differ from one manufacturer to another and may not always indicate the same cutting length, so be careful when purchasing these items. Traditionally, the 0000 blade has produced the closest cut, but today's balding clipper blades may cut closer, depending on the manufacturer. The size $3\frac{1}{2}$ clipper blade leaves the hair approximately $\frac{3}{8}$ inches long. A good rule of thumb is to follow the manufacturer's recommendations for the style and size of clipper blades that are appropriate for their clipper models. Manufacturers are constantly improving their clipper blades to permit faster and more precise haircutting so be on the lookout for the newest in haircutting tools (**Figure 6-28**).

Clipper **guards,** also known as attachment combs, are most often made of plastic or hard rubber and can be used with most clipper models. The purpose of a clipper guard is to allow the hair to be left longer than what

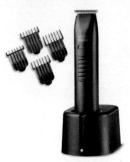

▲ **FIGURE 6-27**

Cordless rechargeable outliner.

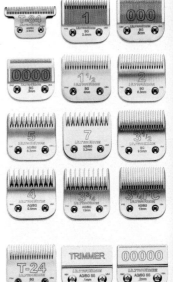
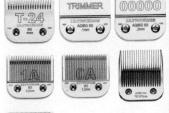

▲ **FIGURE 6-28**

Clipper blades.

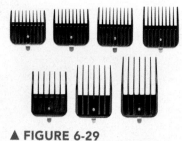

might be achieved from the size of the clipper blades alone. Like clipper blades, guards also help to ensure uniformity within the cut; however, since the guards do not do the actual cutting, they should not be confused with the clipper blades. Instead, guards are simply supplemental implements the barber may choose to use in haircutting services (Figure 6-29).

REMINDER

>> Using clipper guards is not considered a professional barbering technique and is usually not permissible at state board practical exams.

mini PROCEDURE

HOW TO HOLD CLIPPERS

The technique used by a barber to hold the clippers is most often determined by the section of the head he or she is working on. Cutting the back section will necessitate holding the clippers differently than when cutting the top section. A general rule to follow is that the clippers should always be held in a manner that permits freedom of wrist movement. Four methods of holding clippers are explained below, but be guided by your instructor for alternative methods.

1 When a right-handed barber holds the clippers, the thumb is placed on top of the clipper with the fingers supporting it from the underside (Figure 6-30). This position is usually comfortable for tapering in the nape or side areas of a haircut or when the clipper is switched to the left hand while cutting hair sections from a different direction.

2 An alternative method is to place the thumb on the left side of the unit at the switch and the fingers on the right side, with the blades pointing up (Figure 6-31). Like the holding position in Figure 6-30, some may find this a comfortable position for tapering around the hairline.

3 Figures 6-32a and 6-32b show alternative underhand positions that may be used when working haircut sections from side-view and back-view positions.

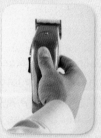

▲ FIGURE 6-30

Clipper-holding position #1.

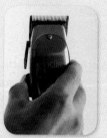

▲ FIGURE 6-31

Clipper-holding position #2.

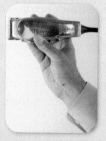

▲ FIGURE 6-32a

Clipper-holding position #3.

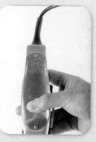

▲ FIGURE 6-32b

Clipper-holding position #4.

CARE OF ELECTRIC CLIPPERS

To take proper care of clippers and trimmers, you will need a clipper brush with stiff bristles, a small container, blade wash, clipper oil, and lubricating or cooling sprays. **CAUTION:** While lubricating sprays may perform well as coolants, they may not contain sufficient oil for thorough lubrication. It is recommended that blades be oiled before, during (as needed), and after each use as important steps in your daily haircutting and clipper-maintenance routine. The following procedures outline some basic clipper-maintenance steps, but always read the manufacturers' directions for specific care of their tools. Your instructor may also guide you in the care of clippers and trimmers.

- *General maintenance before, during, and after haircutting:* Hold the clippers with the blades pointed in a downward position. Use the clipper brush to remove hair particles. Immerse only the teeth of the clipper blades in a shallow container of blade wash and turn the unit on. Run the clippers until all the hair embedded between the blades is removed. Make sure that the clippers remain in a downward position so the blade wash does not accumulate in the motor. Turn the clippers off and wipe off excess blade wash. Again, while maintaining a downward position of the clippers, apply several drops of oil on the front and sides of the blades, then wipe off excess oil with a soft cloth. Remember, even a minimal amount of oil in the motor may reduce the clippers' cutting ability.

- *Rotary motor clippers:* To detach the cutting blade from the still blade, slide the still blade out from under the compression spring. The blades may be washed with hot water, reassembled, and a drop of oil placed in the two holes in the compression plate. Remove the nameplate and check the grease. The grease chamber should be kept about two-thirds full. If the gears should come out, be careful to reassemble them the same way as they were originally. Remove the carbon brush knobs and check the carbon brushes. If they are worn down, replace them with new brushes. Add a few drops of oil weekly to the oiler at the rear of the clippers. Clean the hair from the oil vents surrounding the switch to ensure proper ventilation.

- *Magnetic clippers:* These clippers do not require frequent internal greasing, although one or two drops of oil should be applied routinely between the blades. If vibratory clippers seem to be cutting exceptionally slowly or are pulling the hair, immerse the blades in clipper oil or a prepared clipper cleaner and then turn the clippers on and off. This will clean the blades and oil them at the same time. Clippers may also be immersed in a cleaning solvent followed by a few drops of oil added to the blades.

Properly cared for, electric clippers will last for years. Manufacturer's directions should be followed carefully to assure optimal performance and to maintain the validity of the warranty.

Did You Know...

When using clippers, the amount of hair that remains depends on whether the hair is cut with the grain or against the grain. Generally, cutting against the grain leaves the hair shorter than cutting with the grain.

CAUTION

Never adjust clipper or trimmer blades flush to each other. Doing so can create a cutting edge that can lift the epidermal layers of the skin, causing irritations, abrasions, cuts, and ingrown hairs. Blades should only be set as recommended by the manufacturer. The top or front blade should rest between $\frac{1}{16}$" and $\frac{1}{32}$" below the back blade, depending on the tool. If a client requests a closer cut than what the clipper blade will produce, use balding clippers or a razor to shave the head.

Straight Razors

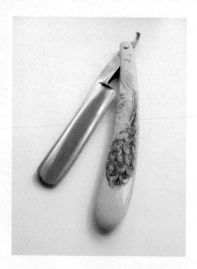

As the sharpest and closest cutting tool, razors are used for facial shaves, neck shaves, finish work around the sideburn and behind-the-ear areas, and haircutting. The razor of choice for professional barbering is the straight razor; safety razors should not be used to render professional services in the barbershop.

There are two types of straight razors typically used in barbering: the **changeable-blade straight razor** and the **conventional straight razor.** Both may be purchased with a razor guard, an attachment that is used in razor-cutting the hair (Chapter 15). The changeable-blade razor generally looks the same as the conventional straight razor and is used in a similar manner. The benefits of using a changeable-blade straight razor are the easy replacement of blades from one client service to another and the maintenance of sanitation standards in the barbershop. The conventional straight razor requires honing and stropping to maintain its cutting edge.

Selecting the right kind of razor is a matter of personal choice. The best guides for buying high-quality razors are as follows:

- Consult with a reliable company representative or salesperson who can recommend the type of razor best suited to your work.

- Consult with more experienced barbers about which razors they have found best for shaving and haircutting.

- Experiment with a variety of razors to determine the most comfortable styles and types for your use.

- Avoid judging a razor simply on color or design. Neither one of these characteristics provides a true indication of the razor's caliber as a cutting tool.

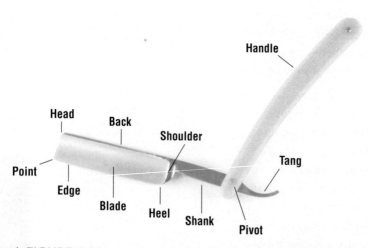

▲ **FIGURE 6-33**

Parts of a razor.

STRUCTURAL PARTS OF A STRAIGHT RAZOR

The structural parts of both conventional and changeable-blade straight razors are the head, back, shoulder, tang, shank, heel, edge, point, blade, pivot, and handle **(Figure 6-33)**.

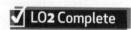

CHANGEABLE-BLADE STRAIGHT RAZORS

The changeable- (or disposable-) blade straight razor closely resembles a conventional straight razor in its overall design. This razor tends to be the most popular because its disposable blade eliminates honing and stropping, saves time, and helps to maintain infection control standards. Additionally, the razor is generally lighter in weight and can be used without the guard for shaving, and with or without the guard for razor haircutting. Blades are available with a square point, rounded point, or a combination, with one end rounded and the other end squared (**Figure 6-34a**).

Razor Shapers

There are a variety of razor shapers (also known as hair shapers) available on the market today. One style is usually made of lightweight stainless steel with a pivot and open-handle construction. Another variety has a stationary handle with a finger rest and stainless steel blade. Razor shapers typically come with a haircutting guard that slides over the exposed blade (**Figure 6-34b**).

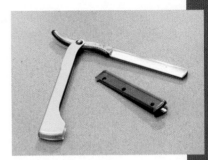

▲ **FIGURE 6-34a**

Changeable-blade razor.

Changing the Blade

Always follow the manufacturer's directions for inserting a new blade or removing an old blade from a changeable-blade razor or razor shaper. Some razor models are designed with a screw mechanism that releases the blade; others require a sliding motion for blade insertion and removal. The following guidelines explain the sliding-motion method of blade replacement for a razor shaper as illustrated in **Figures 6-35** and **6-36**.

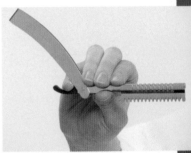

▲ **FIGURE 6-34b**

Razor shaper.

1. Hold razor firmly above the joint of the handle and shank. Use the teeth of the razor guard to catch the blade and push it out of the razor. Always store used blades in a sharps container until ready for hazardous waste disposal (Figure 6-35).

2. To insert a new blade, position the end of the blade into the razor groove. Use the teeth of the razor guard to slide the blade in until it clicks into position (Figure 6-36).

NOTE: Some razor blade packaging is designed to act as a blade dispenser. The razor groove is slid over the top of the blade from the side of the dispenser until the blade is in place.

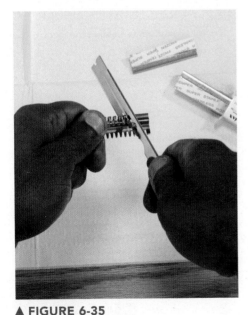

▲ **FIGURE 6-35**

Removing the blade.

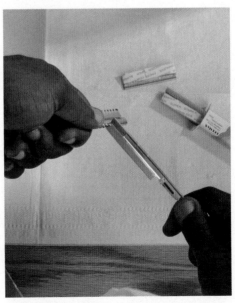

▲ **FIGURE 6-36**

Correct blade insertion.

mini PROCEDURE

HOLDING THE RAZOR

There are several methods of holding the razor, depending on the procedure to be performed. Specific techniques are covered in the shaving and haircutting chapters. Figures 6-37 to 6-39 show two basic methods for holding a razor shaper for haircutting. It is advisable for students to practice and become familiar with the basic holding positions:

1 The ball of the thumb supports the razor at the bottom of the shank between the blade and the pivot. The handle is angled up, allowing the little finger to rest on the tang. The index finger and thumb should rest along the flat side of the shank for control with the two middle fingers resting comfortably along the top of the shank **(Figure 6-37)**.

2 The razor can also be held in a straightened position with the index finger and thumb along the flat side of the shank and the remaining fingers resting around the pivot and handle **(Figure 6-38)**.

3 To palm the razor, curl in the ring finger and little finger around the handle. Hold the comb between the thumb, index, and middle fingers **(Figure 6-39)**.

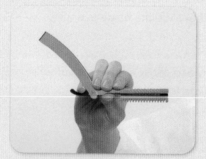

▲ **FIGURE 6-37**

Holding the razor shaper properly.

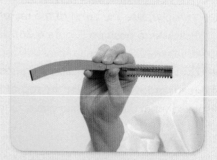

▲ **FIGURE 6-38**

Alternate method of holding the razor shaper.

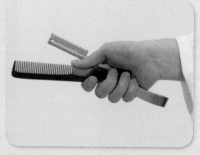

▲ **FIGURE 6-39**

Palming the razor and comb.

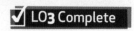
✓ **LO3 Complete**

CONVENTIONAL STRAIGHT RAZORS

The conventional straight razor is composed of a hardened steel blade attached to a handle by means of a pivot. The handle may be constructed of hard rubber, plastic, bone, or new polymer materials, and only the highest-quality conventional straight razors should be used. In order to determine the quality of the razor, the barber must consider the following factors: razor balance, temper, grind, finish, size, and style. In addition, barbers must master the techniques of honing and stropping in order to produce a fine cutting edge (Figure 6-40).

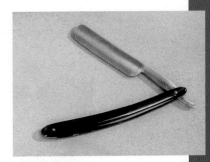

▲ FIGURE 6-40
Conventional straight razor(s).

Straight Razor Balance

Razor balance refers to the weight and length of the blade relative to that of the handle. A straight razor is properly balanced when the weight of the blade and handle are equal. Proper balance of the razor allows for greater ease and safety in handling the razor during shaving. Opening the razor and resting it on the index finger at the pivot will test the balance of the razor. If the head of the razor moves up or down, the razor is not well balanced.

Razor Temper

Tempering the razor involves a special heat treatment included in the manufacturing process. When a razor is properly tempered, it acquires the degree of hardness required for a good cutting edge. Razors can be purchased with a hard, soft, or medium temper. The barber should select the temper that produces the most satisfactory shaving results. While hard-tempered razors will hold an edge longer, they are difficult to sharpen; conversely, soft-tempered razors are easier to sharpen, but the sharp edge does not last long. For those reasons, many barbers prefer a medium-tempered razor.

Razor Grind

The grind of a razor is the shape of the blade after it has been ground. There are two general types: the concave grind and the wedge grind.

- *Concave grind:* The concave grind (often referred to as the hollow ground) is available in full concave, one-half concave, and one-quarter concave forms. The back and edge of the razor looks hollow, being slightly thicker between the hollow part and the extreme edge. Many barbers prefer the hollow-ground razor since the resistance of the beard can be felt more easily and alerts the barber to check the sharpness of the cutting edge. Although the one-half and one-quarter concave grinds are less hollow than the full concave, the outside dimensions of the blade appear the same (Figure 6-41).

- *Wedge grind:* The wedge grind is neither hollow nor concave. Both sides of the blade form a sharp angle at the extreme edge of the razor. Most older razors were made with a wedge grind. Although learning how to sharpen a wedge grind may be a challenge, once mastered, this grind produces an excellent shave. It is especially preferred for men with coarse, heavy beards (Figure 6-41).

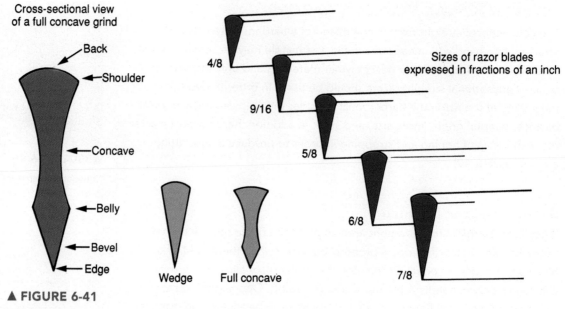

Cross-sectional view of a full concave grind

Back
Shoulder
Concave
Belly
Bevel
Edge

Wedge   Full concave

Sizes of razor blades expressed in fractions of an inch

4/8
9/16
5/8
6/8
7/8

▲ FIGURE 6-41

Razor grinds.

Razor Finish

The finish of a razor is the polish of its surface. This finish may be plain, crocus (polished steel), or plated with nickel or silver. Of these types, the crocus finish is usually the choice of the discriminating barber. Although the crocus finish is more costly, it lasts longer and does not rust as easily as other finishes. Metal-plated razors are undesirable because the finish wears off quickly and may hide poor-quality steel.

Razor Sizes

The size of the razor is measured by the length and width of the blade. The width of the razor is measured either in eighths or sixteenths of an inch, such as $\frac{4}{8}$, $\frac{5}{8}$, $\frac{6}{8}$, $\frac{7}{8}$ and $\frac{9}{16}$. Two of the most common sizes are the $\frac{5}{8}''$ and $\frac{9}{16}''$, with the $\frac{5}{8}''$ being the more popular.

Razor Styles

The style of a razor indicates its shape and design. Modern razors have such features as a back and edge that are straight and parallel to each other; a round heel; a square point; and a flat or slightly round handle. To avoid scratching the skin, the barber usually rounds off the square point of the razor slightly by drawing the point of the razor along the edge of the hone.

Razor Care

Razors will maintain their quality if care is taken to prevent corrosion of the extremely fine edge. After use, a razor should be cleaned, stropped, and a little oil applied to the cutting edge. Be careful not to drop the razor as doing so may damage the blade. When closing the razor, be careful that the cutting edge does not strike the handle. If the cutting edge strikes the handle when closing the razor, it may indicate that the handle is warped or that the pivot is too tightly riveted. The barber's tool kit should include several high-grade razors so that a damaged razor can be replaced immediately.

CONVENTIONAL STRAIGHT RAZOR ACCESSORIES

There are two vital accessories used with conventional straight razors: the hone and the strop. A **hone** is an abrasive material that has the ability to cut steel. It is used to grind the steel and impart an effective cutting edge to the razor's blade (**Figure 6-42**). A **strop** is a leather and canvas accessory that is used to smooth and align the cutting teeth of the razor edge and polish the blade (**Figure 6-43**).

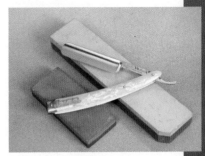

▲ **FIGURE 6-42**

Hones with conventional straight razor.

Hones

There are various types of hones available for the purpose of sharpening razors. Hones are usually manufactured in a rectangular block shape for ease of blade placement on the surface. Since the abrasive material of the hone is harder than steel, it will cut or file the edge on the blade of the razor.

The final choice of hone is based on personal preference. Generally, any type of hone is satisfactory, provided it is used properly and is capable of producing a sharp cutting edge on the razor. Students usually practice with a slow-cutting hone, while experienced practitioners generally prefer a faster-cutting hone. In selecting a hone, remember that the finer the abrasive, the slower its action. There are three main types of hones: natural, synthetic, and combination.

Natural hones are derived from natural rock deposits. Water or shaving lather is usually applied before use to facilitate movement of the razor's blade over the hone surface.

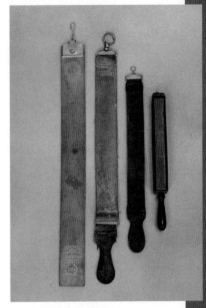

▲ **FIGURE 6-43**

Strops.

The *water hone* is a natural hone cut out of rock formations, usually imported from Germany. Accompanying the water hone is a small piece of slate of the same texture, called the rubber. When the rubber is applied over the hone, which is moistened with water, a proper cutting surface is created.

The water hone is primarily a slow-cutting hone. When used as directed by the manufacturer, a smooth and lasting edge will result. It is gray or brown in color. Of the two colors, the brown water hone is considered to be slightly superior and also exerts a slightly faster cutting action. When honing, care should be taken not to work a bevel into the hone.

The *Belgian hone* is a natural hone cut from rock formations found in Belgium. It is a slow-cutting hone, but a little faster than the water hone, and can create a very sharp edge. Lather is generally applied to the hone to facilitate movement of the razor.

One type of Belgian hone consists of a light yellowish rock top glued on to the back of dark red slate. Its principal advantage is that it yields a keen cutting edge on the razor and can be used either wet or dry.

Synthetic hones, such as the Swaty hone and the carborundum (car-bo-run-dum) hone, are manufactured products. These hones may be used dry or lather may be applied before use. Because they cut faster than water hones, synthetic hones have the advantage of producing a keen cutting edge in less time. The carborundum hone is available in a range of types from slow-cutting to fast-cutting. Many practitioners prefer the fast-cutting type because of its quick sharpening action, although care needs to be taken to avoid producing rough edges.

Combination hones consist of both a water hone and a synthetic hone. The synthetic side is a dark brown and is used first to develop a good cutting edge. To give the razor a finished edge, it is stroked over the side of the water hone.

Choosing a Hone

As with all the other barbering tools and implements, the type of hone used is a matter of personal choice. Most barbers use carborundum or combination hones; however, it is advisable to be familiar with the other types of hones and to understand the benefits of each.

The type of steel in a razor also makes some difference as to whether a good edge can be obtained with a particular type of hone. There are many other hones available in addition to the ones described that will give very satisfactory results. Be guided by your instructor and personal experimentation with different hones.

Care of Hones

Always clean the hone before use. Use water and a pumice stone to remove the tiny steel particles that accumulate on the surface of the hone. If a new hone is very rough, the same method can be used to work it into shape.

When wet honing is done, always wipe the hone dry after use. This aids the cleaning process and also wipes away the particles of steel that adhere to the cutting surface. Disinfect according to manufacturer's directions.

Strops

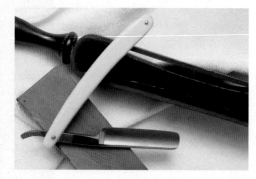

Unlike hones, which are designed to grind the edge of a razor into a sharp cutting edge, strops are used to remove small metal particles from the blade, smooth the edge, and polish the razor. A good strop is made of durable and flexible material, has the proper thickness and texture, and shows a smooth, finished surface. Some barbers like a thin strop; others prefer a thick, heavy strop.

Most strops are made with two layers of material: one side of leather and the other side of canvas (see Figure 6-43). The leather side is made from cowhide, horsehide, or synthetic materials. Depending upon the material used and the style of construction, strops are categorized as follows: French or German, canvas, cowhide, horsehide, and imitation leather. The finer-quality strops are usually "broken in" by the manufacturer and require less breaking in by the barber.

The *French* or *German strop* is a combination strop with leather on one side and a finishing strop on the other. It is used by many barbers for styling razors and provides an all-in-one razor accessory.

The *canvas strop* is made of high-quality linen or silk, woven into a fine or coarse texture. A fine-textured linen strop is most desirable for putting a lasting edge on a razor. To obtain the best results, a new canvas strop should be thoroughly broken in. A daily hand-finish treatment will keep the strop's surface smooth and in readiness for stropping. A canvas strop should be given the following treatment:

1. Attach the swivel end of the strop to a fixed point, such as a nail. (Most of the older barber chairs and some of the newer models have a metal loop attached to the arm of the chair for the purpose of stopping.)

2. Hold the other end tightly over a smooth and level surface.

3. Rub a bar of dry soap over the strop, working it well into the grain of the canvas.

4. Rub a smooth glass bottle over the strop several times, each time forcing the soap into the grain and also removing any excess soap.

The *cowhide strop* was originally imported from Russia. To this day it still bears the name **Russian strop**, even though it may be manufactured in the United States. This name usually implies that the strop is made of cowhide and that the Russian method of tanning was employed. The cowhide or Russian strop is considered to be one of the best. When new, it requires a daily hand finish until it is thoroughly broken in. There are several ways to break in a Russian strop. A method frequently used is as follows:

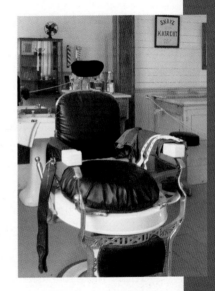

1. Rub dry pumice stone over the strop in order to remove the outer nap and develop a smooth surface.

2. Rub stiff lather into the strop.

3. Rub dry pumice stone over the strop until smooth.

4. Clean off the strop.

5. Rub fresh, stiff lather into the strop.

6. Rub a smooth glass bottle over the strop several times until a smooth surface is developed.

Another method to break in a Russian strop omits the pumice stone. Instead, stiff lather is rubbed into the strop with the aid of a smooth glass bottle or with the palm of the hand.

Horsehide strops are divided into two main groups: the ordinary horsehide strop and the shell strop.

- An ordinary horsehide strop is of medium grade, has a fine grain, and tends to be very smooth. In this condition it does not readily impart the proper edge to a razor. For this reason, it is not recommended for professional use. However, it is suitable for private use.

- The second type of horsehide strop is called a shell or Russian **shell strop**. This is a high-quality strop taken from the muscular rump area of a horse. Although it is quite expensive, it makes one of the best strops for barbers and stylists. It tends to remain smooth and requires very little, if any, breaking in.

The *imitation leather strop* has not proven very satisfactory for use in the barbershop. Because of the availability of high-quality strops, it is wise to avoid strops made of imitation leather.

Strop Dressing

Strop dressing cleans the leather strop, preserves its finish, and also improves its draw and sharpening qualities. For proper use, apply a very small amount of dressing to the leather strop. Rub it into the pores well and remove any surplus. Always wait at least 24 hours between applications.

Honing and Stropping Procedures

Honing (hone-ing) is the process of sharpening a blade on a hone; the primary purpose is to obtain a perfect cutting edge on the razor. The blade is sharpened by honing the razor with smooth, even strokes of equal number and pressure on both sides of the blade. In addition, the angle at which the blade is stroked must be the same for both of its sides. Student barbers should use an old, damaged razor for practicing the honing process.

mini PROCEDURE

HONING THE RAZOR

1 The first step in honing is to practice holding the hone firmly in a perfectly flat position in the hand (see Figure 6-44).

2 Next, practice rolling the razor against the hone with no pressure. Use the thumb and index finger to turn the razor from one side to another without turning the wrist. Practice this rolling motion against the hone with no pressure until it is mastered. This will help to keep the razor in good condition and to maintain the equal pressure required in the honing process.

3 Prepare the hone. Both the razor and the hone should be kept at room temperature. Depending on the type of hone used, it may need to be moistened with water or lather, or kept dry. Be guided by the manufacturer's directions and your instructor.

4 Position the hone by placing it firmly and flatly in the palm of the hand or by laying it on a hard, smooth surface. **CAUTION:** Make sure that the fingertips do not project above the hone to avoid cutting them; allow for sufficient space to permit freedom of movement in a safe manner (Figure 6-44).

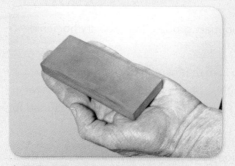

▲ **FIGURE 6-44**
Hold the hone firmly and flat.

(Continued)

5 Grasp the razor handle comfortably in the right hand as follows:

a Rest the index finger on top of the side part of the shank.

b Rest the ball of the thumb at the joint.

c Place the second finger at the back of the razor near the edge of the shank.

d Fold the remaining fingers around the handle to permit easy turning of the razor.

FYI Position the index finger along the top of the shank to ensure even pressure against the blade while honing.

6 *First position and stroke:* Place the razor on its back on the upper far left corner of the hone. Roll the razor, using the thumb and index finger to position the blade edge flat against the hone and facing toward you. The blade must be stroked diagonally across the hone from heel to point as shown in **Figures 6-45a** and **6-45b**. Turn the razor on its back and slide it toward the bottom left corner of the hone to position it for the second position and stroke (**Figure 6-45c**).

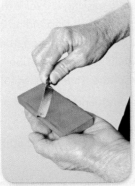

▲ **FIGURE 6-45a**

Begin at upper left corner of the hone.

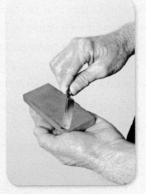

▲ **FIGURE 6-45b**

Draw blade diagonally to lower right corner of hone.

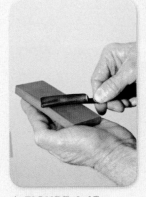

▲ **FIGURE 6-45c**

Use a rolling motion to turn the razor on its back for second stoke.

7 *Second position and stroke:* Finish the turn of the razor so the blade edge is flat against the hone and facing away from you. Stroke the blade diagonally toward the upper right corner of the hone (**Figures 6-46a** and **6-46b**). Turn the razor on its back, slide it toward the upper left corner of the hone, and roll it into position it for the next stroke (**Figure 6-46c**).

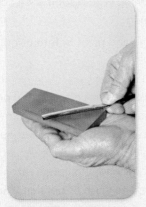

▲ **FIGURE 6-46a**

Begin at lower left corner of the hone.

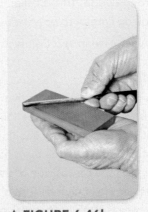

▲ **FIGURE 6-46b**

Stroke blade diagonally to upper right corner of hone.

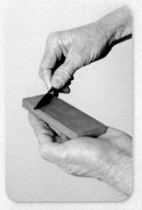

▲ **FIGURE 6-46c**

Roll razor to position for next stroke.

8 Repeat the strokes in a slow and rhythmic manner with equal pressure. If the razor is very dull, firm pressure may be used during the first honing strokes followed by a decrease in the pressure as the razor takes an edge.

Some general guidelines to remember when honing a razor are as follows:

1. The razor is stroked *edge-first* diagonally across the hone. This produces teeth with a cutting edge.

2. The blade should be kept flat on the hone with no rocking or lifting off from the hone.

3. The razor must be stroked with equal pressure from heel to point and from side to side.

4. An equal number of strokes should be made on both sides of the blade.

5. When honing, try to maintain four distinct movements, rather than a sweeping movement.

6. As the blade edge is sharpened, gradually lighten the pressure and test frequently.

7. The number of strokes required in honing depends on the condition of the razor's edge.

8. A honed razor may be tested by lightly passing it over a thumbnail moistened with water or lather (Figure 6-47). Depending on the hardness of the hone and the number of strokes taken, the razor edge may be keen, blunt, coarse, or rough. Different sensations are felt when the razor is passed lightly across the thumbnail as follows:

   - A perfect or keen edge has fine teeth and tends to dig into the nail with a smooth, steady grip.

   - A blunt or dull razor edge passes over the nail smoothly without any cutting power.

   - A coarse razor edge digs into the nail with a jerky feeling.

   - A rough (coarse) or over-honed edge has large teeth that stick to the nail and produce a harsh, grating sound.

   - A nick in the razor produces the feeling of a slight gap or unevenness when drawn across the nail.

9. To correct an over-honed edge, draw the razor backward in a diagonal line across the hone, using the same movement and pressure as in regular honing. One or two strokes each way will usually remove the rough edge. This is called *back honing*. The razor is then honed again, being careful to prevent over-honing.

10. Always clean and disinfect the hone and razor before using.

Stropping The Razor

Stropping a razor is a fine art that is developed through repeated practice. Its aim is to smooth and shape the razor into a keen cutting implement. A conventional straight razor should never be used for shaving without first being stropped. Once the razor has been properly honed, it should not need stropping on the canvas side of the strop. Instead, the honed razor is stropped directly over the leather surface of the strop to finish or polish it. The time to use the canvas strop is when the razor has developed a smooth edge from continued use and requires the mild honing effect of the canvas.

The strop is usually attached to the arm of the barber chair by a closed clip. This allows the barber to maintain a firm, taut grip without the strop accidentally coming off during the stropping process.

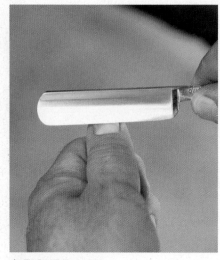

▲ FIGURE 6-47

Testing a honed razor.

Did **You** Know...

The direction of the razor's edge used in stropping is the reverse of the direction used in honing.

FYI Stropping may also be performed from the chair to the hand. Be guided by your state barber board rules and instructor.

STROPPING THE RAZOR

From a technical standpoint, the razor may be stropped from the barber's hand toward the chair or from the chair to the hand. When performed correctly, both methods will achieve the same results; however, some instructors recommend that students begin from the hand to chair for safety reasons. The stropping method used may also depend on the barber board regulations in your state and the performance requirements for state board exams. Be guided by your instructor when practicing the following stropping procedures.

1 Hold the end of the strop firmly in the left hand so it cannot sag. Hold it on a slight diagonal from the chair and as high as is comfortable. Grasp the razor firmly in the right hand so that the index finger is on the shank, the subsequent fingers are on the handle, and the thumb rests lightly on both parts. The index finger of the right hand should rest at the edge of the strop.

2 Position of the razor. The direction of the blade edge in stropping is the reverse of that used in honing. When stropping the razor, the back of the razor will lead, rather than the blade edge.

3 Practice turning the razor. Place the razor on the strop and turn it with the index finger and thumb. Practice the turning action until it is mastered.

4 *First stroke:* Start the stroke at the top edge of the strop closest to the hand. Using a long, diagonal stroke with even pressure from the heel to the point, draw the razor perfectly flat, with back leading, straight over the surface. Bear down just heavily enough to feel the razor draw. Do not worry about speed; a moderate speed between fast and slow is preferred and will occur with practice **(Figure 6-48)**.

5 *Second stroke:* When the first stroke is completed, turn the razor on the back of the blade by rolling it between the fingers without turning the hand **(Figure 6-49)**. Draw the razor away from the chair toward you to complete the second stroke **(Figure 6-50)**. Repeat strokes about 20 times or as necessary.

6 Make a final test of the razor prior to shaving on the moistened tip of the thumb. **CAUTION:** This testing technique requires a great deal of practice and experience. Be very cautious of the amount of pressure and speed with which the test is performed. Touch the razor's edge lightly, and note the reaction. A dull edge does not produce a drawing sensation. A proper cutting edge will have a sharp drawing sensation. If the razor's edge yields a smooth feeling upon testing, finish it again on the canvas strop, followed by a few more strokes on the leather strop.

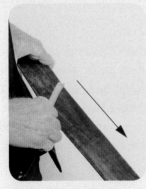

▲ FIGURE 6-48

Placement of hand and razor on strop. Stroke toward chair.

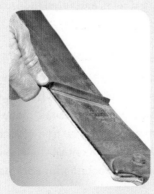

▲ FIGURE 6-49

Roll razor for second stroke.

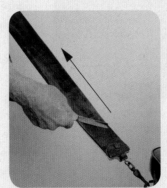

▲ FIGURE 6-50

Begin second stroke. Stroke toward hand.

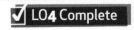
✓ LO4 Complete

Additional Barbering Implements, Tools, and Equipment

In addition to shears, clippers, combs, razors, hones, and strops, there are a number of other items that are traditionally found in the barbershop. Review the following descriptions to become familiar with these implements, tools, and equipment that you may use in the practice of barbering.

LATHER RECEPTACLES

Lather receptacles are containers used to hold or dispense lather for shaving. The most basic and commonly used types are the electric latherizer, the press-button can latherizer, and the lather mug with paper lining (Figure 6-51).

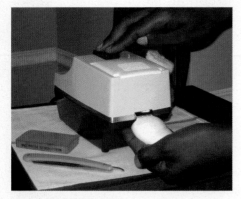

▲ **FIGURE 6-51**
The electric latherizer is far superior to other lather receptacles.

Electric latherizers are lather-making devices that are far superior to the lather mug. These appliances are sanitary, convenient, and easy to operate. The clean and preheated lather coming from these modern machines impresses most clients favorably. For satisfactory performance, follow the manufacturer's instructions on their proper use and care.

NOTE: The electric latherizer is employed to such an extent that other methods are seldom used in today's barbershops.

Press-button can latherizers are convenient and sanitary, but they are not as professional as electric latherizers.

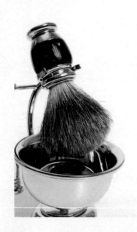

Lather mugs are receptacles made out of glass, earthenware, rubber, or metal. When the lather mug is used, shaving soap and warm water are mixed thoroughly with the aid of a lather brush. Since the lather mug is exposed and collects dirt easily, it requires thorough cleansing and disinfection after each client. To maintain sanitary conditions, a clean lather brush and paper lining should be used with the lather mug for each client. Check your state barber board rules and regulations concerning the use of lather mugs and brushes.

> **REMINDER**
>
> ▶ ▶ ▶ Check your state barber board rules and regulations concerning the use and disinfection of lather mugs and brushes.

Lather brushes are used to apply the soap lather used to soften the beard. Most barbers favor the number 3 size of lather brush. The vulcanized type is the most durable, since its bristles will not fall apart in hot water. To guard against contaminated brushes, many states have laws requiring that brushes made from animal hair be free of anthrax germs at the time of purchase. These brushes must contain the imprint "Sterilized." Lather brushes must be cleaned and disinfected after each use.

Shaving soaps can be purchased in various forms and shapes. These soaps usually contain animal and vegetable oils, alkaline substances, and water. The presence of coconut oil improves the lathering qualities of the shaving soap, which helps to keep the hair erect while the alkalinity of the soap softens the hair for shaving.

Hard shaving soaps include those sold in cake, stick, or powdered form and are similar in composition to toilet soaps. Soft soap is available as shaving cream in a tube, jar, or press-button container, and a liquid cream soap is used in electric latherizers.

HAIR REMOVAL METHODS

Hair removal methods have changed over the years. The neck duster, once a traditional implement in barbershops, is no longer considered a safe and sanitary option for hair removal unless disinfected after each use. Since a number of states have forbidden the use of hair dusters, other methods are now used to remove loose hair. Some methods that are in compliance with state and local health codes include the following:

- A paper or cloth towel folded around the barber's hand and used to dust off loose hair

- Paper neck strips; these may not facilitate a thorough enough dusting

- Small electric hand vacuums and air hoses

NOTE: The electric hair vacuum provides quick clean-up service after a haircut. It can remove hair clippings and loose dandruff, and is particularly suitable for going over the forehead and around the neck and ears. Be sure to clean the nozzle applicator after each use and empty the container as hair accumulates within it.

BLOW-DRYERS

Blow-dryers are designed for drying and styling hair in a single operation. Standard parts include a handle, air-directional nozzle, small fan, heating element, and controls. Comb, brush, and air diffuser attachments may also be available on some models. The blow-dryer produces a steady stream of temperature-controlled air at various speeds. The controls permit the barber to make heat and air-speed adjustments while operating the dryer. Some blow-dryers offer an automatic cool-down feature. In addition to the particular features of the unit, always check the warranty and service agreements when purchasing a blow-dryer (**Figures 6-52a** and **6-52b**).

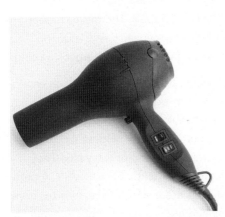

▲ **FIGURE 6-52a**

Blow-dryer.

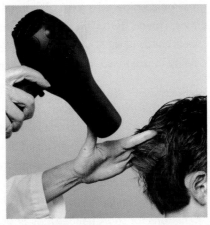

▲ **FIGURE 6-52b**

Holding a blow dryer.

HOW TO HOLD THE BLOW-DRYER

The blow-dryer should be balanced and fit the barber's hand comfortably. The dryer is usually held just above the area being dried, with the nozzle pointing downward at an angle as the hair is dried from the scalp to the ends. Free-style drying can be performed by moving the dryer back and forth sideways, allowing the hair to fall naturally into place; see Chapter 15.

BLOW-DRYER SAFETY

To ensure the safety of the barber and the client, the following precautions should be observed:

1 Apply a protective setting or blow-drying agent to the hair to shield it from the heat of the dryer.

2 Check the comb teeth and brush bristles on attachments for sharp points.

3 Test the temperature controls.

4 Keep the air and the hair moving to prevent burns. Do not concentrate dryer heat too close to the scalp.

5 Follow the styling brush or comb with the blow-dryer, working in the direction of the desired style, blowing damp hair onto dry hair.

6 Avoid dropping the dryer.

7 Never use the dryer near water.

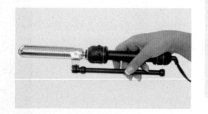

▲ **FIGURE 6-53a**

Electric thermal iron.

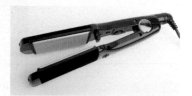

▲ **FIGURE 6-53b**

Electric flat iron.

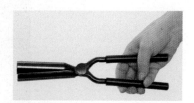

▲ **FIGURE 6-54**

Conventional (Marcel) iron.

THERMAL STYLING TOOLS

Thermal styling tools use heat to wave or curl straight hair or to press curly hair into a straightened form. Any form of styling with a heated tool or appliance may be considered a form of thermal styling. This includes the use of Marcel irons, stoves, hot rollers, flat irons, and other heated tools. Thermal hairstyling tools are used most often in women's and African American hairstyling. The ability to use these tools correctly is an important aspect of the barber's training.

Thermal irons are available in a variety of styles, sizes, and weights, with small to large barrel diameters, and may be electric or require heating on a stove. Electric thermal irons are available with or without a vaporizing action feature and can be purchased with a stationary or rotating handle (**Figure 6-53a**). Electric flat irons are used to temporarily straighten curly or wavy hair. They can also be used to give direction to straighter hair texture styles while imparting a glossy, finished look to the hair. Flat irons are available in many sizes from mini-irons for short hair lengths or tight styling areas to larger irons suitable for long hair styling (**Figure 6-53b**). The *conventional (Marcel) iron* requires the use of a stove to heat it (**Figure 6-54**).

Pressing combs also require the use of the stove and are used for straightening or pressing hair. Electric pressing combs are also available. Both types of combs are constructed in high-quality steel or brass.

The *electric stove* heats conventional irons and metal pressing combs. Stoves become very hot and must be handled carefully (**Figure 6-55**).

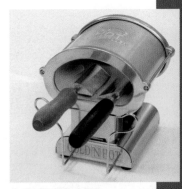

▲ **FIGURE 6-55**
Electric heater for pressing combs and conventional irons.

mini PROCEDURE

HOLDING MARCEL IRONS

Hold the iron in a comfortable position that gives you complete control.

1 Grasp the handles with the right hand, far enough away from the joint to avoid the heat.

2 Place the three middle fingers on the back of the lower handle, the little finger in front of the lower handle, and the thumb in front of the upper handle. Using only the fingers, practice rolling the iron forward and backward.

3 Next, practice opening and closing the iron while performing the rolling motion.

4 When you are comfortable with steps 1 and 2, practice the techniques on a mannequin (**Figure 6-56**). See Chapter 17.

TESTING THERMAL IRONS

After heating the irons to the desired temperature, test them on a piece of tissue paper. Clamp the heated irons over the tissue and hold for 5 seconds. If the paper scorches or turns brown, the irons are too hot. Let them cool before using. Remember that fine, lightened, or badly damaged hair withstands less heat than normal hair (**Figure 6-57**).

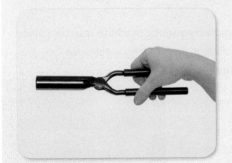

▲ **FIGURE 6-56**
Rolling the iron.

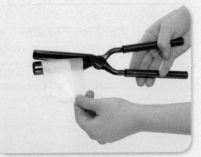

▲ **FIGURE 6-57**
Testing the heat of thermal irons.

(Continued)

Care of Thermal Irons

Thermal irons should be kept clean and free from rust and carbon. To remove dirt or grease, wash the irons in a soap solution containing a few drops of ammonia. This cuts the oil and grease that usually adhere to the irons. Fine sandpaper, or steel wool with a little oil, helps to remove rust and carbon. It also polishes the irons. To permit greater facility in movement, oil the joint of the irons.

Safety Precautions

● Use thermal irons only after receiving instruction on their use.

● Keep irons clean.

● Always test the temperature of the iron before using it on a client.

● Do not overheat irons.

● Handle and remove heated irons and stoves carefully.

● Do not place heated stoves near the station mirror as the heat can cause breakage.

● Place a hard rubber comb between the client's scalp and the iron. Never use a metal comb.

● Place heated stoves and irons in a safe place to cool.

FYI

New thermal irons are tempered at the factory in order to hold heat uniformly. If the irons are overheated, the temper of the steel can be compromised and ruined.

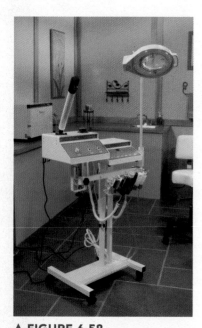

▲ **FIGURE 6-58**

"Five-in-one" machine, including galvanic electrodes.

OTHER EQUIPMENT

Some additional appliances and implements that may be used in the barbering profession are as follows.

- *Galvanic machine:* This is an apparatus with attachments designed to produce galvanic current. The main function of the galvanic machine is to introduce water-soluble products into the skin during a facial (**Figure 6-58**). See Chapter 13.

- *High-frequency machine:* A **high-frequency machine** uses electricity to produce a high rate of oscillation within glass electrodes that are used in facial and scalp treatments (**Figure 6-59**). See Chapters 11 and 12.

- *Hot-towel cabinet:* The hot-towel or steam-towel cabinet is the ideal method for maintaining a ready supply of warm towels for barbering services. Warm towels will be used during facials and shaves, but they are also appreciated during a manicure or scalp treatment or after a neck shave (**Figure 6-60**).

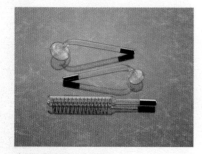

▲ **FIGURE 6-59**

Electrodes for high-frequency machine.

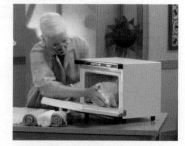

▲ **FIGURE 6-60**

A hot towel cabinet provides a good suppy of warm towels.

- *Comedone extractor:* The **comedone extractor** is a metallic implement with a screwed attachment at each end. A fine needle point or lancet is situated at one end and the opposite end has a blunt prong with a hole in the center that is used to press out blackheads (**Figure 6-61**).

- *Tweezer:* A tweezer is a metallic implement with two blunt prongs at one end that is used to pluck unsightly or ingrown hair. To remove a hair, pull it in the same direction in which it grows. For added comfort, the area can be pre-steamed to open the hair follicle for easier extraction.

- *Electric massager:* The massager (vibrator) is an electric appliance used in facial, scalp, and shoulder massage services (**Figure 6-62**).

- *Hydraulic chair:* The hydraulic barber chair is an essential fixture for rendering services to clients. It can be easily adjusted in both height and position. Generally, such chairs are spaced about 6 feet apart from center to center. For effective operation, follow the manufacturer's instructions at all times and use the guidelines listed below (**Figure 6-63**).

To use the chair properly:

▶ Lower and lock the chair before a client gets in or out of it.

▶ Rotate the chair to the proper position and lock it.

▶ Operate the chair's hand pump in a skillful and quiet way.

▶ Always lock the chair after repositioning during a service.

▶ Press the release when removing or adjusting the headrest.

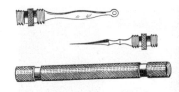

▲ **FIGURE 6-61**

Comedone extractor.

⬛STATE

Be guided by your state barber board rules and regulations regarding the use of comedone extractors.

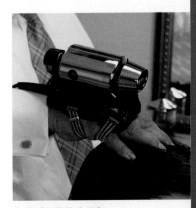

▲ **FIGURE 6-62**

Electric scalp massager.

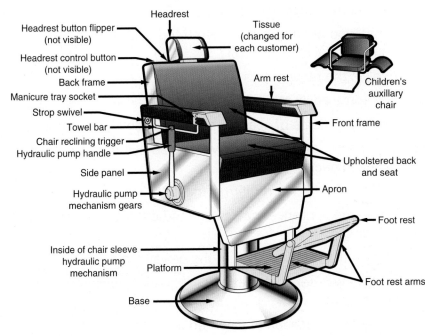

▲ **FIGURE 6-63**

Hydraulic chair.

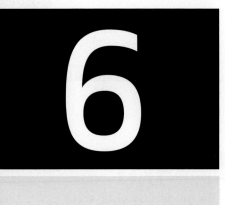

6 Review Questions

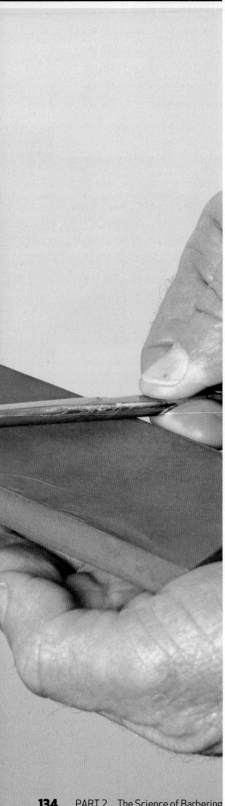

1. List the principal tools and implements used in barbering.
2. What style of comb is generally used for haircutting?
3. Name three services in which tapering combs may be used.
4. Identify the parts of haircutting shears.
5. What is the difference between German and French shears?
6. How are the lengths of shears usually measured? Which sizes are used most often?
7. Identify the two main types of shear grinds.
8. What are thinning shears used for?
9. List three types of clipper motors.
10. List the visible parts of electric clippers.
11. Identify two size clipper blades that produce the shortest cut.
12. Name two types of straight razors.
13. List the 11 parts of a razor.
14. Explain the purpose of a hone.
15. List three types of hones.
16. Explain the movements used in honing.
17. Explain the purpose of a strop.
18. What type of strop is considered the best for stropping a conventional straight razor?
19. Explain the movements used in stropping.
20. List some advantages of using an electric latherizer.
21. Identify the type of soap that is used in an electric latherizer.
22. List three methods of removing loose hair from the client's face and neck.
23. What does the word *thermal* mean?
24. Name the appliance that is used to heat thermal irons and pressing combs.
25. Explain the main function of the galvanic machine.
26. Identify two services that high-frequency machines might be used for.
27. What is the function of a comedone extractor?
28. What is the best type of chair for performing barbering services?

Chapter
Glossary

blades the cutting parts of the clippers, usually manufactured from high-quality carbon steel and available in a variety of styles and sizes

changeable-blade straight razor a type of straight razor that uses changeable, disposable blades

clippers electric haircutting tools with a single adjustable blade or detachable blade system; used in freehand or clipper-over-comb cutting to shape, blend, or taper the hair

comedone extractor an implement used to extract blackheads

conventional straight razor a razor made of a hardened steel blade that requires honing and stropping to produce a cutting edge

guards plastic or hard rubber comb attachments that fit over clipper blades to minimize the amount of hair being cut with the clippers; or metal shields applied over a haircutting razor for protection

high-frequency machine a machine that produces a high rate of oscillation or Tesla current for the purpose of stimulating scalp, facial, and body tissues

hone a sharpening block manufactured from rock or synthetic materials and used to create a cutting edge on conventional straight razors

palming the comb the technique used to hold the comb in the hand opposite of the hand that is cutting with the shears; should allow for holding and controlling the hair to be cut between the first and second fingers of the same hand

palming the shears the technique used to hold shears in a safe manner while combing through or otherwise working with hair

Russian strop a type of cowhide strop that is considered to be one of the best and that requires "breaking in"

set of the shears the manner in which the blades and shanks of the shears align with each other and are joined at the tension screw or rivet

shell strop a type of horsehide strop made from the muscular rump area of the horse and considered to be the best strop for use by barbers

strop an elongated piece of leather or other materials used to finish the edge of conventional straight razors to a smooth, whetted cutting edge

taper comb used for cutting or trimming hair when a gradual blending from short to longer is required within the haircut

thermal styling tools used to denote types of tools that use heat for the purpose of hairstyling.

thinning shears also known as serrated or texturizing shears; used to remove excess bulk from hair or to create texture and special effects

trimmers small clippers, also known as outliners and edgers, used for detail, precision design, and fine finish work after a haircut or beard trim

7 Anatomy and Physiology

☑ Learning Objectives

AFTER COMPLETING THIS CHAPTER, YOU SHOULD BE ABLE TO:

1 Explain the importance of anatomy and physiology to the barbering profession.

2 Describe the structure and reproduction of cells.

3 Describe the structure of the skull, face, and neck and their relationship to barbering.

4 Identify important muscles of the head, face, and neck that relate to barbering services.

5 Identify important nerves of the head, face, and neck that relate to barbering services.

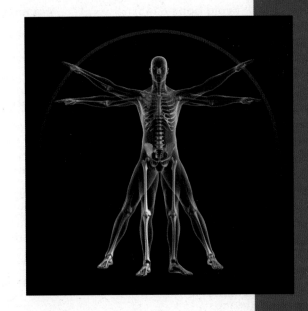

Key Terms

PAGE NUMBER INDICATES WHERE IN THE CHAPTER THE TERM IS USED.

abductor muscles / 151

adductor muscles / 151

anabolism / 140

anatomy / 139

angular artery / 160

anterior auricular artery / 160

aorta / 158

aponeurosis / 149

arteries / 158

atrium / 157

auricularis anterior / 151

auricularis posterior / 151

auricularis superior / 151

auriculotemporal nerve / 155

autonomic nervous system (ANS) / 153

belly of a muscle / 148

blood / 158

blood vascular system / 156

brain / 153

buccal nerve / 156

buccinator / 150

capillaries / 158

carpus / 146

catabolism / 140

cell membrane / 140

cells / 140

central nervous system (CNS) / 152

cervical cutaneous nerve / 156

cervical nerve / 156

cervical vertebrae / 145

circulatory system / 156

common carotid arteries / 159

corrugator / 150

cranium / 143

cytoplasm / 140

depressor labii inferioris / 150

diaphragm / 163

digestive system / 162

eleventh cranial nerve / 156

endocrine system / 162

epicranius / 148

ethmoid bone / 143

excretory system / 162

external carotid artery / 159

external jugular vein / 161

facial artery / 160

facial bones / 144

fifth cranial nerve / 154

frontal artery / 160

frontal bone / 143

frontalis / 149

glands / 162

greater auricular nerve / 156

greater occipital nerve / 156

gross anatomy / 139

heart / 157

histology / 139

humerus / 146

hyoid bone / 145

indirect division / 140

inferior labial artery / 160

infraorbital artery / 160

infraorbital nerve / 155

infratrochlear nerve / 155

insertion of a muscle / 147

integumentary system / 164

internal carotid artery / 159

internal jugular vein / 161

lacrimal bones / 144

levator anguli oris / 150

levator labii superioris / 150

lungs / 163

lymph / 161

lymphatic-immune
   system / 161

lymph nodes / 161

lymph vascular system / 157

mandible bone / 145

mandibular nerve / 156

masseter / 151

maxillary bones / 145

mental nerve / 155

mentalis / 150

metabolism / 140

metacarpus / 146

middle temporal artery / 160

mitosis / 140

mixed nerves / 154

motor nerves / 154

muscular system / 147

myology / 147

nasal bones / 144

nasal nerve / 155

nucleus / 140

occipital artery / 161

occipital bone / 143

occipitalis / 149

opponent muscles / 151

orbicularis oculi / 150

orbicularis oris / 150

organs / 141

origin of a muscle / 147

parietal artery / 160

parietal bones / 143

pericardium / 157

peripheral nervous
   system (PNS) / 153

phalanges / 146

physiology / 139

plasma / 159

platelets / 159

platysma / 151

posterior auricular artery / 161

posterior auricular nerve / 156

procerus / 150

radius / 146

red blood cells / 159

reflex / 154

reproductive system / 164

respiratory system / 163

risorius / 150

sensory nerves / 154

seventh cranial nerve / 156

skeletal system / 143

smaller occipital nerve / 156

sphenoid bone / 143

spinal cord / 153

sternocleidomastoideus / 151

submental artery / 160

superficial temporal
   artery / 160

superior labial artery / 160

supraorbital artery / 160

supraorbital nerve / 155

supratrochlear nerve / 155

systems / 142

temporal bones / 143

temporal nerve / 156

temporalis / 151

thorax / 146

tissues / 141

transverse facial artery / 160

trapezius / 151

triangularis / 151

ulna / 146

veins / 158

ventricle / 157

white blood cells / 159

zygomatic (or malar)
   bones / 144

zygomatic nerve / 155

zygomaticus / 150

An overview of human anatomy and physiology will provide you with a basic knowledge of the structure and functions of the human body to assist your performance in the barbering field. Knowledge of the anatomical structure of the head form provides a foundation for designing haircut and beard styles or performing a proper shave. The study of human physiology is important for understanding the proper application of facial or scalp manipulations and the benefits that can be derived from these services.

Introduction of Terms

Anatomy and physiology are branches of the larger science of biology, which is the study of all forms of life. The human body is composed of cells, tissues, organs, and systems. Collectively, these structures amount to approximately one-fourth solid matter and three-fourths liquid in the human organism. This chapter will introduce you to three primary studies of the human body that should be of interest to barbers: anatomy, physiology, and histology.

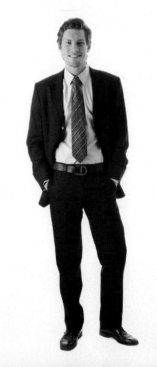

Anatomy is the study of the shape and structure of an organism's body and the relationship of one body part to another. **Gross anatomy** is the study of the anatomical structures of an organism that are easily observable through inspection with the naked eye. Different body parts and regions are studied with regard to their general shape, external features, and main divisions. Barbers practice a form of gross anatomical study during hair, skin, and scalp analyses or when envisioning hairstyles and facial hair designs. In general, barbers are concerned with those anatomical parts receiving services in the barbershop, such as the head, face, neck, and hands.

Physiology studies the mechanical, physical, and biochemical functions and activities of each body part and the way in which these actions coordinate or interact to form a complete living organism. Barbers should be aware of the ways in which massage manipulations, heat, or absorptive products used in the practice of barbering might affect physiological activities of the body, such as increasing the circulation. Barbers should also be aware of certain physiological stresses caused by prolonged standing or repetitive movements that may affect their own skeletal or circulatory systems, as well as the preventative measures that can help minimize the occurrence of associated occupational disorders (see Chapter 3).

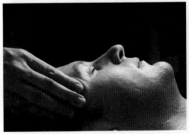

Histology is the microscopic study of the structure of the various tissues and organs that make up the entire body of an organism. Barbers are particularly concerned with the histology of the skin and its appendages (hair, nails, sweat glands, and oil glands).

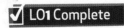
✓ **LO1 Complete**

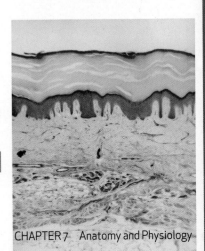

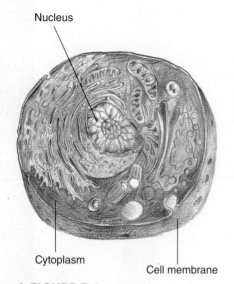

Nucleus

Cytoplasm

Cell membrane

▲ FIGURE 7-1
Anatomy of the cell.

Cells

Cells are the basic units of structure and function of all living things and, as such, are responsible for carrying on all life processes within an organism. The human body is composed of cells that differ in size, shape, structure, and purpose, with millions of specialized cells that perform a variety of functions required for living.

STRUCTURE OF THE CELL

A cell is a microscopic unit of a living organism that contains protoplasm (a colorless, jellylike substance) in which food elements such as proteins, fats, carbohydrates, mineral salts, and water are present. Most cells also contain the following important structures (**Figure 7-1**):

- The **nucleus** is the most important organelle, or structure, within the cell. Situated in the center of the cell and consisting of dense and active protoplasm, the functions of the nucleus are to control cell activity and to facilitate cell division.

- The **cytoplasm** is found outside of the nucleus. It is made up of protoplasm less dense than that of the nucleus. It contains food materials necessary for the growth, reproduction, and self-repair of the cell.

- The **cell membrane** encloses the protoplasm and permits soluble substances to enter and leave the cell.

CELL GROWTH AND REPRODUCTION

Cells have the ability to reproduce, thereby providing new cells for growth and the replacement of worn or injured cells. When a cell reaches maturity in the human body, reproduction takes place through **indirect division.** This is a process in which a series of changes occur in the nucleus before the entire cell divides in half.

Most cells reproduce by dividing into two identical cells called daughter cells. This reproduction process is known as **mitosis.** As long as there is adequate food, oxygen, water, proper temperatures, and an ability to eliminate waste products, the cell will continue to grow and thrive for the duration of its life cycle. If these requirements are not fulfilled, or the presence of toxins is evident, the growth and health of the cell become impaired. Most body cells are capable of growth and self-repair during their life cycle.

CELL METABOLISM

Metabolism is a complex chemical process whereby the body's cells are nourished and supplied with the energy needed to carry out their many activities.

There are two phases to metabolism:

1. **Anabolism** is constructive metabolism that builds up cellular tissues. During anabolism, the body cells absorb and store water, food, and oxygen for the purpose of growth and repair.

2. **Catabolism** is the metabolic phase that involves the breaking down of complex compounds within cells into smaller ones. During catabolism, the cells consume what they have absorbed in order to release the

energy needed to perform specialized functions such as muscular contractions, body secretions, digestion, or heat production.

Anabolism and catabolism are carried out simultaneously and continually within the cells to facilitate the processes required for life.

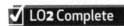 ✓ LO2 Complete

Tissues

Tissues are composed of groups of cells that are similar in shape, size, structure, and function. Each tissue has a specific function and can be recognized by its characteristic appearance. There are four main types of tissues:

1. Connective tissue serves to support, protect, and bind together the tissues of the body. Bone, cartilage, ligament, tendon, and fat tissue are examples of connective tissue.
2. Epithelial (ep-ih-THEE-lee-ul) tissue is a protective covering on body surfaces such as the skin, mucous membranes, and linings of the heart, digestive and respiratory organs, and glands.
3. Muscular tissue contracts and moves various parts of the body.
4. Nerve tissue carries messages to and from the brain, and controls and coordinates all body functions.

Organs

Organs are structures containing two or more different tissues that are combined to accomplish a specific function. **Table 7-1** lists the most important organs of the body and their functions.

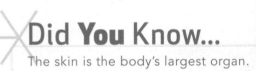
Did **You** Know...
The skin is the body's largest organ.

> TABLE **7-1** Important Body Organs and Their Functions

ORGAN	FUNCTION
brain	controls the body
eyes	control vision
heart	circulates the blood
kidneys	excrete water and other waste products
lungs	supply oxygen to the blood
liver	removes toxic products of digestion
skin	forms the external protective covering of the body
stomach and intestines	digest food

Systems

Systems are groups of organs that act together to perform one or more functions within the body. While each system forms a unit specially designed to perform a specific function, that function cannot be performed without the complete cooperation of other systems. The human body is composed of 11 major systems as defined in **Table 7-2**.

> **TABLE 7-2** Body Systems and Their Functions

SYSTEM	FUNCTION
circulatory	controls the steady circulation of the blood through the body by means of the heart and blood vessels
digestive	changes food into nutrients and wastes; consists of the mouth, stomach, intestines, salivary and gastric glands, and other organs
endocrine	affects the growth, development, sexual activities, and health of the entire body; consists of specialized glands
excretory	purifies the body by the elimination of waste matter; consists of the kidneys, liver, skin, intestines, and lungs
integumentary	serves as a protective covering and helps in regulating the body's temperature; consists of skin and its accessory organs such as oil and sweat glands, sensory receptors, hair, and nails
lymphatic/immune	works to protect the body from disease; develops immunities and destroys disease-causing microorganisms
muscular	covers, shapes, and supports the skeletal tissue; also contracts and moves various parts of the body; consists of muscles
nervous	controls and coordinates all other systems and makes them work harmoniously and efficiently; consists of the brain, spinal cord, and nerves
reproductive	responsible for processes by which humans produce offspring
respiratory	enables breathing, supplying the body with oxygen, and eliminating carbon dioxide as a waste product; consists of lungs and air passages
skeletal	physical foundation of the body; consists of the bones and are connected by movable and immovable joints

The Skeletal System

The **skeletal system** is the physical foundation of the body. It is composed of 206 differently shaped bones that are connected by movable and immovable joints. The scientific study of bones and their structure, functions, and diseases is called *osteology*. *Os* is the technical term for bone and is used as a prefix in bone-related terminology.

Except for the tissue that forms the major part of the teeth, bone is the hardest tissue of the body. It is composed of connective tissue consisting of about one-third animal matter such as cells and blood, and two-thirds mineral matter, mainly calcium carbonate and calcium phosphate.

The primary functions of the skeletal system are to:

- give shape and support to the body.
- protect various internal structures and organs.
- serve as attachments for muscles and act as levers to produce body movement.
- produce red and white blood cells in the red marrow of the bone.
- store minerals such as calcium, phosphorus, magnesium, and sodium.

A *joint* is the connection between two or more skeletal bones. There are two types of joints: movable, such as elbows, knees, and hips; and immovable, such as the pelvis or skull, which allows little or no movement.

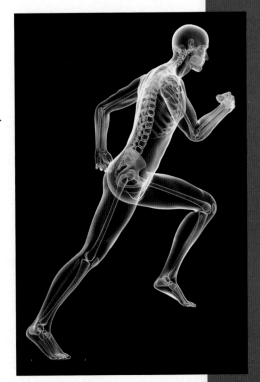

BONES OF THE SKULL

The skull is the skeleton of the head. It is an oval, bony case that shapes the head and protects the brain. Divided into two parts, the skull consists of 8 bones in the **cranium** and 14 facial bones **(Figure 7-2)**.

Bones of the Cranium

An understanding of the positioning of the cranial bones assists barbers in hair design and scalp massage services. The eight bones of the cranium are as follows:

- The **occipital bone** is the hindmost bone of the skull and is located below the parietal bones to form the back of the cranium above the nape.
- Two **parietal bones** form the sides and top of the cranium.
- The **frontal bone** forms the forehead and portions of the eye sockets and nasal cavities.
- Two **temporal bones** form the sides of the head in the ear region, below the parietal bones.
- The **ethmoid bone** is a light, spongy bone between the eye sockets that forms part of the nasal cavities.
- The **sphenoid bone** joins all of the bones of the cranium together.

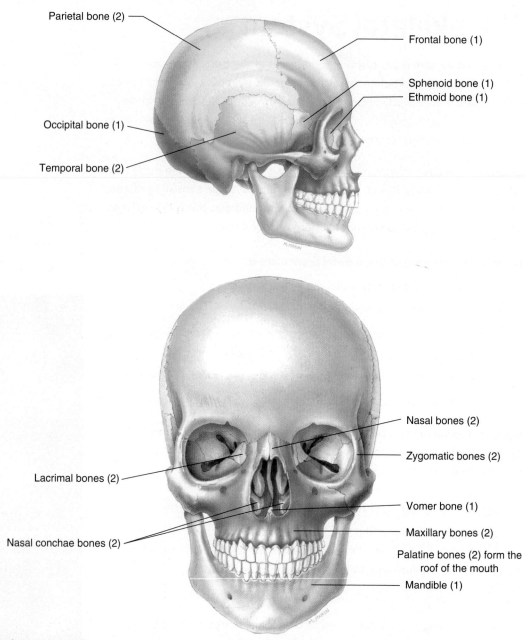

▲ FIGURE 7-2
The skull and facial bones.

Bones of the Face

Barbers benefit from an understanding of facial skeletal structure when performing hair, mustache, and beard design, facials, and shaving services. The 14 **facial bones** include the following:

- Two **nasal bones** form the bridge of the nose.

- Two **lacrimal bones** are small, fragile bones located at the front part of the inner wall of the eye sockets.

- Two **zygomatic** (or **malar**) **bones** form the prominence of the cheeks.

- Two **maxillary bones** are the upper jawbones that join to form the whole upper jaw.

- The **mandible bone** is largest and strongest bone of the face; forms the lower jaw.

- Two *turbinal* bones, thin layers of spongy bone situated on the outer walls of the nasal depression.

- The *vomer*, a single bone that forms part of the dividing wall of the nose.

- Two *palatine* bones, which form the floor and outer wall of the nose, the roof of the mouth, and the floor of the eye socket.

BONES OF THE NECK

The skeleton of the neck supports the head and consists of the following bones (See **Figure 7-3**):

- The **hyoid bone** is a U-shaped bone located in the front part of the throat.

- **Cervical vertebrae** refer to the seven bones that form the top part of the spinal column located in the neck region.

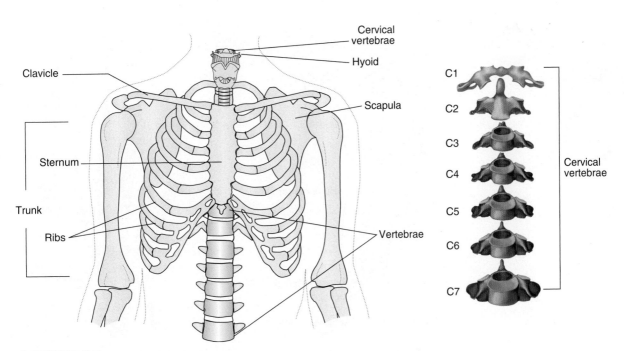

▲ FIGURE 7-3

Bones of the neck, chest, shoulder, and back.

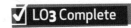

✔ LO**3** Complete

BONES OF THE CHEST, SHOULDER, AND BACK

The **thorax**, or chest, is an elastic, bony cage consisting of the sternum, clavicle, scapula, and 12 pairs of ribs. This framework serves as a protective covering for the heart, lungs, and other delicate internal organs (Figure 7-3).

BONES OF THE SHOULDER, ARM, AND HAND

The important bones of the shoulders, arms, and hands that barbers should know about include the following (**Figures 7-4** and **7-5**):

- The **humerus** is the largest bone of the arm and extends from shoulder to elbow.

- The **ulna** is the inner and larger bone of the forearm, forms the elbow, and is located along the same side of the arm as the little finger.

- The **radius** is the smaller bone on the thumb side of the forearm.

- The **carpus** or wrist is a flexible joint composed of eight small, irregular bones held together by ligaments.

- The **metacarpals** are the bones of the palm, consisting of five slender bones between the carpus and phalanges.

- The **phalanges** are the bones of the fingers, consisting of three in each finger and two in the thumb, totaling 14 bones in each hand.

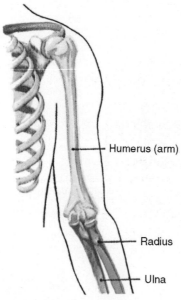

▲ FIGURE 7-4

Bones of the shoulder and arm.

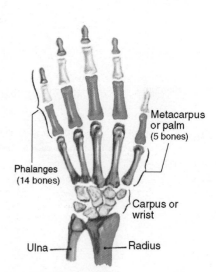

▲ FIGURE 7-5

Bones of the hand.

The Muscular System

The **muscular system** covers, shapes, and supports the skeleton, and its function is to help produce movement within the body. **Myology** is the study of the structure, functioning, and diseases of the muscles.

The muscular system consists of over 600 large and small muscles that comprise 40 to 50 percent of the body's weight. Muscles are composed of contractile, fibrous tissues that stretch and contract to facilitate the action of various body movements. The muscular system relies upon the skeletal and nervous systems for its activities and proper operation.

There are three types of muscular tissues:

1. Striated (striped) or voluntary muscles contain nerves, are attached to bones, and are controlled by will **(Figure 7-6)**. For example, the face consists of many voluntary muscles that facilitate expression.

2. Non-striated (smooth) or involuntary muscles function without the action of the will. These muscles are found in the internal organs of the body, such as the stomach and intestines **(Figure 7-7)**.

3. Cardiac muscle is the heart itself. An involuntary muscle with striations and centrally located nuclei, it is not duplicated anywhere else in the body **(Figure 7-8)**.

MUSCLE STRUCTURE

When a muscle contracts and shortens, one of its attachments usually remains fixed and the other one moves. A muscle has three parts: origin, belly, and insertion.

- The **origin of a muscle** refers to the more fixed attachment, such as the ends of muscles attached to bones or other muscles. Muscles attached to bones are usually referred to as skeletal muscles.

- The **insertion of a muscle** refers to the more movable attachment, such as the ends of muscles attached to other movable muscles, to movable bones, or to the skin. For example, the masseter and temporalis muscles are the muscles of mastication. They assist in chewing and the side-to-side movement of the mandible (jaw). The masseter originates at the maxilla and zygomatic arch while its insertion is located at the angle of the mandible. The temporalis originates at the parietal bone and its insertion is situated at the

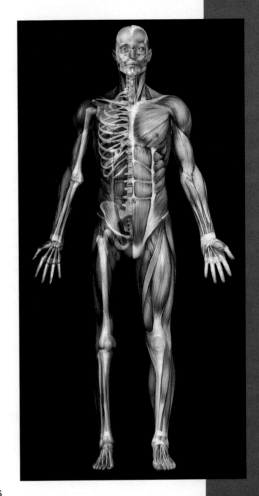

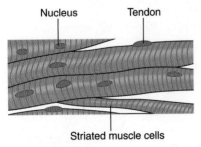

▲ **FIGURE 7-6**

Striated muscle cells.

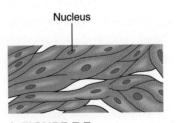

▲ **FIGURE 7-7**

Nonstriated muscle cells.

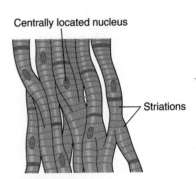

▲ **FIGURE 7-8**

Cardiac muscle cells.

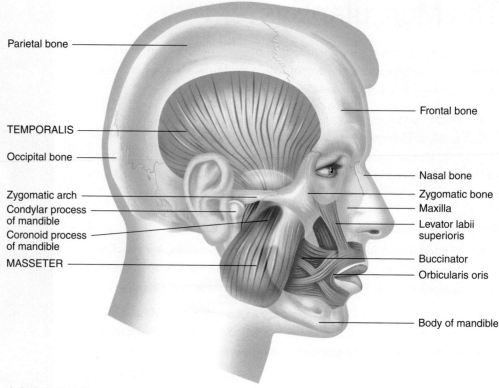

Parietal bone

TEMPORALIS

Occipital bone

Zygomatic arch

Condylar process
of mandible

Coronoid process
of mandible

MASSETER

Frontal bone

Nasal bone

Zygomatic bone

Maxilla

Levator labii
superioris

Buccinator

Orbicularis oris

Body of mandible

▲ **FIGURE 7-9a**

Origin and insertion locations for the muscles of mastication.

coronoid process of the mandible (**Figure 7-9a**). Pressure in massage is usually directed from the insertion of the muscle to its origin.

- The **belly of a muscle** is the middle part of the muscle between the origin and the insertion.

STIMULATION OF MUSCLES

Muscular tissue may be stimulated by any of the following methods:

- massage (hand massage or electric vibrator)
- electric current (high-frequency or faradic current)
- light rays (infrared rays or ultraviolet rays)
- heat rays (heating lamps or heating caps)
- moist heat (steamers or moderately warm steam towels)
- nerve impulses (through the nervous system)
- chemicals (certain acids and salts)

MUSCLES OF THE SCALP, FACE, AND NECK

The performance of professional services such as scalp, facial, and neck massages requires barbers to know the location of the voluntary muscles of the head, face, and neck and the functions these muscles control (**Figures 7-9b** and **7-10**).

Muscles of the Scalp

- The **epicranius** (ep-ih-KRAY-nee-us) or occipito-frontalis is a broad muscle consisting of the occipitalis and frontalis that covers the top of the skull.

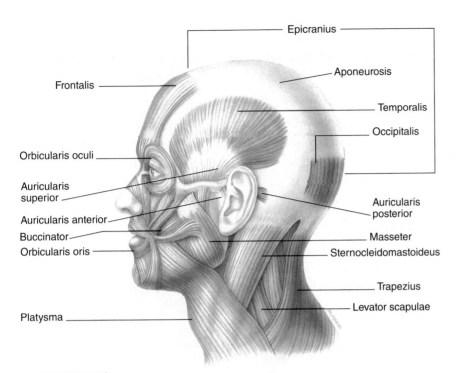

▲ FIGURE 7-9b

Muscles of the head, face, and neck.

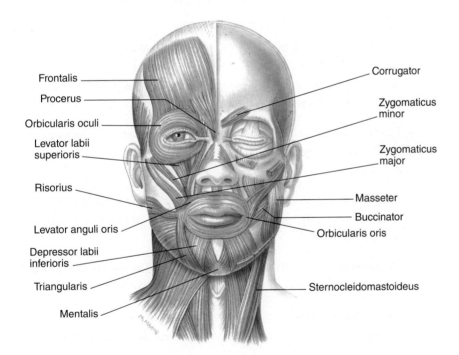

▲ FIGURE 7-10

Muscles of the face.

- The **occipitalis** (ahk-SIP-i-tahl-is) is the muscle at the back part of the epicranius that draws the scalp backward.

- The **frontalis** (frun-TAY-lus) is the front portion of the epicranius that draws the scalp forward and causes wrinkles across the forehead.

- The **aponeurosis** (ap-uh-noo-ROH-sus) is a tendon that connects the occipitalis and the frontalis.

Muscles of the Eyebrows

- The **orbicularis oculi** (or-bik-yuh-LAIR-is AHK-yuh-lye) is a muscle that completely surrounds the margin of the eye socket and closes the eyelid.

- The **corrugator** (KOR-oo-gay-tohr) is the muscle beneath the frontalis and orbicularis oculi that draws the eyebrows down and in, producing vertical lines and causing frowning.

Muscles of the Nose

- The **procerus** (proh-SEE-rus) covers the top of the nose, depresses the eyebrow, and causes wrinkles across the bridge of the nose. The other nasal muscles are small muscles around the nasal openings, which contract and expand the opening of the nostrils.

Muscles of the Mouth

- The **levator labii superioris** (lih-VAYT-ur LAY-bee-eye soo-peer-ee-OR-is), also known as quadratus labii superioris, is a muscle surrounding the upper lip that elevates the upper lip and dilates the nostrils.

- The **depressor labii inferioris** (dee-PRES-ur LAY-bee-eye in-FEER-ee-or-us), also known as quadratus labii inferioris is a muscle that surrounds the lower part of the lip, depressing the lower lip and drawing it a little to one side.

- The **buccinator** (BUK-sih-nay-tur) is the muscle between the upper and lower jaws that compresses the cheeks and expels air between the lips.

- The **levator anguli oris** (lih-VAYT-ur ANG-yoo-ly OH-ris), also known as caninus (kay-NY-us) muscle, raises the angle of the mouth and draws it inward.

- The **mentalis** (men-TAY-lis) is a muscle situated at the tip of the chin that raises and pushes up the lower lip, wrinkling the chin.

- The **orbicularis oris** (or-bik-yuh-LAIR-is OH-ris) forms a flat band around the upper and lower lips to compress, contract, pucker, and wrinkle the lips.

- The **risorius** (rih-ZOR-ee-us) extends from the masseter muscle to the angle of the mouth and draws the corner of the mouth out and back.

- The **zygomaticus** (zy-goh-MAT-ih-kus) extends from the zygomatic bone to the angle of the mouth and elevates the lip.

- The **triangularis** (try-ang-gyuh-LAY-rus) extends along the side of the chin and draws down the corner of the mouth.

Muscles of the Ear

- The **auricularis** (aw-rik-yuh-LAIR-is) **superior** is a muscle above the ear that draws the ear upward.

- The **auricularis posterior** is a muscle behind the ear that draws the ear backward.

- The **auricularis anterior** is a muscle in front of the ear that draws the ear forward.

Muscles of Mastication

- The **masseter** (muh-SEE-tur) and the **temporalis** (tem-poh-RAY-lis) are muscles that coordinate in opening and closing the mouth, and are sometimes referred to as chewing muscles.

Muscles of the Neck

- The **platysma** (plah-TIZ-muh) is a broad muscle extending from the chest and shoulder muscles to the side of the chin and is responsible for depressing the lower jaw and lip.

- The **sternocleidomastoideus** (STUR-noh-KLEE-ih-doh-mas-TOYD-ee-us) is the muscle extending from the collar and chest bones to the temporal bone in back of the ear; this muscle bends and rotates the head.

- The **trapezius** (trah-PEE-zee-us) allows movement of the shoulders and covers the back of the neck.

MUSCLES OF THE HANDS

The hand is one of the most complex parts of the body, with many small muscles that overlap from joint to joint, providing flexibility and strength to open and close the hand and fingers. Important muscles to know include:

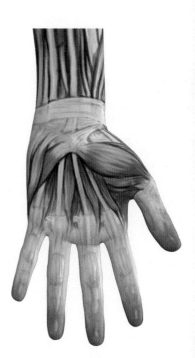

- The **abductor muscles**, which separate the fingers.

- The **adductor muscles**, the muscles at the base of each finger that draw the fingers together.

- The **opponent muscles**, the muscles in the palm that act to bring the thumb toward the fingers.

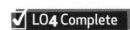

✓ LO**4** Complete

The Nervous System

Neurology is the study of the structure, function, and pathology of the nervous system. The nervous system is one of the most important systems of the body. It controls and coordinates the functions of all the other systems and makes them work harmoniously and efficiently. Every square inch of the human body is supplied with fine fibers known as nerves.

An understanding of how nerves work will help barbers to perform the massage services associated with shampoos, scalp treatments, and facials. It will also help increase awareness of the effects these treatments can have on the skin, the scalp, and on the body as a whole.

DIVISIONS OF THE NERVOUS SYSTEM

The principal components of the nervous system are the brain, the spinal cord, and the nerves themselves. The nervous system is divided into three main subdivisions: the cerebrospinal (ser-ree-bro-SPY-nahl), the peripheral (puh-RIF-uh-rul), and the autonomic (aw-toh-NAHM-ik) systems **(Figure 7-11)**.

1. The cerebrospinal system, or **central nervous system (CNS),** consists of the brain, cranial nerves, spinal cord, and spinal nerves. It controls consciousness and all mental activities, the voluntary functions of the five senses, and voluntary muscle actions including all body movements and facial expressions.

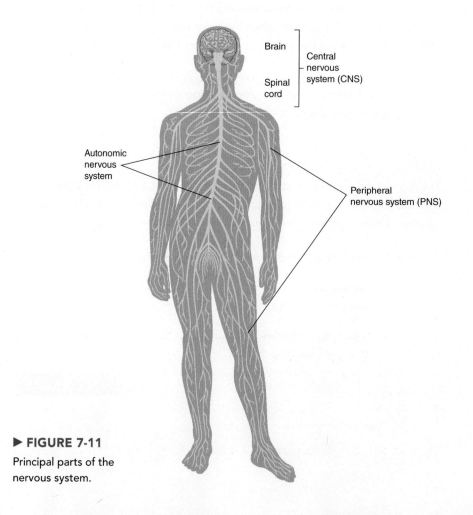

▶ FIGURE 7-11

Principal parts of the nervous system.

2. The **peripheral nervous system (PNS)** is made up of sensory and motor nerve fibers that extend from the brain and spinal cord to all parts of the body. Their function is to carry impulses, or messages, to and from the central nervous system.

3. The **autonomic,** or sympathetic, **nervous system (ANS)** is related structurally to the central nervous system, but its functions are independent of human will. This system is important in the operation of internal body functions such as breathing, circulation, digestion, and glandular activities. Its main purpose is to regulate these internal operations to keep them in balance and working properly.

THE BRAIN AND SPINAL CORD

The **brain** is the largest and most complex nerve tissue in the body. Weighing an average of 44 to 48 ounces, the brain is contained within the cranium and controls sensation, muscles, glandular activity, and the ability to think and feel. It sends and receives messages through 12 pairs of cranial nerves that originate in the brain and extend to various parts of the head, face, and neck.

The **spinal cord** is the portion of the central nervous system that originates in the brain, extends down to the lower extremity of the trunk, and is protected by the spinal column. Thirty-one pairs of spinal nerves extending from the spinal cord are distributed to the muscles and skin of the trunk and limbs.

NERVE STRUCTURE AND FUNCTION

A neuron, or nerve cell, is the primary structural unit of the nervous system (**Figure 7-12**). It is composed of a cell body and nucleus with long and short fibers called cell processes. The short processes, called *dendrites*, carry impulses to the cell body. The longer processes, called *axons*, carry impulses away from the cell body to the muscles and organs. The cell body stores energy and food for the cell processes, which convey the nerve impulses throughout the body. Practically all of the nerve cell axons are contained in the brain and spinal cord.

Nerves are long, white cords made up of bundles of nerve fibers, held together by connective tissue, through which impulses are transmitted. Nerves have their origin in the brain and spinal cord, and distribute branches to all parts of the body to facilitate sensation and motion.

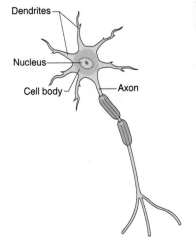

▲ **FIGURE 7-12**
A nerve cell.

Nerve Stimulation

Stimulation of the nerves causes muscles to contract and expand. When heat is applied to the skin the underlying muscles relax; when cold is applied, contraction takes place. Nerve stimulation may be accomplished by any of the following methods:

- Chemicals, such as certain salts or acids
- Massage with the hands, a massage tool, or an electric massager

- Electric current such as Tesla high-frequency current
- Light rays
- Heat rays
- Moist heat, such as warm steam towels

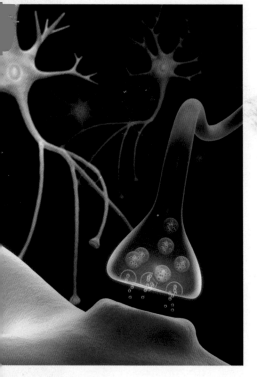

TYPES OF NERVES

All nerves fall into one of the following categories:

- **Sensory nerves,** also called *afferent* nerves, carry (transmit) impulses or messages from sense organs to the brain, where sensations of touch, cold, heat, sight, hearing, taste, smell, and pain are experienced.
- **Motor nerves,** or *efferent* nerves, transmit impulses from the brain to the muscles to produce movement.
- **Mixed nerves** contain both sensory and motor fibers and have the ability to send and receive messages.

Sensory nerves are situated near the surface of the skin. Motor nerves are in the muscles. As impulses pass from the sensory nerves to the brain and back over the motor nerves to the muscles, a complete circuit is established and movements of the muscle result.

A **reflex** is an automatic nerve reaction to a stimulus. It involves the movement of an impulse from a sensory receptor to the spinal cord and a responsive impulse to a muscle causing a reaction (for example, the quick removal of the hand from a hot object). Reflex action does not have to be learned.

NERVES OF THE HEAD, FACE, AND NECK
Cranial Nerves

There are 12 pairs of cranial nerves. All are connected to a part of the brain surface. They emerge through openings on the sides and base of the cranium and reach various parts of the head, face, and neck. They are classified as mixed nerves and contain both motor and sensory fibers.

The most important cranial nerves to consider when massaging the head, face, and neck are the fifth cranial, seventh cranial, and eleventh cranial nerves; and the cervical nerves, which originate in the spinal cord.

The largest of the cranial nerves is the **fifth cranial nerve**, also known as the *trifacial* or *trigeminal* (try-JEM-in-ul) nerve. It is the chief *sensory* nerve of the face and also serves as the motor nerve of the muscles that control chewing. It consists of three primary branches: ophthalmic (ahf-THAL-mik), mandibular (man-DIB-yuh-lur), and maxillary (MAK-suh-lair-ee) **(Figure 7-13)**.

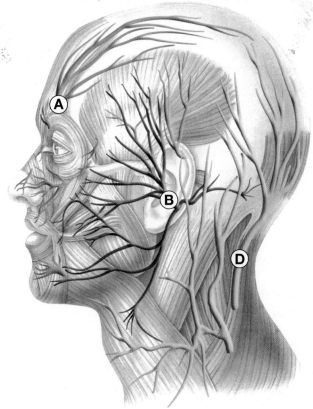

A — Fifth cranial nerve
B — Seventh cranial nerve
C — Eleventh cranial nerve
(not shown)
D — Spinal nerve

▲ **FIGURE 7-13**
Nerves of the face and neck.

Important sensory branches of the fifth cranial nerve affected by massage include:

- The **supraorbital** (soo-pruh-OR-bih-tul) **nerve**, which affects the skin of the forehead, scalp, eyebrows, and upper eyelids.

- The **supratrochlear** (soo-pruh-TRAHK-lee-ur) **nerve**, which affects the skin between the eyes and upper sides of the nose.

- The **infratrochlear** (in-frah-TRAHK-lee-ur) **nerve**, which affects the membrane and skin of the nose.

- The **nasal nerve**, which affects the point and lower sides of the nose.

- The **zygomatic** (zy-goh-MAT-ik) **nerve**, which affects the skin of the temples, sides of the forehead, and upper part of the cheeks.

- The **infraorbital** (in-frah-OR-bih-tul) **nerve**, which affects the skin of the lower eyelids, sides of the nose, upper lip, and mouth.

- The **auriculotemporal** (aw-RIK-yuh-loh-TEM-puh-rul) **nerve**, which affects the external ear and the skin from above the temples to the top of the skull.

- The **mental nerve**, which affects the skin of the lower lip and chin.

The **seventh cranial nerve** or facial nerve is the chief *motor* nerve of the face. It emerges near the lower part of the ear. Its divisions and their branches control all the muscles used for facial expression and extend to the muscles of the neck. The most important branches of the facial nerve are:

- the **posterior auricular nerve**, which affects the muscles behind the ears at the base of the skull
- the **temporal nerve**, which affects the muscles of the temples, sides of the forehead, eyebrows, eyelids, and upper part of the cheeks
- the **zygomatic nerve** (upper and lower), which affects the muscles of the upper part of the cheeks
- the **buccal** (BUK-ul) **nerve**, which affects the muscles of the mouth
- the **mandibular nerve**, which affects the muscles of the chin and lower lip
- the **cervical nerve**, which affects the sides of the neck

The **eleventh cranial nerve,** or accessory nerve, is a spinal nerve branch that affects the muscles of the neck and back.

CERVICAL NERVES

The cervical or spinal nerves originate at the spinal cord. Their branches supply the muscles and scalp at the back of the head and neck, as follows:

- The **greater occipital nerve** is located in the back of the head and affects the scalp as far up as the top of the head.
- The **smaller (lesser) occipital nerve** is located at the base of the skull and affects the scalp and muscles of this region.
- The **greater auricular nerve** is located at the side of the neck and affects the external ears and the areas in front and back of the ears.
- The **cervical cutaneous nerve** is located at the side of the neck and affects the front and sides of the neck as far down as the breastbone.

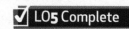 ✓ LO5 Complete

The Circulatory System

The **circulatory system**, also referred to as the cardiovascular or vascular system, controls the steady circulation of the blood through the body by means of the heart and blood vessels. It is essential to proper circulation and the maintenance of good health. The vascular system is made up of two divisions:

1. The **blood vascular system** consists of the heart, arteries, capillaries, and veins for the circulation and distribution of blood throughout the body.

2. The **lymph vascular**, or lymphatic, **system** aids the blood vascular system and consists of lymph, glands, vessels (lymphatics), and other structures. Lymph is a colorless, watery fluid that circulates in the lymphatics of the body, where it helps carry wastes and impurities from the cells, and is then routed back into the circulatory system.

THE HEART

The **heart** is a muscular, conical organ, about the size of a closed fist, that keeps the blood moving within the circulatory system (**Figure 7-14**). It weighs approximately 9 ounces and is located in the chest cavity, where it is enclosed in a membrane known as the **pericardium** (payr-ih-KAR-deeum). The heartbeat is regulated by the vagus (tenth cranial nerve) and other nerves in the autonomic nervous system. A normal adult heart beats about 60 to 80 times per minute, but it can beat as high as 100 times per minute.

The interior of the heart contains four chambers and four valves. The upper, thin-walled chambers are the right **atrium** (AY-tree-um) and left atrium. An atrium is also called an auricle. The lower, thick-walled chambers are the right **ventricle** (VEN- truh-kul) and left ventricle. Valves allow the blood to flow in only one direction. With each contraction and relaxation of the heart, the blood flows in, travels from the atria to the ventricles, and is then driven out to be distributed all over the body.

BLOOD VESSELS

The blood vessels are tube-like structures that include the arteries, capillaries, and veins. The function of these vessels is to transport blood to and from the heart and to various tissues of the body.

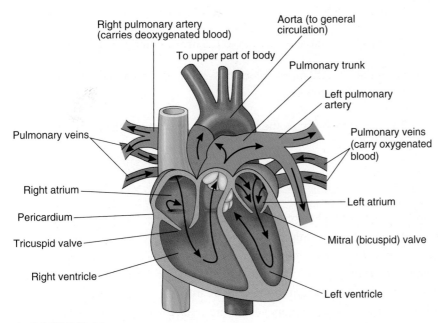

▲ **FIGURE 7-14**

Anatomy of the heart.

Blood flow toward the heart

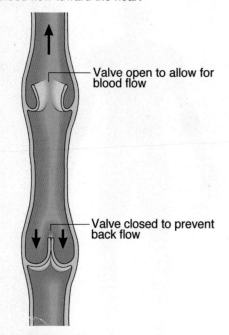

Valve open to allow for blood flow

Valve closed to prevent back flow

▲ FIGURE 7-15
Valves in the veins.

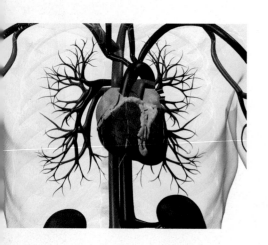

- **Arteries** are thick-walled, muscular, elastic tubes that carry pure blood from the heart to the capillaries. The largest artery in the body is the **aorta.**

- **Capillaries** are minute, thin-walled blood vessels that connect the smaller arteries with the veins. The tissues receive nourishment and eliminate waste products through the capillary walls.

- **Veins** are thin-walled vessels that are less elastic than arteries. They contain cuplike valves to prevent backflow, and carry deoxygenated blood away from the capillaries back to the heart (Figure 7-15). Veins are located closer to the outer surface of the body than are the arteries.

CIRCULATION OF THE BLOOD

The blood is in constant circulation from the moment it leaves the heart until it returns to the heart. There are two systems that control this circulation:

1. Pulmonary circulation is the blood circulation that goes from the heart to the lungs to be purified and then returns to the heart.

2. General circulation is the blood circulation from the heart throughout the body and back again to the heart.

These two systems work in the following sequence:

1. Blood flows from the body into the right atrium.

2. From the right atrium, the blood flows through the tricuspid valve into the right ventricle.

3. The right ventricle pumps the blood to the lungs where it releases waste gases and receives oxygen. At this stage, blood is considered to be oxygen rich.

4. The oxygen-rich blood returns to the heart, entering the left atrium.

5. From the left atrium, the blood flows through the mitral valve (MY-trul VALV) into the left ventricle.

6. The blood then leaves the left ventricle and travels to all parts of the body.

BLOOD

Blood is the nutritive fluid circulating throughout the circulatory system. It is a sticky, salty fluid with an alkaline reaction and a normal temperature of 98.6 degrees Fahrenheit that makes up about one-twentieth of the body's weight. The average adult has 8 to 10 pints of blood, which is a bright red color in the arteries (except in the pulmonary artery) and dark red in the veins (except in the pulmonary vein). This color change occurs as a result of the gain or loss of oxygen as the blood passes through the lungs and other tissues of the body.

Composition of Blood

The blood is composed of about one-third red and white corpuscles (cells) and blood platelets, and two-thirds plasma.

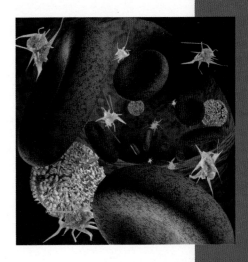

- **Red blood cells,** also called *red corpuscles* or *erythrocytes* (ih-RITH-ruhsyts), are produced in the red bone marrow. They contain hemoglobin, a complex iron protein that gives blood its bright red color. The function of red blood cells is to carry oxygen to the body cells.

- **White blood cells,** also known as white *corpuscles* or *leucocytes,* are produced in the spleen, lymph glands, and red bone marrow. The most important function of white blood cells is to protect the body against disease by fighting harmful bacteria and their toxins.

- **Platelets** are much smaller than the red blood cells and are also formed in the red bone marrow. These colorless bodies are important to the blood-clotting process that stops bleeding in a wound.

- **Plasma** is the fluid part of the blood in which the red and white blood cells and blood platelets flow. Straw-like in color, plasma is about 90 percent water. The main function of plasma is to carry food and secretions to the cells and to take carbon dioxide away from the cells.

Chief Functions of the Blood

Blood performs the following critical functions:

- Carries water, oxygen, food, and secretions to body cells
- Carries carbon dioxide and waste products from the cells to be eliminated through the lungs, skin, kidneys, and large intestine
- Helps equalize body temperature, thus protecting the body from extreme heat and cold
- Helps protect the body from harmful bacteria and infections through the action of the white blood cells
- Closes minute blood vessels that have been injured through the clotting process

ARTERIES OF THE HEAD, FACE, AND NECK

The **common carotid arteries** (kuh-RAHT-ud) are the main sources of the blood supply to the head, face, and neck (**Figure 7-16**). They are located on either side of the neck and each one is divided into an internal and external branch. The **internal carotid artery** supplies blood to the brain, eye sockets, eyelids, and forehead. The **external carotid artery** supplies blood to the front parts of the head, face, and neck.

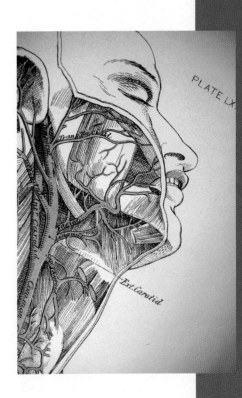

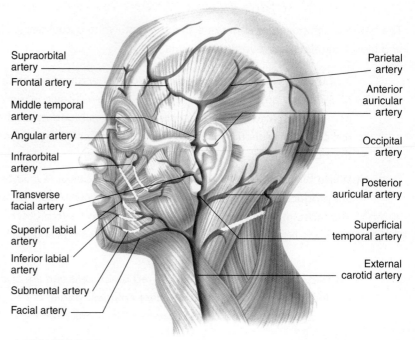

Supraorbital artery
Frontal artery
Middle temporal artery
Angular artery
Infraorbital artery
Transverse facial artery
Superior labial artery
Inferior labial artery
Submental artery
Facial artery

Parietal artery
Anterior auricular artery
Occipital artery
Posterior auricular artery
Superficial temporal artery
External carotid artery

▲ FIGURE 7-16

Arteries of the head, face, and neck.

The external carotid artery subdivides into a number of branches that provide blood supply to the lower region of the face, mouth, and nose. The arterial branches that are most significant to barbers are the facial artery, superficial temporal artery, occipital artery, and posterior auricular artery.

- The **facial artery** or external maxillary supplies blood to the lower region of the face, mouth, and nose through the following branches:

  ▶ The **submental artery** supplies the chin and lower lip.

  ▶ The **inferior labial artery** supplies the lower lip.

  ▶ The **angular artery** supplies the side of the nose.

  ▶ The **superior labial artery** supplies the upper lip, septum, and wings of the nose.

  ▶ The **infraorbital artery** supplies the teeth, lower eyelid, eyes and upper lip.

- The **superficial temporal artery** is a continuation of the external carotid artery and supplies the muscles, skin, and scalp on the front, side, and top of the head. The following are some of its important branches:

  ▶ The **frontal artery** supplies the forehead.

  ▶ The **parietal artery** supplies the crown and sides of the head.

  ▶ The **transverse facial artery** supplies the masseter.

  ▶ The **middle temporal artery** supplies the temples and eyelids.

  ▶ The **anterior auricular artery** supplies the anterior part of the ear.

  ▶ The **supraorbital artery** supplies the scalp and scalp muscle.

- The **occipital artery** supplies the scalp and back of the head up to the crown. Its most important branch is the sterno-cleido-mastoid artery, which supplies the muscle of the same name.

- The **posterior auricular artery** supplies the scalp, behind and above the ear. Its most important branch is the auricular artery, which supplies the skin in back of the ear.

VEINS OF THE HEAD, FACE, AND NECK

The blood returning to the heart from the head, face, and neck flows on each side of the neck in two principal veins: the **internal jugular** and the **external jugular.** The most important veins are parallel to the arteries and take the same names as the arteries.

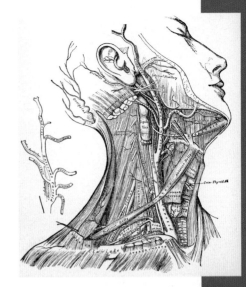

The Lymphatic-Immune System

The **lymphatic-immune system** is made up of lymph, lymph nodes, the thymus gland, the spleen, and the lymph vessels that act as an aid to the blood circulatory system. **Lymph** is a colorless, watery fluid derived from blood plasma as a result of filtration through the capillary walls into the tissue spaces. The function of the lymphatic system is to protect the body from disease by developing immunities, to destroy disease-causing microorganisms, and to drain tissue spaces of excess interstitial fluids (blood plasma found in the spaces between tissue cells) in the blood. It carries waste and impurities away from the cells.

The lymphatic system is closely connected to the blood and the cardiovascular system for the transportation of fluids. The difference is that the lymphatic system transports lymph fluid.

The lymphatic vessels start as tubes that are closed at one end. They can occur individually or in clusters that are called *lymph capillaries.* The lymph capillaries are distributed throughout most of the body, except the nervous system.

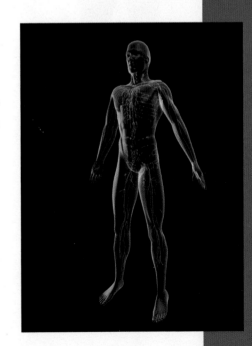

The lymphatic vessels are filtered by the **lymph nodes,** which are gland-like structures found inside the vessels. This filtering process helps detoxify and fight infection before the lymph is reintroduced into the bloodstream.

The primary functions of the lymphatic system are:

- to act as a defense against invading bacteria and toxins.
- to remove waste material from the body cells to the blood.
- to provide a suitable fluid environment for the cells.

The Endocrine System

The **endocrine (EN-duh-krin) system** consists of a group of specialized glands that affect the growth, development, sexual function, and health of the entire body. **Glands** are specialized organs that vary in size and function and have the ability to remove certain elements from the blood and convert them into new compounds. There are two main types of glands: exocrine and endocrine.

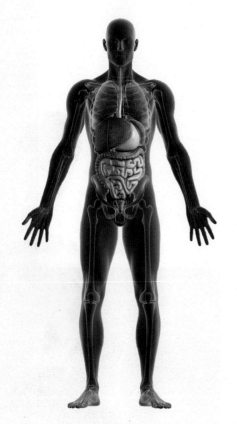

- Exocrine glands (EK-suh-krin GLANDZ), or duct glands, possess canals that lead from the gland to a particular part of the body. Sweat and oil glands of the skin and intestinal glands belong to this group.

- Endocrine glands, or ductless glands, release secretions called hormones (HOR-mohnz) directly into the bloodstream. This influences the welfare of the entire body since hormones such as insulin, adrenaline, and estrogen stimulate functional activity or secretion in other parts of the body.

The Digestive System

The **digestive system (dy-JES-tiv SIS-tum)**, also known as the *gastrointestinal system*, is responsible for changing food into nutrients and waste. Digestive enzymes (EN-zymz) are chemicals that change certain kinds of food into a form that can be used by the body. When the food is in a soluble form, it is transported by the bloodstream and used by the body's cells and tissues. The entire digestive process takes about 9 hours to complete.

The Excretory System

The **excretory system** (EK-skre-tor-ee) is responsible for purifying the body by eliminating waste matter. Cellular metabolism produces various toxic substances that if retained could poison the body. Each of the following organs plays a crucial role in the excretory system:

- The kidneys excrete urine.
- The liver discharges bile pigments.
- The skin eliminates perspiration.
- The large intestine evacuates decomposed and undigested food.
- The lungs exhale carbon dioxide.

The Respiratory System

The **respiratory system** enables breathing (respiration) and consists of the lungs and air passages (Figure 7-17). The **lungs** are spongy tissues composed of microscopic cells into which the inhaled air penetrates and the oxygen it contains is exchanged for carbon dioxide during one breathing cycle. The respiratory system is located within the chest cavity and is protected on both sides by the ribs. The **diaphragm** is a muscular partition that separates the thorax from the abdominal region and helps control breathing.

With each respiratory or breathing cycle, an exchange of gases takes place between the blood and air sacs. During inhalation the chest expands and the diaphragm is pulled down, causing the lungs to draw in air for oxygen absorption into the blood. The chest contracts and draws the diaphragm up to force the expulsion of carbon dioxide from the lungs.

Oxygen is more essential than either food or water. Although a human being may live more than 60 days without food or a few days without water, life cannot continue without air for more than a few minutes.

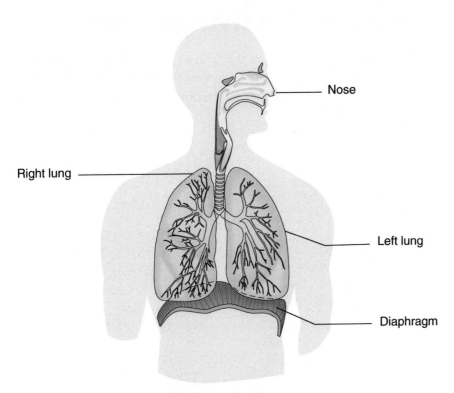

Respiratory System

▲ **FIGURE 7-17**

The respiratory system.

The rate of breathing depends on the activity of the individual. Muscular activities and energy expenditures increase the body's demands for oxygen. As a result, the rate of breathing is increased. A person requires about three times as much oxygen when walking as when standing.

Nose breathing is healthier than mouth breathing because skin surface capillaries warm the air as the hairs lining the mucous membranes of the nasal passages catch airborne bacteria.

Abdominal breathing is of value in building health. Abdominal breathing means deep breathing, which brings both the ribs and diaphragm into action. The greatest exchange of gases is accomplished through abdominal breathing. *Chest breathing* involves light, or shallow, breathing without action of the diaphragm.

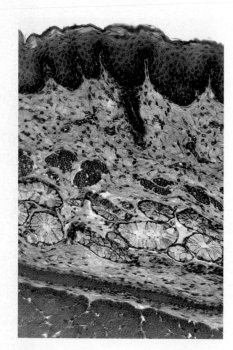

The Integumentary System

The **integumentary system** consists of the skin and its various appendages, such as sweat and oil glands, hair, and nails, and sensory receptors. The histology of skin is discussed in detail in Chapter 10.

The Reproductive System

The **reproductive system** performs the function of reproducing and perpetuating the human race. Although important for the continuation of the human species, it is not of major importance to the practice of barbering.

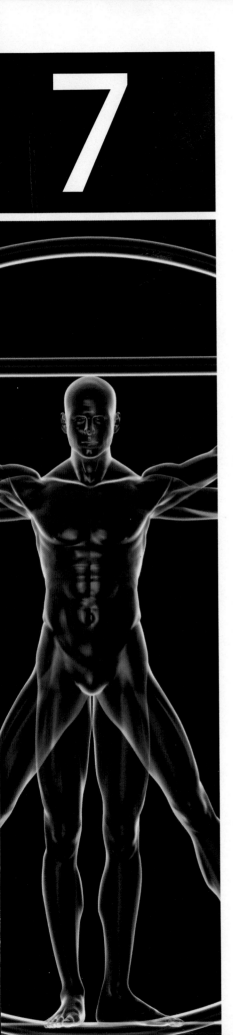

Review
Questions

1. Define *anatomy*, *physiology*, and *histology*.

2. Identify the anatomical parts of the body that barbers are most concerned with.

3. What is a cell?

4. Define *mitosis*.

5. Explain the two phases of cell metabolism.

6. Describe the composition of body tissues.

7. What is an organ?

8. List eight important organs of the body and their functions.

9. What are systems?

10. Name the 11 body systems and their main functions.

11. List the primary functions of the skeletal system.

12. Name the two parts of the skull and the number of bones in each.

13. List the bones of the cranium.

14. Identify the bone that joins all the cranial bones together.

15. List the facial bones with their locations and functions.

16. Where is the hyoid bone located?

17. Describe the function and composition of muscles.

18. List and describe the parts of a muscle.

19. List the ways in which muscles may be stimulated.

20. List the scalp, facial, and neck muscles with their locations and functions.

21. List and describe the functions of the three main divisions of the nervous system.

22. List and describe three types of nerves found in the human body.

23. List the ways in which nerves may be stimulated.

24. Give an example of a nerve reflex.

25. Name the cranial nerves most important in massage services and their functions.

26. Identify the two divisions of the circulatory system.

27. What is the function of the heart? What does it look like?

28. List three kinds of vessels found in the blood-vascular system.

29. What is the composition of blood?

30. Explain the functions of red blood cells and white blood cells.

31. Identify and describe the two main types of glands in the human body.

32. List the five important organs of the excretory system.

33. Describe a respiratory cycle.

34. What structures are included in the integumentary system?

Chapter
Glossary

abductor muscles muscles that separate the fingers

adductor muscles muscles at the base of each finger that draw the fingers together

anabolism constructive metabolism; the process of building up larger molecules from smaller ones

anatomy the science of the structure of organisms and of their parts

angular artery artery that supplies blood to the sides of the nose

anterior auricular artery artery that supplies blood to the front part of the ear

aorta largest artery in the body

aponeurosis tendon that connects the occipitalis and the frontalis

arteries muscular, flexible tubes that carry oxygenated blood from the heart to the capillaries throughout the body

atrium one of the two upper chambers of the heart through which blood is pumped to the ventricles

auricularis anterior muscle in front of the ear that draws the ear forward

auricularis posterior muscle behind the ear that draws the ear backward

auricularis superior muscle above the ear that draws the ear upward

auriculotemporal nerve nerve that affects the external ear and skin

above the temple, up to the top of the skull

autonomic nervous system (ANS) the part of the nervous system that controls the involuntary muscles; regulates the action of the smooth muscles, glands, blood vessels, and heart

belly of a muscle middle part of a muscle

blood nutritive fluid circulating through the circulatory system that supplies oxygen and nutrients to cells and tissues and removes carbon dioxide and waste from them

blood vascular system group of structures (heart, veins, arteries, and capillaries) that distribute blood throughout the body

brain largest and most complex nerve tissue; part of the central nervous system contained within the cranium

buccal nerve nerve that affects the muscles of the mouth

buccinator thin, flat muscle of the cheek between the upper and lower jaws

capillaries thin-walled vessels that connect the smaller arteries to the veins

carpus the bones of the wrist

catabolism the phase of metabolism that breaks down complex compounds within the cells; releases energy to perform functions

cell membrane part of the cell that encloses the protoplasm; permits soluble substances to enter and leave the cell

cells basic units of all living things

central nervous system (CNS) cerebrospinal nervous system consisting of the brain, spinal cord, spinal nerves, and cranial nerves

cervical cutaneous nerve nerve located at the side of the neck; affects the front and sides of the neck to the breastbone

cervical nerve nerve that originates at the spinal cord, affecting the scalp and back of the head and neck

cervical vertebrae seven bones that form the top part of the spinal column in the neck region

circulatory system system that controls the steady circulation of blood through the body by means of the heart and blood vessels

common carotid arteries arteries that supply blood to the head, face, and neck

corrugator facial muscle that draws eyebrows down and wrinkles the forehead vertically

cranium oval, bony case that protects the brain

cytoplasm all of the protoplasm of a cell except that in the nucleus

depressor labii inferioris muscle surrounding the lower lip

diaphragm muscular wall that separates the thorax from the abdominal region and helps control breathing

digestive system the mouth, stomach, intestines, and salivary and gastric glands that change food into nutrients and wastes

eleventh cranial nerve spinal nerve branch that affects the muscles of the neck and back

endocrine system group of specialized glands that affect growth, development, sexual function, and general health

epicranius broad muscle that covers the top of the skull; also know as *occipito-frontalis*

ethmoid bone a light, spongy bone between the eye sockets forming part of the nasal cavities

excretory system group of organs including the kidneys, liver, skin, large intestine, and lungs that purify the body by the elimination of waste matter

external carotid artery artery that supplies blood to the anterior parts of the scalp, face, neck, and side of the head

external jugular vein vein located at the side of the neck that carries blood returning to the heart from the head, face, and neck

facial artery artery that supplies blood to the lower region of the face, mouth, and nose

facial bones two nasal bones; two lacrimal bones; two zygomatic bones; two maxillae; the mandible; two turbinal bones; two palatine bones; and the vomer

fifth cranial nerve chief sensory nerve of the face; controls chewing

frontal artery artery that supplies blood to the forehead and upper eyelids

frontal bone bone that forms the forehead

frontalis anterior or front portion of the epicranius; muscle of the scalp

glands specialized organs varying in size and function that have the ability to remove certain elements from the blood and to convert them into new compounds

greater auricular nerve nerve at the sides of the neck affecting the face, ears, and neck

greater occipital nerve nerve located at the back of the head, affecting the scalp

gross anatomy the study of large and easily observable structures on an organism as seen through inspection with the naked eye

heart muscular, cone-shaped organ that keeps blood moving through the circulatory system

histology the study of the minute structure of the various tissues and organs that make up the entire body of an organism

humerus uppermost and largest bone in the arm

hyoid bone U-shaped bone at the base of the tongue at the front part of the throat

indirect division the method by which a mature cell reproduces in the body

inferior labial artery artery that supplies blood to the lower lip

infraorbital artery artery that supplies blood to the eye muscles

infraorbital nerve nerve that affects the skin of the lower eyelid, side of the nose, upper lip, and mouth

infratrochlear nerve nerve that affects the membrane and skin of the nose

insertion of a muscle the more moveable attachment of a muscle

integumentary system the skin at its appendages

internal carotid artery artery that supplies blood to the brain, eyes, eyelids, forehead, nose, and ear

internal jugular vein vein located at the side of the neck; collects blood from the brain and parts of the face and neck

lacrimal bones small bones located in the wall of the eye sockets

levator anguli oris muscle that raises the angle of the mouth and draws it inward

levator labii superioris muscle surrounding the upper lip

lungs organs of respiration; spongy tissues composed of microscopic cells into which inhaled air penetrates and its oxygen is exchanged for carbon dioxide

lymph colorless, watery fluid that circulates in the lymphatic system; carries waste and impurities from cells

lymphatic (immune) system consists of lymph, lymph nodes, the thymus gland, the spleen, and lymph vessels that act as an aid to the blood system

lymph nodes gland-like structures found inside lymphatic vessels that filter lymph

lymph vascular system also known as the lymphatic system; consists of lymph, lymph nodes, the thymus gland, the spleen, and lymph vessels that act as an aid to the blood system

mandible bone lower jawbone

mandibular nerve branch of the fifth cranial nerve that supplies the muscles and skin of the lower part of the face

masseter one of the jaw muscles used in chewing

maxillary bones bones of the upper jaw

mental nerve nerve that affects the skin of the lower lip and chin

mentalis muscle that elevates the lower lip and raises and wrinkles the skin of the chin

metabolism a complex chemical process whereby cells are nourished and supplied with the energy needed to carry out their activities

metacarpus contains the metacarpal bones in the palm of the hand

middle temporal artery artery that supplies blood to the temples

mitosis cells dividing into two new cells (daughter cells)

mixed nerves nerves that contain both sensory and motor nerve fibers; can send and receive messages

motor nerves nerves that carry impulses from the brain to the muscles

muscular system body system that covers, shapes, and supports the skeletal tissue

myology study of the structure, function, and diseases of the muscles

nasal bones bones that form the bridge of the nose

nasal nerve nerve that affects the point and lower sides of the nose

nucleus dense, active protoplasm found in the center of a cell; important to reproduction and metabolism

occipital artery artery that supplies the scalp and back of the head up to the crown

occipital bone hindmost bone of the skull; located below the parietal bones

occipitalis back of the epicranius; muscle that draws the scalp backward

opponent muscles muscles in the palm that bring the thumb toward the fingers

orbicularis oculi ring muscle of the eye socket

orbicularis oris flat band around the upper and lower lips

organs structures composed of specialized tissues performing specific functions

origin of a muscle more fixed part of a muscle that does not move

parietal artery artery that supplies blood to the side and crown of the head

parietal bones bones that form the sides and top of the cranium

pericardium membrane enclosing the heart

peripheral nervous system (PNS) system that connects the peripheral parts of the body to the central nervous system

phalanges bone of the fingers or toes

physiology study of the functions or activities performed by the body's structures

plasma fluid part of blood and lymph

platelets blood cells that aid in forming clots

platysma muscle that extends from the chest and shoulder to the side of the chin; depresses lower jaw and lip

posterior auricular artery artery that supplies blood to the scalp, behind and above the ear

posterior auricular nerve nerve that affects the muscles behind the ear at the base of the skull

procerus muscle that covers the bridge of the nose, depresses the eyebrows, and wrinkles the nose

radius smaller bone in the forearm on the same side as the thumb

red blood cells cells that carry oxygen from the lungs to the body cells and transport carbon dioxide from the cells back to the lungs

reflex automatic nerve reaction to a stimulus

reproductive system body system responsible for processes by which plants and animals produce offspring

respiratory system consists of the lungs and air passages; enables breathing

risorius muscle of the mouth that draws the corner of the mouth out and back as in grinning

sensory nerves nerves that carry impulses or messages from the sense organs to the brain

seventh cranial nerve chief motor nerve of the face

skeletal system physical foundation of the body; composed of bones and movable and immovable joints

smaller occipital nerve nerve that affects the scalp and muscles behind the ear

sphenoid bone bone that connects all the bones of the cranium

spinal cord portion of the central nervous system that originates in the brain and runs downward through the spinal column

sternocleidomastoideus muscle of the neck that depresses and rotates the head

submental artery artery that supplies blood to the chin and lower lip

superficial temporal artery artery that supplies blood to the muscles of the front, sides, and top of the head

superior labial artery artery that supplies blood to the upper lip and lower region of the nose

supraorbital artery artery that supplies blood to the upper eyelid and forehead

supraorbital nerve nerve that affects the skin of the forehead, scalp, eyebrows, and upper eyelids

supratrochlear nerve nerve that affects the skin between the eyes and the upper side of the nose

systems groups of body organs acting together to perform one or more functions

temporal bones bones that form the sides of the head in the ear region

temporal nerve nerve that affects the muscles of the temple, side of the forehead, eyelid, eyebrow, and upper cheek

temporalis muscle that aids in opening and closing the mouth and chewing

thorax the chest

tissues collections of similar cells that perform a particular function

transverse facial artery artery that supplies blood to the skin and the masseter

trapezius muscle that covers the back of the neck and upper and middle region of the back

triangularis muscle that extends alongside the chin and pulls down the corner of the mouth

ulna inner and larger bone of the forearm

veins blood vessels that carry deoxygenated blood back to the heart from the capillaries

ventricle one of the two lower chambers of the heart

white blood cells perform the function of destroying disease-causing germs

zygomatic bones bones that form the prominence of the cheeks

zygomatic nerve nerve that affects the skin of the temple, side of the forehead, and upper cheek

zygomaticus muscle extending from the zygomatic bone to the angle of the mouth; elevates the lip as in laughing

8 Chemistry

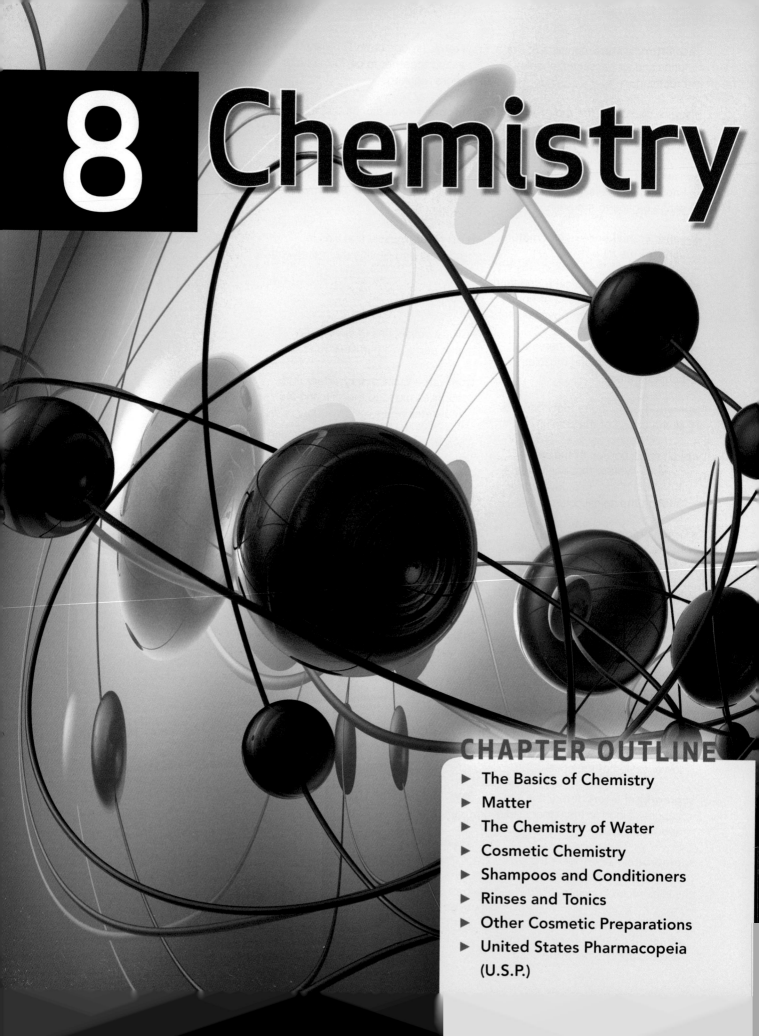

☑ Learning Objectives

AFTER COMPLETING THIS CHAPTER, YOU SHOULD BE ABLE TO:

1 Define *organic* and *inorganic chemistry*.

2 Define *matter* and its states.

3 Define *pH* and understand the pH scale.

4 Explain the characteristics of emulsions, suspensions, and solutions.

5 Understand how the pH level of hair products affect the hair and scalp.

6 Discuss cosmetic preparations used in barbering including shampoos, conditioners, rinses, and tonics.

Key Terms

PAGE NUMBER INDICATES WHERE IN THE CHAPTER THE TERM IS USED.

acid-balanced shampoos / 190

acids / 178

alkalis / 178

atoms / 175

balancing shampoos / 190

bases / 178

bluing rinses / 193

chemical change / 177

chemical properties / 177

chemistry / 174

clarifying shampoos / 190

color-enhancing
    shampoos / 190

compounds / 178

conditioners / 191

deep-conditioning
    treatments / 192

dry or powder
    shampoos / 190

element / 175

emulsions / 185

inorganic chemistry / 174

instant conditioners / 191

ion / 180

ionization / 180

leave-in conditioners / 192

liquid-dry shampoos / 190

matter / 174

medicated rinses / 193

medicated shampoos / 191

moisturizing
    conditioners / 192

moisturizing or conditioning
    shampoos / 191

molecule / 175

organic chemistry / 174

organic shampoos / 191

oxidation / 182

oxides / 178

pH (potential hydrogen) / 180

pH scale / 180

physical change / 177

physical mixture / 179

physical properties / 176

protein conditioners / 192

pure substance / 177

redox / 183

reduction / 183

rinses / 193

salts / 179

scalp conditioners / 192

shampoo / 187

surfactants / 185

suspensions / 184

synthetic polymer
    conditioners / 192

tonic / 194

If you are wondering why you need to study chemistry in the pursuit of your barbering training, pause a moment to consider the many ways in which barbers use chemicals in the barbershop. From glass cleaners to shampoos to color formulations, barbers use chemical products on a daily basis.

One of the most important uses of chemicals in the barbershop is the application of disinfectant and cleaning solutions to maintain an effective program of infection control. In most cases, barbers prepare their own solutions because it is more economical to purchase concentrated products.

Chemicals are also involved in the performance of services when a permanent change to the structure of the hair is desired. These changes are created through the use of haircoloring formulations, permanent waving lotions, and chemical hair-relaxing products. In fact, without chemicals, a permanent change in the hair is not possible!

This chapter provides a general overview of chemistry along with more specific applications to the field of barbering. As a professional barber, it is important to know how to use chemical preparations safely and effectively in the performance of your work.

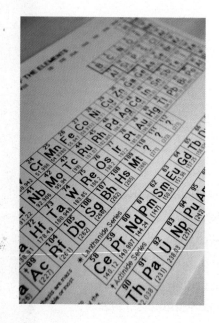

The Basics of Chemistry

Chemistry is the science that deals with the composition, structure, and properties of matter and how matter changes under different chemical conditions. The field is divided into two areas: organic and inorganic chemistry.

Organic chemistry is the study of substances that contain the element carbon; all living things are made of compounds that contain carbon. The term *organic* applies to all living things and those things that were once alive. Gasoline, synthetic fabrics, plastics, and pesticides are all considered organic because they are manufactured from natural gas and oil, which are the remains of plants and animals that died millions of years ago. Most organic substances will burn.

Inorganic chemistry is the study of substances that do not contain carbon but may contain hydrogen. Inorganic substances are not, and never were, alive; therefore, they will not burn. Metals, minerals, water, air, and ammonia are inorganic substances.

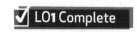

Matter

Matter may be defined as anything that occupies space and has physical and chemical properties. It exists in the states of solids, liquids, and gases.

To further understand the concept of matter, look around your classroom and note what can be seen: people, desks, chairs, walls, and so forth. These are all matter in a solid state. In the clinic area of the school, water, shampoos, lotions, and hair tonics can be seen. These solutions are matter in a liquid state. Take a deep breath. The air you have just brought into your lungs is also matter. It is in a gaseous state.

Although matter has physical properties that we can touch, taste, see, or smell, not everything we see is matter. For example, we can see visible light and color, but these are forms of energy, and energy is not matter.

ELEMENTS

An **element** is a pure chemical substance that cannot be separated into simpler substances by chemical means. Chemical elements are the basic materials that make up all matter and each one has its own kind of atom. As of 2008, 94 of the 117 known elements have been found to occur naturally on Earth. All the matter in the known universe is made from these elements. Each element is given a letter symbol such as O for oxygen, S for sulfur, or H for hydrogen, and an atomic number that indicates how many protons are in one atom of an element. The full periodic table of elements can be found in any chemistry book.

Atoms are the basic building blocks of all matter and the smallest part of an element that retains the characteristics of that element. Although the word *atom* comes from the Greek word atomos, meaning *indivisible*, physicists have proven the existence of subatomic components within atoms. Atoms consist of *protons* (positive electrical charge), *neutrons* (no electrical charge), and *electrons* (negative electrical charge). The number of protons identifies an atom and also provides the atom with its atomic number. For example, the atomic number of oxygen is 8 because oxygen has eight protons; it also commonly has eight neutrons and eight electrons.

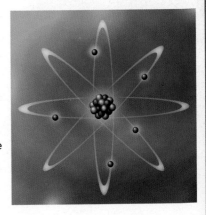

A **molecule** is formed when two or more atoms are joined by a chemical bond. *Elemental molecules* are chemical combinations of two or more atoms of the same element. An example is the oxygen (O_2) in the air we breathe **(Figure 8-1)**. *Compound molecules* are chemical combinations of two or more atoms of different elements **(Figure 8-2)**. Sodium chloride, or common table salt, is a compound molecule that is a chemical combination of one atom of sodium (Na) and one atom of chlorine (Cl).

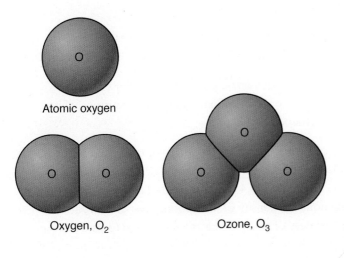

Atomic oxygen

Oxygen, O_2

Ozone, O_3

◄ FIGURE

Elem

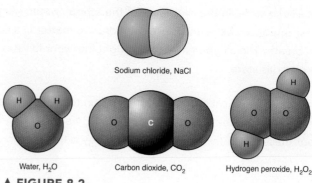

Sodium chloride, NaCl

Water, H₂O

Carbon dioxide, CO₂

Hydrogen peroxide, H₂O₂

▲ FIGURE 8-2

Compound molecules.

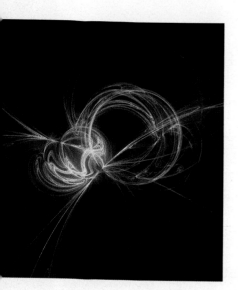

STATES OF MATTER

All matter exists in one of three different physical forms: solid, liquid, or gas (Figure 8-3). When energy is added through increased temperature or pressure, or taken away through decreased temperature or pressure, changes in the states of matter occur. For example, the form of water changes according to changes in the temperature, but it is still water. As ice, water is in a solid state with definite shape and volume. When water is liquid, it has volume, but no definite shape. As steam, it is an example of a gas, which does not have volume or shape.

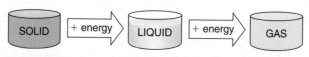

SOLID + energy LIQUID + energy GAS

▲ FIGURE 8-3

States of matter.

PHYSICAL AND CHEMICAL PROPERTIES OF MATTER

Every substance has unique properties that facilitate identification. The two different types of properties are *physical* and *chemical*.

Physical properties are those characteristics that can be determined without a chemical reaction and without a chemical change in the identity of the substance. Physical properties include color, odor, density, weight, melting point, boiling point, and hardness.

- *Color* helps in the identification of many substances; for instance, gold, silver, copper, brass, and coal are identified in part by their color.

- The *odor* of a substance can help to identify it. For example, the characteristic odor of ammonium thioglycolate is one of its distinguishing characteristics.

- The *density* of a substance refers to its *weight* divided by its volume. For example, 1 cubic foot of water weighs 62.4 pounds. Therefore, its density is its weight (62.4 pounds) divided by its volume (1 cubic foot), which equals a density of 62.4 pounds per cubic foot. The degree of hardness of a substance can also relate to its density.

- *Melting* and *boiling points* are the degrees at which a substance will melt or boil.

- *Hardness* refers to a substance's ability to resist being deformed, such as by scratching or indentation.

Chemical properties are those characteristics that can only be determined with a chemical reaction and that cause a change in the identity of the substance. Rusting iron and burning wood are examples of a change in chemical properties. In both these examples, the chemical reaction of oxidation creates a chemical change: iron is chemically changed to rust, and wood is chemically changed to ash.

PHYSICAL AND CHEMICAL CHANGES OF MATTER

As can be seen from the discussion of the states of matter, matter can be changed in two different ways: physically and chemically.

- A **physical change** does not form a new substance; therefore there are no chemical reactions or new chemicals formed in the process (Figure 8-4). An example of physical change is ice melting to water. Temporary haircolor is another example of physical change because it physically adds color to the surface of the hair, but does not create a chemical change in the hair's structure or color.

- A **chemical change** occurs when there is a change in the chemical composition of a substance, as with the iron-to-rust example (Figure 8-5). Chemical changes in the hair can be created with permanent haircolor because the chemical reaction of oxidation takes place to develop the dye in the color. Oxidation creates chemical changes in the hair's structure and in its color, forming new chemicals in the process.

PURE SUBSTANCES AND PHYSICAL MIXTURES

All matter can be classified as either a pure substance or a physical mixture (Figure 8-6). A **pure substance** is matter that has a fixed chemical

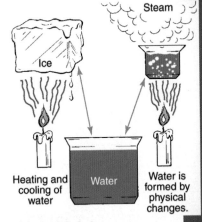

▲ **FIGURE 8-4**

Physical changes.

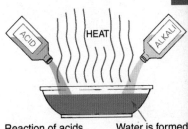

Reaction of acids with alkalis (neutralization)   Water is formed by chemical change.

▲ **FIGURE 8-5**

Chemical changes.

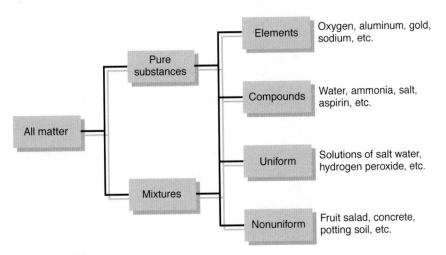

		Elements	Oxygen, aluminum, gold, sodium, etc.
All matter	Pure substances		
		Compounds	Water, ammonia, salt, aspirin, etc.
		Uniform	Solutions of salt water, hydrogen peroxide, etc.
	Mixtures		
		Nonuniform	Fruit salad, concrete, potting soil, etc.

▲ **FIGURE 8-6**

Pure substances and mixtures.

TABLE 8-1 Chemical Compounds and Physical Mixtures

CHEMICAL COMPOUNDS	PHYSICAL MIXTURES
Involve a chemical reaction	Do not involve a chemical reaction
Change the chemical properties	Change only the physical properties
Mixed in definite proportions	Mixed in any proportions
Water (H_2O) or salt ($NaCl$) are examples	Salt water is an example
Pure hydrogen peroxide is an example	Solutions of hydrogen peroxide are examples

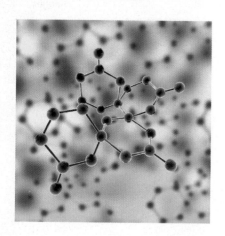

composition, definite proportions, and distinct properties. Elements and compounds are pure substances.

Elemental molecules contain two or more atoms of the same element that unite chemically. Aluminum foil is an example of a pure substance; it is composed only of atoms of the element aluminum.

Chemical compounds are combinations of two or more atoms of different elements united chemically with fixed chemical composition, definite proportions, and distinct properties. Chemical compounds are the result of a chemical reaction. Water is a chemical compound consisting of two atoms of hydrogen and one atom of oxygen. Table 8-1 summarizes the differences between chemical compounds and physical mixtures.

Compounds can be divided into four classifications of importance to barbering:

1. **Oxides** are compounds of any element combined with oxygen. For example, one part carbon and two parts oxygen create carbon dioxide. One part carbon and one part oxygen create carbon monoxide.

2. **Acids** are compounds of hydrogen, a nonmetal such as nitrogen, and, sometimes, oxygen. For example, hydrogen, sulphur, and oxygen combine to form sulphuric acid. Acids turn blue litmus paper red, providing a quick way to test a compound.

3. **Bases,** also known as **alkalis,** are compounds of hydrogen, a metal, and oxygen. For example, sodium, oxygen, and hydrogen form sodium

hydroxide, which is used in the manufacture of soap. Bases will turn red litmus paper blue.

4. **Salts** are compounds that are formed by the reaction of acids and bases, with water also produced by the reaction. Two common salts are sodium chloride (table salt), which contains sodium and chloride, and magnesium sulphate (Epsom salts), which contains magnesium, sulphur, hydrogen, and oxygen.

A **physical mixture** is a combination of two or more substances united physically in any proportions without a fixed composition. Pure air is a physical mixture of mostly nitrogen and oxygen gases. Concrete is another example because it is composed of water, sand, gravel, and cement. It is a mixture that has its own functions, yet does not lose the characteristics of the individual ingredients.

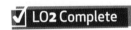

The Chemistry of Water

Water (H_2O) is the most abundant and important of all chemicals, composing about 75 percent of the earth's surface and about 65 percent of the human body. Water is known as the universal solvent, because it dissolves more substances than any other liquid. Distilled or de-mineralized water is used as a nonconductor of electricity, while water containing certain mineral substances is an excellent conductor of electricity.

Water is purified through boiling, filtration, or distillation. Boiling water at 212 degrees Fahrenheit destroys most microbes and renders it suitable for drinking. During filtration, water passes through a porous substance, such as filter paper or charcoal, to remove organic material. Distillation is the process whereby water is heated to a vapor in a closed vessel. The vapors are captured and passed off through a tube into another vessel, where they are cooled and condensed to a liquid. This process purifies water used in the manufacturing of cosmetics.

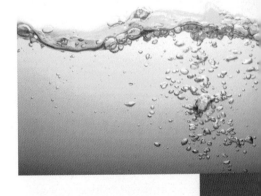

Soft water is rainwater or chemically treated water that has low levels of mineral substances such as calcium and magnesium salts. Lesser amounts of such minerals in soft water allow for soaps and shampoos to lather freely. It is the best choice for use in the barbershop.

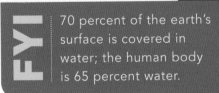

FYI 70 percent of the earth's surface is covered in water; the human body is 65 percent water.

Hard water contains mineral substances, such as calcium and magnesium salts, that curdle or precipitate soap instead of permitting a permanent lather to form. Hard water may be softened by distillation or by the use of sodium carbonate (washing soda) or sodium phosphate.

WATER AND pH

The letters **pH** denote **potential hydrogen,** the relative degree of acidity or alkalinity of a substance. The **pH scale** measures the concentration of hydrogen ions in acidic and alkaline water-based solutions. Notice that pH is written with a small *p*, which represents quantity, and a capital *H*, which represents the hydrogen ion.

A basic understanding of ions is important to an understanding of pH. An **ion** is an atom or molecule that carries an electrical charge. **Ionization** is the separation of a substance into ions that have opposite electrical charges. A negatively charged ion is called an anion, and a positively charged ion is called a cation.

In pure water, some of the water molecules ionize naturally into hydrogen ions and hydroxide ions. The pH scale measures those ions. The hydrogen ion is acidic and the hydroxide ion is alkaline. The ionization of water is what makes pH possible because only aqueous (water) solutions have pH. Non-aqueous solutions, such as alcohol or oil, do not have pH. In pure water, every water molecule that ionizes produces one hydrogen ion and one hydroxide ion **(Figure 8-7)**. Pure water contains the same number of hydrogen ions as hydroxide ions, which makes it neutral. Pure water is 50 percent acidic and 50 percent alkaline, as denoted by the number 7 on the pH scale **(Figure 8-8)**.

The pH scale

The pH values are arranged on a scale ranging from 0 to 14. A pH of 7 indicates a neutral solution, a pH below 7 indicates an acidic solution, and a pH above 7 indicates an alkaline solution **(Figure 8-9)**.

The pH scale is a logarithmic scale, which means that a change of one whole number represents a tenfold change in pH. For example, a pH of 8 is 10 times more alkaline than a pH of 7. A change of two whole numbers indicates a change of 10 times 10, or a hundredfold change. A pH of 9 is 100 times more alkaline than a pH of 7.

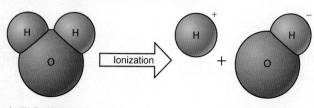

▲ **FIGURE 8-7**

The ionization of water.

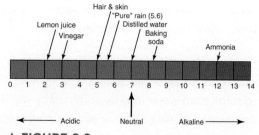

▲ **FIGURE 8-8**

The pH scale (horizontal).

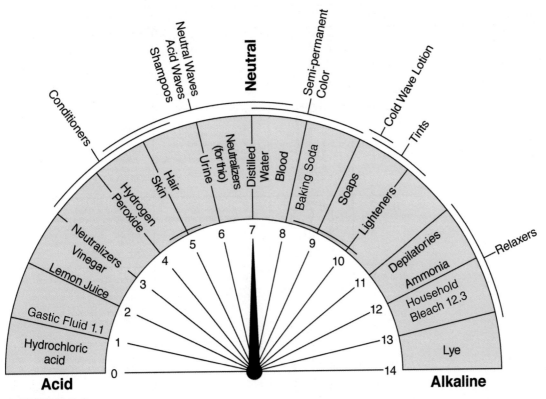

▲ FIGURE 8-9

The pH scale.

The pH range of hair and skin is 4.5 to 5.5, with an average of 5, on the pH scale. That means that pure water is 100 times more alkaline than hair and skin, even though it has a neutral pH. In fact, pure water can cause the hair to swell up to 20 percent.

Acids and Alkalis

All acids owe their chemical reactivity to the hydrogen ion (H+). Acids have a pH below 7.0, taste sour, and turn litmus paper from blue to red. Acidic solutions tend to contract and harden the hair **(Figure 8-10)**. As toners or skin fresheners, they also tighten the skin.

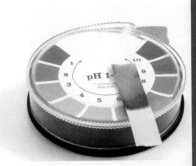

All alkalis owe their chemical reactivity to the hydroxide (OH–) ion. The terms *alkalis* and *bases* are interchangeable. Alkalis have a pH above 7.0, taste bitter, feel slippery on the skin, and turn litmus paper from red to blue. Alkalis soften and swell the hair (Figure 8-10). Sodium hydroxide (lye) is a very strong alkali used in chemical drain cleaners and chemical hair relaxers.

Acid-Alkali Neutralization Reactions

When acids and alkalis are mixed together in equal proportions, they neutralize each other to form water and a salt. For example, because hydrochloric acid is a strong acid and sodium hydroxide is a strong alkali, they will neutralize each other when mixed in equal amounts and form a solution of pure water and table salt. Acid-balanced shampoos and normalizing lotions

Solution	Effect on Hair		Important Features
Very Strong Acid (pH 0.0—1.0)	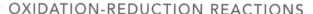	Dissolves hair completely.	Must not be applied to hair or scalp.
Strong to Mild Acid (pH 1.0—4.5)		Hair shrinks and hardens. Body is increased. Cuticle imbrications close up. Porosity is reduced. Sheen of hair is improved. Soap residues are removed. Neutralizes traces of alkalis.	Acid or cream rinses restore body to bleached, porous hair. Conditioners and fillers overcome the excess porosity of damaged hair. Special shampoos reduce tangling and matting of hair and prevent color loss. Hair creams increase sheen. Color rinses provide temporary effect. Neutralizers remove residual waving lotion.
Neutral (pH 4.5—5.5)		Hair is normal diameter. Texture and luster standard.	Neutral solutions are designed to prevent excess swelling of normal and damaged hair. Mild shampoos for normal cleaning and manageability of hair.
Mild Alkali (pH 5.5—10.0)		Hair swells. Porosity increases as imbrications open. Hair has a dry, drab appearance.	Tints and bleaches penetrate easier and chemical action increases. Cold wave solutions for resistant hair. Soap shampoos to overcome acidity of tap water. Activators for hydrogen peroxide.
Stronger Alkali (pH 10.0—14.0)		Dissolves hair completely.	Must not be applied to hair or scalp unless used as relaxers or depilatories.

▲ **FIGURE 8-10**

The effect of pH on hair.

associated with hydroxide hair relaxers work to create a similar acid–alkali neutralization reaction.

OXIDATION-REDUCTION REACTIONS

Oxidation is a chemical reaction that combines an element or compound with oxygen to produce an oxide. When oxygen combines with another element, some heat is usually produced. Chemical reactions that are characterized by the giving off of heat are called *exothermic*. For example, exothermic permanent waving lotions produce heat because of an oxidation reaction. *Slow oxidation* occurs in oxidation haircolors and permanent wave neutralizers. When hydrogen peroxide is added to oxidation haircolors, there will be an increase in the temperature due to the process of oxidation.

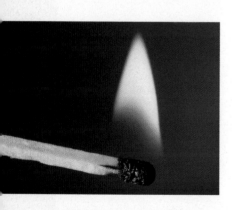

NOTE: To provide a frame of reference for slow oxidation, it might be helpful to know that combustion is a form of *rapid oxidation* reaction that produces a high quantity of heat and light. For instance, lighting a match is an example of rapid oxidation.

When oxygen is combined with a substance, the substance is *oxidized*. When oxygen is removed from a substance, the substance is *reduced*. Oxidizing agents are substances that release oxygen. Hydrogen peroxide is an oxidizing agent because it contains extra oxygen. When hydrogen peroxide is mixed with an oxidation haircolor, the haircolor gains oxygen. At the same time the hydrogen peroxide loses oxygen and is therefore reduced.

Oxidation and **reduction** always occur simultaneously and are referred to as **redox** reactions. In a redox reaction, the oxidizer is always reduced and the reducing agent is always oxidized.

Many oxidation reactions do not involve oxygen. Oxidation also results from the loss of hydrogen, and reduction is the result of the addition of hydrogen. Permanent waving is an example of this type of redox reaction. Permanent waving solution contains thioglycolate acid. The waving solution breaks the disulfide bonds in the hair through a reduction reaction that adds hydrogen ions to the hair. In this reaction, the hair is reduced and the permanent waving solution is oxidized. After processing and rinsing, the neutralizer is used to oxidize the hair by removing the hydrogen that was previously added with the waving solution. When the hair has oxidized, the neutralizer will have been reduced in the process.

When performing chemical services, the term *oxidation* is used to define either the addition of oxygen or the loss of hydrogen. Conversely, the term *reduction* is used to define either the loss of oxygen or the addition of hydrogen. Refer to Chapters 18 and 19 for more detailed information about pH and the products used to effect chemical changes in the hair.

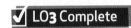
✓ **LO3 Complete**

Cosmetic Chemistry

Cosmetic chemistry is the scientific study of the cosmetic products used in the barbering and cosmetology industries. An understanding of the different types of products that are available will better equip barbers to service their clientele in the barbershop. The principal physical and chemical classifications of cosmetics are powders, solutions, suspensions, emulsions, soaps, and ointments.

POWDERS
Powders consist of a uniform mixture of insoluble substances, inorganic, organic, and colloidal, that have been properly blended, perfumed, and/or tinted.

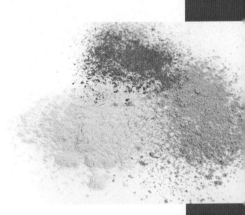

SOLUTIONS
A *solution* is a mixture of two or more substances that is made by dissolving a solid, liquid, or gaseous substance in another substance. A solute is any substance that is dissolved into a solvent to form a solution. A solvent is any substance, usually a liquid, that dissolves the solute to form a solution. The components of a solution are illustrated in **Figure 8-11**. When a gas or

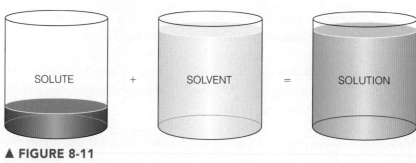

▲ FIGURE 8-11
Components of a solution.

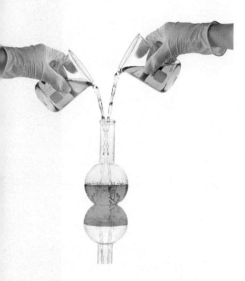

a solid is dissolved in a liquid, the gas or solid is the solute and the liquid is the solvent.

Solutions are usually clear or transparent permanent mixtures of a solute and a solvent that do not separate upon standing. The particles in solutions are invisible to the naked eye. Salt water and hydrogen peroxide are two examples of solutions. Salt water is a solution of a solid dissolved in a liquid. Water is the solvent that dissolves the salt and holds it in a solution. Solutions can also be prepared by dissolving a powdered solute in a warm solvent and stirring at the same time.

Water is a universal solvent. It is capable of dissolving more substances than any other liquid. Grain alcohol and glycerin are also used frequently as solvents. Water, glycerin, and alcohol readily mix with each other; therefore they are *miscible* (mixable). On the other hand, water and oil do not mix with each other; hence they are *immiscible* (unmixable).

The solute may be either a solid, liquid, or gas. For example, boric acid solution is a mixture of a solid in a liquid; glycerin and rose water is a mixture of two miscible liquids; and ammonia water is a mixture of a gas in water.

NOTE: Solutions containing volatile substances such as ammonia and alcohol should be stored in a cool place to avoid evaporation.

Solutions may be classified as dilute, concentrated, or saturated solutions. A *dilute solution* contains a small quantity of the solute in proportion to the quantity of solvent. A *concentrated solution* contains a large quantity of the solute in proportion to the quantity of solvent. A *saturated solution* will not dissolve or take up more solute than it already holds at a given temperature.

SUSPENSIONS

Suspensions are uniform mixtures of two or more substances. The particles in suspensions can be seen with the naked eye because they are larger than the particles in solutions. Suspensions are not usually transparent, may be colored, and tend to separate over time. Many of the products used by barbers, such as hair tonics, are suspensions and should be shaken or mixed well before use. Salad dressing, calamine lotion, paint, and aerosol hair spray are also examples of suspensions.

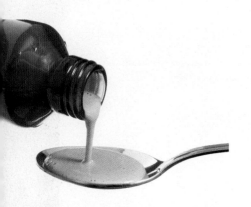

EMULSIONS

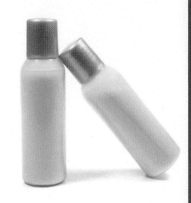

Emulsions are suspensions (mixtures) of two immiscible liquids held together by an emulsifying agent. An emulsion is a suspension of one liquid dispersed in another. Although emulsions tend to separate over time, with proper formulation and storage an emulsion may remain stable for at least three years. Mayonnaise is an oil-in-water emulsion of two immiscible liquids. The egg yolk in mayonnaise emulsifies the oil droplets and disperses them uniformly in the water. Mayonnaise should not separate upon standing. Review Table 8-2 for a summary of the differences between solutions, suspensions, and emulsions.

A **surfactant** is a substance that acts as a bridge to allow oil and water to mix or emulsify by reducing surface tension. A surfactant molecule has two distinct parts: the head of the molecule is hydrophilic (water-loving) and the tail is lipophilic (oil-loving) (Figure 8-12). Since "like dissolves like," the hydrophilic head dissolves in water and the lipophilic tail dissolves in oil.

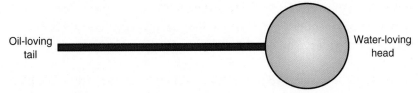

Oil-loving tail   Water-loving head

▲ FIGURE 8-12

Surfactant molecules.

> TABLE **8-2** Solutions, Suspensions, and Emulsions

SOLUTIONS	SUSPENSIONS	EMULSIONS
Miscible	Slightly miscible	Immiscible
No surfactant	No surfactant	Surfactant
Small particles	Larger particles	Largest particles
Usually clear	Usually cloudy	Usually a solid color
Stable mixture	Unstable mixture	Limited stability
Solution of hydrogen peroxide	Calamine lotion	Shampoos and conditioners

Thus, the surfactant molecule dissolves in both water and oil and joins them together to form an emulsion. Surfactants are used in thousands of products that result in an emulsion.

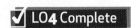

SOAPS

Soaps are compounds made by mixing plant oils or animal fats with strong alkaline substances. Glycerin is also formed in the process. Potassium hydroxide produces a soft soap, whereas sodium hydroxide forms a hard soap. A mixture of the two alkalis will yield a soap of intermediate consistency. A good soap does not contain excess free alkali and is made from pure oils and fats. Soaps used in the industry may be categorized as deodorant soaps, beauty soaps, medicated soaps, and shaving soaps.

Deodorant soaps include a bactericide that remains on the body to kill the bacteria responsible for odors. One of the most common antiseptic and anti-bacterial agents used in these soaps is triclocarban. Triclocarban, often listed in the ingredients as TCC, is prepared from aniline. Aniline additives have been known to increase the skin's sensitivity to the sun.

Beauty soaps are intended for the more delicate tissues of the face. They have a more acid pH and are less drying to the skin, yet are able to remove dirt and oil from the skin's surface. Many beauty soaps are transparent and contain large quantities of glycerin. Other beauty soaps contain larger amounts of oils that leave an emollient film on the skin.

Medicated soaps are designed to treat skin problems such as rashes, pimples, and acne. Many contain small percentages of cresol, phenol, or other antiseptics. Resorcinol is often used as a drying agent in medicated products designed to treat oily conditions. The strongest medicated soaps can be obtained only with a doctor's prescription.

Shaving soaps can be purchased in various forms and shapes. Hard shaving soaps include those sold in cake, stick, or powdered form, and are similar in composition to toilet soaps. They are also available as soft soaps, such as shaving cream in a tube, jar, or press-button container. Liquid soaps are another option that barbers and stylists can utilize. Whatever form of shaving soap is used, it usually contains animal and/or vegetable oils, alkaline substances, and water. The presence of coconut and other plant oils tends to improve the lathering qualities of shaving soap.

OINTMENTS

Ointments are semisolid mixtures of organic substances, such as lard, petrolatum, or wax, and a medicinal agent. No water is present. For the ointment to soften, its melting point should be below body temperature (98.6 degrees Fahrenheit). Ointments are prepared by melting an organic substance and mixing it with a medicinal agent.

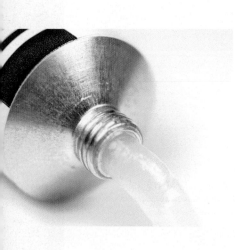

Shampoos and Conditioners

Most shampoo products are emulsions, and there are many different types on the market. As a professional barber, you will need to become skilled at selecting products that best serve the condition of the client's hair and scalp. Make it a standard operating procedure to read manufacturer's labels so that an informed choice can be made. In addition, display and use the barbershop's retail products at the workstation or shampoo sink back bar. Doing so not only promotes product sales, but also demonstrates to clients that the barber endorses the product and its effectiveness inside and outside the barbershop.

To be effective, a **shampoo** must remove all dirt, oil, perspiration, and skin debris, without adversely affecting either the scalp or the hair. The hair collects dust particles, natural oils from the sebaceous glands, perspiration, and dead skin cells that can accumulate on the scalp. This accumulation creates a breeding ground for disease-producing bacteria, which can lead to scalp disorders. The hair and scalp should be thoroughly shampooed as frequently as is necessary to keep them clean, healthy, and free from bacteria.

An effective shampoo product should:

- cleanse the hair of oils, debris, and dirt.

- work efficiently in hard as well as soft water.

- not irritate the eyes or skin.

- leave the hair and scalp in their natural condition.

SHAMPOO CHEMISTRY

The acidity or alkalinity of a shampoo is important because it influences how the product will affect various layers of the hair and skin. Acidic solutions (below pH 7.0) shrink, constrict, and harden the cuticle scales of the hair shaft. An alkaline solution (above pH 7.0) softens, swells, and expands the cuticle scales. Remember, the lower the pH of a solution, the greater the degree of acidity; the higher the pH of a solution, the greater the degree of alkalinity (See Figure 8-9).

Shampoo emulsions usually range between 4.5 and 7.5 on the pH scale. Since the normal pH range for hair and skin is 4.5 to 5.5, mild or more acidic shampoos are found closer to this range. Conversely, stronger or more alkaline shampoos are found beyond 6.0 on the pH scale.

SHAMPOO MOLECULES

Shampoos consist of two main ingredients: water and surfactants. Next to water, surfactants are the second most common ingredient found in shampoos and acts as cleansing, emulsifying, or foaming agents. Shampoo molecules are created by combining water and at least one surfactant. These molecules are composed of a head and tail, each with its own special

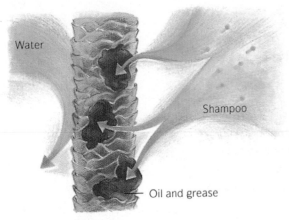

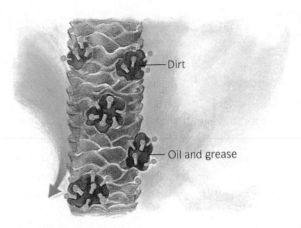

▲ FIGURE 8-13

The tail of the shampoo molecule is attracted to oil and dirt.

▲ FIGURE 8-14

Shampoo causes oils to run up into small globules.

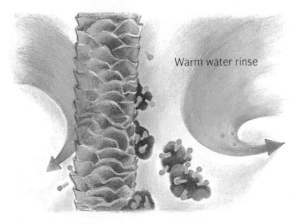

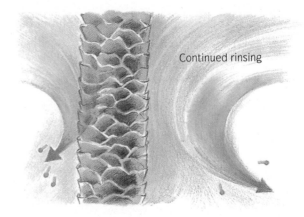

▲ FIGURE 8-15

During rinsing, the heads of the shampoo molecules attach to water molecules and cause debris to roll off.

▲ FIGURE 8-16

Thorough rinsing washes away debris and excess shampoo.

function. In a shampoo molecule the tail attracts dirt, grease, debris, and oil, but repels water. The head of the shampoo molecule attracts water, but repels dirt. Working together, both parts of the molecule effectively cleanse the hair (**Figures 8-13** to **8-16**).

The base surfactant or combination of surfactants determines the classification of a shampoo. These classifications include *anionic, cationic, nonionic,* and *amphoteric* surfactants. Most manufacturers use detergents from more than one classification. It is customary to use a secondary surfactant to complement, or offset, the negative qualities of the base surfactant. For example, an amphoteric that is nonirritating to the eyes can be added to a harsh anionic to create a product that is more comfortable to use.

- *Anionics* (negatively charged), such as sodium lauryl sulfate and sodium laureth sulfate, are the most commonly used detergents. Sodium lauryl sulfate is a relatively harsh cleanser that produces a rich foam. It is suitable for use in hard or soft water because it rinses easily from the hair. Sodium laureth sulfate is also a strong, rich, foaming detergent but, because it is less alkaline than lauryl sulfates, it is often used in shampoos that are designed to be milder or less drying to the hair shaft.

- *Cationics* (positively charged) are made up almost entirely of quaternary ammonium compounds, or quats. Practically all quaternary compounds have some antibacterial action so they are sometimes included in the chemical composition of dandruff shampoos.

- *Nonionics* (no charge) are valued as surfactants for their versatility, stability, and ability to resist shrinkage, particularly in cold temperatures. They have a mild cleansing action and low incidence of irritation to human tissues. Cocamide (DEA, MEA) is one of the most widely used nonionics in the industry, not only in shampoos but also in lipsticks and permanent waving lotions.

- *Amphoterics* (positively or negatively charged) can behave as an anionic or a cationic substance, depending on the pH of the solution. Amphoteric surfactants have a slight tendency to cling to hair and skin, which aids in hair manageability. They also possess germicidal properties that vary between derivatives. Amphoteric surfactants are used in several baby shampoos because they do not sting the eyes. Many amphoterics are identified on the ingredient list as *Amphoteric I-20*.

A familiarity with these surfactant classifications and their use in shampoo products should assist the barber in making professional decisions when selecting the appropriate product for use on a client's hair and scalp.

Additional ingredients in the forms of moisturizers, preservatives, foam enhancers, perfumes, and others are added to create a variety of shampoo formulations. Along with water and base surfactants, these ingredients are listed on product labels in descending order according to the percentage of each ingredient in the shampoo.

CATEGORIES OF SHAMPOOS

Shampoo products account for the highest dollar expenditure in haircare products and are available in liquid, liquid-dry, and dry or powder formulations. Until a few decades ago, shampoo (and conditioner) choices were limited to a few types and brands. The standard shampoos then included plain, liquid cream, castile, egg, and green soap shampoos.

Today, barbers have a wide variety of products that are suitable for most hair and scalp conditions. There are shampoos for dry, oily, normal, fine, coarse, limp, or chemically treated hair. There are shampoos that add a slight amount of color to hair and those that cleanse the hair of mineral deposits and product buildup. Many manufacturers have become more "hair condition conscious" so that even medicated shampoos are less drying to the hair and scalp.

A visit to your local barber supply store will introduce you to a wide variety of products for use in the barbershop. The following provides basic information that may be needed to make an informed choice concerning the categories of shampoos.

Liquid shampoos are available in cream or clear (plain) forms. *Liquid cream shampoos* are usually fairly thick liquids that contain either soap or soap jelly. Magnesium stearate may be used as a whitening agent. These shampoos often contain oily compounds to make the hair feel silky and softer. Use this type of shampoo as directed by your instructor or the manufacturer. *Plain shampoos* are usually translucent and may be clear or tinted. These shampoos seldom have lanolin or other special agents used to leave a gloss on the hair. A plain shampoo may be used on hair that is in good condition, but not on color-treated hair because it may strip or fade the color.

Liquid-dry shampoos are cosmetic products used for cleansing the scalp and hair when the client is prevented from having a regular shampoo. Some have an astringent quality that allows the product to evaporate quickly.

Dry or powder shampoos can be used when the client's health will not permit a wet shampoo or the service is too uncomfortable. Powder or dry shampoos may contain orris root powder and cleanse the hair without the use of water. The shampoo is sprinkled onto the hair, where it picks up dirt and oils as it is brushed through the hair. Always follow the manufacturer's directions and never give a dry shampoo prior to a chemical service.

TYPES OF SHAMPOOS

Most of today's shampoos can be classified as belonging to one of the following shampoo types.

Acid-balanced shampoos are balanced to the pH level of hair and skin and usually contain citric, lactic, or phosphoric acid. These shampoos are mild formulations designed to prevent the stripping of haircolor from the hair. They have a low alkaline content, which makes them a good choice for normal, chemically treated, and fragile hair. Follow the manufacturer's directions, but most acid-balanced shampoos can be used daily.

Balancing shampoos are designed for oily hair and scalps. These shampoos wash away excess oiliness while keeping the hair from drying out.

Clarifying shampoos contain an acidic ingredient such as cider vinegar to cut through product buildup that can coat and flatten hair. They provide thorough cleansing and should be used only when buildup is evident. Once- or twice-weekly applications should suffice, depending on how much styling product the client uses. These shampoos are also helpful in preparing the hair for chemical services or to remove medication or hard-water mineral buildup from the hair.

Color-enhancing shampoos are created by combining the surfactant with basic colors. They are attracted to porous hair and provide only slight color changes, which are removed with plain shampooing. Color shampoos are used to brighten the hair, add slight color, and eliminate unwanted color tones.

Medicated shampoos contain a medicinal or antiseptic agent such as sulfur, tar, cresol, or phenol. They are usually effective in reducing dandruff or relieving scalp conditions. Although sold without a prescription, they may be strong enough to affect the color of tinted or lightened hair. *Therapeutic medicated shampoos* contain special chemicals or drugs that are very effective in reducing excessive dandruff. They must be used only by prescription and instructions should be followed carefully.

Moisturizing or conditioning shampoos are usually mild cream shampoos that contain moisturizing agents (*humectants*) designed either to "lock in" the moisturizing properties of the product or to draw moisture into the hair. They are formulated to make the hair smooth and shiny and to avoid damaging chemically treated hair. Protein and biotin are conditioning agents that help restore moisture and elasticity, strengthen the hair shaft, and add volume. Like acid-balanced shampoos, moisturizing shampoos will not remove artificial color from the hair.

Organic shampoos are some of the most recent to be available on the market, yet their origins are centuries old. True organic formulations will contain natural, organic substances such as herbs, flowering or other plants, and/or minerals. Aloe vera, nettles, chamomile, or jojoba are just some of the ingredients that may be formulated into these shampoos, which are usually pH balanced.

CONDITIONERS

Much like shampoos, in past decades the availability of commercial conditioners was limited. Products such as olive oil preparations, cholesterol, and cream rinses represented the usual choice range.

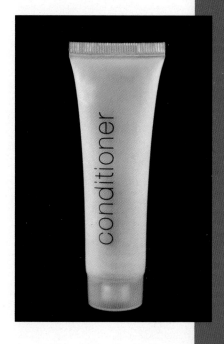

Conditioners are special chemical agents that are applied to hair to deposit protein or moisture, restore hair strength and body, or protect against possible damage. Conditioners typically range from 3.0 to 5.5 on the pH scale. They are temporary remedies for hair that feels dry or is damaged. Conditioners cannot actually repair damaged hair, nor can they permanently improve the quality of new hair growth.

Excessive use of conditioners, or using the wrong type of conditioner, can lead to a heavy or oily buildup of product on the hair. For this reason, the barber needs to be able to select the right product, for example, a cream rinse for detangling or a reconstructor for damaged hair.

Conditioners are available in three basic types: instant (or rinse-out), treatment or repair, and leave-in. The barber must decide the type to use based on the texture and condition of the hair and the desired results.

Instant conditioners are applied to the hair following a shampoo and are rinsed out after 1 to 5 minutes. They usually have a lower pH than the hair, which helps to close the cuticle scales. The typical instant conditioner does not penetrate into the hair shaft but may add oils, moisture, and sometimes protein to the cuticle scales of the hair. Finishing rinses, detangling rinses, and cream rinses are examples of instant conditioners.

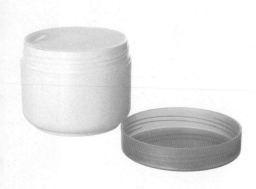

Moisturizing conditioners contain chemical compounds called *humectants* that absorb and promote the retention of moisture in the hair. They can also seal moisture inside damp hair by coating the cuticle. Moisturizing conditioners are usually heavier than instant conditioners and have a longer application time of 10 to 20 minutes. They often contain the same ingredients as instant conditioners, but are formulated to be more penetrating. Some require the use of heat for deeper penetration and longer-lasting results. Quaternary ammonium compounds are included in the formulation of moisturizers for their ability to attach to hair fibers. Natural moisturizing ingredients may include oils, essential fatty acids, sodium PCA, and sometimes botanicals. Coating moisturizers usually contain wax or glycerin in addition to other ingredients.

Protein conditioners are available in a cream form with moisturizers and oils and in a concentrated liquid-protein form. Both utilize hydrolized protein for its ability to pass through the cuticle to penetrate the cortex, where the keratin has been lost from the hair. These conditioners improve texture, equalize porosity, and help to increase elasticity in the hair. The hair should be well rinsed prior to cutting, setting, or drying, as excess conditioner may coat or weigh down the hair.

Deep-conditioning treatments, also known as hair masks or conditioning packs, are chemical mixtures of concentrated protein in the heavy cream base of a moisturizer. They penetrate several layers of the cuticle and are the preferred therapy when an equal degree of moisturizing and protein treatment is desired. As with the previously discussed conditioners, deep-conditioning treatments require thorough rinsing prior to other services.

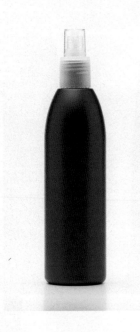

Synthetic polymer conditioners are special formulations for use on badly damaged hair. A polymer is a compound consisting of many repeating units that form a chain. Hair is a natural polymer and when it is so severely damaged that normal protein conditioners cannot recondition it, a synthetic polymer may be necessary to prevent breakage and correct excessive porosity.

Leave-in conditioners, such as spray-on thermal protectors (blow-drying sprays), are products that should not be rinsed out of the hair. Some are designed for use with thermal tools, while others are included with some chemical service products to equalize the porosity of the hair shaft.

Scalp conditioners are available in a variety of formulations and for different purposes. Cream-based products with moisturizers and emollients are usually used to soften and improve the health of the scalp. *Medicated scalp lotions* are conditioners that promote the healing of the scalp. *Astringent scalp tonics* help to remove oil accumulation on the scalp and are used after a scalp treatment.

It is the barber's responsibility to be knowledgeable about the products used in the shop or salon. Basic product knowledge can be easily obtained from product labels, distributors, trade show demonstrations, and manufacturer representatives. See **Table 8-3** for shampoo and conditioning products suitable for different hair types.

HAIR TYPE	FINE	MEDIUM	COARSE
Straight	Volumizing shampoo Detangler, if necessary Protein treatments	Acid-balanced shampoo Finishing rinse Protein treatments	Moisturizing shampoo Leave-in conditioner Moisturizing treatments
Wavy, Curly, Extremely Curly	Fine-hair shampoo Light leave-in conditioner Protein treatments Spray-on thermal protectors	Acid-balanced shampoo Leave-in conditioner Moisturizing treatment	Moisturizing shampoo Leave-in conditioner Protein and moisturizing treatments
Dry & Damaged (Perms, Color, Relaxers, Blow-drying, Sun, Hot Irons)	Gentle cleansing shampoo Light leave-in conditioner Protein and moisturizing repair treatments Spray-on thermal protection	Shampoo for chemically treated hair Moisturizing conditioner Protein and moisturizing repair treatments	Deep-moisturizing shampoo for damaged hair Leave-in conditioner Deep-conditioning treatments and hair masks

Rinses and Tonics

RINSES

Although the application of a conditioning agent is usually the second step in a shampoo service, the application of color or bluing rinses is a profitable service that can be easily learned and applied at the shampoo bowl.

A hair **rinse** is an agent that is used to cleanse or condition the hair and scalp, bring out the luster of the hair, or add highlights.

Water rinses are obviously used to wet and rinse the hair during the shampoo service. Warm water should be used to thoroughly rinse and remove any shampoo residue on the hair.

Medicated rinses are formulated to control minor dandruff and scalp conditions. A dandruff rinse is a commercial product that is applied following a shampoo to remove and control dandruff. Some rinses are used in a prepared form while others are diluted with water. Always follow the manufacturer's directions.

Bluing rinses are preparations that contain a blue base color. The bluing counteracts yellowish or dull gray tones in the hair, neutralizing them to silvery gray or white tones. These rinses are available in cream shampoo form or as a temporary hair color rinse in liquid form. Both are applied at the shampoo bowl. The cream shampoo type is rinsed from the hair, but temporary color rinses are not.

NOTE: The porosity of the hair must be taken into consideration to avoid a two-toned effect on the porous ends or shaft of the hair. Follow the manufacturer's directions when mixing to achieve the desired silver or slate tone.

TONICS

The term **tonic** usually applies to a cosmetic solution that stimulates the scalp, helps to correct a scalp condition, or that is used as a grooming aid. There are numerous hair tonics on the market so it is important to understand the ingredients, specific actions, and use of each type. The barber should also be prepared to advise clients concerning the use of tonics and the specific purpose of each.

Hair tonics are available in nonalcoholic, alcoholic, emulsion, and oil mixture formulations.

- *Nonalcoholic tonics* usually contain an antiseptic solution, with hair-grooming ingredients added.
- *Alcoholic tonics* consist of an antiseptic and alcohol combination that acts as a mild astringent.
- *Cream tonics* are emulsions containing lanolin and mineral oils for use in styling.
- *Oil mixture tonics* contain considerable amounts of alcohol with a small portion of oil floating on the top. These tonics are used as a grooming agent.

NOTE: For maximum benefit, a scalp massage should be used in conjunction with tonic applications..

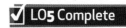
✓ LO5 Complete

Other Cosmetic Preparations

Astringents may have an alcohol content of up to 35 percent. Astringents cause contraction of tissues and may be used to remove oil accumulation on the skin or to close the pores after a facial or shave. Due to the high alcohol content of astringent lotions, some skin types may be sensitive and react with a slight swelling or redness of the skin. Additional astringent ingredients may include one or more of the following: alum, boric acid, sorbitol, water, camphor, and perfumes.

Cake or pancake makeup is generally composed of kaolin, zinc, talc, titanium oxide, mineral oil, fragrances, precipitated calcium carbonate, finely ground pigments, and inorganic pigments such as iron oxides. Cake makeup is used to cover scars and pigmentation defects.

Cleansing creams are used during facials and shaves in the barbershop. The action of a cleansing cream is caused in part by the oil content of the cream, which has the ability to dissolve other greasy substances. Older formulas, such as cold cream, contain relatively few ingredients that may include vegetable or mineral oil, beeswax, water, preservatives, and emulsifiers. The newer cleansing formulations are more skin condition–specific and may contain additional degreasers such as lemon juice, synthetic surfactants, emollients, or humectants.

Cleansing lotions serve the same purposes as cleansing creams but are of a lighter consistency and are usually water-based emulsions. They are available in dry-, normal-, and oily-skin formulations. Some ingredients common to cleansing lotions are cetyl alcohol, cetyl palmitate, and sorbitol; perfumes and colorings are added to enhance lotions' marketing value.

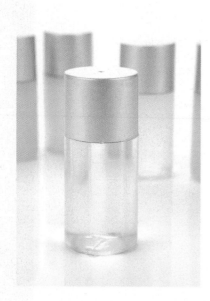

Depilatories are preparations used for the temporary removal of superfluous hair by dissolving it at the skin line. Depilatories contain detergents to strip the sebum from the hair and adhesives to hold the chemicals to the hair shaft for the 5 to 10 minutes necessary to remove the hair. During the short processing time, swelling accelerating agents such as urea or melamine expand the hair, helping to break the hair bonds. Finally, chemicals such as sodium hydroxide, potassium hydroxide, thioglycolic acid, or calcium thioglycolate destroy the disulfide bonds. These chemicals turn the hair into a soft, jelly-like mass of hydrolyzed protein that can be scraped from the skin. Although depilatories are not commonly used in barbershops, knowing about them is necessary because your customers may use them at home.

Epilators remove hair by pulling it out of the follicle. Two types of wax are currently used for professional epilation: cold and hot. Both products are made primarily of resins and beeswax. Beeswax has a relatively high incidence of allergic reaction; therefore, it is advisable to do a small patch test of the product to be used. Recently, an electrical apparatus made for the home hair-removal market has become available.

Eye lotions or toners are generally formulas of boric acid, bicarbonate of soda, zinc sulfate, glycerin, and herbs. They are designed to soothe and brighten the eyes.

Fresheners, also known as skin freshening lotions, have the lowest alcohol content (0 to 4 percent) of the tonic lotions. They are designed for dry, mature, and sensitive skin types. The formulation of a freshener typically includes some or all of the following: witch hazel, alcohol and camphorated alcohol, citric acid, boric acid, lactic acid, phosphoric acid, aluminum salts, menthol, chamomile, and floral scents.

Greasepaint is a mixture of fats, petrolatum, and a coloring agent that is used for theatrical purposes.

Hair spray is used to hold the finished style. Many new formulations for hair spray contain a variety of polymers, such as acrylic/acrylate copolymer, vinyl acetate, crotonic acid copolymer, PVM/MA copolymer, and polyvinylpyrrolidone (PVP), and plasticizers such as acetyl triethyl citrate, benzyl alcohol, and silicones as stiffening agents. Additional ingredients might include silicone, shellac, perfume, lanolin or its derivatives, vegetable gums, alcohol, sorbitol, and water.

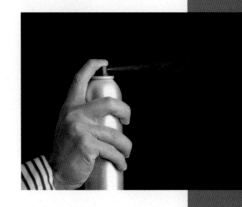

Hairdressings, such as pomades, give shine and manageability to dry or curly hair. They may be applied to either wet or dry hair. Such dressings typically consist of lanolin or its derivatives, petrolatum, oil emulsions, fatty acids, waxes, mild alkalis, and water.

Masks and *packs* are available to serve many purposes and skin conditions including deep cleansing, pore reduction, tightening, firming, moisturizing, and wrinkle reduction. Clay masks typically contain varying combinations of kaolin (china clay), bentonite, purified siliceous (fuller's) earth or colloidal clay, petrolatum, glycerin, proteins, SD alcohol, and water. The primary ingredients typically found in peel-off masks are SD alcohol 40, polysorbate-20, and polymers such as polyvinyl alcohol or vinyl acetate.

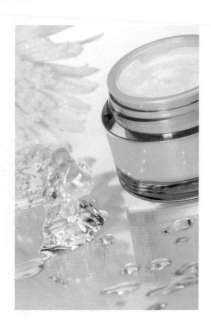

Massage creams are used to help the hands to glide over the skin. They contain formulations of cold cream, lanolin or its derivatives, and sometimes casein (a protein found in cheese).

Medicated lotions are available by prescription for skin problems such as acne, rashes, or other eruptions.

Moisturizing creams are designed to treat dryness. They contain humectants, which create a barrier that allows the natural water and oil of the skin to accumulate in the tissues. This barrier also works to protect the skin from air pollution, dirt, and debris. Moisturizers contain a variety of emollients ranging from simple ingredients such as peanut, coconut, or a variety of other oils, to more complex chemical compounds such as cetyl alcohol, cholesterol, dimethicone, or glycerin derivatives.

Pastes are soft, moist cosmetics with a thick consistency. They are bound together with the aid of gum, starch, and water. If oils and fats are present, water is absent. The colloidal mill assists in the removal of grittiness from the paste.

Scalp lotions and ointments usually contain medicinal agents for active correction of a scalp condition such as itching or flakiness. An astringent lotion may be applied to the scalp before shampooing to control oiliness as well as the itching and flakiness of dry scalp conditions. Medicated lotions and ointments for severe scalp conditions must be prescribed by a physician.

Sticks are made from a mixture of organic substances (oils, waxes, or petrolatum) that is poured into a mold to solidify or from pressed chemical compounds. Eyebrow pencils and styptic pencils are examples of stick cosmetics.

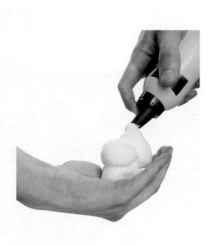

Styling aids, such as gels and mousses, typically consist of polymer and resin formulations that are designed to give the hair body and texture. Many incorporate the same ingredients found in hair sprays but add moisturizers and humectants, such as cetyl alcohol, panthenol, hydrolyzed protein, quats, or a variety of oils to the ingredient list.

Suntan lotions are designed to protect the skin from the harmful ultraviolet rays of the sun. They are rated with a sun protection factor (SPF) that enables sunbathers to calculate the time they can remain in the sun before the skin begins to burn. Suntan lotions are emulsions that might contain para-aminobenzoic acid (PABA), a variety of oils, petrolatum, sorbitan stearate, alcohol, ultraviolet inhibitors, acid derivatives, preservatives, and perfumes.

Toners usually have an alcohol content of 4 to 15 percent and are designed for use on normal and combination skin types.

Wrinkle treatment creams are designed to conceal lines on aging skin either via a crease-filling capacity or through a "plumping up" of the tissues. Among the many possible ingredients in these treatments are hormones and collagen. Some are made of herbs and other natural ingredients while others are entirely synthetic.

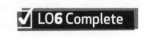

United States Pharmacopeia (U.S.P.)

The *United States Pharmacopeia* is a public health organization that sets standards for food ingredients, health-care products, and drugs sold or manufactured in the United States and used by the public. Some of the most common chemical ingredients used in the formulation of hair and skin products are as follows.

Alcohol is a colorless liquid obtained from the fermentation of starch, sugar, and other carbohydrates. Isopropyl (rubbing) and ethyl (beverage or grain) alcohol are both volatile (readily evaporated) alcohols. These alcohols function as solvents and can be found in shampoos, conditioners, hair colorants, hair sprays, tonics, and styling aids. Fatty alcohols, such as cetyl and cetearyl alcohol, are nonvolatile oils that are used as conditioners. The alcohols most often used in the barbershop are ethyl alcohol and isopropyl alcohol. Fifty to sixty percent isopropyl alcohol is an effective antiseptic that can be applied to the skin.

Alkanolamines (al-kan-all-AM-eenz) are substances used to neutralize acids or raise the pH of hair products. They are often used in place of ammonia because there is less odor associated with their use. Alkanolamines are used as alkalizing agents in hair lighteners and permanent wave solutions.

Alum is an aluminum potassium or ammonium sulphate supplied in the form of crystals or powder; it has a strong astringent action. For this reason, alum can be found in some skin tonics and lotions. The use of styptic powder or liquid is permissible in some states to stop the bleeding of small nicks and cuts.

Ammonia, a colorless gas composed of hydrogen and nitrogen, has a pungent odor. Ammonia is used to raise the pH in permanent waving, haircoloring, and lightening substances. Ammonium hydroxide and ammonium thioglycolate are examples of ammonia compounds that are used to raise solution pH levels for better penetration into the hair.

Ammonia water, as commercially used, is a colorless liquid with a pungent, penetrating odor. It is a by-product of the manufacture of coal gas. As it readily dissolves grease, it is used as a cleansing agent and is also used with hydrogen peroxide in hair lighteners. A 28 percent solution of ammonia gas dissolved in water is available commercially.

Boric acid is used for its bactericidal and fungicidal properties in baby powders, eye creams, mouthwashes, soaps, and skin fresheners. It is a mild healing and antiseptic agent, although the American Medical Association warns of possible toxicity. Severe irritation and poisonings have occurred after application to open skin wounds.

Ethyl methacrylate (ETH-il meth-u-KRYE-layt) is an ester (compound) of ethyl alcohol and methacrylic acid used in the chemical formulation of many sculptured nails. Inhalation of the fumes is not recommended.

Formaldehyde is a colorless gas manufactured by an oxidation process of methyl alcohol. It is used as a disinfectant, fungicide, germicide, and preservative as well as an embalming solution. In the cosmetics industry, small amounts of formaldehyde are used in soaps, cosmetics, and nail hardeners and polishes.

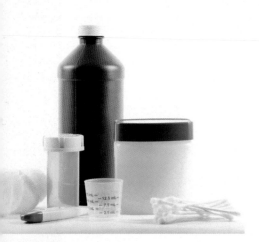

Formaldehyde and its derivatives, such as *formalin*, should be used with caution because National Cancer Institute studies indicate that it is toxic, can lead to DNA damage, and is known to react with other chemicals to become a carcinogen.

Glycerin is a sweet, colorless, odorless, oily substance formed by the decomposition of oils, fats, or fatty acids. It is used as a solvent and as a skin moisturizer in cuticle oils and facial creams.

Hydrogen peroxide is a compound of hydrogen and oxygen. It is a colorless liquid with a characteristic odor and a slightly acidic taste. Organic matter, such as silk, hair, feathers, and nails, is bleached by hydrogen peroxide because of its oxidizing power. A hydrogen peroxide solution is used as a bleaching agent for the hair in solutions of 20 to 40 volume. A 3 to 5 percent solution of hydrogen peroxide possesses antiseptic qualities.

Petrolatum, commonly known as Vaseline, petroleum jelly, or paraffin jelly, is a yellowish to white, semisolid, greasy mass that is almost insoluble in water. It is used in wax epilators, eyebrow pencils, lipsticks, protective creams, cold creams, and many other cosmetics for its ability to soften and smooth the skin.

Phenol, or carbolic acid, is not actually an acid but rather a slightly acidic coal tar derivative. A 5 percent solution is used to sanitize metallic implements.

Phenylenediamine, derived from coal tar, has a succession of derivatives known to penetrate the skin. It is believed to cause cancer.

Potassium hydroxide (caustic potash) is prepared by electrolysis of potassium chloride. It may be used for its emulsifying abilities in formulas for hand lotions, liquid soaps, protective creams, and cuticle softeners.

Quaternary ammonium compounds (quats) are found in many antiseptics, surfactants, preservatives, sanitizers, and germicides. Quats are synthetic derivatives of ammonium chloride. Although quats can be toxic, they are considered safe in the proportions used in the industry.

Silicones are a special type of oil used in hair conditioners and as water-resistant lubricants for the skin. Silicones are less greasy than plain oils and have the ability to form a "breathable" film that does not cause comedones.

Sodium bicarbonate (baking soda) is a precipitate made by passing carbon dioxide gas through a solution of sodium carbonate. The resulting white powder is used as a neutralizing agent and, when mixed in shampoo, to remove hair spray buildup.

Sodium carbonate (soda ash or washing soda) is found naturally in ores and lake brines or seawater. It is used in shampoos and permanent wave solutions. Sodium carbonate absorbs water from the air.

Witch hazel is a solution of alcohol, water, and powder ground from the leaves and twigs of *Hamamelis virginiana*. It works as an astringent and skin freshener. Because of the alcohol content, it should not be applied directly to an open wound or to the delicate membranes of the eye.

Zinc oxide is a heavy white powder that is insoluble in water. It is used cosmetically in face powder, foundation cream, and sunscreen products for its ability to impart opacity.

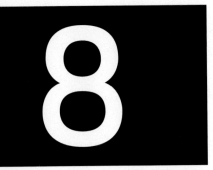

Review Questions

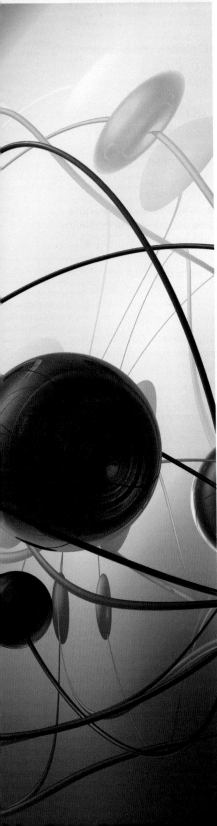

1. Define *organic* and *inorganic chemistry*.

2. List the three states of matter.

3. Define *elements*, *compounds*, and *mixtures*.

4. Describe the differences between solutions, suspensions, and emulsions.

5. Define *pH* and draw a pH scale.

6. What effect does a strong-to-mild acidic solution have on hair?

7. What effect does a mild alkaline solution have on hair?

8. Explain oxidation and reduction reactions. Give an example of each.

9. Why is the acidity or alkalinity of hair care products important to the barber?

10. Identify the parts and functions of the shampoo molecule.

11. List three general shampoo categories.

12. What type of shampoo is generally recommended for normal, chemically treated, or fragile hair?

13. What type of conditioner is generally applied to the hair for 1 to 5 minutes?

14. Identify the hair condition that may require a synthetic polymer.

15. List four types of hair tonics.

Chapter
Glossary

acid-balanced shampoos shampoos that are balanced to the pH of hair and skin (4.5 to 5.5)

acids solutions that have a pH below 7.0

alkalis solutions that have a pH above 7.0

atoms smallest particles of an element that still retain the properties of that element

balancing shampoos designed for hair and scalp conditions

bases also known as alkalis

bluing rinses temporary colors or shampoo products with a blue base used to offset yellow and gray tones in hair

chemical change change in the chemical composition of a substance by which new substances are formed

chemical properties characteristics that can only be determined with a chemical reaction

chemistry the science that deals with the composition, structure, and properties of matter

clarifying shampoos shampoos containing an acidic ingredient that cuts through product buildup

color-enhancing shampoos created by combining surfactant bases with basic dyes

compounds two or more atoms of different elements united chemically with fixed chemical composition, definite proportions, and distinct properties

conditioners chemical agents used to deposit protein or moisturizers in the hair

deep-conditioning treatments chemical mixtures of concentrated protein and moisturizers

dry or powder shampoos shampoos that cleanse the hair without water

element the simplest form of matter

emulsions mixtures of two or more immiscible substances united with the aid of a binder or emulsifier

inorganic chemistry chemistry dealing with compounds lacking carbon

instant conditioners conditioners that typically remain on the hair from one to five minutes and are rinsed out

ion an atom or molecule that carries an electrical charge

ionization the separating of a substance into ions

leave-in conditioners conditioners and thermal protectors that can be left in the hair without rinsing

liquid-dry shampoos liquid shampoos that evaporate quickly and do not require rinsing

matter any substance that occupies space, has physical and chemical properties, and exists in the form of a solid, liquid, or gas

medicated rinses rinses formulated to control minor dandruff and scalp conditions

medicated shampoos shampoos containing medicinal agents for control of dandruff and other scalp conditions

moisturizing conditioners contain humectants to absorb and promote the retention of moisture in the hair

moisturizing or conditioning shampoo products formulated to add moisture to dry hair

molecules two or more atoms joined chemically

organic chemistry the study of substances that contain carbon

organic shampoos formulated from natural organic ingredients

oxidation chemical reaction that combines an element or compound with oxygen to produce an oxide

oxides compounds of any element combined with oxygen

pH (potential hydrogen) relative degree of acidity or alkalinity of a substance

pH scale a measure of the concentration of hydrogen ions in acidic and alkaline solutions

physical change change in the form of a substance without the formation of a new substance

physical mixture combination of two or more substances united physically

physical properties characteristics of matter that can be determined without a chemical reaction

protein conditioners products designed to slightly increase hair diameter with a coating action and to replace lost proteins in hair

pure substance matter that has a fixed chemical composition, definite proportions, and district properties

redox contraction for reduction—oxidation

reduction the subtraction of oxygen from, or the addition of hydrogen to, a substance

rinse an agent used to cleanse or condition the hair and scalp

salts compounds that are formed by the reaction of acids and bases

scalp conditioners cream-based products and ointments used to soften and improve the health of the scalp

shampoo removes dirt, oil, perspiration, and skin debris from the hair and scalp

surfactant a substance that acts as a bridge to allow oil and water to mix or emulsify by reducing surface tension.

suspensions formulations in which solid particles are distributed throughout a liquid medium

synthetic polymer conditioners formulated to prevent breakage and correct excessive porosity on badly damaged hair

tonic cosmetic solution that stimulates the scalp, helps to correct a scalp condition, or is used as a grooming aid

9 Electricity and Light Therapy

☑ Learning Objectives

AFTER COMPLETING THIS CHAPTER, YOU SHOULD BE ABLE TO:

1 Identify and define common electrical terms.

2 Discuss and recognize electrical safety devices.

3 Explain different electrical modalities and their uses.

4 Explain the effects of ultraviolet and infrared light on the skin.

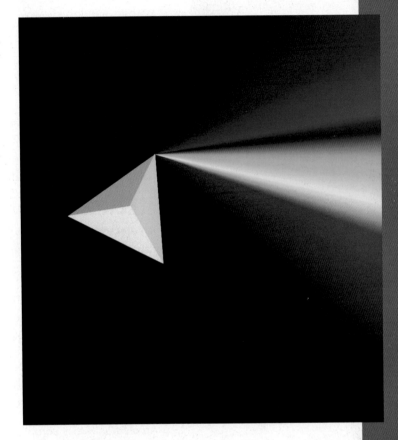

Key Terms

PAGE NUMBER INDICATES WHERE IN THE CHAPTER THE TERM IS USED.

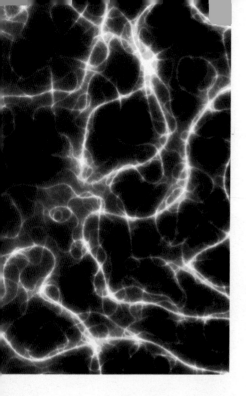

In today's barbershop, haircutting and other services would be very uncomfortable without electricity. It is probably safe to say that most barbers would not like to return to the days of the hand clipper or a lack of air-conditioning! In this chapter, you will learn some important safety precautions regarding the use of electricity in the barbershop. You will also be introduced to different electrical currents that can be used for scalp and facial electrotherapy treatments.

Light therapy treatments are another service that barbers can offer their clients. Different light rays have different effects on the skin. For this reason, barbers need to know when it is appropriate to apply the thermal and chemical properties associated with light therapy to the skin.

Electricity

Electricity (ee-lek-TRIS-ih-tee) is a valuable tool for the barber, provided it is used carefully and intelligently. Electricity is the directional flow of electrons (negatively charged subatomic particles) between atoms that creates a form of energy capable of producing magnetic, chemical, or thermal effects while in motion.

ELECTRICAL TERMS

An **electric current** is the flow of electricity along a conductor. All substances can be classified as *conductors* or *insulators*, depending on the ease with which an electric current can be transmitted through them.

A **conductor** (kahn-DUK-tur) is any substance, material, or medium that conducts electricity. Most metals, carbon, the human body, and watery solutions of acids and salts are good conductors of electricity.

An **insulator** (IN-suh-layt-ur), or nonconductor (nahn-kun-DUK-tur), is a substance that does not easily transmit electricity. Rubber, silk, dry wood, glass, and cement are good insulators.

An *electric wire* is composed of fine, twisted metal threads, which act as a conductor, and a covering of silk or rubber, which is the insulator.

A **complete circuit** (kahm-PLEET SUR-kit) is the path of an electric current from the generating source through conductors and back to its original source (**Figure 9-1**).

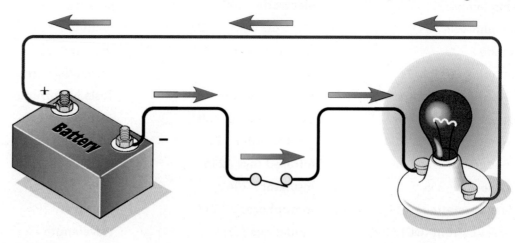

▲ **FIGURE 9-1**
A complete electrical circuit.

A **rheostat** is an adjustable resistor, such as a light dimmer, that is used for controlling the current in a circuit.

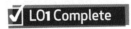 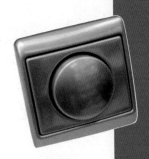

TYPES OF ELECTRIC CURRENT

There are two kinds of electric current: direct current and alternating current.

1. **Direct current** (DC) is a constant, even-flowing current that travels in one direction only and produces a chemical reaction. Battery-operated instruments such as flashlights, cell phones, and certain tools use direct current. A **converter** is an apparatus that changes direct current to alternating current. Some cars have converters that allow the use of appliances that would normally be plugged into an electrical wall outlet to be powered by the car's battery.

2. **Alternating current** (AC) is a rapid and interrupted current, flowing first in one direction and then in the opposite direction, that produces a mechanical action. A wall socket utilizes alternating current. Electric clippers, hair-dryers, and other tools that plug into a wall outlet use alternating current. A **rectifier** is an apparatus that changes alternating current to direct current. Rechargeable cordless clippers and battery chargers use a rectifier to convert the AC current from an electrical wall outlet to the DC current needed to recharge the batteries.

ELECTRICAL MEASUREMENTS

In the flow of electric current, individual electrons flow through a wire in the same way that individual water molecules flow through a garden hose.

A **volt** (V) is a unit of electrical pressure that pushes the flow of electrons forward through a conductor, much as water pressure pushes water molecules through a hose. A higher voltage indicates more pressure, more force, and more power. If the voltage is lower, the current is weaker **(Figure 9-2)**.

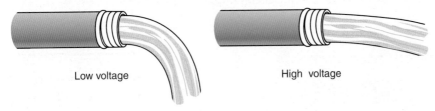

Low voltage   High voltage

▲ **FIGURE 9-2**
Volts measure the pressure or force that pushes electrons forward.

An **amp or ampere** (A), often called an amp, is the standard unit for measuring the strength of an electric current and also the rate of flow of charge in a conductor. Just as a water hose must be able to expand as the amount of water flowing through it increases, so a wire must expand with an increase in the number of electrons (amps). A cord must be heavy-duty enough to handle the amps put out by the appliance. For example, a hair-dryer rated at 10 amps requires a cord that is twice as thick as one rated at 5 amps. If the current, or number of amps, is too strong, the cord can overheat and cause a fire. If the current is not strong enough, the appliance will not operate correctly.

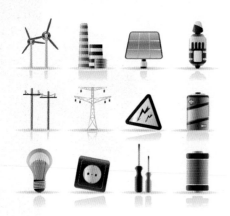

A *milliampere* (mil-ee-AM-peer) is one-thousandth of an ampere. The current for facial and scalp treatments is measured in milliamperes as an ampere current would be much too strong.

An **ohm** (O) is the unit of electrical resistance in an electric current. Unless the force (volts) is stronger than the resistance (ohms), the current will not flow through the wire.

A **watt** (W) (WAHT) is the unit of power (amperes multiplied by volts) and indicates how much electric energy is being used in one second. A 40-watt bulb uses 40 watts of energy per second. A *kilowatt* (kW) is 1,000 watts. The electricity in a house is measured in kilowatt-hours (kWh).

SAFETY DEVICES

A **fuse (F-YOOZ)** is a safety device that prevents the overheating of electrical wires by preventing excessive current from passing through a circuit. It blows or melts when the wire becomes too hot from overloading the circuit with too much current from too many appliances, for example, or if faulty equipment is used. To re-establish the circuit, the appliance must be unplugged or disconnected and a new fuse inserted in the fuse box (**Figure 9-3**).

A **circuit breaker** is a switch that automatically interrupts or shuts off an electric circuit at the first indication of an overload (**Figure 9-4**). In modern electric circuits, circuit breakers have replaced fuses. Circuit breakers supply the same safety control as fuses against overloaded lines and faulty electrical apparatus, but they do not require replacement. They can also be reset. When wires become too hot because of overloading or a faulty piece of equipment, the breaker will click off or disengage, thus breaking the circuit. If an electric appliance malfunctions while in operation, disconnect the appliance from the wall socket immediately and check all connections and insulations before resetting.

A **ground fault circuit interrupter** (GFCI) is a life-saving device that senses imbalances within an electric circuit (**Figure 9-5**). When it "pops" open,

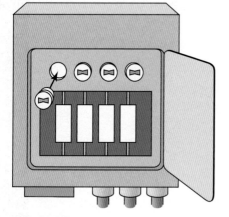

▲ FIGURE 9-3
Fuse box.

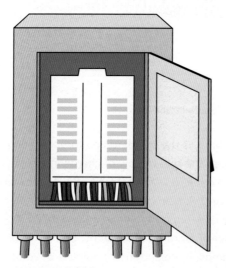

▲ FIGURE 9-4
Circuit breakers.

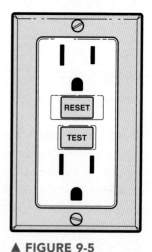

▲ FIGURE 9-5
Ground fault circuit interrupter (GFCI).

it means that it has sensed a ground fault or current leaking to ground. These devices must be installed properly to operate as intended; otherwise, although the outlet may work, the protection function of their design will be lost.

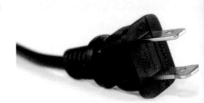

The principle of *grounding* is another important way of promoting electrical safety. All electrical appliances must have at least two electrical connections. These two "live" connections supply current and complete the circuit. A ground connection is a third connection that carries the current safely away to the ground in the event of a short circuit.

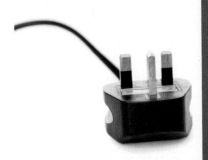

The different sizes of the prongs on modern electrical plugs guarantee that the plugs can only be inserted one way. This feature provides protection from electrical shock in the event of a short circuit. Some appliance cords have a third, circular prong that provides a connection to the ground. This extra prong is designed to guarantee a safe path for electricity if the circuit fails or is interrupted. See Table 9-1 for a summary of electrical terms.

> TABLE **9-1** Basics of Electricity

TERM	DESCRIPTION
Alternating current	Current that moves in an alternating direction, from A to B and B back to A. There is no fixed polarity in alternating current. The current that comes out of a wall socket is an example of alternating current.
Amp or Ampere	A standard unit for measuring the strength of an electric current; also the rate of flow of charge in a conductor.
Conductor	A material that electric current flows through without much resistance.
Direct current	A current where electrons flow in the same direction. Direct current has fixed polarity. Iontophoresis is an example of a use of direct current.
Electric charge	A basic feature of certain particles of matter that causes them to attract or repel other charged particles.
Electric circuit	The path that an electric current follows.
Electric field	The influence a charged body has on the space around it that causes other charged bodies in that space to experience electric forces.
Electrode	A piece of metal, glass, or other conductor through which current enters or leaves an electrical device.
Electromagnetism	A basic force in the universe that involves both electricity and magnetism.
Electron	A subatomic particle with a negative electric charge.

TERM	DESCRIPTION
Insulator	A material that opposes the flow of an electric current.
Ion	An atom or group of atoms that has either gained or lost electrons and so has an electric charge.
Kilowatt-hour	The amount of electric energy a 1,000-watt device uses per hour.
Milliampere meter	An instrument for measuring the rate of flow of an electric current.
Neutron	A subatomic particle in the nucleus of an atom that has no electric charge.
Ohm	The unit of electrical resistance in an electric current.
Plug	A two- or three-prong connector at the end of an electrical cord that connects an apparatus into an electrical outlet.
Polarity changer	A switch that reverses with the direction of the current from positive to negative and vice versa.
Proton	A subatomic particle with a positive electric charge, located in the nucleus.
Resistance	A material's opposition to the flow of electric current.
Rheostat	A specific control regulating the strength of the current used; a variable resistor.
Static electricity	An electric charge that is not moving.
Volt	A unit of electrical pressure.
Watt	A unit of power indicating how much electric energy is being used in one second.

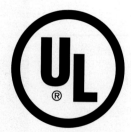

▲ **FIGURE 9-6**

A UL symbol as it appears on electrical devices.

ELECTRICAL EQUIPMENT SAFETY

The protection and safety of the client should be the primary concern of barbers and stylists. All electrical equipment should be inspected regularly to determine that it is in safe working condition. Careful attention to electrical safety helps to eliminate accidental shocks, fires, and burns. A review of the following reminders will help ensure the safe use of electricity in the barbershop.

- All electrical appliances should be UL-certified (Figure 9-6).
- Study the instructions *before* using any electrical equipment.
- Disconnect appliances when not in use.

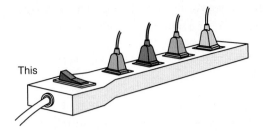
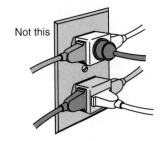

▲ FIGURE 9-7
One plug per outlet.

- Keep all wires, plugs, and equipment in good repair.
- Inspect all electrical equipment frequently.
- Do not overload outlets (**Figure 9-7**).
- Avoid getting electrical cords wet.
- When using electrical equipment, protect the client at all times.
- Do not touch any metal while using an electrical appliance.
- Do not handle electrical equipment with wet hands.
- Do not allow the client to touch any metal surfaces while being treated with electrical equipment.
- Do not leave the room while a client is connected to an electrical device.
- Do not attempt to clean around an electric outlet while equipment is plugged in.
- Do not touch two metallic objects at the same time if either is connected to an electric current.
- Do not step on, or set objects on, electrical cords.
- Do not allow electrical cords to become twisted or bent; the fine wires inside the cord will break and the insulation will wear away from the wires.
- Disconnect appliances by pulling on the plug, not on the cord.
- Do not repair electrical appliances unless you are qualified to do so.

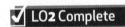
✓ LO2 Complete

Electrotherapy

Electronic facial and scalp treatments are commonly referred to as **electrotherapy.** Different types of electric currents are used for facial and scalp treatments. These different types of currents are called **modalities** and each one produces a different effect on the skin.

An **electrode** is an applicator used to direct the electric current from the machine to the client's skin. Electrodes are available in many shapes and are usually made of carbon, glass, or metal (**Figure 9-8**).

POLARITIES

Polarity indicates the negative or positive pole of an electric current. The positive pole is called an **anode,** is usually red, and may be marked with a

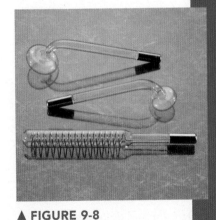

▲ FIGURE 9-8
Electrodes come in a variety of shapes.

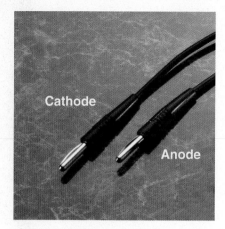

▲ FIGURE 9-9

Anode and cathode.

"P" or a plus (+) sign **(Figure 9-9)**. The negative electrode is called a **cathode.** It is usually black and marked with an "N" or a minus (–) sign (Figure 9-9).

If the electrodes are not marked, either of the following tests will help to determine the anode from the cathode.

- Separate the tips of two conducting cords from each other and immerse them in a glass of salt water. Turn the selector switch of the appliance to galvanic current, and then turn up the intensity. As the water is decomposed, more active bubbles will accumulate at the negative pole than at the positive pole.

- Place the tips of two conducting cords on two separate pieces of blue, moistened litmus paper. The paper under the positive pole will turn red, while the paper under the negative pole will stay blue. If you use red litmus instead of blue, the positive pole will keep the red litmus the same and the negative pole will turn the red litmus blue.

MODALITIES

Modalities are the currents used in electronic facial and scalp treatments. The four main modalities are the *galvanic, sinusoidal, faradic,* and *Tesla high-frequency* currents. The two primary modalities used in barbering are the galvanic and Tesla high-frequency currents.

Galvanic Current

The most commonly used modality is the **galvanic current.** It is a constant and direct current, using a negative and positive pole, that is reduced to a safe, low-voltage level. Galvanic current produces chemical changes when passed through body tissues and fluids, and is used to create chemical and ionic reactions in the skin. These reactions depend on the negative or positive polarity that is used **(Table 9-2)**. Note that the effects produced

CAUTION

Polarity tests can be dangerous and should not be performed without an instructor's supervision. Do not allow the tips of the conduction cords to touch, which can cause a short circuit.

TABLE **9-2** Effects of Galvanic Current

POSITIVE POLE (ANODE)	NEGATIVE POLE (CATHODE)
Produces acidic reactions	Produces alkaline reactions
Closes the pores	Opens the pores
Soothes nerves	Stimulates and irritates the nerves
Decreases blood supply	Increases blood supply
Contracts blood vessels	Expands blood vessels
Hardens and firms tissues	Softens tissues

by the positive pole are the exact opposite of those produced by the negative pole.

Desincrustation is used to facilitate deep pore cleansing. During this process galvanic current is used to create a chemical reaction that acts to emulsify the sebum and waste in the pores. An electropositive solution is applied to the skin, and the negative pole is used to make direct contact with the solution while the client holds the positive pole (see Chapter 13).

Iontophoresis means the introduction of ions. It is a process in which galvanic current is used to introduce water-soluble products into the deeper layers of the skin. Both the positive and negative poles are used in the process. Ionic penetration takes place in two ways: **cataphoresis,** which forces acidic substances into the tissues from the positive toward the negative pole, and **anaphoresis,** which forces liquids into the tissues from the negative toward the positive pole (see Chapter 13).

Faradic Current

Faradic current is an alternating and interrupted current capable of producing a mechanical reaction without a chemical effect. Two electrodes are required to complete the faradic circuit. Faradic current causes muscular contractions and may be used in scalp and facial treatments (see Chapter 13). Some of the benefits of using faradic current include:

- Improved muscle tone
- Increased blood circulation
- Increased metabolism
- Removal of waste products
- Stimulation of hair growth
- Invigoration of the area being treated
- Increased glandular activity
- Relief of blood congestion

CAUTION

The use of faradic or sinusoidal current by anyone other than a licensed physician is prohibited in some states. Refer to your state barber board regulations regarding the use of these modalities.

Sinusoidal Current

Sinusoidal current, which is similar to faradic current, may be used during scalp and facial manipulations. It is an alternating current that produces mechanical contractions in the muscles and also requires the use of two electrodes (see Chapter 13). Sinusoidal current has the following advantages:

- Supplies greater stimulation, deeper penetration, and is less irritating than faradic current.
- Soothes the nerves and penetrates into deeper muscle tissue.

CAUTION

Do not use a sinusoidal current if the face is flushed or if the client has broken capillaries in the skin, high blood pressure, or a skin condition with pustules.

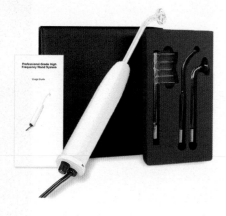

Tesla High-Frequency Current

Tesla high-frequency current is characterized by a high rate of oscillation that produces heat. It is commonly called the "violet ray" and is used for both scalp and facial treatments. Due to its rapid oscillation, Tesla current does not cause muscular contractions. Instead, the physiological effects are either stimulating or soothing, depending on the method of application.

The electrodes are made of glass or metal and only one electrode is used to perform a service. The shapes of the electrodes vary depending on the service: the facial electrode is flat and the scalp electrode is rake-shaped. As the current passes through the glass electrode, tiny violet sparks are emitted. All treatments given with high-frequency current should be started with mild current and gradually increased to the required strength. Approximately 5 minutes should be allowed for a general facial or scalp treatment, depending upon the condition being treated (see Chapters 12 and 13). As with all other tools and implements, follow the manufacturer's directions. The potential benefits of using Tesla high-frequency current include:

- Stimulated blood circulation
- Improved glandular activity
- Increased metabolism
- Increased absorption of nutrients and elimination of wastes
- Improved germicidal action
- Relief of congestion

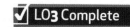
✓ **LO3 Complete**

Light Therapy

Light therapy, also known as *phototherapy*, is the application of light waves to the skin for the treatment of disorders such as dry skin or mild skin eruptions. Light therapy machines are designed to emit specific wavelengths of the light spectrum. In the human body, this light is changed into electrochemical energy that creates biochemical reactions in the cells that can stimulate the immune system. Different light rays will produce heat, chemical reactions, or germicidal effects.

Visible light is electromagnetic radiation that we can see. Electromagnetic radiation is also called *radiant energy* because it radiates energy through space in waves. The distance between two successive peaks is called the **wavelength.** Long wavelengths have low frequency, meaning the waves pass a point less frequently within a given length of time. Short wavelengths have a higher frequency because the waves pass more frequently within a given length of time (**Figure 9-10**).

The entire range of electromagnetic radiation wavelengths is called the *electromagnetic spectrum*. Visible light is the part of the spectrum that we can see and makes up 35 percent of natural sunlight.

Ultraviolet rays and infrared rays are also forms of electromagnetic radiation, but they are invisible to the human eye. Invisible rays make up 65 percent of natural sunlight at the earth's surface.

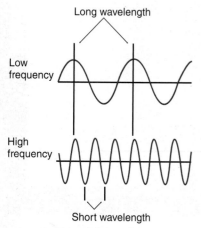

▲ **FIGURE 9-10**

Long and short wavelengths.

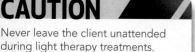

CAUTION

Never leave the client unattended during light therapy treatments.

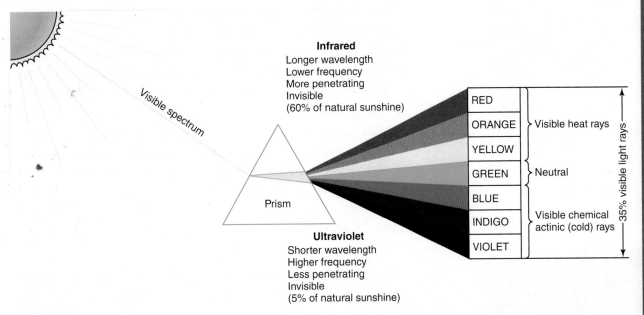

Infrared
Longer wavelength
Lower frequency
More penetrating
Invisible
(60% of natural sunshine)

Visible spectrum

Prism

RED	⎫
ORANGE	⎬ Visible heat rays
YELLOW	
GREEN	⎫ Neutral
BLUE	⎬
INDIGO	⎫ Visible chemical
VIOLET	⎬ actinic (cold) rays

35% visible light rays

Ultraviolet
Shorter wavelength
Higher frequency
Less penetrating
Invisible
(5% of natural sunshine)

▲ **FIGURE 9-11**
The visible spectrum.

When light passes through a glass prism, it produces the seven colors of the rainbow, arrayed in the following manner: red, orange, yellow, green, blue, indigo, and violet **(Figure 9-11)**. Within the visible spectrum of light, violet has the shortest wavelength and red has the longest. In the field of barbering, we are concerned with the rays that produce heat (infrared rays) and those that produce chemical and germicidal reactions (ultraviolet rays).

In the barbershop, artificial light waves are produced through the use of therapeutic lamps. The bulbs in these lamps are capable of producing the same rays that are created by the sun. Therapeutic lamps that produce infrared and ultraviolet rays are available in either separate or combination units. They are also available in several different styles, which include tabletop and floor models **(Figure 9-12)**.

VISIBLE LIGHT RAYS

Visible light rays are the primary light sources used for scalp and facial treatments. The bulbs used for visible light therapy are white, red, and blue. *White light* is referred to as a *combination light* because it consists of all the visible rays of the spectrum. *Red light* produces the most heat and penetrates the deepest. It is used on dry skin in combination with oils and creams. *Blue light* contains few heat rays, is the least penetrating, and provides germicidal and chemical benefits. Blue light should be used only on bare, clean skin.

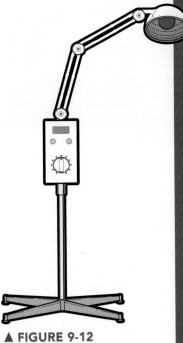

▲ **FIGURE 9-12**
Therapeutic lamp.

The lamp used to reproduce visible light is usually a dome-shaped reflector mounted on a pedestal with a flexible neck. The dome is finished with a highly polished metal lining capable of reflecting heat rays. The bulbs used with this lamp come in various colors for different purposes. As with all other lamps, the client's eyes must be protected from the glare and heat of the light. For proper eye protection, the client's eyes are covered with cotton pads saturated with dilute boric acid or witch hazel solution.

- *White light* relieves pain, especially in congested areas, and more particularly around the nerve centers, such as the back of the neck and across the shoulders. It also relaxes the muscles and produces some chemical and germicidal effects.

- *Blue light* produces little heat and has a tonic effect on bare skin and a soothing effect on the nerves. Blue light should be used only over clean skin, without any cream, oil, or powder present on the skin.

- *Red light* has strong heat rays, creates a stimulating effect, can be used over creams and ointments to soften and relax body tissue, and penetrates the skin more deeply than does blue light. Heat rays aid the penetration of lanolin creams into the skin and are recommended for dry, scaly, or wrinkled skin.

INVISIBLE LIGHT RAYS

Ultraviolet Rays

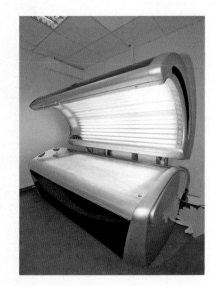

Ultraviolet (UV) **rays,** also known as cold rays or actinic rays, make up 5 percent of natural sunlight. UV rays have short wavelengths, produce chemical effects, kill germs, and are the least penetrating rays. There are three general types of ultraviolet lamps: the glass bulb, the hot quartz, and the cold quartz.

- The glass bulb lamp is used mainly for cosmetic or tanning purposes.

- The hot quartz lamp is a general, all-purpose lamp suitable for tanning, tonic, cosmetic, or germicidal purposes.

- The cold quartz lamp produces mostly short ultraviolet rays. It is used primarily in hospitals.

UV rays are divided into three categories: UVA, UVB, and UVC. The farther away from the visible light spectrum, the shorter and less penetrating the ultraviolet rays.

- *UVA rays* are the tonic UV rays. UVA rays are closest to the visible spectrum and are the longest of all the UV rays. These rays are used in tanning booths and penetrate deeply into skin tissue. Overexposure can destroy the elasticity of the skin, causing premature aging and wrinkling.

- *UVB rays* are the therapeutic rays in the middle of the UV range, which produce some effects from both ends of ultraviolet rays. Long exposure to UVB rays will burn the skin.

- *UVC rays* are the most germicidal and chemically active of the ultraviolet rays, as well as being the farthest away from the visible spectrum. These rays don't penetrate far into the skin but can burn the surface. UVC rays are destructive to bacteria, as well as to skin tissue if the skin is exposed to them for too long a period of time.

Ultraviolet rays are used to treat acne, tinea, and seborrhea and to combat dandruff due to their germicidal and antibacterial effects. They also promote healing and can stimulate the growth of hair, as well as produce a tan by increasing skin pigment if the skin is exposed in short doses over a long period of time. **Table 9-3** summarizes the pros and cons of UV ray treatments.

Ultraviolet rays are applied with a lamp at a distance of 30 to 36 inches from the skin. Average exposure can produce skin redness, and overdoses will

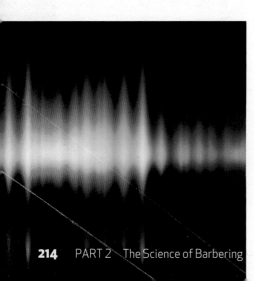

TABLE **9-3** Benefits and Disadvantages of Ultraviolet Rays

BENEFITS OF ULTRAVIOLET RAY TREATMENTS	DISADVANTAGES OF ULTRAVIOLET RAYS
Increases resistance to disease by promoting the production of vitamin D in the skin and increasing the number of red and white cells in the blood.	May destroy hair pigment.
Increases the elimination of waste products and restores nutrition where needed.	Continued exposure to UV light causes premature aging of the skin.
Stimulates the circulation by improving the flow of blood and lymph.	Continued exposure to UV light causes painful sunburn.
Increases the fixation of calcium in the blood.	Continued exposure to UV light causes a higher risk of skin cancer, especially for fair- or light-skinned individuals.

cause blistering. It is best to start with a short exposure of 2 to 3 minutes and gradually increase the exposure over a period of days to 7 to 8 minutes. To receive full benefit from ultraviolet rays, the area to be treated should be clean, with no cream or lotion applied to the skin.

Infrared Rays

Beyond the red rays of the spectrum are the **infrared rays.** These are pure heat rays, comprising about 60 percent of sunshine. Infrared rays are long, penetrate more than 2" into the body, and can produce the most heat. Infrared rays produce no light whatsoever, and the lamps have only a rosy glow when active. Special glass bulbs, which can be red or white, are used to produce infrared rays. Most moisturizing skin creams may be used, but check the ingredients for possible contraindications. The lamp should be operated at an average distance of 30 inches and the client's comfort checked frequently.

Infrared ray treatments will heat and relax the skin without increasing the temperature of the body as a whole. These rays will dilate blood vessels in the skin, thereby increasing blood circulation, and increase metabolism and chemical changes within skin tissues. Infrared rays will also soothe nerves, relieve muscular pain, and increase the production of perspiration and oil on the skin.

Electrotherapy and light therapy treatments are special client services that new and established barbers should consider offering. When the services discussed in this chapter are performed professionally and marketed effectively, the barbershop will benefit from increased revenue, client retention, and new-client referrals that can elevate the shop's reputation "a cut above" the rest.

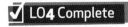 LO**4** Complete

CAUTION

The client's eyes should always be protected when ultraviolet rays are used. Goggles or eye pads saturated with dilute boric acid or witch hazel should be provided for clients, and protective eyewear or sunglasses for the barber.

CAUTION

When performing infrared treatments, the length of exposure should not exceed 5 minutes. It is important to break the path of the rays every few seconds to prevent overexposure. This can be accomplished by moving a hand back and forth across the ray's path between the lamp and the client's skin.

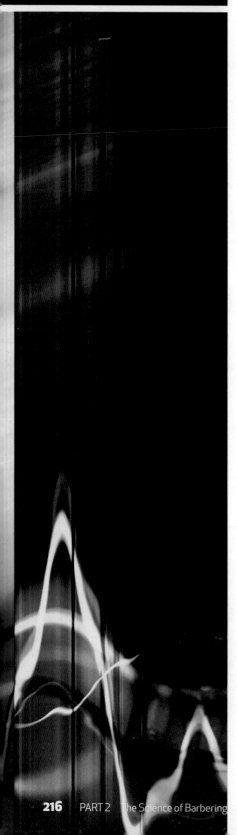

Review
Questions

1. Describe two types of electrical current.

2. Explain the differences between a fuse, circuit breaker, and a GFCI.

3. List and define four electrical modalities used in scalp and facial treatments.

4. Discuss the effects of visible and invisible light rays.

5. Explain the differences between ultraviolet and infrared rays.

6. Explain the effects of ultraviolet and infrared rays.

Chapter
Glossary

alternating current (AC) rapid and interrupted current, flowing first in one direction then the opposite direction *amp* a unit measures the strength of an electric current

amp (ampere) standard unit for measuring the strength of an electric current or the rate of flow of charge in a conductor; also called an amp

anaphoresis process of forcing substances into tissues using galvanic current from the negative toward the positive pole

anode positive electrode

cataphoresis process of forcing acidic substances into tissues using galvanic current from the positive toward the negative pole

cathode negative electrode

circuit breaker switch that automatically interrupts or shuts off an electric circuit at the first sign of overload

complete circuit the path of an electric current from the generating source through the conductor and back to its original source

conductor any substance, medium, or material that conducts electricity

converter an apparatus that changes direct current to alternating current

desincrustation process used to soften and emulsify oil and blackheads in the hair follicles

direct current (DC) constant current that travels in one direction only and produces a chemical reaction

electric current the flow of electricity along a conductor

electrode an applicator used to direct electric current from a machine to the skin

electrotherapy electronic scalp and facial treatments

faradic current alternating current that produces a mechanical reaction without chemical effect

fuse device that prevents excessive current from passing through a circuit

galvanic current constant and direct current, having a positive and negative pole, that produces chemical changes in tissues and body fluids

ground fault circuit interrupter a device that senses imbalances in an electric current

infrared rays invisible rays with long wavelengths and deep penetration; produce the most heat of any therapeutic light

insulator substance that does not easily transfer electricity

iontophoresis process of introducing water-soluble products into the skin through the use of electric current

modalities currents used in electric facial and scalp treatments

ohm (O) the unit of electrical resistance in an electric current

polarity negative or positive pole of an electric current

rectifier apparatus that changes alternating current to direct current

rheostat an adjustable resistor used for controlling current in a circuit

sinusoidal current alternating current used in scalp and facial manipulations that produces mechanical contractions

Tesla high-frequency current thermal or heat-producing current with a high oscillation rate; also known as the violet ray

ultraviolet light invisible rays, with short wavelengths and minimal skin penetration, that produce chemical effects and kill germs; also called actinic or cold rays

visible light electromagnetic radiation that can be seen by the human eye

volt (V) a unit of electrical pressure that pushes the flow of electrons forward through a conductor

watt (W) the unit of power (amperes multiplied by volts), indicating how much electric energy is being used in one second

wavelength distance between two successive peaks of electromagnetic waves

10

PROPERTIES AND DISORDERS OF

The Skin

☑ Learning Objectives

AFTER COMPLETING THIS CHAPTER, YOU SHOULD BE ABLE TO:

1 Describe the structure and divisions of the skin.

2 List the functions of the skin.

3 Identify recognizable skin disorders.

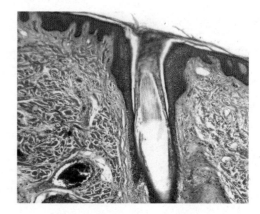

Key Terms

PAGE NUMBER INDICATES WHERE IN THE CHAPTER THE TERM IS USED.

acne / 233

adipose tissue / 222

albinism / 232

anhidrosis / 235

anthrax / 232

asteatosis / 234

basal cell carcinoma / 235

blackheads / 234

bromhidrosis / 235

bulla / 229

chloasma / 231

cicatrix / 230

collagen / 224

comedones / 234

corium / 221

crust / 230

cuticle / 220

cutis / 221

cyst / 229

derma / 221

dermatitis / 232

dermatitis venenata / 232

dermatology / 220

dermis / 221

eczema / 232

elastin / 224

epidermis / 220

excoriation / 230

fissure / 231

herpes simplex / 233

hyperhidrosis / 235

hypertrophy / 231

ivy dermatitis / 233

keloid / 231

keratoma / 231

lentigines / 231

lesion / 229

leukoderma / 231

macule / 229

malignant melanoma / 236

melanin / 224

milia / 234

miliaria rubra / 235

mole / 231

motor nerve fibers / 223

nevus / 232

papillary layer / 222

papule / 230

psoriasis / 233

pustule / 230

reticular layer / 222

rosacea / 234

scale / 231

scarf skin / 220

sebaceous glands / 225

seborrhea / 235

sebum / 225

secretory nerve fibers / 223

sensory nerve fibers / 223

squamous cell carcinoma / 236

stain / 232

steatoma / 235

stratum corneum / 220

stratum germinativum / 221

stratum granulosum / 220

stratum lucidum / 220

stratum spinosum / 221

subcutaneous tissue / 222

sudoriferous glands / 225

symptoms / 226

tan / 232

true skin / 221

tubercule / 230

tumor / 230

ulcer / 231

verruca / 231

vesicle / 230

vitiligo / 232

wheal / 230

whiteheads / 234

Dermatology is the scientific study of the skin—its nature, structure, functions, diseases, and treatment. A study of the skin and scalp is important to barbers because it forms the basis for effective treatment programs. The barber who has mastered a thorough understanding of the skin is in a more knowledgeable position to provide clients with professional advice on scalp and facial care.

Histology of the Skin

The skin is the largest and one of the most important organs of the body because it is the body's first line of defense against disease. Healthy skin is slightly moist, soft, and flexible with a smooth, fine-grained texture. The slightly acidic pH of healthy skin provides a protective response against organisms that touch or try to enter it. Ideally, the skin should be free of blemishes and other disorders and have the ability to renew itself.

Skin varies in thickness. It is thinnest on the eyelids and thickest on the palms of the hands and soles of the feet. Continued pressure over any part of the skin can cause it to thicken and become calloused. The skin of the scalp is constructed similarly to the skin elsewhere on the human body, but the scalp has larger and deeper hair follicles to accommodate the longer hair on the head. The appendages of the skin are hair, nails, sweat glands, and oil glands.

The skin is constructed of two clearly defined divisions: the epidermis and the dermis (**Figure 10-1**).

EPIDERMIS

The **epidermis** (ep-uh-DUR-mis) is the outermost protective layer of the skin. It is the thinnest layer of the skin and is also known as the **cuticle** or **scarf skin**. The epidermis contains no blood vessels, but has many small nerve endings. The layers, or *strata*, of the epidermis are as follows:

- The **stratum corneum** (STRAT-um KOR-nee-um), or *horny layer*, is the outer layer of the epidermis. It consists of tightly packed, scale-like cells that are continually shed and replaced by cells coming to the surface from the underlying layers. These cells are made up of a chemical protein called *keratin*, which combines with a thin layer of oil (sebum) to help make the stratum corneum a protective, waterproof layer.

- The **stratum lucidum** (LOO-sih-dum), or *clear layer*, lies beneath the stratum corneum and consists of small, transparent cells through which light can pass.

- The **stratum granulosum** (gran-yoo-LOH-sum), or *granular layer*, consists of cells that look like distinct granules. These cells are almost dead and are pushed to the surface to replace cells that are shed from the stratum corneum.

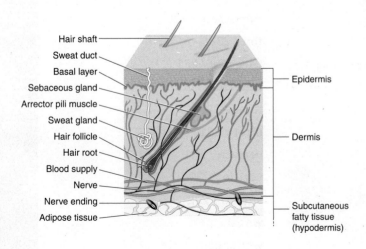

Hair shaft
Sweat duct
Basal layer
Sebaceous gland
Arrector pili muscle
Sweat gland
Hair follicle
Hair root
Blood supply
Nerve
Nerve ending
Adipose tissue

Epidermis
Dermis
Subcutaneous fatty tissue (hypodermis)

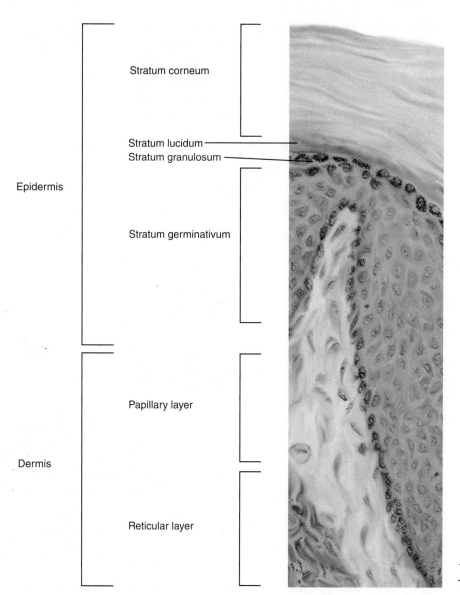

Stratum corneum

Stratum lucidum

Stratum granulosum

Epidermis

Stratum germinativum

Papillary layer

Dermis

Reticular layer

◀ FIGURE 10-1

The layers of the skin.

- The **stratum spinosum,** or *spiny layer,* often classified as part of the germinativum, is a sublayer that lies above the basal strata and beneath the stratum granulosum. It is in the spiny layer that the beginning of the process that causes skin cells to shed begins.

- The **stratum germinativum** (jer-mih-nah-TIV-um), also known as the *Malpighian* or *basal cell layer,* is the deepest layer of the epidermis. This layer is responsible for the growth of the epidermis and contains a dark pigment called *melanin,* which protects the sensitive cells below from the destructive effects of excessive exposure to ultraviolet light.

FYI The stratum spinosum (spiny layer) may be classified as part of the stratum germinativum.

DERMIS

The **dermis** (DUR-mis) is the underlying, or inner layer of the skin. It is also called the **derma, corium, cutis,** or **true skin.** The dermis is about 25 times thicker than the epidermis and consists of a highly sensitive vascular layer of connective tissue. Within its structure are numerous blood vessels, nerves, lymph and oil glands, hair follicles, arrector pili muscles, and papillae. The

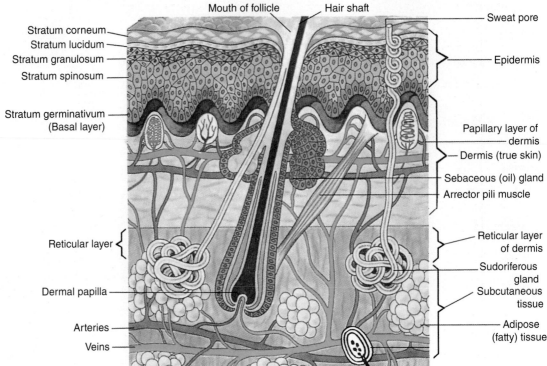

FIGURE 10-2

Structures of the skin.

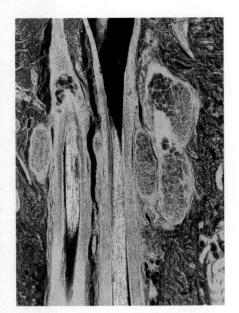

dermis consists of two layers: the papillary or superficial layer; and the reticular or deeper layer (**Figure 10-2**).

- The **papillary** (PAP-uh-lair-ee) **layer** lies directly beneath the stratum germinativum of the epidermis. It contains small, cone-shaped projections of elastic tissue called papillae (puh-PIL-eye) that point upward into the epidermis. Some of these papillae contain looped capillaries or small blood vessels. Others contain small structures called tactile corpuscles with nerve fiber endings that are sensitive to touch and pressure. This layer also contains some melanin (skin pigment).

- The **reticular** (ruh-TIK-yuh-lur) **layer** is the deeper layer of the dermis, which supplies the skin with oxygen and nutrients. It contains the following structures within its network:

  - ▶ Fat cells
  - ▶ Sweat glands
  - ▶ Blood vessels
  - ▶ Hair follicles
  - ▶ Lymph glands
  - ▶ Arrector pili muscles
  - ▶ Oil glands

Subcutaneous (sub-kyoo-TAY-nee-us) **tissue,** also known as **adipose tissue,** is a layer of fatty tissue found below the dermis that some specialists regard as a continuation of the dermis. Subcutaneous tissue varies in thickness according to age, gender, and general health. It gives smoothness and contour to the body, contains fats for use as energy, and also acts as a protective cushion for the outer skin.

HOW THE SKIN IS NOURISHED

Blood and lymph supply nourishment to the skin. From one-half to two-thirds of the body's blood supply is distributed to the skin. As the blood and lymph circulate through the skin, they contribute essential materials for the growth, nourishment, and repair of the skin, hair, and nails. Networks of arteries and lymphatics in the subcutaneous tissue send their smaller branches to hair papillae, hair follicles, and skin glands.

NERVES OF THE SKIN

The skin contains the surface endings of many nerve fibers, which are classified as follows:

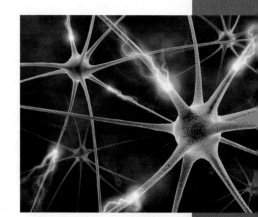

- **Motor nerve fibers** are distributed to the arrector pili muscles attached to the hair follicles. These muscles trigger "goose bumps" when a person is frightened or cold.

- **Sensory nerve fibers** react to heat, cold, touch, pressure, and pain **(Figure 10-3)**. These receptors send messages to the brain.

- **Secretory nerve fibers** are distributed to the sweat and oil glands of the skin. Secretory nerves regulate the excretion of perspiration from the sweat glands and the flow of sebum from the oil glands.

Sense of Touch

The papillary layer of the dermis houses the nerve endings that provide the body with the sense of touch. These nerve endings register basic sensations such as touch, pain, heat, cold, pressure, or deep touch. Nerve endings are most abundant in the fingertips. Complex sensations, such as vibrations, seem to depend on the sensitivity of a combination of these nerve endings.

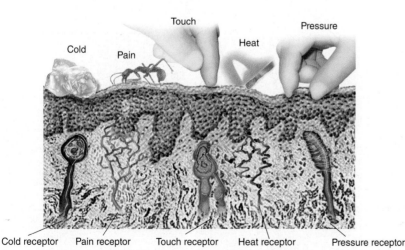

▲ **FIGURE 10-3**
Sensory nerve endings in the skin.

SKIN ELASTICITY

The skin gets its strength, form, and flexibility from protein fibers within the dermis called collagen and elastin. **Collagen** fibers make up a large portion of the dermis and help to give support to the many structures found in this layer. When collagen fibers become weakened, wrinkles and sagging of the skin can occur. **Elastin** gives the skin its elasticity and flexibility and the ability to regain its shape after stretching. When healthy skin expands, it regains its former shape almost immediately. Conversely, one of the most prominent characteristics of aged skin is its loss of elasticity.

SKIN COLOR

The color of the skin, whether fair or dark, depends on two factors: blood supply and melanin. Of the two, blood supply to the skin is least influential to skin color. Melanin, however, is the primary source of skin color; the grains of pigment are deposited in the stratum germinativum of the epidermis and the papillary layer of the dermis (Refer to Figure 10-2).

Special cells called *melanocytes* produce the pigment granules that are scattered throughout the germinativum and papillary layers. These granules are called *melanosomes* and they produce the complex protein called **melanin,** a brown-black pigment that serves as the skin's protective screen from the sun's rays. The color of pigment is a hereditary trait that varies among races and nationalities and from person to person. Dark skin contains more melanin than light skin.

THE GLANDS OF THE SKIN

The skin contains two types of duct glands, the *sudoriferous* (sood-uh-RIF-uh- rus) *glands* or *sweat glands* and the *sebaceous* (sih-BAY-shus) *glands* or *oil glands*, which extract material from the blood to form new substances **(Figure 10-4).**

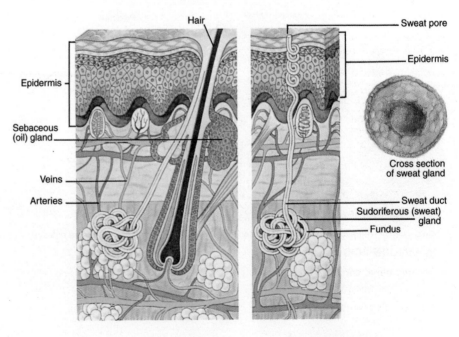

► **FIGURE 10-4**

Sweat gland and oil production.

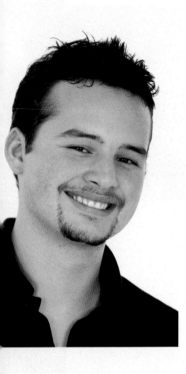

Sudoriferous (Sweat) Glands

The **sudoriferous glands** consist of a coiled base (called a *fundus*) and a tube-like duct that terminates at the skin surface to form the sweat pore. Practically all parts of the body are supplied with sweat glands, although they are more numerous on the palms, soles, forehead, and armpits.

The sweat glands regulate body temperature and help to eliminate waste products from the body. Because the excretion of sweat is under the control of the nervous system, sweat gland activity is greatly increased by heat, exercise, emotion, and certain drugs.

Normally, one or two pints of liquid containing salts are eliminated daily through the sweat pores in the skin.

Sebaceous (Oil) Glands

The sebaceous or oil glands of the skin are connected to the hair follicles. These glands consist of little sacs with ducts that open into the hair follicle where they secrete **sebum,** which lubricates the skin and preserves the softness of the hair. With the exception of the palms and soles, these glands are found in all parts of the body, particularly the face.

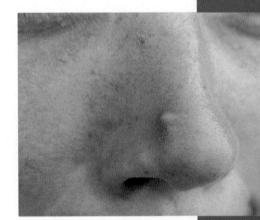

Sebum is a semi-fluid, oily substance produced by the oil glands. Ordinarily it flows through the oil ducts leading to the mouths of the hair follicles. However, when the sebum becomes hardened and the duct becomes blocked, a blackhead is formed. The primary function of sebum is to act as a shield that prevents moisture from evaporating from the skin surface.

ABSORPTION LEVEL OF THE SKIN

Although the skin serves as a protective barrier against microorganisms and chemical absorption, some topical products and creams are designed to penetrate this barrier for medicinal purposes. Limited absorption occurs through the skin cells, hair follicles, **sebaceous glands,** and sudoriferous glands and facilitates the entry of special drugs or chemicals into the body. For example, antiseptics may be used to combat skin infections, or vitamin creams to support skin repair. The amount or level of absorption that takes place is dependent upon the thickness and location of the skin on the body, the concentration of the product, and the frequency of the application.

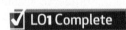

LO1 Complete

FUNCTIONS OF THE SKIN

The principal functions of the skin are sensation, heat regulation, absorption, protection, excretion, and secretion.

- *Sensation:* The skin responds to heat, cold, touch, pressure, pain, and movement through its sensory nerve endings. Stimulation of a sensory nerve ending sends a message to the brain, which then stimulates a response. When you scratch an itch or pull away from a hot object, you are responding to the stimulation of sensory nerve endings and the message they conveyed to the brain. Sensory endings responsive to touch and pressure lie in close relation to hair follicles.

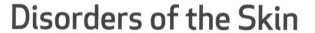

FYI

Use the acronym SHAPES to remember the functions of the skin: Sensation, Heat regulation, Absorption, Protection, Excretion, and Secretion.

- *Heat regulation:* Heat regulation is a function of the skin that protects the body from the environment. A healthy body maintains a constant internal temperature of about 98.6 degrees Fahrenheit. As changes occur in the outside temperature, the blood and sweat glands of the skin make necessary adjustments to facilitate the cooling of the body through the evaporation of sweat.

- *Absorption:* Absorption is limited, but does occur. Some female hormone creams can enter the body through the skin and influence it to some degree. Fatty materials, such as lanolin creams, are absorbed largely through the hair follicles and sebaceous gland openings.

- *Protection:* The skin protects the body from injury and bacterial invasion. The outermost layer of the epidermis is covered with a thin layer of sebum, which renders it waterproof. The skin is resistant to variations in temperature, minor injuries, chemical substances, and many forms of bacteria.

- *Excretion:* Perspiration is excreted from the skin. Water lost by perspiration carries salt and other chemicals with it.

- *Secretion:* Sebum is secreted by the sebaceous glands and lubricates the skin, keeping it soft and pliable. Sebum also lubricates the hair. Emotional stress may increase the flow of sebum.

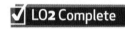

Disorders of the Skin

Although barbers are not licensed to perform treatments for medical conditions, providing facials and shaves are traditional services well within the barber's scope of expertise. This includes addressing certain skin conditions, such as oily or dry skin, or alleviating minor acne conditions. Before proceeding with services, barbers need to be able to recognize *hypertrophies*, such as moles and warts on the face, or scalp and skin conditions that may be aggravated by facial or shaving procedures. The following section has been compiled to familiarize you with some common skin disorders to ensure that barbering services are carried out in a knowledgeable and skillful manner.

Symptoms are signs or indications of disease. Symptoms of skin disorders are generally divided into two groups: *subjective symptoms*, such as itching, burning, or pain that can be felt only by the individual; and *objective symptoms*, such as pimples or boils, which can be observed by anyone. *Lesions*, in the form of scales, pimples, or pustules, are symptoms that may characterize the skin conditions that barbers see in the performance of their work. Since these symptoms may be similar in appearance to certain contagious disorders, it is important to be able to differentiate between common or non-contagious skin conditions and more serious or communicable ones. This knowledge helps the barber to know which services may or may not be performed in the barbershop.

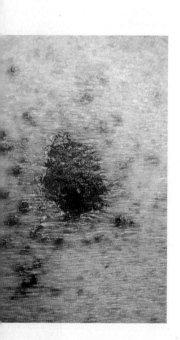

Did **You** Know...

Barbers often recognize changes in their client's skin and scalp. Report any changes in a lesion or growth to the client so they can pursue diagnosis and treatment.

Some skin and scalp disorders may be treated in cooperation with, or under the supervision of, a physician or dermatologist. To protect both the barber and client, the client should provide the barber with a copy of the prescription directions. Medicinal preparations must be applied as directed by the physician and treatment should not extend beyond the number of applications or date indicated. If a client has a skin or scalp condition you do not recognize, refer the client to a physician.

CAUTION: In order to safeguard personal and public health, it is crucial that barbers do not perform services on a client who has an infectious or contagious disorder. This includes parasitic conditions such as pediculosis and scabies as discussed in Chapter 11. It is also very important not to perform services on inflamed skin, whether it is infectious or not. Certain products and services that are applied on inflamed or irritated skin may intensify and worsen the condition. Barbers should be able to recognize such conditions and tactfully suggest that the client seek appropriate medical treatment before receiving services.

The skin is a durable but sensitive organ that may be affected by a variety of internal or external conditions. The general terms relating to disease you were introduced to in Chapter 4, as well as some new terms, are reviewed in **Table 10-1**.

> ### TABLE **10-1** General Terms Relating to Disease

TERM	DEFINITION
acute disease	disease having a rapid onset, severe symptoms, and a short course or duration
allergy	reaction due to extreme sensitivity to certain foods, chemicals, or other normally harmless substances
chronic disease	disease of long duration, usually mild but recurring
congenital disease	disease that exists at birth
contagious disease	disease that is communicable or transmittable by contact
contraindication	any condition or disease that makes an indicated treatment or medication inadvisable
diagnosis	determination of the nature of a disease from its symptoms
disease	abnormal condition of all or part of the body or mind that makes it incapable of carrying on normal function

> TABLE **10-1** (Continued)

TERM	DEFINITION
epidemic	appearance of a disease that simultaneously attacks a large number of persons living in a particular locality
etiology	study of the causes of diseases and their modes of operation
infectious disease	disease caused by pathogenic microorganisms or viruses that are easily spread
inflammation	condition of some part of the body as a protective response to injury, irritation, or infection, characterized by redness, heat, pain, and swelling
objective symptoms	symptoms that are visible, such as pimples, pustules, or inflammation
occupational disease	illness resulting from conditions associated with employment, such as coming in contact with certain chemicals or tints
parasitic disease	disease caused by vegetable or animal parasites, such as pediculosis and ringworm
pathogenic disease	disease produced by bacteria, such as staphylococci and streptococci (pus-forming bacteria), or viruses
pathology	science that investigates modifications of the functions and changes in structure caused by disease
prognosis	foretelling of probable course of a disease
seasonal disease	disease influenced by the weather
subjective symptoms	symptoms that can be felt, such as itching, burning, or pain
systemic disease	disease that affects the body generally, often due to under- or over-functioning of the internal glands
venereal disease	contagious disease commonly acquired by contact with an infected person during sexual intercourse

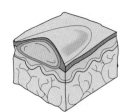

Bulla:
Same as a vesicle only greater than 0.5 cm
Example:
Contact dermatitis, large second-degree burns, bulbous impetigo, pemphigus

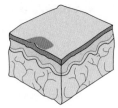

Macule:
Localized changes in skin color of less than 1 cm in diameter
Example:
Freckle

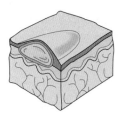

Tubercle:
Solid and elevated; however, it extends deeper than papules into the dermis or subcutaneous tissues, 0.5-2 cm
Example:
Lipoma, erythema, nodosum, cyst

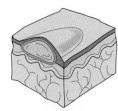

Papule:
Solid, elevated lesion less than 0.5 cm in diameter
Example:
Warts, elevated nevi

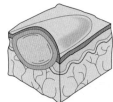

Pustule:
Vesicles or bullae that become filled with pus, usually described as less than 0.5 cm in diameter
Example:
Acne, impetigo, furuncles, carbuncles, folliculitis

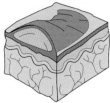

Vesicle:
Accumulation of fluid between the upper layers of the skin; elevated mass containing serous fluid; less than 0.5 cm
Example:
Herpes simplex, herpes zoster, chickenpox

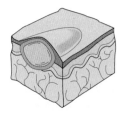

Nodule/Tumor:
The same as a nodule only greater than 2 cm
Example:
Carcinoma (such as advanced breast carcinoma); **not** basal cell or squamous cell of the skin

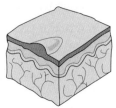

Wheal:
Localized edema in the epidermis causing irregular elevation that may be red or pale
Example:
Insect bite or a hive

▲ **FIGURE 10-5**
Primary skin lesions.

LESIONS OF THE SKIN

A **lesion** is a structural change in the tissues caused by injury or disease. There are three types of lesions: primary, secondary, and tertiary. The barber is concerned with primary and secondary lesions only.

Primary Lesions

Primary lesions are characterized by flat, non-palpable changes in skin color, such as a macule; elevations formed by fluid in a cavity, such as pustules; or by elevated, palpable solid masses, as in papules **(Figure 10-5)**. The following are common primary lesions:

- A **bulla** (BULL-uh) is a large blister containing a watery fluid, similar to a vesicle, but larger in size **(Figure 10-6)**.

- A **cyst** (SIST) is a closed, abnormally developed sac containing fluid, semi-fluid, or morbid matter above or below the skin.

- A **macule** (MAK-yool) is a small, discolored spot or patch on the surface of the skin. Macules are neither raised nor sunken.

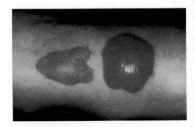

▲ **FIGURE 10-6**
Bullae.

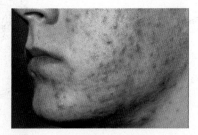

▲ FIGURE 10-7

Papules and pustules.

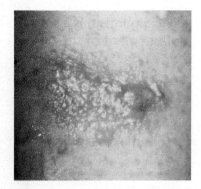

▲ FIGURE 10-8

Poison oak vesicles.

- A **papule** (PAP-yool) is a small, elevated pimple that contains no fluid, but that may develop pus (**Figure 10-7**).

- A **pustule** (PUS-chool) is an inflamed pimple containing pus (**Figure 10-7**).

- A **tubercule** (TOO-bur-kul) is an abnormal rounded, solid lump larger than a papule that projects above the surface or lies within or under the skin.

- A **tumor** (TOO-mur) is an abnormal cell mass varying in size, shape, and color that results from the excessive multiplication of cells. *Nodules* are also referred to as tumors, but they are smaller.

- A **vesicle** (VES-ih-kel) is a small blister or sac containing clear fluid lying within or just beneath the epidermis. Poison ivy and poison oak produce small vesicles (**Figure 10-8**).

- A **wheal** (WHEEL) is an itchy, swollen lesion that lasts only a few hours. Hives and insect bites are examples of wheals.

Secondary Lesions

Secondary lesions are characterized by a collection of material on the skin, such as a scale, crust, or keloid; or by a loss of skin surface, as with an ulcer or fissure (**Figure 10-9**).

- A **cicatrix** (SIK-uh-triks), or scar, is a light-colored, slightly raised mark that is formed after an injury or skin lesion has healed.

- A **crust** or scab is an accumulation of dead cells that forms over a wound or blemish while it is healing or an accumulation of sebum and pus, sometimes mixed with epidermal material.

- An **excoriation** (ek-skor-ee-AY-shun) is a skin sore produced by scratching or scraping. The skin's surface becomes raw due to the loss of superficial skin after an injury.

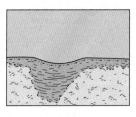

Scar

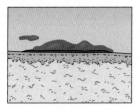

Crust

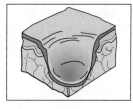

Ulcer

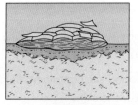

Scale

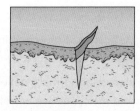

Fissure

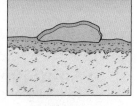

Excoriation

▲ FIGURE 10-9

Secondary skin lesions.

- A **fissure** (FISH-ur) is a crack in the skin that penetrates into the dermis, such as with chapped hands or lips.

- A **keloid** (KEE-loyd) is a thick scar resulting from excessive growth of fibrous tissue **(Figure 10-10)**.

- A **scale** is any accumulation of dry or greasy flakes, such as abnormal or excessive dandruff.

- An **ulcer** (UL-sur) is an open lesion on the skin or mucous membrane of the body, accompanied by pus and loss of skin depth; a deep erosion or depression in the skin, normally due to infection or cancer.

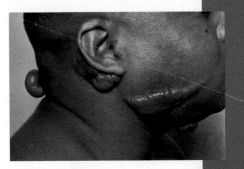

▲ **FIGURE 10-10**
Keloids.

HYPERTROPHIES OF THE SKIN

A **hypertrophy** (hy-PUR-truh-fee) of the skin is an abnormal growth of skin tissue that is usually benign or harmless.

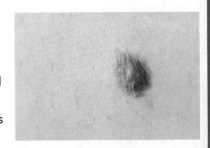

- A **keratoma** (kair-uh-TOH-muh) is an acquired, superficial, thickened patch of skin, commonly known as a *callus*, that is caused by continued pressure or friction; keratomas frequently occur in regions subject to friction, such as the hands and feet.

- A **mole** is a small, brownish spot or blemish on the skin ranging in color from pale tan to brown to bluish black. Some moles are small and flat, resembling freckles, while others are more deeply seated and darker in color. Large, dark hairs often grow in moles. If a mole grows in size, gets darker, or becomes sore or scaly, medical attention is needed.

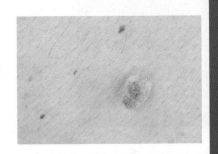

- A **verruca** (vuh-ROO-kuh) is commonly called a wart, and is a hypertrophy of the papillae and epidermis. Caused by a virus, it is infectious to the person who has one and can spread from one location to another, particularly along a scratch in the skin.

CAUTION

Do not treat or remove hair from moles.

PIGMENTATIONS OF THE SKIN

Pigment may be affected by internal factors within the body or by external conditions such as prolonged sun exposure. Abnormal colors are seen in every skin disease and in many systemic disorders. A change in pigmentation can be observed when certain substances and drugs are being taken internally. The following conditions or disorders relate to changes in the pigmentation of the skin.

- **Chloasma** (kloh-AZ-mah), also called *liver spots*, are caused by increased pigment deposits in the skin. They are found mainly on the forehead, nose, and cheeks.

- **Lentigines** (len-TIJ-e-neez), is the technical term for freckles, small yellow- to brown-colored spots appearing on the skin when exposed to sunlight and air.

- **Leukoderma** (loo-koh-DUR-muh) is a skin disorder characterized by abnormal white patches, caused by a burn or congenital pigmentation defects.

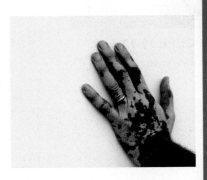

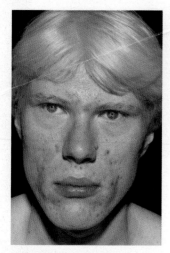

▲ **FIGURE 10-11**
Albinism.

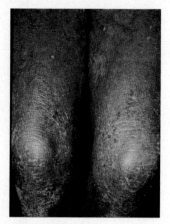

▲ **FIGURE 10-12**
Vitiligo.

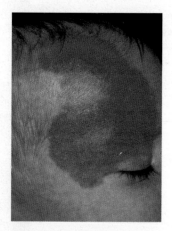

▲ **FIGURE 10-13**
Port wine stain.

▶ **Albinism** (AL-bi-niz-em) is congenital leukoderma or absence of melanin pigments in the body, including the skin, hair, and eyes. This condition may be partial or complete. The hair is silky and white or pale yellow. The skin is pinkish-white, and will not tan **(Figure 10-11)**.

▶ **Vitiligo** (vit-I-LEE-goh) is an acquired condition of leukoderma affecting the hair or skin in patches **(Figure 10-12)**.

• A **nevus** (NEE-vus) is a small or large malformation of the skin due to abnormal pigmentation or dilated capillaries, commonly known as a birth-mark.

• A **stain** is an abnormal brown or wine-colored skin discoloration with a generally circular and irregular shape. Its permanent color is due to the presence of darker pigment. Stains occur during aging, after certain diseases, and after the disappearance of moles, freckles, and liver spots. The cause is unknown **(Figure 10-13)**.

• A **tan** is a change in the pigmentation of the skin caused by exposure to ultraviolet rays from the sun or from tanning lamps.

INFLAMMATIONS OF THE SKIN

• **Anthrax** (AN-thraks) is an inflammatory bacterial skin disease characterized by the presence of a small, red-brown papule, followed by the formation of a pustule, vesicle, and hard swelling. It is accompanied by itching and burning at the point of infection and is contagious. Sometimes flu-like symptoms are present.

Skin anthrax is usually transmitted to humans from infected animals or animal products, and therein rests its connection with the barbershop. The disease can be spread through the use of infected shaving or hair brushes made from animal hair that was not sterilized during manufacture or disinfected on a regular basis. Inhalation anthrax, caused by inhaling anthrax spores, is the most serious form, resulting in death for about half of those afflicted. Gastrointestinal anthrax is rare but can be transmitted from eating contaminated meat.

• **Dermatitis** (dur-muh-TY-tis) is the general term for an inflammatory condition of the skin. The lesions may appear in various forms, such as vesicles or papules.

• **Dermatitis venenata** (VEN-uh-nah-tuh) is an eruptive skin infection that is characteristic of the abnormal conditions resulting from occasional or frequent contact with chemicals or tints. Individuals may develop allergies to certain ingredients in cosmetics, antiseptics, disinfectants, and aniline derivative tints used in the barbering profession. This occupational disorder or disease may be minimized by using rubber gloves or protective creams whenever possible.

• **Eczema** (EG-zuh-muh) is an inflammatory skin disease that may be acute or chronic in nature and present in many forms of dry or moist lesions. Eczema is frequently accompanied by itching or burning and all cases should be referred to a physician for treatment. Its cause is unknown (**Figure 10-14**).

- **Herpes simplex** (HER-peez SIM-plex) is a recurring viral infection that produces fever blisters or cold sores characterized by a single vesicle or group of vesicles with red, swollen bases. The blisters usually appear on the lips, nostrils, or other parts of the face, and rarely last more than a week. Herpes simplex is contagious (**Figure 10-15**).

- **Ivy dermatitis** is a skin inflammation caused by exposure to poison ivy, poison oak, or poison sumac leaves. Blisters and itching develop soon after contact occurs. The condition can be spread to other parts of the body by contact with contaminated hands, clothing, objects, or anything that was exposed to the plant itself. If the irritating plant oil remains on the skin, it also can be spread from one person to another by direct contact. Serious cases should be referred to a physician.

- **Psoriasis** (suh-RY-us-sis) is a chronic inflammatory skin disease characterized by dry red patches covered with coarse, silvery scales. Psoriasis usually occurs on the scalp, elbows, knees, chest, or lower back, but rarely on the face. If irritated, bleeding points occur. It is not contagious and the cause is unknown (**Figure 10-16**).

DISORDERS OF THE SEBACEOUS GLANDS

There are several common disorders of the sebaceous glands that barbers should be able to identify and understand.

- **Acne** (AK-nee) is a skin disorder characterized by chronic inflammation of the sebaceous glands from retained secretions and bacteria, occurring most frequently on the face, back, and chest. Acne, or common pimples, is also known as *acne vulgaris*. Although the cause of acne is generally held to be microbial in nature, factors such as heredity, hormones, stress, and digestive disturbances can trigger inflammations.

  Acne conditions are rated in four grades (**Figures 10-17a through 10-17d**):

  ▶ Grade I: Minor breakouts, mostly open comedones, some closed comedones, and a few papules and pustules

  ▶ Grade II: Many closed comedones, more open comedones, and more papules and pustules

  ▶ Grade III: Redness and inflammation with many papules and pustules

  ▶ Grade IV: Cysts with comedones, papules, pustules, and inflammation (cystic acne)

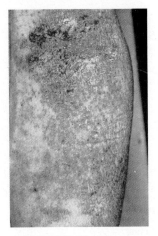

▲ **FIGURE 10-14**
Eczema.

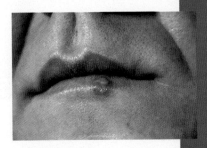

▲ **FIGURE 10-15**
Herpes simplex.

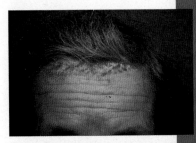

▲ **FIGURE 10-16**
Psoriasis.

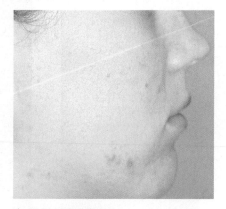

▲ FIGURE 10-17a

Grade I Acne.

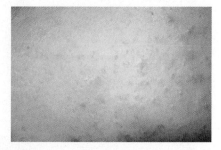

▲ FIGURE 10-17b

Grade II Acne.

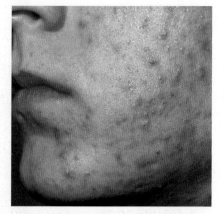

▲ FIGURE 10-17c

Grade III Acne.

It is always advisable for the client to seek diagnosis and treatment by a competent physician before any acne facial service is given in the barbershop.

- **Asteatosis** (as-tee-ah-TOH-sis) is a condition of dry, scaly skin, characterized by the absolute or partial deficiency of sebum. It can be the result of old age, exposure to cold or alkalies, or bodily disorders.

- **Comedones** (KAHM-uh-dohns) are masses of hardened sebum and dead cells in a hair follicle. *Open* comedones **(blackheads)** occur when excess oil in the follicles is exposed to oxygen and oxidizes to a dark color. *Closed* comedones **(whiteheads)** do not have a follicular opening to be exposed to oxygen, so the sebum remains a whitish color and produces a whitehead. Comedones appear most frequently on the face, forehead, and nose and sometimes on the chest, back, or shoulders. They should be removed under aseptic conditions by using proper extraction procedures, and barbers should limit this service to the facial area only. Severe conditions require medical attention and treatment (Figure 10-18).

- **Milia** (MIL-ee-uh), also known as milk spots, are small, benign, whitish bumps that occur when dead skin is trapped in the surface of the skin. Commonly seen in infants, milia usually disappear after a few weeks. Adult milia may develop due to inflammation or injury and is more common to dry skin types. Milia can occur on any part of the face and neck and occasionally on the chest and shoulders with no lasting negative effect (Figure 10-19).

- **Rosacea** (roh-ZAY-shee-uh), formerly called *acne rosacea*, is a chronic inflammatory congestion of the cheeks and nose. It is characterized by redness, dilation of the blood vessels, and the formation of

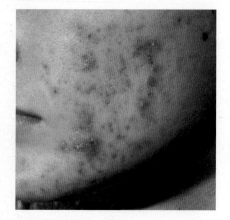

▲ FIGURE 10-17d

Grade IV Acne.

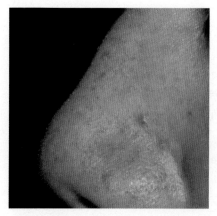

▲ FIGURE 10-18

Comedones.

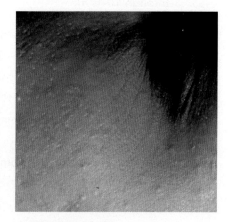

▲ FIGURE 10-19

Milia.

papules and pustules. The cause of rosacea is unknown, but certain factors are known to aggravate the condition in some individuals. These include consumption of hot liquids, spicy foods, or alcohol; exposure to extremes of heat and cold; exposure to sunlight; and stress (Figure 10-20).

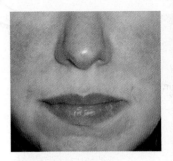

▲ FIGURE 10-20
Rosacea.

- **Seborrhea** (seb-oh-REE-ah) is a skin condition due to over-activity and excessive secretion of the sebaceous glands. An itching or burning sensation may accompany it. An oily or shiny nose, forehead, or scalp indicates the presence of seborrhea. On the scalp, it is readily detected by the presence of an unusual amount of oil on the hair (Figure 10-21).

- **Steatoma** (stee-ah-TOH-muh): a sebaceous cyst or fatty tumor that is filled with sebum. It is a subcutaneous tumor of the sebaceous glands that can range in size from a pea to an orange. A steatoma usually occurs on the scalp, neck, or back and is sometimes called a *wen* (Figure 10-22).

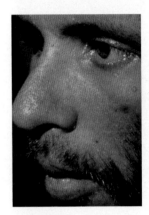

▲ FIGURE 10-21
Seborrhea.

DISORDERS OF THE SUDORIFEROUS (SWEAT) GLANDS

- **Anhidrosis** (an-hih-DROH-sis) is a lack of perspiration, often as a result of a fever or certain skin diseases. It requires medical attention.

- **Bromhidrosis** (broh-mih-DROH-sis) refers to foul-smelling perspiration, usually noticeable in the armpits or on the feet.

- **Hyperhidrosis** (hy-per-hi-DROH-sis) is excessive perspiration caused by excessive heat or general body weakness. The parts of the body most commonly affected are the armpits, joints, and feet. It requires medical treatment.

- **Miliaria rubra** (mil-ee-AIR-ee-ah ROOB rah), or *prickly heat*, is an acute inflammatory disorder of the sweat glands characterized by the eruption of small, red vesicles, accompanied by burning and itching of the skin. It is caused by exposure to excessive heat.

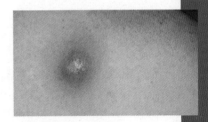

▲ FIGURE 10-22
Steatoma.

SKIN CANCER

Skin cancer from overexposure to the sun comes in three distinct forms that vary in severity. Each is named for the type of body cells that it affects.

- **Basal cell carcinoma** is the most common and the least severe type of skin cancer, and is often characterized by light or pearly nodules (Figure 10-23).

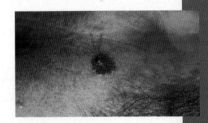

▲ FIGURE 10-23
Basal cell carcinoma.

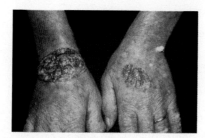

▲ **FIGURE 10-24**
Squamous cell carcinoma.

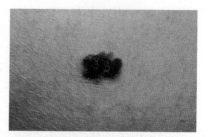

▲ **FIGURE 10-25**
Malignant melanoma.

- **Squamous cell carcinoma** is a skin cancer that is more serious than basal cell carcinoma and is often characterized by scaly red papules or nodules (**Figure 10-24**).

- **Malignant melanoma** is the most serious form of skin cancer, often characterized by dark brown or black patches on the skin. The patches may appear jagged, raised, or uneven in texture. Malignant melanomas often appear on individuals who do not receive regular sun exposure and are sometimes termed the "city person's cancer." Although the least common, malignant melanoma is the most dangerous type of skin cancer (**Figure 10-25**).

If detected early, most cases of skin cancer respond to medical treatment. Barbers should not attempt to diagnose skin disorders, but they should be aware of changes in their clients' skin. If and when a change is noticed, barbers can tactfully suggest to the client to seek the advice of a dermatologist.

Did **You** Know...

MAINTAINING THE HEALTH OF THE SKIN

Diet is the major factor involved in maintaining the skin's overall health and appearance. Proper and beneficial dietary choices help to regulate hydration, oil production, and the function of cells.

- Foods: Eating a well-balanced diet of the three basic food groups of fats, carbohydrates, and proteins is the best way to support the health of the skin.

- *Vitamins and supplements:* Various nutrients aid in healing, softening, and fighting diseases of the skin. Vitamin A supports the overall health of the skin, vitamin C is important to skin and tissue repair, vitamin D promotes healthy and rapid healing of the skin, and vitamin E helps to fight against the harmful effects of the sun's rays.

- *Water:* Ingesting plenty of fluids sustains the health of the cells, aids in the elimination of toxins and waste, helps to regulate the body's temperature, and aids in proper digestion.

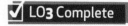
✓ **LO3 Complete**

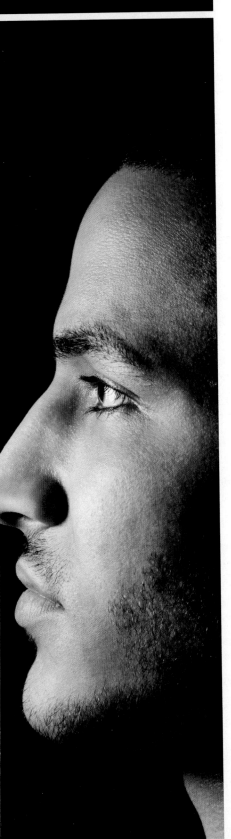

Review Questions

1. Briefly describe healthy skin.

2. Name the two main divisions of the skin and describe the layers within each division.

3. Identify the appendages of the skin.

4. How is the skin nourished?

5. Name three types of nerve fibers found in the skin.

6. What determines the color of the skin?

7. Identify two types of glands found in the skin and describe their functions.

8. List the six important functions of the skin.

9. What is a lesion?

10. What are the characteristics of primary skin lesions?

11. Describe the characteristics of secondary skin lesions.

12. List the characteristics of the following: eczema, herpes simplex, psoriasis, and dermatitis venenata.

13. What are some characteristics of seborrhea that distinguish it from acne?

14. Which two disorders of the sudoriferous glands require medical attention?

15. What is the most common and least severe type of skin cancer?

Chapter
Glossary

acne skin disorder characterized by chronic inflammation of the sebaceous glands from retained secretions

adipose tissue also know as subcutaneous tissue; lies beneath the dermis

albinism congenital leukoderma or absence of melanin pigment in the body

anhidrosis deficiency or lack of perspiration

anthrax inflammatory skin disease characterized by the presence of a small, red papule, followed by the formation of a pustule, vesicle, and hard swelling

asteatosis condition of dry, scaly skin due to lack of sebum

basal cell carcinoma most common and least severe type of skin cancer

blackhead an open comedone; consists of an accumulation of excess oil (sebum) that has been oxidized to a dark color

bromhidrosis foul-smelling perspiration

bulla large blister containing a watery fluid

chloasma non-elevated spots due to increased pigmentation in the skin

cicatrix technical term for a scar

collagen fibrous protein that gives the skin form and strength

comedones a mass of hardened sebum and skin cells in a hair follicle that may be open (blackhead) or closed (whitehead)

corium another name for the dermis

crust dead cells that have accumulated over a wound

cuticle another name for the epidermis

cutis another name for the dermis

cyst a closed, abnormally developed sac containing fluid or morbid matter, above or below the skin

derma technical name for skin; also another name for the dermis

dermatitis an inflammatory condition of the skin

dermatitis venenata an eruptive skin condition due to contact with irritating substances such as tints or chemicals

dermatology medical science that deals with the study of the skin

dermis second or inner layer of the skin; also known as the derma, corium, cutis, or true skin

eczema inflammatory skin condition characterized by painful itching; dry or moist lesion forms

elastin protein base similar to collagen that forms elastic tissue

epidermis outermost layer of the skin; also called the cuticle or scarf skin

excoriation skin sore or abrasion caused by scratching or scraping

fissure a crack in the skin that penetrates to the dermis

herpes simplex fever blister or cold sore; a recurring viral infection

hyperhidrosis excessive perspiration or sweating

hypertrophy abnormal skin growth

ivy dermatitis a skin inflammation caused by exposure to poison ivy, poison oak, or poison sumac

keloid thick scar resulting from excessive tissue growth

keratoma technical name for a callus, caused by pressure or friction

lentigines technical name for freckles

lesion a structural change in the tissues caused by injury or disease

leukoderma skin disorder characterized by abnormal white patches

macule spot or discoloration of the skin such as a freckle

malignant melanoma most severe form of skin cancer

melanin coloring matter or pigment of the skin; found in the stratum germinativum of the epidermis and in the papillary layers of the dermis

milia technical name for milk spots; small, benign, whitish bumps that occur when dead skin is trapped in the surface of the skin, commonly seen in infants

miliaria rubra technical name for prickly heat

mole small brownish spot on the skin

motor nerve fibers nerve fibers distributed to the arrector pili muscles, which are attached to the hair follicles

nevus technical name for a birthmark

papillary layer outer layer of the dermis, directly beneath the epidermis

papule pimple

psoriasis skin disease characterized by red patches and silvery-white scales

pustule inflamed pimple, containing pus

reticular layer deeper layer of the dermis

rosacea chronic congestion of the skin characterized by redness, blood vessel dilation, papules, and pustules

scale an accumulation of dry or greasy flakes on the skin

scarf skin another name for the epidermis

sebaceous glands oil glands of the skin connected to hair follicles

seborrhea skin condition caused by excessive sebum secretion

sebum an oily substance secreted by the sebaceous glands

secretory nerve fibers regulate the excretion of perspiration from the sweat glands and the flow of sebum from the oil glands

sensory nerve fibers react to heat, cold, touch, pressure, and pain, and send messages to the brain

squamous cell carcinoma type of skin cancer more serious than basal cell carcinoma, but not as serious as malignant melanoma

stain abnormal brown or wine-colored skin discoloration

steatoma sebaceous cyst or fatty tumor

stratum corneum outermost layer of the epidermis; the horny layer

stratum germinativum innermost layer of the epidermis, also known as the basal or Malpighian layer

stratum granulosum granular layer of the epidermis beneath the stratum lucidum; the grainy layer

stratum lucidum clear layer of the epidermis, directly beneath the stratum corneum

stratum spinosm spiny layer of the epidermis, often considered part of the stratum germinativum

subcutaneous tissue fatty tissue layer that lies beneath the dermis; also called adipose tissue

sudoriferous glands sweat glands of the skin

symptoms signs of disease that can be felt (subjective) or seen (objective)

tan darkening of the skin due to exposure to ultraviolet rays

true skin another name for the dermis

tubercule abnormal solid lump above, within, or below the skin

tumor abnormal cell mass resulting from excessive multiplication of cells

ulcer open skin lesion accompanied by pus and loss of skin depth; a deep erosion; a depression in the skin, normally due to infection or cancer

verruca technical name for a wart

vesicle small blister or sac containing clear fluid

vitiligo an acquired leukoderma characterized by milky-white spots

wheal itchy, swollen lesion caused by insect bites or plant irritations, such as nettle

whitehead a closed comedone; consists of accumulated sebum that remains a whitish color because it does not have a follicular opening for exposure to oxygen

11 Properties and Disorders

OF THE HAIR AND SCALP

☑ Learning Objectives

AFTER COMPLETING THIS CHAPTER, YOU SHOULD BE ABLE TO:

1 Name and describe the structures of the hair root.

2 Name and describe the layers of the hair shaft.

3 Describe the structure of hair protein.

4 Describe the growth cycle of hair.

5 List the characteristics of hair important to hair analysis.

6 Identify different types of hair loss and treatments.

7 Identify common scalp disorders.

8 Identify common hair disorders.

Key Terms

PAGE NUMBER INDICATES WHERE IN THE CHAPTER THE TERM IS USED.

alopecia / 256

alopecia areata / 258

alopecia prematura / 257

alopecia senilis / 258

alopecia syphilitica / 258

amino acids / 246

anagen phase / 251

androgenic alopecia / 256

arrector pili / 244

canities / 265

carbuncle / 265

catagen phase / 251

cortex / 245

cowlick / 251

cuticle / 244

dermal papilla / 243

disulfide bond / 248

end bonds / 246

eumelanin / 248

follicle / 243

folliculitis barbae / 263

furuncle / 265

hair bulb / 243

hair density / 254

hair elasticity / 255

hair porosity / 254

hair root / 242

hair shaft / 242

hair stream / 251

hair texture / 253

hydrogen bond / 247

hypertrichosis / 265

keratin / 242

lanugo / 250

malassezia / 260

medulla / 245

pediculosis capitis / 262

peptide bonds / 246

pheomelanin / 248

pityriasis capitis simplex / 260

pityriasis steatoides / 260

polypeptide chain / 247

primary terminal hair / 250

pseudofolliculitis barbae / 263

salt bond / 248

secondary terminal hair / 250

side bonds / 247

sycosis vulgaris / 264

telogen phase / 252

tinea / 261

tinea capitis / 261

tinea favosa / 262

tinea sycosis / 262

trichology / 242

vellus / 250

wave pattern / 249

whorl / 251

Barbers need a technical understanding of hair structure so they will be able to provide knowledgeable and professional service to clients. To keep hair in a healthy condition, proper attention must be given to its care and treatment. Abusing the hair by harmful cosmetic applications or faulty hair treatments can weaken or damage the hair structure. Knowledge and analysis of the client's hair, tactful suggestions for its improvement, and a sincere interest in maintaining its health and appearance should be the concern of every barber and stylist.

The scientific study of hair, its disorders, and its care is called **trichology** (trih-KAHL-uh-jee), which comes from the Greek words *trichos* (hair) and *ology* (study of). In addition to being used as a form of adornment, hair protects the head from heat, cold, and injury.

The Structure of Hair

Hair is an appendage of the skin in the form of a slender, threadlike outgrowth of the skin and scalp. It is composed chiefly of a protein called **keratin,** which is present in all horny growths such as nails, claws, and hoofs. Full-grown human hair is divided into two parts: the hair root and the hair shaft. The **hair root** is that portion of the hair enclosed within the follicle beneath the skin surface. The **hair shaft** is the portion of the hair we see extending above the skin surface.

STRUCTURES OF THE HAIR ROOT

The main structures of the hair root are the follicle, bulb, dermal papilla, sebaceous glands, and arrector pili muscle **(Figure 11-1).**

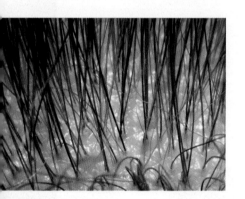

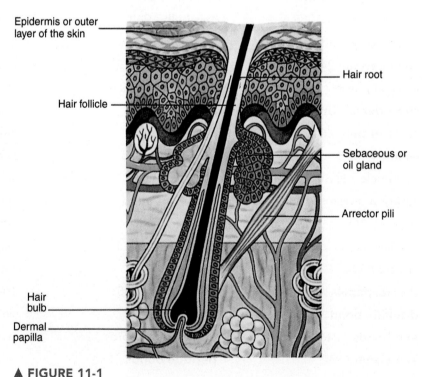

Epidermis or outer layer of the skin

Hair follicle

Hair root

Sebaceous or oil gland

Arrector pili

Hair bulb

Dermal papilla

▲ **FIGURE 11-1**
Structures of the hair root.

The hair **follicle** (FAWL-ih-kul) is a tubelike depression or pocket in the skin or scalp that encases the hair root. Hair follicles are distributed all over the body with the exception of the palms of the hands and the soles of the feet. The follicle extends downward from the epidermis into the dermis, where it surrounds the dermal papilla. Follicles vary in depth, depending on the thickness and location of the skin. They are usually set into the skin at an angle, allowing the hair shaft to flow naturally over the skin surface. There is a follicle for every hair, but it is not uncommon for more than one hair to grow from a single follicle.

NOTE: The funnel-shaped mouths of hair follicles are favorite breeding places for germs and the accumulation of sebum and dirt. Proper shampooing and rinsing procedures help to minimize the occurrence of scalp and hair disorders caused by these conditions.

The **hair bulb** is a thickened, club-shaped structure that forms the lower part of the hair root. The lower part of the hair bulb is hollow and fits over and covers the dermal papilla (Figure 11-2).

The **dermal papilla** (puh-PIL-uh) is a small, cone-shaped elevation at the base of the hair follicle that fits into the hair bulb. It consists of many tiny capillaries that are responsible for supplying oxygen and nutrients to the epidermal tissue that lines the hair follicle. Eventually, the epidermal tissue completely surrounds the papilla and forms the hair bulb. This rich blood and nerve supply is vital to the growth and regeneration of the hair, since it is through the papilla that nourishment reaches the hair bulb. As long as the papilla is healthy and well nourished, new hair will grow.

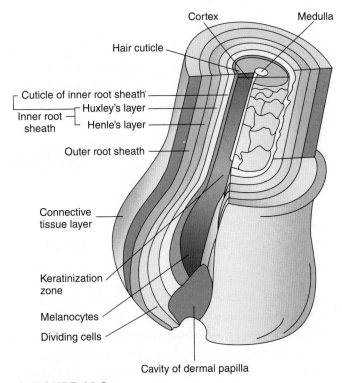

▲ **FIGURE 11-2**

Structure of the hair bulb.

The sebaceous glands consist of small, saclike structures with ducts that are attached to each hair follicle. They secrete an oily substance called sebum that gives the hair luster and pliability. The overproduction of sebum can bring on a common form of oily dandruff, which in turn may become a contributing factor to hair loss or baldness.

Some of the factors that influence sebum production are subject to personal control. These factors are diet, blood circulation, emotional disturbance, stimulation of the endocrine glands, and certain drugs.

- *Diet* influences the general health of the hair. Overindulgence in sweet, starchy, and fatty foods may cause the sebaceous glands to become over-active and to secrete too much sebum.

- *Blood circulation* is a factor because the hair derives its nourishment from the blood supply, which in turn depends upon the foods eaten for certain elements. In the absence of necessary food elements, the health of the hair declines.

- *Emotional disturbance*s are linked with the health of the hair through the nervous system. The hair's condition is affected by stress. Healthy hair is an indication of a healthy body.

- *Endocrine glands* are ductless glands. Their secretions go directly into the bloodstream, which in turn influences the welfare of the entire body. The condition of the endocrine glands influences their secretion. During adolescence, endocrine glands are very active; after middle age, their activity usually decreases. Endocrine gland disturbances influence the hair as well as other aspects of health.

- *Drugs*, such as hormones and certain medications, may adversely affect the hair.

The **arrector pili** (ah-REK-tor PY-ly) is a minute, involuntary muscle fiber in the skin attached to the underside and base of the hair follicle. Strong emotions or cold causes it to contract, which makes the hair stand up straight, resulting in "goose bumps." Eyelash and eyebrow hairs lack arrector pili muscles.

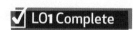

STRUCTURES OF THE HAIR SHAFT

The three main layers of the hair shaft are the cuticle, cortex, and medulla **(Figure 11-3)**.

The term **cuticle** is also used to identify the outermost layer of hair and should not be confused with the cuticle of the skin. The cuticle of the hair consists of a single overlapping layer of transparent, scale-like cells that point away from the skin or scalp toward the hair ends. A healthy, compact cuticle layer is the hair's primary defense against damage, protecting the inner structure of the hair, and is responsible for the shine and silkiness of the hair. Conversely, heat

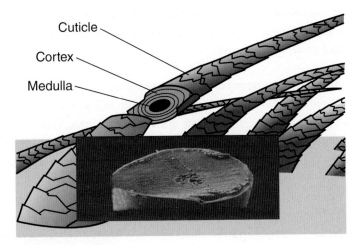

▲ FIGURE 11-3

Cross section of hair.

and certain chemical solutions can raise these scales to allow for penetration and absorption of substances into the cortex.

A lengthwise cross-section of hair shows that although the cuticle scales overlap, each individual cuticle scale is attached to the cortex, thereby creating only one cuticle layer (Figure 11-4). Swelling the hair with high pH products, such as oxidation tints, permanent waving solutions, or chemical hair relaxers, raises the cuticle layer and opens the spaces between the scales, allowing liquids to penetrate into the cortex. The **cortex** is the middle layer of the hair. It is a fibrous protein core formed by elongated cells that contain melanin pigment. About 90 percent of the total weight of the hair comes from the cortex. Its unique protein structure provides strength, elasticity, and natural color to the hair. The changes that take place in the hair during chemical services occur within the cortex.

The **medulla** is the innermost layer and is sometimes referred to as the *pith* or *marrow* of the hair. It is composed of round cells. Although mature male beard hair contains a medulla, this layer of the hair may be absent in very fine and naturally blond hair.

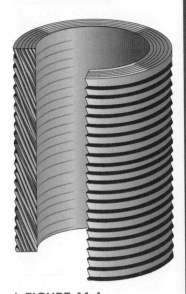

▲ FIGURE 11-4

The cuticle layer.

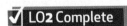

The Chemical Composition of Hair

Hair is composed of protein that grows from cells that originate within the hair follicle. This is where the hair shaft begins. When these living cells form they begin a journey upward through the follicle, where they mature through a process called keratinization. As the newly formed cells mature, they fill up with a fibrous protein called keratin, move upward, lose their nuclei, and die. By the time the hair shaft emerges from the scalp, the cells are completely keratinized and no longer living. The hair shaft that we see is a nonliving fiber composed of keratinized protein.

Proteins are essential organic compounds necessary for life. The protein in human hair is made of chemical units called **amino acids** and the amino acids are made of elements. These elements are carbon, oxygen, hydrogen, nitrogen, and sulfur. They are often referred to as the COHNS elements because of their scientific abbreviations, and are also found in skin and nails. As illustrated in Table 11-1, the chemical composition of average hair is 51 percent carbon, 21 percent oxygen, 6 percent hydrogen, 17 percent nitrogen, and 5 percent sulfur. The chemical composition varies with color. Light hair contains less carbon and hydrogen and more oxygen and sulfur. Conversely, dark hair has more carbon and less oxygen and sulfur.

> TABLE **11-1** The COHNS Elements	
ELEMENT	**PERCENTAGE IN NORMAL HAIR**
Carbon	51%
Oxygen	21%
Hydrogen	6%
Nitrogen	17%
Sulfur	5%

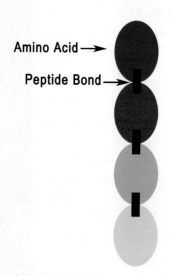

Amino Acid →

Peptide Bond →

▲ FIGURE 11-5

Amino acids joined by peptide bonds.

THE NATURE OF HAIR PROTEIN

Hair is a complex structure that varies greatly from one person to another. The diameter, elasticity, and configuration of the bonds of each strand all help to determine what the keratinized protein we call hair will look and feel like. Although there are many variations, all hair types have certain common factors that include proteins, amino acids, polypeptide chains, and bonds.

Human hair is approximately 91 percent protein. Proteins are made of long chains of amino acids. The amino acids are joined end-to-end in a definite order by chemical bonds known as **peptide bonds** or **end bonds** (Figure 11-5).

The peptide bonds are the strongest chemical bonds in the cortex as they join each amino acid to form the polypeptide chain. Most of the strength and elasticity of the hair is attributed to these chemical bonds. When even a few bonds are broken through overstretching or the use of strong acidic or alkaline solutions, the hair can become weakened or damaged to the point of breakage. Once the end bonds are broken, there is no way of re-forming them. This is just one reason why barbers need to be aware of the potential structural damage that may occur to the hair as a result of rough treatment or chemical over-processing. A long chain of amino acids joined by peptide bonds is called a *polypeptide* or **polypeptide chain.** The polypeptide chains intertwine around each other to create a coil or spiral of protein called a *helix* (Figure 11-6).

SIDE BONDS OF THE HAIR CORTEX

Within the hair cortex, a more complex structure is formed when millions of polypeptide chains are cross-linked by three types of **side bonds** (formerly known as cross-bonds) to form a ladder-like structure (Figure 11-7). The side bonds consist of hydrogen, salt, and disulfide bonds, which account for the strength and elasticity of human hair. They are also essential to blow-drying, wet sets, thermal styling, and chemical processes. Table 11-2 summarizes the properties of the types of bonds found within the protein structure of hair.

A **hydrogen bond** is a special type of ionic side bond that is easily broken by water or heat. Although individual hydrogen bonds are weak, they are so numerous in the hair that they account for about one-third of the hair's overall strength.

Hydrogen bonds add body to the hair and also help to keep the parallel chains of polypeptides together. The physical breaking of the hydrogen bonds when shampooing and rinsing causes the cuticle to swell. When the hair is set on rollers, the cortex shrinks into a new position as it dries around the rollers. This is also true of blow-drying techniques when the barber works with a comb or brush to style the hair into place while drying.

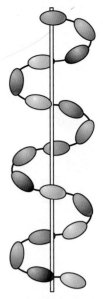

▲ FIGURE 11-6
A polypeptide chain.

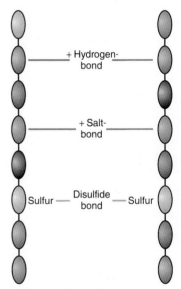

▲ FIGURE 11-7
Side bonds.

> ## TABLE **11-2** Bonds of the Hair

BOND	TYPE	STRENGTH	BROKEN BY	RE-FORMED BY
hydrogen	side bond	weak physical	water or heat	drying or cooling
salt	side bond	weak physical	changes in pH	normalizing pH
disulfide	side bond	strong chemical	1. thio perms and thio relaxers 2. hydroxide relaxers	1. oxidation with neutralizer 2. converted to lanthionine bonds
peptide	end bond	strong chemical	chemical depilatories	not re-formed; hair dissolves

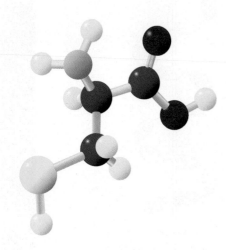

Since hydrogen bonds reflect physical changes in the hair fiber, they are also referred to as physical bonds or H-bonds. Water, dilute alkali, neutral, and acid solutions will break hydrogen bonds. Drying and dilute acids will re-form them.

A **salt bond** is also a physical, ionic bond, but it reacts to changes in pH. Salt bonds depend on pH and account for another one-third of the hair's total strength. These bonds are easily broken by strong acidic or alkaline solutions.

A **disulfide** (dy-SUL-fyd) **bond,** also known as a sulfur bond, is a strong covalent bond, which is different from the ionic bonds of hydrogen or salt bonds. Disulfide bonds join the sulfur atoms of two neighboring cysteine amino acids to create cystine. Although there are fewer disulfide bonds in the hair, they are stronger than hydrogen or salt bonds and account for the final third of the hair's total strength.

Unlike hydrogen and salt bonds, disulfide bonds are not broken by heat or water. Because the disulfide bonds create chemical side bonds between the polypeptide chains, chemical solutions are required to change or restructure them. For example, ammonium thioglycolate permanent waves break disulfide bonds, which are then re-formed with neutralizers. Sodium hydroxide chemical hair relaxers also break disulfide bonds, which are converted to lanthionine bonds when the relaxer is rinsed from the hair. Disulfide bonds broken by hydroxide relaxers are permanently broken and cannot be re-formed. The more disulfide bonds in the hair, the more resistant it will be to chemical processes. Disulfide or sulfur bonds are also known as S-bonds and may sometimes be referred to as cystine bonds.

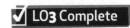
✓ **LO3 Complete**

HAIR PIGMENT

Natural hair color is the result of the melanin pigment found within the cortex. There are two different types of melanin: eumelanin and pheomelanin.

Eumelanin (yoo-MEL-uh-nin) provides brown and black color to hair. **Pheomelanin** (fee-oh-MEL-uh-nin) provides natural hair colors that range from red and ginger to yellow and light blond tones. All natural color is dependent on the ratio of eumelanin to pheomelanin, along with the total number and size of the pigment granules.

The number of hairs on the head varies with the color of the hair. The approximate amounts for different hair colors are: blond, 140,000; brown, 110,000; black, 108,000; and red, 80,000.

WAVE PATTERN

The **wave pattern** of the hair refers to the amount of movement in the hair strand and is described as straight, wavy, curly, and extremely curly or coiled (**Figure 11-8**). Although an individual's particular wave pattern is the result of genetics and racial background, the four wave patterns can all be found in each racial or ethnic group. Wave patterns may also vary from strand to strand on the same head of hair, with a combination of straight, wavy, and/or curly sections throughout.

Other than the genetic factor, scientific study has yet to determine why hair grows straight, wavy, or curly. Theories include the following potentially influencing factors:

- Angle or shape of the follicle
- Shape of the hair's cross-section
- Rate of growth along the sides of the hair
- Position or condition of the bulb in the follicle
- Arrangement of the keratin bundles

Generally speaking, a magnified cross-section of an individual hair is elliptical in shape. Asian hair is closest to being round and Caucasian hair is more oval. Both straight and wavy hair possesses a fairly uniform diameter along the hair strand. African American black hair has a more elliptical or flatter oval shape with varying diameters along the strand and a tendency to grow in twisted spirals. However, there is no strict rule regarding cross-sectional shapes of straight, wavy, or curly hair, and all hair types have been found within different ethnic cultures (**Figure 11-9**).

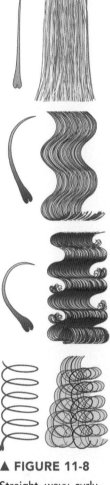

▲ FIGURE 11-8
Straight, wavy, curly, and coiled strands.

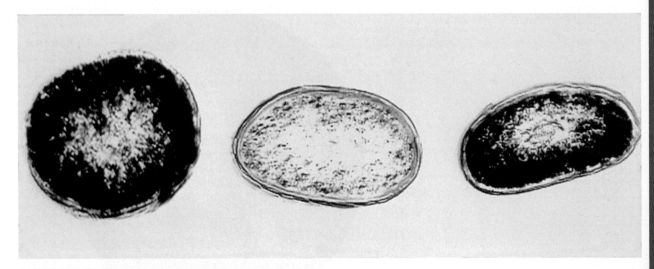

▲ FIGURE 11-9
Cross-section of three hairs: Asian (left) Caucasian (center) African (right).

Hair Growth

Hair is found all over the body except on the palms, soles, lips, and eyelids. The two main types are vellus or lanugo hair and terminal hair (**Figure 11-10**).

1. **Vellus** or **lanugo** hair is the short, fine, soft, downy hair found on the cheeks, forehead, and nearly all areas of the body. It almost never has a medulla or melanin and helps in the efficient evaporation of perspiration.

2. Terminal hair is coarse hair that has a medulla. The short, thick hairs that grow on the eyebrows and eyelashes are **primary terminal hair.** Eyebrows divert sweat from the eyes and eyelashes help protect the eyes from foreign bodies and light. **Secondary terminal hair** is the long hair found on the scalp, beard, chest, back, legs, and pubic area that replaces some vellus hair after puberty. The same follicle is capable of producing both types of hair. In cases of male pattern baldness, the follicles stop making terminal hair and revert back to producing the vellus type.

The average growth of healthy hair on the scalp is about $\frac{1}{2}$" per month. The rate of growth will differ on specific parts of the body, between sexes, among races, and with age. The growth of scalp hair occurs more rapidly between the ages of 15 and 30 and declines sharply between 50 and 60. Hair growth is also influenced by such factors as the seasons of the year, nutrition, and hormonal changes within the body. Temporary climatic conditions also affects the hair: Moisture in the air deepens the natural wave, cold air causes the hair cuticle to contract, and heat causes the hair to swell or expand and absorb moisture.

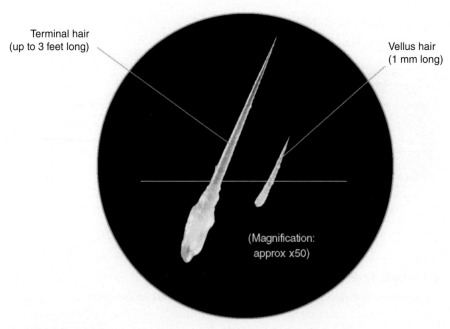

Terminal hair
(up to 3 feet long)

Vellus hair
(1 mm long)

(Magnification:
approx x50)

▲ **FIGURE 11-10**
Terminal and vellus hair.

Hair growth is not increased by shaving, trimming, cutting, singeing, or by the application of ointments or oils. Oils act as lubricants to the hair shaft, but do not feed the hair.

NORMAL HAIR SHEDDING

It is normal to lose an average of 75 to 100 hairs per day. This shedding process makes room for new hair that is in the process of growing. Hair loss beyond this estimated average indicates some problem. Eyebrow hairs and eyelashes are replaced every four to five months.

GROWTH PATTERNS

It is important when cutting and styling hair to consider the hair's natural growth patterns. Doing so will produce a more natural-looking haircut and a style that the client will have less trouble duplicating for everyday wear. Growth patterns result in hair streams, whorls, and cowlicks.

- A **hair stream** is hair that flows in the same direction. It is the result of follicles being arranged and sloping in a uniform manner. When two such streams slope in opposite directions, they form a natural part in the hair.

- A **whorl** is hair that grows in a circular or swirl pattern. Whorls are most often seen at the crown.

- A **cowlick** is a tuft of hair that stands straight up. Cowlicks are usually more noticeable at the front hairline, but they may be located anywhere on the scalp. Styles should be chosen to minimize their upright effects.

THE GROWTH CYCLES OF HAIR

In normal, healthy hair, each individual strand goes through a cycle of growth, fall, and replacement. These three phases are known as the anagen, catagen, and telogen phases **(Figure 11-11)**.

Anagen: The Growth Phase

During the **anagen** (AN-uh-jen), or growth, **phase,** new hair is produced. The stem cells actively manufacture new keratinized cells in the hair follicle at a rapid rate. About 90 percent of scalp hair is growing in the anagen phase at any one time. This part of the cycle generally lasts from three to five years, but can last as long as 10 years and determines how long the hair will grow before shedding.

Catagen: The Transition Phase

The **catagen** (KAT-uh-jen) **phase** is a transition period between the growth and resting phases of a hair strand. During this phase the follicle shrinks, the hair bulb disappears, and the shrunken root end forms a rounded club. Also during the catagen phase, the follicle is preparing for new growth by making germ cells. They surround the club and await the signal to renew the anagen phase. Lasting from one to three weeks, less than 1 percent of the hair is in the catagen phase at any one time.

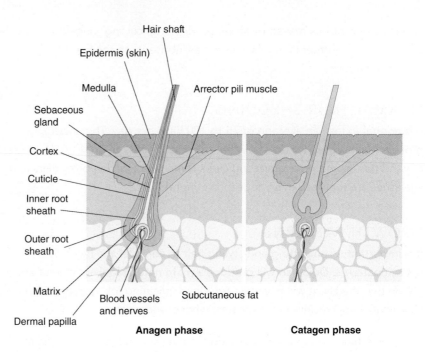

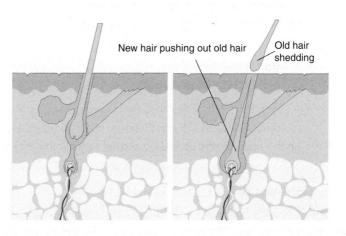

▲ **FIGURE 11-11**

Cycles of hair growth.

Telogen: The Resting Phase

The **telogen** (TEL-uh-jen), or resting, **phase** is the final phase of the hair cycle. The hair is either shed during this phase or remains in place until it is pushed out by the growth of a new hair in the next anagen phase. About 10 percent of scalp hair is in the telogen phase at any one time, and this lasts for approximately three to six months. On average, the entire growth process repeats itself once every four or five years.

In summary, new hair replaces old hair in the following ways:

1. The new hair is formed by cell division from a growing point at the root around the papilla.

2. The bulb loosens and separates from the papilla.

3. The bulb moves upward in the follicle.

4. The hair moves slowly to the surface, where it is shed.

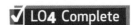

Hair Analysis

Barbering services include a variety of applications that benefit from a barber's ability to analyze the condition of a client's hair. In addition to wave and growth patterns, barbers should be able to analyze the hair's texture, density, porosity, and elasticity.

Knowledge and skill in performing a hair analysis can be acquired by observation and practice using the senses of sight, hearing, smell, and touch.

- *Sight*: Observation will impart some knowledge immediately, such as whether the hair looks dry or oily. Sight alone, however, will not provide an accurate judgment of the hair's quality. The sense of sight comprises approximately 15 percent of the process of hair analysis.

- *Hearing*: Some clients will volunteer information about their hair, health problems, or experiences with products and medications. Since all of these factors are important when deciding how to treat the hair, it is advisable to listen carefully.

- *Smell*: Certain scalp disorders will create an odor. If the client is in general good health and the scalp is clean, the hair should be odor-free.

- *Touch*: The sense of touch is key to analyzing hair condition and texture. This sense needs to be developed to its fullest capacity for the barber to provide truly professional services.

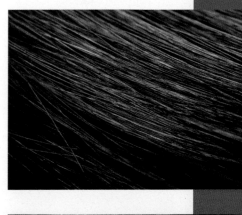

HAIR TEXTURE

Hair texture refers to the degree of coarseness or fineness of individual hair strands, which may vary on different parts of the head. Hair texture is measured by the diameter of the hair strand and is classified as coarse, medium, or fine.

Coarse hair has the largest diameter and tends to be stronger than fine hair. It also has a stronger structure that may require more processing or stronger products during chemical services than medium or fine hair. Generally, it is more difficult for hair lighteners, haircolors, waving solutions, and relaxing creams to penetrate coarse hair.

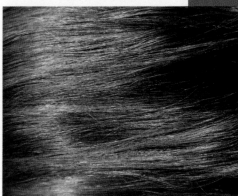

Medium hair texture is the most common and is the standard to which other hair is compared. Medium hair is considered normal and does not usually pose any special problems or concerns.

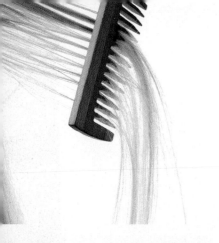

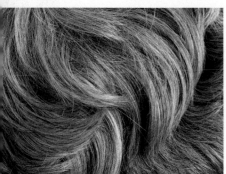

Fine hair has the smallest diameter and is generally more fragile, easier to process, and more susceptible to damage from chemical services than is coarse or medium hair. Some fine or very fine hair does not possess a medulla, which helps to account for a smaller diameter of the strand.

Wiry hair, whether coarse, medium, or fine, has a hard, glassy finish because the cuticle scales lie flat against the hair shaft. It usually takes longer to give this type of hair a chemical service.

Hair texture can be determined by feeling a single strand of dry hair between the fingers. Hold the strand securely with one hand while rolling it between the thumb and forefinger of the other hand. With practice, you will be able to feel the difference between coarse, medium, and fine hair textures.

HAIR DENSITY

Hair density measures the number of individual hair strands per square inch of scalp area. It can be classified as thick, average, or thin; or as high, medium, or low density. Hair density is different from hair texture in that individuals with the same hair texture can have different densities or different amounts of hair per square inch. For example, one person may have thick, fine hair while another has thin, fine hair.

The average hair density is approximately 2,200 strands per square inch, with the average head of hair containing about 100,000 individual strands. The number of hairs on the head varies with the color of the hair—blonds usually have the highest density and redheads the least density per square inch.

HAIR POROSITY

Hair porosity is the ability of the hair to absorb moisture. The degree of porosity is directly related to the condition of the cuticle layer of the hair. A compact cuticle layer is naturally more resistant to penetration, whereas porous hair has a raised cuticle layer that easily absorbs water. The porosity level of hair can be classified as moderate, poor, and porous; or as average, low, and high porosity.

Hair that has moderate or average porosity is considered normal. This hair type presents no special problems and chemical applications usually process as expected.

Hair with a high porosity level is considered overly porous and is usually the result of previous over-processing. Hair in this condition absorbs liquids quickly and requires special care.

Hair that is classified as having poor or low porosity is considered resistant. This hair type absorbs the least amount of moisture and may require a more alkaline solution than other hair types.

The porosity of the hair can be checked by holding multiple strands of dry hair between the fingers while sliding the thumb and forefinger of the other hand down toward the scalp (Figure 11-12). If the hair feels smooth and the cuticle is compact, it is considered resistant. If you can feel a slight roughness or the imbrications of the cuticle scales, the hair is porous. Should the hair break or feel very rough, the hair is probably over-porous.

HAIR ELASTICITY

Hair elasticity is the ability of the hair to stretch and return to its original length without breaking. Hair with normal elasticity is springy and has a live and lustrous appearance. Wet hair with normal elasticity, especially curly or wavy hair, will stretch up to 50 percent of its original length and return to that length without breaking. Test for hair elasticity by gently tugging a few strands of hair as shown in Figure 11-13.

Hair elasticity is an indication of the strength of the side bonds in the hair. Hair with normal elasticity tends to hold the curl from sets and permanent waves without excessive relaxing of the curl. Hair with low or poor elasticity is brittle and breaks easily. Hair in this condition may have been over-processed during previous chemical applications or may be the result of poor nutrition or internal disorders.

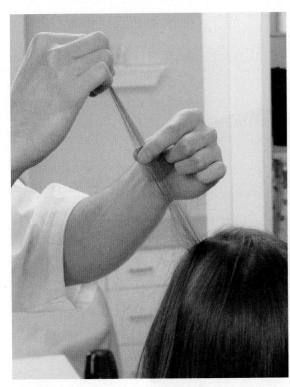

▲ **FIGURE 11-12**
Testing for hair porosity.

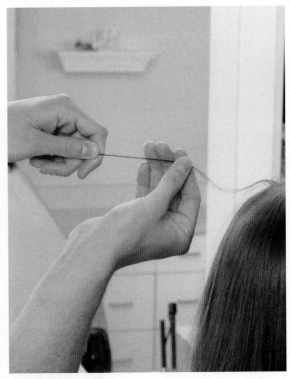

▲ **FIGURE 11-13**
Testing for hair elasticity.

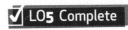

☑ **LO5 Complete**

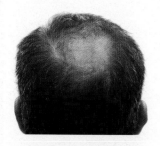

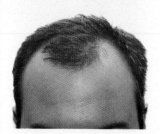

Hair Loss

As previously discussed, we all lose some hair every day as a result of the normal shedding that takes place during the hair's natural growth and replacement cycle. Over 63 million men and women in the United States suffer from **alopecia** (al-oh-PEE-shah), the technical term for abnormal hair loss. Understandably, hair loss for either sex can be a traumatic experience, so conversations about it should be handled tactfully.

TYPES OF ABNORMAL HAIR LOSS

Alopecia may appear in different forms as a result of a variety of abnormal conditions. These forms include androgenic alopecia, alopecia areata, alopecia senilis, and alopecia syphilitica.

Androgenic Alopecia

Androgenic (an-druh-JEN-ik) **alopecia** is hair loss that occurs as a result of genetics, age, and hormonal changes that cause the miniaturization of terminal hair, converting it to vellus hair **(Figure 11-14)**. Hair growth is controlled by androgens and one of the most well known androgens is testosterone. Testosterone is converted to dihydrotestosterone (DHT) by the enzyme 5-alpha-reductase. At sexual maturity, DHT causes the conversion of vellus hair to terminal hair. Latter in life, a genetic hypersensitivity of the

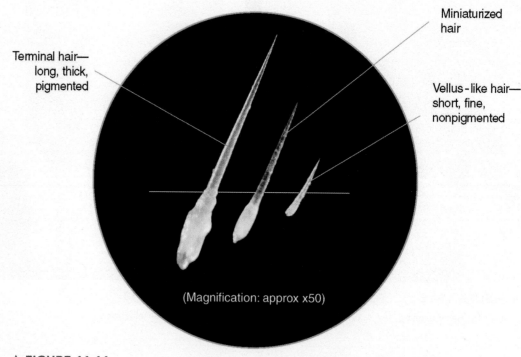

Terminal hair—long, thick, pigmented

Miniaturized hair

Vellus-like hair—short, fine, nonpigmented

(Magnification: approx x50)

▲ **FIGURE 11-14**
Miniaturization of the hair follicle.

dermal papilla to DHT may develop, causing the miniaturization of terminal scalp hair and the conversion back to vellus hair. Androgenic alopecia can begin as early as the teens (**alopecia prematura**) and is frequently seen by the age of 40. Almost 40 percent of men and women show some degree of hair loss by age 35.

In men, androgenic alopecia is known as male pattern baldness, which usually progresses to the familiar horseshoe-shaped pattern or fringe of hair (**Figure 11-15**). In women, it shows up as a generalized thinning in the crown area.

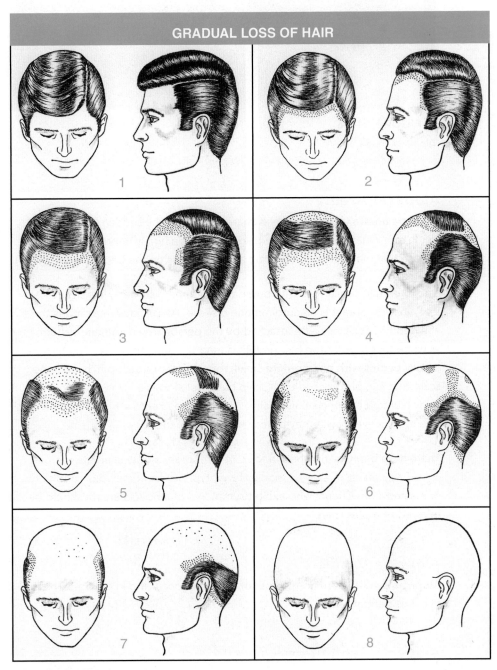

GRADUAL LOSS OF HAIR

▲ **FIGURE 11-15**

Gradual balding process.

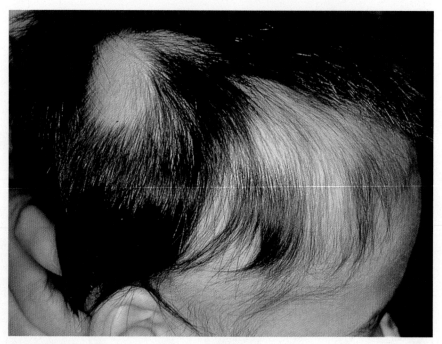

▲ FIGURE 11-16
Alopecia areata.

Alopecia Areata

Alopecia areata (air-ee-AH-tah) is characterized by the sudden falling out of hair in round patches that create bald spots. It is a highly unpredictable skin disease that may occur on the scalp and elsewhere on the body **(Figure 11-16)**.

Due to certain similarities with other autoimmune disorders, it is suggested that alopecia areata is an autoimmune disease. Alopecia areata causes the affected hair follicles to be attacked by the person's own immune system, as white blood cells stop hair growth during the anagen phase. The hair loss usually begins with one or more small, round, smooth bald patches on the scalp that can progress to total scalp hair loss (alopecia totalis) or complete body hair loss (alopecia universalis). Although hair regrowth may occur within a year, the new growth may or may not be permanent.

There have been cases where a form of temporary alopecia areata has occurred as a result of anemia, scarlet fever, typhoid fever, nervous conditions, or malnutrition. Clients who exhibit symptoms of alopecia areata should be referred to a physician.

Alopecia Senilis

Alopecia senilis is the normal loss of scalp hair occurring in old age. The loss of hair is permanent.

Alopecia Syphilitica

Alopecia syphilitica is caused by syphilis. The non-inflamed bald areas look molted or moth-eaten and may also affect the beard and eyebrow areas. The hair usually grows back.

HAIR LOSS TREATMENTS

The only two FDA-approved hair loss treatments that have been proven to stimulate hair growth are Minoxidil and Finasteride.

Minoxidil is a topical treatment that has been proven to stimulate hair growth. Applied to the scalp twice a day, it is sold over the counter as a nonprescription drug under the brand name Rogaine. Minoxidil is available for both men and women and comes in two different strengths: 2 percent (regular) and 5 percent (extra strength). It is not known to have any negative side effects.

Finasteride is an oral prescription medication for men only sold under the brand name Propecia. This drug inhibits the production of 5-alpha-reductase, the enzyme that reacts with DHT (dihydrotestosterone) to cause male pattern baldness. Although Finasteride is considered more effective and convenient than Minoxidil, its possible side effects include weight gain and loss of sexual function.

In addition to the medicinal treatments described above, there are also several surgical options available. Transplants, or hair plugs, are probably the most common permanent hair replacement technique. The process consists of removing small sections of hair that include the follicle, papilla, and bulb from areas of thick hair growth and transplanting them into the bald area. Only licensed surgeons may perform this procedure and several surgeries are usually necessary to achieve the desired results. The cost of each surgery ranges from about $8,000 to over $20,000.

With proper training, barbers can offer several non-medical options to camouflage hair loss. These include hair replacement systems, wigs, hair weaves, and hair extensions (see Chapter 16).

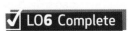 **LO6 Complete**

Disorders of the Scalp

The common disorders of the scalp include dandruff, fungal infections (tinea), animal parasitic infestations, and staphylococci infections.

DANDRUFF

Dandruff is the presence of small, white scales that usually appear on the scalp and hair. It can be easily mistaken for dry scalp because the symptoms of both conditions are a flaky, itchy, irritated scalp, but a dry scalp does not have the oily scalp that is common to dandruff.

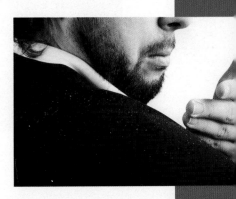

The medical term for dandruff is pityriasis (pit-ih-RY-uhsus) capitis. Just as the skin on other parts of the body is continually being shed and replaced, the uppermost layer of the scalp goes through the same process. Skin cells in the outer layer of the scalp flake off and are replaced by new cells from below.

Ordinarily, these scales loosen and fall off freely, so the natural shedding of the scalp's dead scales should not be mistaken for dandruff.

Dandruff is characterized by the excessive production, shedding, and accumulation of surface cells. Instead of growing to the surface and falling off, these horny scales accumulate on the scalp. A sluggish scalp due to poor circulation, infection, injury, improper diet, or poor personal hygiene can contribute to this accumulation, as does the use of strong shampoos and/or insufficient rinsing of the hair.

Although the cause of dandruff has been debated for over 150 years, current research confirms that dandruff is the result of a fungus called **malassezia** (mal-uh-SEEZ-ee-uh), formerly named *pityrosporum*. Malassezia is a naturally occurring fungus that is present on all human skin, but develops the symptoms of dandruff when it grows out of control. Factors including stress, age, hormones, and hygiene can cause the fungus to multiply and dandruff symptoms to worsen. Anti-dandruff shampoos containing anti-fungal ingredients such as pyrithione zinc, selenium sulfide, or ketoconazole help control dandruff by suppressing the growth of malassezia.

The two principal types of dandruff are pityriasis capitis simplex and pityriasis steatoides.

- **Pityriasis capitis simplex** is the technical term for classic dandruff, characterized by scalp irritation, large flakes, and an itchy scalp (**Figure 11-17a**). The scales may be attached to the scalp in masses or scattered loosely throughout the hair. Topical treatments for controlling dandruff include the use of anti-dandruff shampoos, scalp massage and treatments, and medicated scalp ointments.

- **Pityriasis steatoides** (stee-uh-TOY-deez) is a more severe form of dandruff that is characterized by an accumulation of greasy or waxy scales mixed with sebum (**Figure 11-17b**). This excessive shedding mixed with sebum causes the scales to adhere to the scalp in patches, where they can cause itching and irritation. If the greasy scales are torn off, bleeding or oozing of sebum may follow. Medical treatment is advisable for clients with this condition.

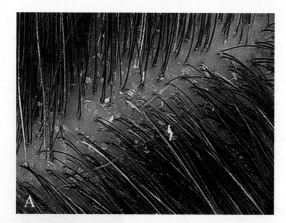

▲ **FIGURE 11-17a**

Pityriasis capitis simplex.

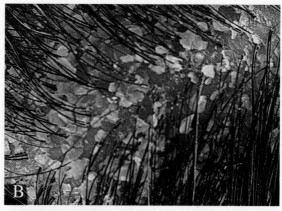

▲ **FIGURE 11-17b**

Pityriasis steatoides.

At one time, dandruff was thought to be contagious; however, the latest research has determined that it is not. Regardless of whether or not dandruff is contagious, the common use of tools and implements from one client to another is prohibited. Barbers must always practice approved cleaning and disinfection procedures in the barbershop before and after each client service. It is also advisable to wear gloves when shampooing a client with a dandruff condition.

FUNGAL INFECTIONS (TINEA)

Tinea (TIN-ee-uh) is the medical term for ringworm. Ringworm is caused by fungal organisms and is characterized by itching, scales, and, sometimes, painful circular lesions. A case usually starts with a small, reddened patch of little blisters that spreads outward and then heals in the middle, with a scale-like appearance. If the ringworm has spread, several patches may be present at one time.

All forms of tinea are contagious and can be easily transmitted from one person to another. Infected skin scales or hair containing the fungi are known to spread the disease; public showers, swimming pools, and unsanitary articles are also sources of transmission. Proper sanitation and disinfection procedures must be used to help prevent the spread of ringworm. Clients with a suspected or confirmed case of tinea should not receive services in the barbershop and should be referred to a physician for medical treatment.

- **Tinea capitis** is commonly known as ringworm of the scalp
  (Figure 11-18). It is characterized by red papules or spots at the openings of the hair follicles. As the patches spread, the hair becomes brittle and lifeless and breaks off, leaving a stump, or falls from the enlarged, open follicles.

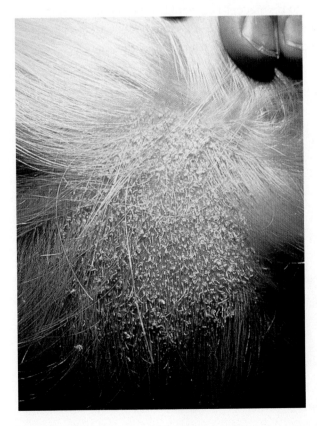

◀ **FIGURE 11-18**

Tinea capitis.

- **Tinea sycosis** (SIGH-koh-sis), or tinea barbae, is a fungal infection occurring chiefly over the bearded area of the face. Beginning as small, round, slightly scaly, inflamed patches, the areas enlarge, clearing up somewhat at the center with elevation at the borders. As the parasites invade the hairs and follicles, hard, lumpy swellings develop. In severe cases, pustules form around the hair follicles and rupture, forming crusts. In the later stage, the hairs become dry, break off, and fall out or are readily extracted. Tinea sycosis is highly contagious and medical treatment is required.

- **Tinea favosa** (fah-VOH-suh) is also known as tinea favus (FAY-vus) or honeycomb ringworm. It is characterized by dry, sulfur-yellow, cuplike crusts on the scalp having a peculiar, musty odor. Scars from favus are bald patches that are pink or white and shiny. Tinea favosa is very contagious and should be referred to a physician.

PARASITIC INFESTATIONS

The two most common parasitic infestations barbers may see in the barbershop are pediculosis capitis and scabies.

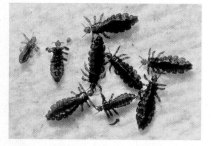

▲ **FIGURE 11-19**
Head lice.

- **Pediculosis** (puh-dik-yuh-LOH-sis) **capitis** is the infestation of the hair and scalp with head lice (**Figures 11-19** and **11-20**). The parasites feed on the scalp and cause severe itching. The head louse is transmitted from one person to another by contact with infested hats, combs, brushes, and other personal items.

  There are several commercially prepared products sold over the counter for the treatment of head lice. Head lice are tenacious creatures that can live away from the human body for up to 48 hours, so it is important to disinfect all household and personal items to avoid re-infestation. Cases of head lice should not be treated in the barbershop—the client should be referred to a physician.

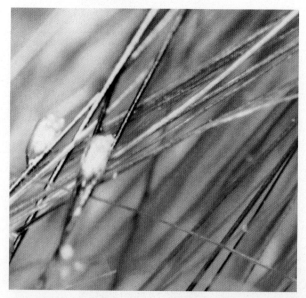

▲ **FIGURE 11-20**
Nits (lice eggs).

NOTE: Remember to thoroughly disinfect the barber chair, capes, tools, the workstation, and the reception area when a case of pediculosis capitis has been recognized in the barbershop.

- *Scabies* is a highly contagious skin disease caused by the itch mite. Vesicles and pustules usually form from the irritation caused by the parasites or from scratching the affected areas **(Figure 11-21)**. A client with this condition should be referred to a physician for medical treatment. As with all disorders and diseases, the practice of approved cleaning and disinfection procedures will help to limit the spread of scabies.

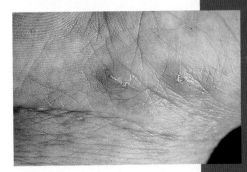

▲ **FIGURE 11-21**
Scabies.

STAPHYLOCOCCI INFECTIONS

Barbers may also encounter bacterial staphylococci infections in the barbershop in the form of different types of folliculitis. Folliculitis can occur anywhere on the body as a result of bacterial or viral infection and is characterized by the inflammation or infection of one or more hair follicles. Some of its more common forms are folliculitis barbae, pseudofolliculitis barbae, sycosis vulgaris, furuncles, and carbuncles.

- *Folliculitis barbae* and *pseudofolliculitis barbae* are inflammations of the follicle caused by bacterial or viral infection, irritation, or ingrown hairs. The cause of the inflammation is what differentiates the two conditions, but both can be triggered from damaged follicles caused by friction, blockages, or improper shaving methods that include close shaving, too much pressure, dull blades, or shaving against the grain.

  Folliculitis barbae, or barber's itch, is an infection of the hair follicles characterized by inflamed pustules in the bearded areas of the face and neck that may have hairs growing through the pustule. Staphylococcus bacteria most often cause the infection; however, a herpes simplex virus can spread to other hair follicles during shaving, resulting in similar pustule formation and infection. Treatments include topical or oral antibiotics as prescribed by a physician.

  Pseudofolliculitis barbae, also referred to as "razor bumps," is a chronic inflammatory condition that resembles folliculitis in terms of papules and pustules but is generally accepted to be caused by ingrown hair. The disorder is most often seen in men and women of Mediterranean, African, Hispanic, and Jewish ethnicity, but can occur to anyone with curly or coiled hair textures. Pseudofolliculitis barbae can be caused by improper shaving or by broken hair below the skin surface that grows into the side of the follicle, causing irritation and swelling that cuts off oxygen to the bottom of the follicle. Bacteria then have a perfect environment for growth, which can lead to the development of pus and, if left untreated, folliculitis. Non-medical treatments include the use of proper shaving techniques, antibiotic or anti-fungal preparations, and the use of electric razors or razors designed to cut hair above the skin to minimize outbreaks and irritation. Warm compresses and clear gel masks that soothe and heal may also help to relieve symptoms **(Figure 11-22)**.

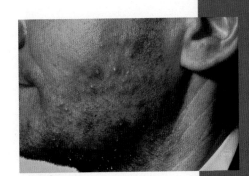

▲ **FIGURE 11-22**
Regular facial treatments incorporating masks can help rid clients of folliculitis.

With an understanding of folliculitis and pseudofolliculitis, barbers can help clients to determine if the condition is caused by chemical or mechanical means. Preparations that contain salicylic acid to break up impactions and kill bacteria are available for the prevention of ingrown hairs. Physicians may prescribe topical and oral antibiotics for more serious conditions. When mechanical causes, such as improper shaving, are the source of the condition, the barber can offer the client some instruction in proper shaving techniques.

- **Sycosis vulgaris,** also known as sycosis barbae, is a chronic bacterial infection involving the areas surrounding the follicles of the beard and mustache areas. It may be contracted through the use of contaminated towels or implements or by contact with public resting areas. The condition can be worsened by irritation caused by shaving or continual nasal discharge. The main lesions are papules and pustules pierced by hairs and crusts that form after eruption. The surrounding skin is tender, reddened, swollen, and itchy. Medical treatment is required and a client with this condition should be referred to a physician.

NOTE: This infection should not be confused with tinea sycosis, which is due to ringworm fungus.

- A **furuncle** (FYOO-rung-kul), or boil, is an acute bacterial infection of a hair follicle, producing constant pain.
  A furuncle is the result of an active inflammatory process limited to a definite area that subsequently produces a pustule perforated by a hair (Figure 11-23). A client with this condition should be referred to a physician.

- A **carbuncle** (KAHR-bung-kul) is the result of an acute, deep-seated bacterial infection in the subcutaneous tissue. It is similar to a furuncle but is larger. A client with this condition should be referred to a physician.

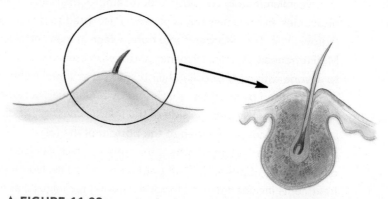

▲ **FIGURE 11-23**
Furuncle (boil).

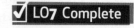

Disorders of the Hair

Hair disorders are usually non-contagious conditions and include disorders such as canities, hypertrichosis, trichoptilosis, trichorrhexis nodosa, monilethrix, and fragilitas crinium.

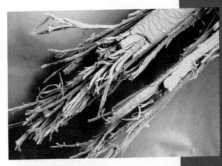

▲ FIGURE 11-24
Trichoptilosis.

- **Canities** (kah-NISH-ee-eez) is the technical term for gray hair. Canities is due mainly to the loss of the hair's natural melanin pigment in the cortical layer. Other than the absence of pigment, gray hair is the same as pigmented hair. Gray hair is really mottled hair; spots of white or whitish-yellow are scattered about in the hair shafts. Normally, gray hair grows out in this condition from the hair bulb; therefore, graying does not take place after the hair has grown. The two main types of canities are congenital and acquired; a third form is known as ringed hair.

  Congenital canities exists at or before birth. It occurs in albinos and occasionally in persons with otherwise normal hair. The patchy type of congenital canities may develop slowly or rapidly, depending on the cause of the condition.

  Acquired canities may be due to the natural aging process and genetics, or it may be premature. Other causes of acquired grayness are worry, anxiety, nervous strain, prolonged illness, and heredity.

  Ringed hair is a third form of canities that is characterized by alternating bands of gray and pigmented hair throughout the length of the hair strand.

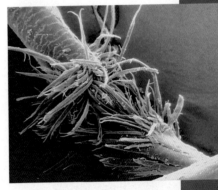

▲ FIGURE 11-25
Trichorrhexis nodosa.

- **Hypertrichosis** (hi-pur-trih-KOH-sis) or hirsuties (hur-SOO-shee-eez) is a condition of abnormal hair growth. It is characterized by the development and growth of terminal hair in those areas of the body that would normally grow only vellus hair. A mustache or light beard on a woman is an example of hypertrichosis. Treatments include tweezing, depilatories, waxing, shaving, mechanical epilators, and electrolysis.

  Trichoptilosis (trih-kahp-tih-LOH-sus) is the technical term for split ends (Figure 11-24). The split ends may be removed by cutting, or conditioning treatments may be used to soften and lubricate dry ends.

- *Trichorrhexis nodosa* (trik-uh-REK-sis nuh-DOH-suh) is the technical term for knotted hair (Figure 11-25). It is characterized by brittleness and the formation of nodular swellings along the hair shaft. Treatments include softening the hair with conditioners and moisturizers.

- Monilethrix (mah-NIL-ee-thrixs) is the technical term for beaded hair (Figure 11-26). The hair breaks easily between the nodes; treatments include hair and scalp conditioning.

- Fragilitas crin*ium* (fruh-JIL-ih-tus KRI-nee-um) is the technical term for brittle hair. The hairs may split along any part of their length. Treatments include hair and scalp conditioning.

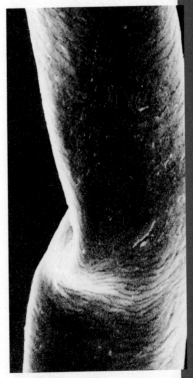

▲ FIGURE 11-26
Monilethrix.

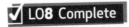
✓ **LO8 Complete**

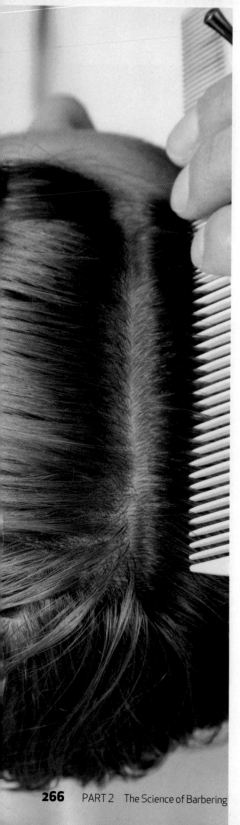

11 Review Questions

1. Why is the study of hair important to the barber?

2. Identify the technical term for the study of hair.

3. Describe the differences between the hair root and hair shaft.

4. List the structures of the hair root.

5. Identify the layers of the hair shaft.

6. What are amino acids?

7. What are peptide bonds?

8. List the side bonds in the hair.

9. Identify ways in which peptide bonds and side bonds can be broken.

10. What is melanin?

11. Define *wave pattern.*

12. Define *hair stream, whorl,* and *cowlick.*

13. Define and explain the anagen, catagen, and telogen phases of hair growth.

14. List and define the characteristics of hair used in hair analysis.

15. List and describe different types of hair loss.

16. List and describe common disorders of the scalp.

17. Explain the similarities and differences associated with folliculitis barbae and pseudofolliculitis barbae.

18. List and describe disorders of the hair.

Chapter
Glossary

alopecia the technical name for hair loss

alopecia areata the sudden falling out of hair in patches or spots

alopecia prematura hair loss that occurs before middle age

alopecia senilis hair loss occurring in old age

alopecia syphilitica hair loss as a result of syphilis

amino acids the building blocks or units of structure in protein

anagen phase growth phase in the hair cycle

androgenic alopecia hair loss that occurs as a result of genetics, age, and hormonal changes; male pattern baldness

arrector pili involuntary muscle fiber attached to the follicle

canities technical term for gray hair

carbuncle the result of an acute, deep-seated bacterial infection in the subcutaneous tissue

catagen phase transition phase of the hair growth cycle

cortex middle layer of the hair shaft

cowlick tuft of hair that stands straight up

cuticle outermost layer of the hair shaft

dermal papilla small, cone-shaped elevation located at the base of the hair follicle that fits into the hair bulb

disulfide bond also known as a sulfur bond; a type of chemical cross bond found in the hair cortex

end bonds also known as peptide bonds; chemical bonds that join amino acids end to end

eumelanin melanin that gives brown and black color to hair

follicle tubelike depression in the skin that contains the hair root

folliculitis barbae also known as barber's itch; a bacterial infection of the hair follicles with inflamed pustules in the bearded areas of the face and neck; may have hairs growing through the pustule

furuncle an acute bacterial infection of a hair follicle, producing constant pain; also known as a boil

hair bulb club-shaped structure that forms the lower part of the hair root

hair density the amount of hair per square inch of scalp

hair elasticity the ability of the hair to stretch and return to its original length

hair porosity the ability of the hair to absorb moisture

hair root the part of the hair that is encased in the hair follicle

hair shaft the part of the hair that extends beyond the skin

hair stream hair that flows in the same direction

hair texture measures the diameter of a hair strand; coarse, medium, fine

hydrogen bond a physical side bond in the hair cortex

hypertrichosis a condition of abnormal hair growth

keratin the protein of which hair is formed

lanugo vellus hair

malassezia fungus that causes dandruff

medulla innermost or center layer of the hair shaft

pediculosis capitis the infection of the hair and scalp with head lice

peptide bonds end bonds; chemical bonds that join amino acids end to end

pheomelanin melanin that gives red to blond colors to hair

pityriasis capitis simplex dry dandruff type

pityriasis steatoides waxy or greasy dandruff type

polypeptide chain long chain of amino acids linked by peptide bonds

primary terminal hair short, thick hairs that grow on the eyebrows and lashes

pseudofolliculitis barbae a chronic inflammatory form of folliculitis known as "razor bumps" resembling folliculitis papules and pustules; generally accepted to be caused by ingrown hair

salt bond a physical side bond within the hair cortex

secondary terminal hair long hair found on the scalp, beard, chest, back, and legs

side bonds also known as cross bonds; hydrogen, salt, and sulfur bonds in the hair cortex

sycosis vulgaris chronic bacterial infection of the bearded areas of the face

telogen phase resting phase of the hair growth cycle

tinea technical name for ringworm

tinea capitis ringworm of the scalp

tinea favosa ringworm characterized by dry, sulfur-yellow crusts on the scalp

tinea sycosis ringworm of the bearded areas on the face

trichology the science dealing with the hair, its diseases, and its care

vellus soft, downy hair that appears on the body

wave pattern amount of movement in the hair strand; straight, wavy, curly, and coiled

whorl hair that grows in a circular pattern

PART 3

PROFESSIONAL BARBERING

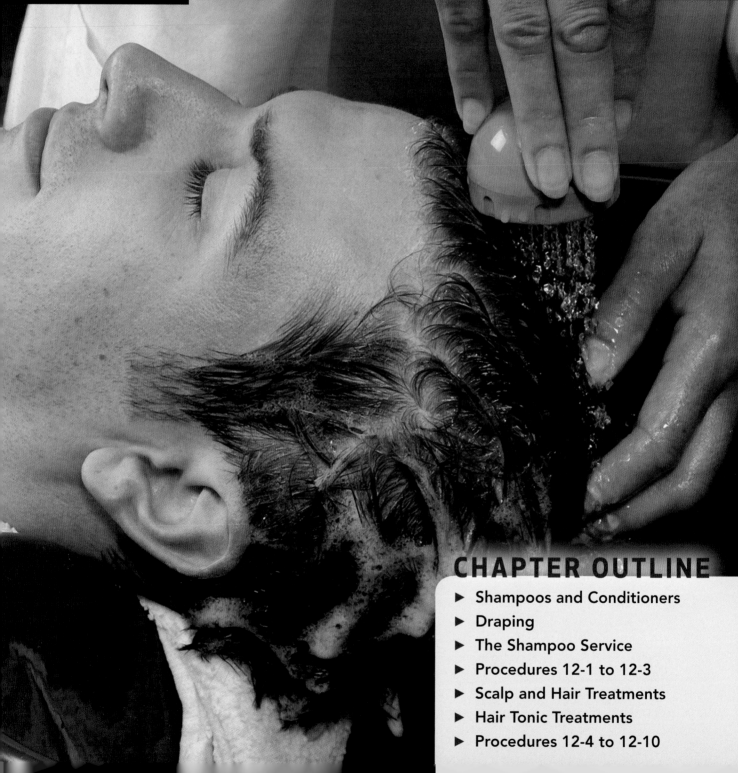

12 Treatment
OF THE HAIR AND SCALP

CHAPTER OUTLINE

AFTER COMPLETING THIS CHAPTER, YOU SHOULD BE ABLE TO:

1 Identify services associated with the treatment of the hair and scalp.

2 Demonstrate proper draping procedures for hair services.

3 Demonstrate the shampoo service.

4 Demonstrate scalp massage techniques and treatments.

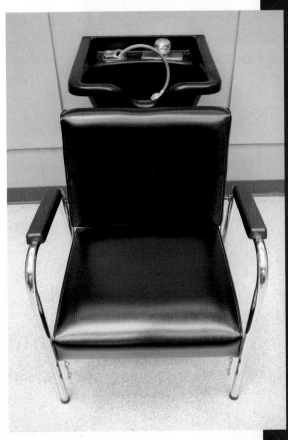

Key Terms

PAGE NUMBER INDICATES WHERE IN THE CHAPTER THE TERM IS USED.

conditioners / 272

draping / 273

hair conditioners / 272

scalp conditioners / 272

scalp steam / 284

shampoos / 272

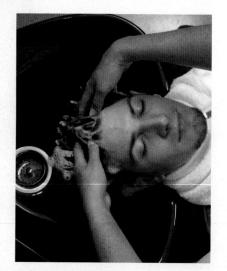

▲ FIGURE 12-1

The shampoo service.

The treatment of the hair and scalp includes regular shampoo and scalp massage services as well as special treatments for hair and scalp conditions. These services can be relaxing and effective in helping to ensure the health of the client's hair and scalp from one shop visit to another.

An analysis of the client's hair and scalp during the client consultation helps to identify their condition. Shampoo services ensure that the barber is working with clean hair that is free from oils or hair products that can interfere with cutting tools and haircut results. Professionally delivered scalp massage during the shampoo offers hygienic, circulatory, and relaxation benefits to the client. Follow-up conditioning treatments after the shampoo help to keep hair in a healthy and manageable condition for the client and the barber (**Figure 12-1**).

Special services, such as electrotherapy or light therapy treatments, can help to maintain healthy scalp and hair. These services may help to increase circulation, which can also help the overall health of the scalp.

Many of today's barbershop owners are aware of the positive impact and results that these services can provide for their patrons from both physiological and psychological standpoints. In addition, the performance of professional hair and scalp treatments can increase client retention and referral, while promoting a positive reputation for the barber and the barbershop.

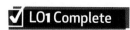

Shampoos and Conditioners

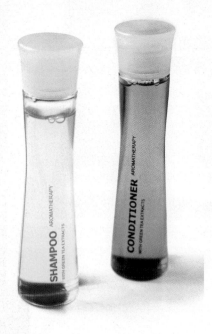

As you know, the purpose of a shampoo product and service is to cleanse the scalp and hair. This may seem obvious, but some barbers still encounter clients who use bar soap or other detergent products that can leave the hair dry or coated with soap residues. Conversely, **shampoos** are specially formulated oil-in-water emulsions for the hair and scalp; they do not contain the harsh alkalis found in soaps and detergents and therefore tend to leave the hair in a more manageable condition.

Conditioners can refer to either hair conditioners or scalp conditioners. Generally, **hair conditioners** moisturize the hair and help to restore some of the oils and/or proteins. **Scalp conditioners**, usually in cream or ointment form, are available for overall scalp maintenance or to treat conditions requiring a medicinal product.

It is the barber's responsibility to be knowledgeable about the products used in the shop or salon. Basic product knowledge can be easily obtained from product labels, distributors, trade show demonstrations, or manufacturer representatives or websites. Refer to **Figure 12-2** and **Table 12-1** for a review of the pH scale and products for different hair types.

REMINDER

Display and use the shop's retail products at the workstation or shampoo sink to promote product sales and convey your endorsement of the products.

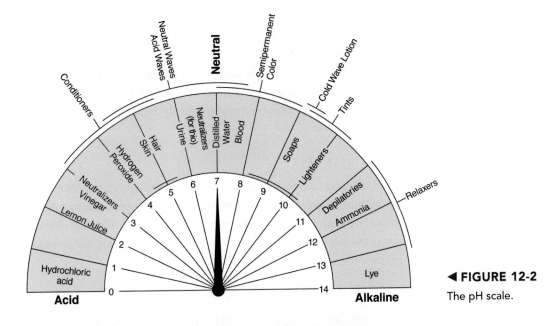

◄ FIGURE 12-2

The pH scale.

TABLE **12-1** Matching Products to Hair Types

HAIR TYPE	FINE	MEDIUM	COARSE
Straight	Volumizing shampoo Detangler, if necessary Protein treatments	Acid-balanced shampoo Finishing rinse Protein treatments	Moisturizing shampoo Leave-in conditioner Moisturizing treatments
Wavy, Curly, Extremely Curly	Fine-hair shampoo Light leave-in conditioner Protein treatments Spray-on thermal protectors	Acid-balanced shampoo Leave-in conditioner Moisturizing treatment	Moisturizing shampoo Leave-in conditioner Protein and moisturizing treatments
Dry and Damaged (Perms, Color, Relaxers, Blow-drying, Sun, Hot Irons)	Gentle cleansing shampoo Light leave-in conditioner Protein and moisturizing repair treatments Spray-on thermal protectors	Shampoo for chemically treated hair Moisturizing conditioner Protein and moisturizing repair treatments	Deep-moisturizing shampoo for damaged hair Leave-in conditioner Deep-conditioning treatments and hair masks

Draping

The comfort and protection of the client must always be considered during barbering services. **Draping** protects the clients' skin and clothing and assures clients that the barber is conscientious about their comfort and safety.

There are two main types of drapes used to perform barbering services: shampoo capes and haircutting capes (also known as chair cloths).

- *Shampoo capes* are typically waterproof drapes made of vinyl used to protect the client's skin and clothing from water, liquids, and chemical processes.

- The preferred *haircutting capes* are made of nylon or other synthetic materials. These draping fabrics are usually more comfortable for the client because they do not hold in as much body heat as vinyl capes. From the barber's standpoint, these fabrics are also more effective in shedding wet or dry hair. Wet hair has a tendency to stick to vinyl capes, making it more difficult to shake loose hairs off the drape.

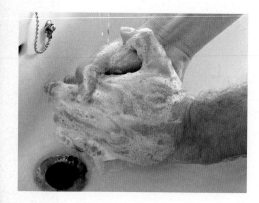

DRAPING METHODS

The method of draping to be used depends on the service to be performed. Several draping methods are presented in this text, although those taught by your instructor are also correct. Regardless of the draping method or the service to be provided, consideration for the client should always be one of your highest priorities.

Important steps for draping a client for any type of service are as follows:

1. Prepare materials and supplies for the service.

2. Sanitize your hands.

3. Ask the client to remove all neck and hair jewelry and store it in a safe place.

4. Turn the client's collar to the inside.

5. Proceed with the appropriate draping method.

mini PROCEDURE

DRAPING FOR WET AND CHEMICAL SERVICES

Wet hair services include shampooing, hair and scalp treatments, and all chemical applications.

1 Hold the towel lengthwise in front of you. Grasp the towel by opposite diagonal corners and fold on the diagonal (**Figures 12-3a** and **12-3b**). This folding technique utilizes the maximum length that can be achieved from the towel. Place the towel lengthwise around the client's neck and shoulders, crossing the ends beneath the chin (**Figure 12-4**).

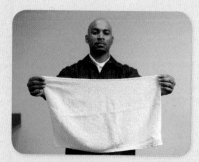

▲ FIGURE 12-3a

Grasp towel by opposite corners.

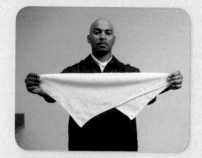

▲ FIGURE 12-3b

Fold on the diagonal.

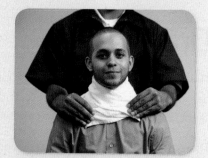

▲ FIGURE 12-4

Cross the towel ends beneath the client's chin.

(Continued)

2 Drape a waterproof cape over the towel and fasten it at the back so that the cape does not touch the client's skin. Position and flatten the top edge of the towel down over the neckline of the cape (**Figures 12-5** and **12-6**).

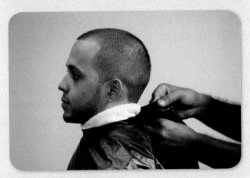

▲ **FIGURE 12-5**

Drape cape over the towel.

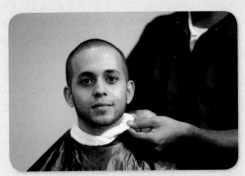

▲ **FIGURE 12-6**

Position and flatten top edge of towel over cape neckline.

3 Optional: Place another towel over the cape and secure it in front with a chair cloth clip (**Figure 12-7**).

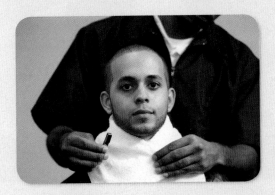

◀ **FIGURE 12-7**

Optional: Place second towel over cape and secure with clip.

Step 3 above is optional for the *shampoo* service. If two towels are too bulky at the shampoo bowl, fold the second towel in thirds and place it in the neck rest of the shampoo bowl to create a barrier between the client and the sink (**Figures 12-8** and **12-9**). Two towels, one under the cape and one over the cape as in Figure 12-7, should always be used for *chemical* services. A third towel from a clean, closed cabinet is used at the shampoo bowl for blotting purposes after rinsing the hair.

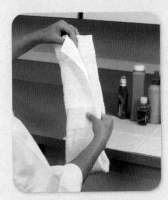

▲ **FIGURE 12-8**

Fold towel in thirds.

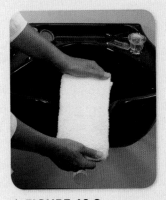

▲ **FIGURE 12-9**

Create a barrier in the neck rest of the shampoo bowl.

DRAPING FOR HAIRCUTTING SERVICES

Haircut draping requires a towel or neck strip and a nylon cape or chair cloth. If a shampoo service precedes the haircut, remove the waterproof cape and towel. Replace the towel with a neck strip, as this allows the hair to fall more naturally without obstruction. Replace the vinyl cape with a nylon cape. Follow the steps below, as illustrated in **Figures 12-10** through **12-12**.

1 Drape the nylon cape loosely across the client's chest and shoulders. Place the neck strip around the client's neck from front to back. Hold one end of the neck strip against the client's skin at the back or side of the neck while wrapping the rest of the strip. Secure the second neck strip end by tucking it neatly into the band of the neck strip **(Figure 12-10)**.

2 Lift the cape from across the client's shoulders, slide it into place around the neck, and fasten it at the back of the neck **(Figure 12-11)**.

3 Fold and flatten the top edge of the neck strip over the neckline of the cape to prevent the client's skin from touching the drape **(Figure 12-12)**.

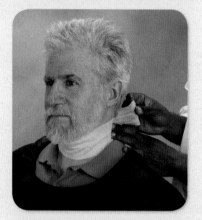

▲ **FIGURE 12-10**
Drape cape loosely and position neck strip around the neck.

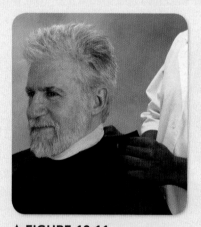

▲ **FIGURE 12-11**
Fasten drape.

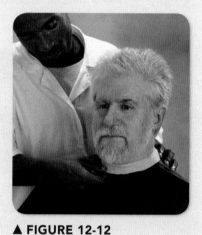

▲ **FIGURE 12-12**
Fold and smooth neck strip.

☑ **LO2 Complete**

FYI

The purpose of the towel or neck strip in draping procedures is to prevent the cape from having direct contact with the client's skin and to maintain sanitation standards. The application of this barrier between the client's skin and the drape is a requirement of every state's barber law, rules, and regulations.

The Shampoo Service

The shampoo service requires proper draping and positioning of the client, scalp manipulations to facilitate the shampoo procedure, and proper body positioning of the barber. Most barbershops are equipped with shampoo bowls either within a working booth area or in a separate section of the shop. Typically, the barber stands beside the client and shampoo bowl while performing the shampoo. Some shops, however, are equipped with the European-style shampoo bowl, which is a freestanding unit that allows the barber to stand in back of the client's head.

METHODS OF SHAMPOOING AND RINSING

Two methods are used for shampooing and rinsing: reclined and inclined.

- The *reclined method* of shampooing is the most commonly used. The hydraulic or shampoo chair is reclined, with the client's head positioned in the neck rest of the shampoo bowl **(Figure 12-13)**. This method is favored because it is more comfortable for the client and permits greater speed and efficiency by the barber.

- The *inclined method* can be used when a standard shampoo bowl is not available or when the client cannot use the reclined method. This method requires the client to bend his head forward over the shampoo bowl or sink **(Figure 12-14)**. The client may also sit on a stool or chair positioned close to the sink.

Physical Presentation

To prevent muscle aches, back strain, and fatigue, it is important to maintain good posture at the shampoo bowl. Review the following suggestions to maintain a good posture while shampooing.

- Stand as close as possible to the back of the client's head.

- Flex the knees slightly and position your body directly over your feet to maintain good balance.

- Try to keep your chin parallel to the floor to avoid neck strain. The head should be raised, with the chest up, abdomen flat, and shoulders relaxed.

- Do not bend or twist sideways from the waist or lean too far forward.

SUPERIOR SHAMPOO SERVICE

Excellence in performing the shampoo service requires barbers and stylists to give individual attention to each client's needs. In addition to selecting the shampoo best suited to the condition of the scalp and hair, the effectiveness of the shampoo will depend on the manner in which the shampoo is applied and rinsed, the quality of the scalp massage, and the temperature of the water used.

A client may find fault with the shampoo service for any of the following reasons:

- Improper shampoo selection

- Insufficient scalp massage

- Extreme water temperatures, either too hot or too cold

- Shampoo or water that runs onto the client's face, ears, or eyes

- Wetting or soiling the client's clothing

- Scraping or scratching the client's scalp with fingernails

- Improper hair blotting

- Insufficient cleansing and rinsing

In addition to learning what a superior shampoo service requires, you will also need to become familiar with such aspects of the shampoo service as the set-up, selection of products, water temperature, application of shampoo, and shampoo massage manipulations.

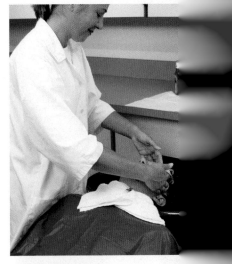

▲ **FIGURE 12-13**
Reclined method.

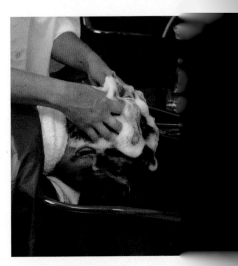

▲ **FIGURE 12-14**
Inclined method.

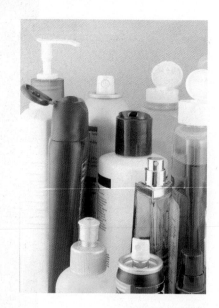

Set-Up and Preparation

Adequate preparation is the first step in performing a good shampoo. Before starting, the barber should assemble all necessary supplies or have them stored in an area convenient to the shampoo bowl. Shampoo service supplies include cleansing and conditioning products, waterproof drapes, and terry cloth towels.

Product Selection

It is essential that the barber be knowledgeable about the products used in the shop. Always read product labels and follow the manufacturer's directions. To determine which product to use, the barber *must* perform a hair and scalp analysis. Six characteristics of the hair and scalp should be considered before choosing products:

1. *Condition of the scalp:* dry, oily, normal, abrasions or disorders present

2. *Condition of the hair:* dry, brittle, fragile, oily, normal, or chemically treated

3. *Hair density:* thin, medium, thick

4. *Hair texture:* fine, average, coarse

5. *Hair porosity:* average porosity, porous, nonporous

6. *Hair elasticity:* poor, average, very good

With practice and experience, barbering students learn the effects of certain products on the hair and scalp. For example, moisturizing shampoos are not alkaline enough to cleanse an oily scalp and hair condition. Also, heavy, cuticle-coating conditioners can weigh down fine hair, leaving it flat or oily, while coarse hair may require a humectant-rich moisturizing conditioner to increase manageability (refer to Table 12-1).

Water Temperature

The water should be comfortably warm for the client. Cold water, in addition to causing discomfort, tends to reduce lathering. Hot water can cause the scalp to flake or become dry. Warm water is not only comfortable and relaxing for the client, it also reacts favorably during the foaming process.

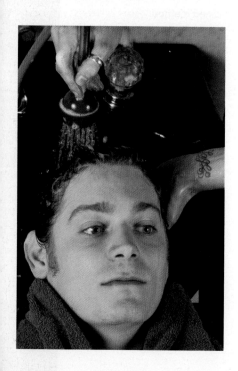

Application of Shampoo

Following a warm-water rinse to dampen the hair, the shampoo product should be dispensed into the barber's hand and then dispersed over both palms to facilitate spreading it throughout the client's hair. Spread sections of the hair apart with the thumbs and fingers to apply the shampoo directly onto the scalp. Make sure that the entire scalp is covered. The shampoo should be massaged completely into the scalp and hair. Warm water is added gradually to work up a rich, creamy lather. As the lather is created and the scalp manipulated, be careful to avoid getting shampoo lather on the client's face.

SHAMPOO MASSAGE MANIPULATIONS

The proper way to massage the scalp during a shampoo is as follows:

1 Stand behind or to the side of the client at the shampoo bowl as the style of sink allows.

2 Wet the hair, protecting the client's face, ears, and neck (**Figures 12-15** through **12-17**).

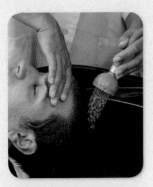

▲ **FIGURE 12-15**

Protecting the face.

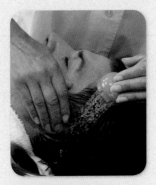

▲ **FIGURE 12-16**

Protecting the ears.

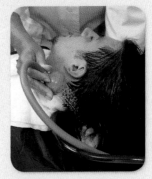

▲ **FIGURE 12-17**

Supporting and protecting the neck.

3 Lather the hair, starting at the front hairline and working along the sides toward the back and nape areas (**Figure 12-18**).

4 Use rotary movements over the entire head area (**Figures 12-19** through **12-21**).

5 Repeat these movements for each section several times.

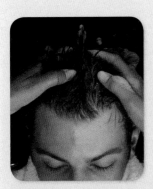

▲ **FIGURE 12-18**

Lathering the hair.

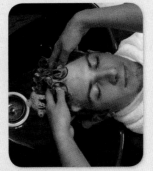

▲ **FIGURE 12-19**

Rotary movements on top of head.

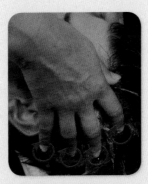

▲ **FIGURE 12-20**

Rotary movements at sides of head.

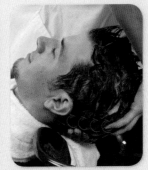

▲ **FIGURE 12-21**

Rotary movements at back of head.

All shampoo movements must be executed with the cushion tips of the fingers. The scalp manipulations are repeated several times until the lather is completely worked into the hair and scalp. The excess lather is then removed by a sweep of the palm from the front of the head to the back and rinsed from the barber's hand. The hair is then rinsed thoroughly with a strong spray.

Shampoo Service

SUPPLIES

- Shampoo bowl
- Waterproof cape
- Towels
- Shampoo
- Conditioner or hair rinse
- Terry cloth towels
- Comb

PREPARATION

1. Assemble supplies.
2. Wash your hands.

PROCEDURE

1 Seat the client in a comfortable and relaxed position.

2 Drape the client according to textbook or instructor's procedures.

3 Consult with the client about products, hair and scalp problems, or any questions they have about their hair or scalp.

4 Examine the condition of the client's hair and scalp. Briefly massage the scalp to loosen epidermal scales, debris, and scalp tissues.

5 Decide on the type of products to be used.

6 Position the client for the shampoo service. Recline the client while draping the back of the cape over the back of the chair.

7 Wet the hair with warm water.

8 Apply shampoo to all parts of the scalp.

9 Massage the scalp for several minutes as shown in Figures 12-19 to 12-21.

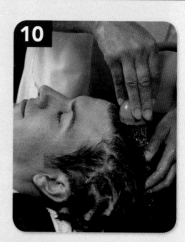

10 Rinse the hair thoroughly with warm water and repeat the lathering step if necessary. Suggest a hair rinse or conditioner at this time.

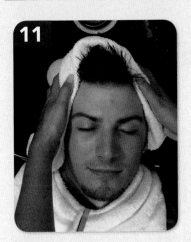

11 Blot the hair

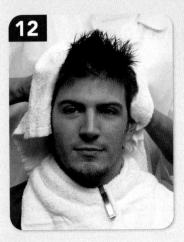

12 Raise client to a sitting position and lightly towel dry the hair; wipe the face and ears if necessary.

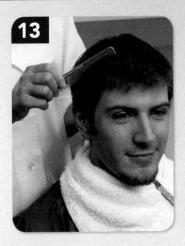

13 Comb hair into position for cutting.

NOTE: With practice, you will develop a set-up routine for the shampoo service and become comfortable with asking clients questions that relate to the service.

CLEAN-UP AND DISINFECTION

1. Cleanse and disinfect all implements; store soiled towels in appropriate container.

2. Sanitize work area.

3. Wash your hands.

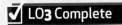 **LO3 Complete**

Liquid-Dry Shampoo

SUPPLIES

- Waterproof cape
- Towels
- Liquid-dry shampoo
- Brush
- Comb
- Cotton pledget

PREPARATION

1. Assemble supplies.
2. Wash your hands.

PROCEDURE

1 Seat the client in a comfortable and relaxed position.

2 Drape the client.

3 Perform hair and scalp analysis.

4 Brush the hair thoroughly and comb it lightly.

5 Part the hair into small sections.

6 Saturate a piece of cotton with the liquid-dry shampoo, squeeze it out lightly, and apply to the scalp along each part line. Follow by swiftly rubbing the scalp with a towel along the same area. Repeat this procedure over the entire head.

7 Saturate more cotton with the product and apply down the length of the hair strands.

8 Rub the hair strands with a towel to remove the soil.

9 Remoisten the hair lightly with liquid and comb it into the desired style.

CLEAN-UP AND DISINFECTION

1. Cleanse and disinfect all implements; store products and soiled towels appropriately.
2. Sanitize work area.
3. Wash your hands.

Dry or Powder Shampoo

A dry or powder shampoo is usually given when the client's health will not permit a wet shampoo.

SUPPLIES

- Shampoo bowl
- Waterproof cape
- Towel or neck strip
- Dry or powder shampoo
- Brush
- Comb

PREPARATION

1. Assemble supplies.
2. Wash your hands.

PROCEDURE

1 Seat the client in a comfortable and relaxed position.

2 Drape the client.

3 Perform hair and scalp analysis.

4 Sprinkle the product into the hair, working it in one section at a time.

5 Brush hair thoroughly to remove the powder.

CLEAN-UP AND DISINFECTION

1. Cleanse and disinfect all implements; store soiled towels in appropriate container.
2. Sanitize work area.
3. Wash your hands.

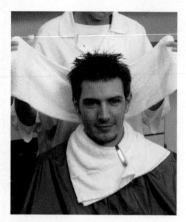

▲ FIGURE 12-22

Towel wrap for scalp steam—step 1.

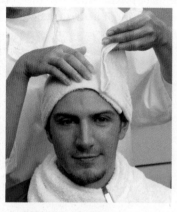

▲ FIGURE 12-23

Towel wrap for scalp steam—step 2.

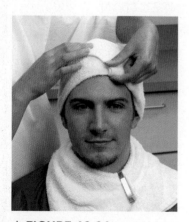

▲ FIGURE 12-24

Towel wrap for scalp steam—step 3.

Scalp and Hair Treatments

The purpose of scalp and hair treatments is to preserve the health and appearance of the hair and scalp. These treatments also help to prevent or combat disorders such as dandruff, dry hair or scalp, and oily hair or scalp.

Cleanliness and stimulation are the essential requirements for healthy hair and scalp. Because the scalp and hair are so interrelated, many scalp disorders need correction in order to maintain the health of the hair. A healthy scalp will help to maintain a healthy head of hair.

Scalp treatments may be given separately or combined with hair treatments. In many cases, a product that is good for the scalp is also good for the hair. In other cases, separate products may need to be used. Conditions caused by neglect, such as a tight scalp, overactive or under-active oil glands, and tense nerves may be corrected by proper scalp treatments. Depending on the client's needs, the scalp treatment may include:

- Cleansing with a suitable shampoo.
- Massage with the hands or electrical appliance.
- Use of electrical appliances such as an electric steamer, infrared lamp, ultraviolet lamp, high-frequency current, or dermal lamp.
- The application of cosmetic preparations such as hair tonics, astringents, antiseptics, or ointments.

SCALP STEAM

The **scalp steam** is effective in preparing the scalp for scalp massage manipulations and treatments. Steam relaxes the pores, softens the scalp and hair, and increases blood circulation. A scalp steamer assures a constant and controlled source of steam; however, steam towels can also be used effectively. To use a scalp steamer, fill the container with water, fit the hood over the client's head, and turn on the current. Many hoods have openings on the side so the barber's hands can be inserted to perform a scalp massage during the scalp steam.

Steam towels are used in the absence of a scalp steamer (**Figures 12-22** through **12-24**). They are prepared, one at a time, by soaking the towel in hot water. The excess water is wrung out and the towel is wrapped around the client's head. When the towel cools, another one is applied in its place. If a hot-towel cabinet is available, prepared steam towels may be stored until needed.

SCALP MASSAGE MANIPULATIONS

Although you have already learned how to perform a shampoo massage, the massage techniques used to perform scalp treatments may be more thorough, requiring additional steps and time. The manipulations should be performed with continuous, even motion and pressure as illustrated in **Procedure 12-4**. A thorough scalp massage is beneficial in the following ways:

- Blood and lymph flow are increased.
- Nerves are rested and soothed.
- Scalp muscles are stimulated.

- The scalp is made more flexible.
- Hair growth is promoted and the hair is made lustrous.

Scalp massage should be performed as a series of treatments, once a week for a normal scalp and more frequently for scalp disorders under the direction of a dermatologist.

Refer to **Table 12-2** to review the muscles, nerves, and arteries affected by scalp massage.

> ### TABLE **12-2** Massage and Its Influence on the Scalp

MASSAGE MOVEMENTS	MUSCLES	NERVES	ARTERIES
Sliding Movement	Auricularis superior	Posterior auricular	Frontal and parietal
Behind Ears and Neck-to-Crown Movement	Auricularis posterior	Greater occipital	Occipital
Forehead-to-Crown Movement	Frontalis	Supra-orbital	Frontal
Front Hairline Movement	Frontalis	Supra-orbital	Frontal and parietal
Rotary Movement	Auricularis posterior	Greater occipital	Posterior auricular and parietal
Ear-to-Crown Movement	Auricularis anterior and superior	Temporal auricular	Frontal and parietal

SCALP TREATMENT WITH AN ELECTRIC MASSAGER

An electric massager, sometimes called a vibrator or hand massager, is an electrical tool that is used to perform a stimulating scalp massage. Before using, adjust the vibrator on the back of the hand, leaving the thumb and fingers free; then turn on the current. The vibrations are transmitted through the cushions of the fingertips. The same movements are followed as for a regular hand scalp massage. When using the vibrator on the scalp, be careful to regulate the intensity and duration of the vibrations, as well as the pressure applied (**Figure 12-25**).

Scalp massage is most effective when given in a series of treatments and may be advised for general scalp maintenance, to promote hair growth, or to correct a scalp condition.

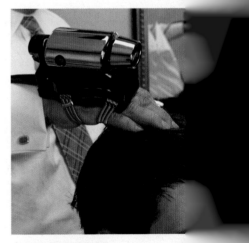

▲ FIGURE 12-25

Hand-held electric massager.

Hair Tonic Treatments

Scalp steamers, steam towels, vibrators, and scalp manipulations may all be used with hair tonics. During scalp steams, apply the tonic after the scalp has been steamed and before combing the hair into the desired style. The order of procedures for a hair tonic treatment is as follows: apply the hair tonic, massage the scalp, apply scalp steam, massage again with hands or a vibrator, and comb the hair into the desired style.

CAUTION

Barbers should not treat scalp diseases caused by parasitic or staphylococcus infections. Clients with abnormal scalp conditions should be referred to a physician.

Scalp Massage

When performing scalp massage, apply firm pressure on the upward strokes. Firm rotary movements loosen the scalp tissues and help to improve the health of hair and scalp by increasing the blood's circulation to the scalp and hair papillae. Massage manipulations should be slow and rhythmic, and care should be taken to avoid pulling the hair in any way. With each movement, the hands are placed under the hair with the fingertips resting on the scalp. The length of the fingers, the balls of the fingertips, and the cushions of the palms all help to stimulate muscles, nerves, and blood vessels in the scalp area.

NOTE: The following is one method of scalp massage. Your instructor may have developed a different procedure, however, that is equally correct. Prepare the client as for a shampoo service.

SUPPLIES

- Waterproof cape
- Towel or neck strip

PREPARATION

1. Assemble supplies.
2. Wash your hands.

PROCEDURE

1 Seat the client in a comfortable and relaxed position.

2 Drape the client.

3 Perform hair and scalp analysis.

4 Perform massage manipulations.

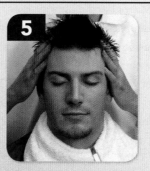

5 Place the fingertips of each hand at the hairline on each side of the client's head, hands pointing upward. Firmly slide the fingers upward, spreading the fingertips. Continue until the fingers meet at the center or top of the scalp. Repeat three or four times.

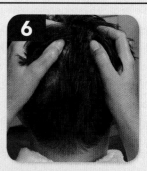

6 Place the fingers of each hand on the sides of the head, behind the ears. Use a rotary movement and the thumbs to massage from behind the ears toward the crown. Repeat four or five times. Move the fingers until both thumbs meet at the hairline at the back of neck. Rotate the thumbs upward toward the crown.

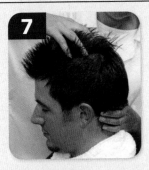

7 Move to the right of the client. Place the left hand at the back of the head. Place the thumb and fingers of the right hand against and over the forehead, just above the eyebrows. With the cushion tips of the thumb and fingers of the right hand, use a sliding movement to massage slowly and firmly across the top of the head toward the crown while keeping the left hand in a fixed position at the back of the head. Repeat four or five times.

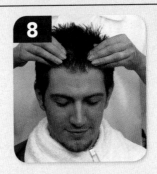

8 Move behind the client. Place the hands on each side of the head at the front hairline. Rotate the fingertips three times. On the fourth rotation, apply a quick, upward twisting motion, firm enough to move the scalp. Continue this movement on the sides and top of the scalp. Repeat three or four times.

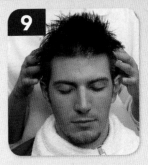

9 Place the fingers of each hand below the back of each ear. Rotate the fingers upward from behind the ears to the crown. Repeat three or four times. Move the fingers toward the back of the head and repeat the movement with both hands. Apply rotary movements in an upward direction toward the crown.

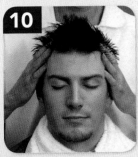

10 Place one hand at either side of the head. Keep fingers close together and position at the hairline above the ears. Firmly move the hands directly upward to the top of the head in a sliding movement. Repeat four times. Move the hands to above the ears and repeat the movement. Move the hands to back of ears and repeat the movement.

CLEAN-UP AND DISINFECTION

1. Cleanse and disinfect all implements; store soiled towels in appropriate container.

2. Sanitize work area.

3. Wash your hands.

Scalp Treatment for Normal Scalp and Hair

The purpose of a general scalp treatment is to keep the scalp and hair clean and healthy. Regular scalp treatments can also help to prevent baldness.

SUPPLIES

- Shampoo bowl
- Infrared lamp
- High-frequency current appliance (optional)
- Waterproof cape
- Towels
- Cotton pledget or swab
- Shampoo for normal hair and scalp
- Scalp conditioner or ointment
- Scalp lotion or tonic
- Brush
- Comb

PREPARATION

1. Assemble supplies.
2. Wash your hands.

PROCEDURE

1 Seat the client in a comfortable and relaxed position.

2 Drape the client.

3 Perform hair and scalp analysis.

4 Brush the hair for a few minutes to loosen dead skin cells.

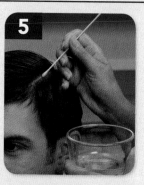

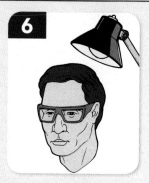

5 Part the hair and apply a scalp conditioner or ointment directly to the scalp with a cotton pledget or cotton swab.

6 Apply infrared lamp for 3 to 5 minutes.

7 Massage the scalp for 10 minutes.

8 Shampoo the hair and towel dry.

9 Optional: Stimulate the scalp with high-frequency current for 2 to 3 minutes.

10 Apply a suitable scalp lotion or tonic and work it into the scalp; comb and style the hair.

CLEAN-UP AND DISINFECTION

1. Cleanse and disinfect all implements; store products and soiled towels appropriately.
2. Sanitize work area.
3. Wash your hands.

Inactivity of the oil glands, or the excessive removal of natural oil, produces dry hair and scalp conditions. Other causes contributing to dry hair and scalp are an indoor lifestyle, frequent washing with strong soaps or shampoos, and the continued use of drying tonics or lotions. Select scalp preparations that contain moisturizing and emollient agents. Avoid the use of strong soaps, preparations containing a mineral or sulfonated oil base, greasy preparations, and lotions with a high alcohol content.

SUPPLIES

- Shampoo bowl
- Scalp steamer (optional)
- Infrared lamp
- High-frequency current appliance
- Waterproof cape
- Towels
- Cotton pledget or swab
- Mild shampoo for dry hair
- Scalp conditioning cream for dry hair and scalp
- Brush
- Comb

PREPARATION

1. Assemble supplies.
2. Wash your hands.

PROCEDURE

1 Seat the client in a comfortable and relaxed position.

2 Drape the client.

3 Perform hair and scalp analysis.

4 Brush the client's hair.

5 Massage and stimulate the scalp for 3 to 5 minutes.

6 Apply a scalp preparation for this condition.

7 Steam the scalp with hot towels or scalp steamer for 7 to 10 minutes.

8 Shampoo the hair using a mild shampoo suitable for dry scalp and hair.

9 Towel dry the hair, making sure the scalp is thoroughly dried.

10 Apply scalp cream sparingly with a rotary, frictional motion.

11 Apply an infrared lamp over the scalp for 3 to 5 minutes.

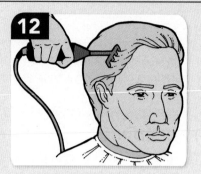

12 Stimulate the scalp with direct high-frequency current, using a glass rake electrode, for about 5 minutes.

13 Rinse hair thoroughly.

14 Comb the hair into the desired style.

CLEAN-UP AND DISINFECTION

1. Cleanse and disinfect all implements; store products and soiled towels appropriately.

2. Sanitize work area.

3. Wash your hands.

CAUTION

Never use a scalp or hair treatment product that contains alcohol *before* applying high-frequency current. Such products can be safely applied only *after* the high-frequency treatment.

Oily Scalp and Hair Treatment

The main cause of an oily scalp is overactive sebaceous glands. Manipulating the scalp will increase circulation and help to release hardened sebum from the follicles.

SUPPLIES

- Shampoo bowl
- Scalp steamer or infrared lamp
- High-frequency current appliance
- Faradic or sinusoidal current appliance (optional)
- Waterproof cape
- Towels
- Cotton pledget or swab
- Shampoo for oily hair and scalp
- Medicated scalp lotion
- Medicated scalp astringent
- Brush
- Comb

PREPARATION

1. Assemble supplies.
2. Wash your hands.

PROCEDURE

1 Seat the client in a comfortable and relaxed position.

2 Drape the client.

3 Perform hair and scalp analysis.

4 Brush the hair gently.

5 Apply a medicated scalp lotion to the scalp only.

6 Apply infrared lamp or scalp steamer for 3 to 5 minutes.

7 Massage the scalp. (Option: Faradic or sinusoidal current may be used.)

8 Shampoo with a product suitable for oily scalp and hair and towel dry the hair.

9 Apply direct high-frequency current for 3 to 5 minutes.

10 Apply a medicated lotion or astringent to the scalp only.

11 Comb the hair into the desired style.

CLEAN-UP AND DISINFECTION

1. Cleanse and disinfect all implements; store products and soiled towels appropriately.
2. Sanitize work area.
3. Wash your hands.

Dandruff Scalp Treatment

The principal signs of dandruff are the appearance of white scales on the hair and scalp accompanied by itching. Dandruff may be associated with either a dry (pityriasis capitis simplex) or a more severe oily condition (pityriasis steatoides). Other contributing causes of dandruff are poor blood circulation to the scalp, improper diet, and lack of hygienic practices.

SUPPLIES

- Shampoo bowl
- Scalp steamer (optional)
- Ultraviolet ray lamp
- Infrared lamp
- Eye protectors for client
- Safety goggles
- Waterproof cape
- Towels
- Cotton pledget or swab
- Antidandruff shampoo
- Antidandruff conditioner or antiseptic lotion
- Medicated scalp astringent
- Brush
- Comb

PREPARATION

1. Assemble supplies.
2. Wash your hands.

PROCEDURE

1 Seat the client in a comfortable and relaxed position.

2 Drape the client.

3 Perform hair and scalp analysis.

4 Shampoo with an antidandruff shampoo according to the type of dandruff and towel dry.

5 Apply antidandruff conditioner or antiseptic lotion to the scalp.

6 Apply steam towels or scalp steamer for 3 to 5 minutes.

7 Massage the scalp.

8 Shampoo again with an antidandruff shampoo.

9 Both the barber and the client should put on tinted safety goggles.

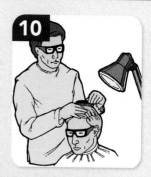

10 Expose the scalp to ultraviolet rays (for its germicidal effects) for 5 to 8 minutes, parting the hair every half inch.

11 Apply leave-in antidandruff conditioner or lotion to the scalp.

12 Expose the scalp to an infrared lamp for 5 minutes to help penetration of the lotion.

13 Comb hair into desired style.

CLEAN-UP AND DISINFECTION

1. Cleanse and disinfect all implements; store products and soiled towels appropriately.

2. Sanitize work area.

3. Wash your hands.

Alternate Step: In place of step 12, high-frequency current may be applied for 3 to 5 minutes. However, be sure the antidandruff conditioner or lotion used in step 11 *does not* contain alcohol.

Scalp Treatment for Alopecia

Alopecia is the term used to describe hair loss. The chief causes of alopecia are heredity, poor circulation, lack of proper stimulation, improper nourishment, certain infectious skin diseases such as ringworm, and constitutional disorders. Conditions of alopecia may benefit from stimulation of the blood supply to the germinal papilla through scalp treatments.

SUPPLIES

- Shampoo bowl
- Scalp steamer (optional)
- Ultraviolet ray lamp
- High-frequency current appliance
- Eye protectors for client
- Safety goggles
- Waterproof cape
- Towels
- Cotton pledget or swab
- Shampoo for normal, dry, or oily hair and scalp
- Prescribed medicated scalp ointment
- Brush
- Comb

PREPARATION

1. Assemble supplies.
2. Wash your hands.

PROCEDURE

1 Seat the client in a comfortable and relaxed position.

2 Drape the client.

3 Perform hair and scalp analysis.

4 Apply regular scalp manipulations.

5 Shampoo the hair and scalp as required (dry or oily).

6 Dry the scalp thoroughly.

7 Protect the client's and barber's eyes with goggles.

8 Expose the scalp to ultraviolet rays for about 5 minutes.

9 Apply a medicated scalp ointment as directed by a physician.

10 Apply indirect high-frequency current (with the client holding the wire glass electrode between both hands) for about 5 minutes.

11 Comb the hair into the desired style.

CLEAN-UP AND DISINFECTION

1. Cleanse and disinfect all implements; store products and soiled towels appropriately.
2. Sanitize work area.
3. Wash your hands.

Corrective Hair Treatment

A corrective hair treatment deals with the hair shaft rather than the scalp. Dry and damaged hair can be greatly improved by reconditioning (corrective) treatments that make the hair soft and pliable. Dry hair may be softened quickly with a reconditioning preparation applied directly on the outside of the hair shaft. The product used for this purpose is usually an emulsion containing cholesterol and related compounds.

SUPPLIES

- Shampoo bowl
- Waterproof cape
- Towels
- Mild shampoo
- Deep conditioner
- Brush
- Comb

PREPARATION

1. Assemble supplies.
2. Wash your hands.

PROCEDURE

1 Seat the client in a comfortable and relaxed position.

2 Drape the client.

3 Perform hair and scalp analysis.

4 Massage and stimulate the scalp for 3 to 5 minutes.

5 Apply a mild shampoo and rinse thoroughly.

6 Blot the hair with a towel.

7 Apply a deep-conditioning agent according to the manufacturer's directions.

8 Rinse conditioner thoroughly; comb hair into the desired style.

CLEAN-UP AND DISINFECTION

1. Cleanse and disinfect all implements; store products and soiled towels appropriately.
2. Sanitize work area.
3. Wash your hands.

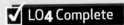
LO**4** Complete

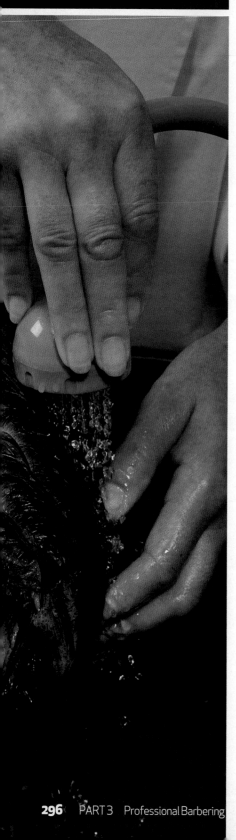

12 Review
Questions

1. Explain the purpose of draping a client.

2. Explain the purpose of the towel or neck strip in draping.

3. Describe the type of cape that should be used for wet and chemical services and why.

4. Describe the type of cape that is preferred for haircutting services and why.

5. List the steps involved in performing a shampoo service.

6. List and describe the massage manipulations applied to the scalp during a shampoo.

7. Compare the massage manipulations used in a shampoo service to the manipulations used in a scalp massage.

8. List the scalp treatments that use ultraviolet rays and infrared rays.

9. Identify three important cautions associated with scalp treatments.

Chapter
Glossary

conditioners refers to either hair conditioners or scalp conditioners

draping covering the client's clothing with a cape or drape for sanitation and protection

hair conditioners products designed to moisturize the hair or restore some of the hair's oils or proteins

scalp conditioners cream or ointment-based products used to soften or treat the scalp

scalp steam process of using steam towels or a steaming unit to soften and open scalp pores

shampoos hair and scalp cleansing products

13 Men's
FACIAL MASSAGE AND TREATMENTS

Learning Objectives

AFTER COMPLETING THIS CHAPTER, YOU SHOULD BE ABLE TO:

1. Describe the benefits of facial massage and treatments.
2. Discuss the location and stimulation of facial muscles.
3. Discuss the location and stimulation of facial nerves.
4. Name and demonstrate massage manipulations.
5. Demonstrate the use of facial treatment equipment.
6. Discuss products used in facial treatments.
7. Identify skin types and appropriate facial treatments and products.

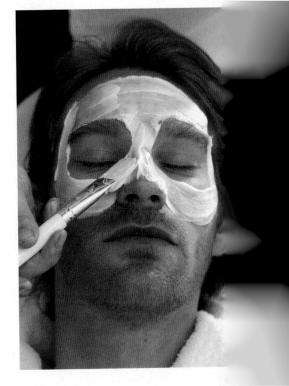

Key Terms

PAGE NUMBER INDICATES WHERE IN THE CHAPTER THE TERM IS USED.

astringent / 320

direct surface
   application / 316

effleurage / 309

electric massager / 313

friction / 309

indirect application / 317

motor point / 308

muscles / 300

percussion / 310

pétrissage / 309

phoresis / 320

rolling cream / 328

tapotement / 310

tonics / 326

vibration / 310

Providing for men's skin care needs is becoming an important and lucrative service in today's personal appearance market. Male clients represent about 20 percent of the skin care clientele in spas and salons, and this percentage is expected to grow in the future. The data, which follows the trend of spas and salons specifically, has identified a market base that may not have been well served in the past few decades by the very branch of the industry that once catered to the male market—barbers and barbershops! Historically, hot steam towels, shaves, and rolling cream facial treatments were standard customer services performed by the barber. Although products and technological options have changed over the years, the concept of providing psychologically and physiologically rewarding services has not. Facial massage and skin care treatments are two such services that the professional barber should master and promote.

A facial massage and treatment is one of the most relaxing and restful services offered in the barbershop. When performed correctly, regularly scheduled facials can produce noticeable improvement in the client's skin tone, texture, and appearance. A facial is also part of the finishing service that follows a facial shave, so barbers need to know the basics of performing facial procedures. In this chapter you will learn about the anatomical structures of the head, face, and neck; primary subdermal systems; and facial massage manipulations. You will also learn how to analyze skin types so that you can recommend the most effective products and treatments to your clients.

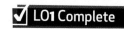

Subdermal Systems and Facial Massage

The muscles, nerves, and arteries of the head, face, and neck are three of the subdermal systems associated with the performance of facial treatments. **Muscles** are fibrous tissues that have the ability to stretch and contract to produce all body movements. *Nerves* are long, white, fibrous cords that act as message carriers from the brain and spinal column to and from all parts of the body. *Arteries* are elastic, muscular, thick-walled blood vessels that transport blood under high pressure.

Since the muscles, nerves, and arteries of the head, face, and neck are all affected by facial massage and treatments, it is the barber's responsibility to perform facial services that may prove beneficial to the client.

STIMULATION OF MUSCLES

Muscular tissue may be stimulated by any of the following actions:

- Massage (hand massage and electric vibrator)
- Electric current (high-frequency and faradic current)
- Light rays (infrared rays and ultraviolet rays)
- Heat rays (heating lamps and heating caps)
- Moist heat (steamers and moderately warm steam towels)

- Nerve impulses (through the nervous system)
- Chemicals (certain acids and salts)

MUSCLES AFFECTED BY MASSAGE

The barber or stylist is concerned with the voluntary muscles of the head, face, and neck. It is essential to know the location of these muscles and what they control. **Figures 13-1a** and **13-1b** and **Table 13-1** provide a review of the muscles of the head, face, and neck from Chapter 7.

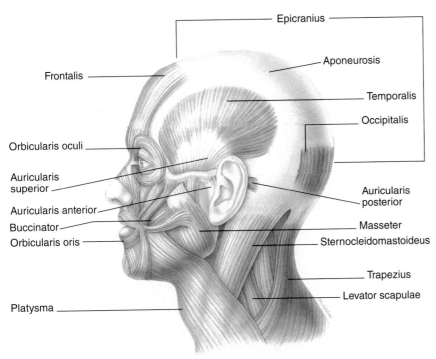

▲ FIGURE 13-1a

Muscles of the head, face, and neck.

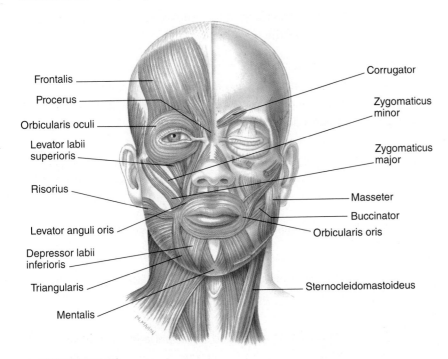

▲ FIGURE 13-1b

Muscles of the face.

TABLE 13-1 Muscles of the Head, Face, and Neck

MUSCLE	LOCATION	FUNCTION
Epicranius (occipito-frontalis)	Scalp	Broad muscle that covers the top of the skull
Frontalis	Scalp	Front portion of the epicranius; draws the scalp forward and causes wrinkles across the forehead
Occipitalis	Scalp	Muscle at the back part of the epicranius; draws the scalp backward
Aponeurosis	Scalp	Tendon that connects the occipitalis and the frontalis
Orbicularis oculi	Eyebrows	Completely surrounds the margin of the eye socket; closes the eyelid
Corrugator	Eyebrows	Muscle beneath the frontalis and orbicularis oculi; draws the eyebrows down and in; produces vertical lines and causes frowning
Procerus	Nose	Covers the top of the nose, depresses the eyebrow, and causes wrinkles across the bridge of the nose; the other nasal muscles are small muscles around the nasal openings that contract and expand the opening of the nostrils
Levator labii superioris (quadratus labii superioris)	Mouth	Muscle surrounding the upper lip; elevates the upper lip and dilates the nostrils
Depressor labii inferioris (quadratus labii inferioris)	Mouth	Muscle that surrounds the lower part of the lip, depressing the lower lip and drawing it a little to one side
Buccinator	Mouth	Muscle between the upper and lower jaws; compresses the cheeks and expels air between the lips
Levator anguli oris (caninus)	Mouth	Raises the angle of the mouth and draws it inward
Mentalis	Mouth	Situated at the tip of the chin; raises and pushes up the lower lip, causing wrinkling of the chin
Orbicularis oris	Mouth	Forms a flat band around the upper and lower lips; compresses, contracts, puckers, and wrinkles the lips

TABLE **13-1** (Continued)

MUSCLE	LOCATION	FUNCTION
Risorius	Mouth	Extends from the masseter muscle to the angle of the mouth; draws the corner of the mouth out and back
Zygomaticus	Mouth	Extends from the zygomatic bone to the angle of the mouth; elevates the lip
Triangularis	Mouth	Extends along the side of the chin; draws down the corner of the mouth.
Auricularis superior	Ears	Muscle above the ear that draws it upward
Auricularis posterior	Ears	Muscle behind the ear that draws it backward
Auricularis anterior	Ears	Muscle in front of the ear that draws it forward
Masseter and the temporalis	Mastication muscles	Muscles that coordinate in opening and closing the mouth; sometimes referred to as chewing muscles
Platysma	Neck, chest, and shoulders	Broad muscle extending from the chest and shoulder muscles to the side of the chin; responsible for depressing the lower jaw and lip
Sternocleidomastoideus	Neck, chest, to back of ear	Extends from the collar and chest bones to the temporal bone in back of the ear; bends and rotates the head
Trapezius	Neck and shoulders	Allows movement of the shoulders and covers the back of the neck

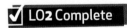
☑ LO2 Complete

STIMULATION OF NERVES

Stimulation of the nerves causes muscles to expand and contract. Heat and moist heat on the skin cause relaxation and cold causes contraction. Nerve stimulation may be accomplished by any of the following means:

- Chemicals (certain acids and salts)
- Massage (hand massage and electric vibrator)
- Electrical current (high-frequency)
- Light rays (infrared)
- Heat rays (heating lamps and heating caps)
- Moist heat (steamers and moderately warm steam towels)

NERVES AFFECTED BY FACIAL MASSAGE

There are 12 pairs of cranial nerves and all are connected to a part of the brain surface. The cranial nerves that are of most interest in the performance of facial and scalp treatments are the fifth, seventh, and eleventh cranial nerves. Cranial nerves are numbered according to the order in which they emerge from the brain and are named by a description of their nature or function. **Figure 13-2** and **Table 13-2** provide a review of the nerves of the head, face, and neck discussed in Chapter 7.

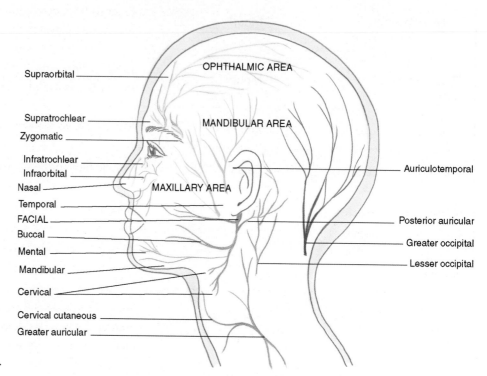

▶ FIGURE 13-2

Nerves of the face and neck.

TABLE 13-2 Cranial Nerves Affected by Facial Massage

CRANIAL NERVE	NAME	TYPE	CONTROLS
First	Olfactory	Sensory	Sense of smell
Second	Optic	Sensory	Sense of sight
Third	Oculomotor	Motor	Motion of the eye
Fourth	Trochlear	Motor	Upward and downward motion of the eye
Fifth	Trigeminal or Trifacial	Sensory-motor	Sensations of the face, tongue, and teeth

TABLE 13-2 (Continued)

CRANIAL NERVE	NAME	TYPE	CONTROLS
Chief sensory nerve of the face and motor nerve to muscles of mastication	*Supraorbital:* affects the skin of the forehead, scalp, eyebrows, and upper eyelids *Supratrochlear:* affects the skin between the eyes and upper sides of the nose *Infratrochlear:* affects the membrane and skin of the nose *Nasal:* affects the point and lower sides of the nose *Zygomatic:* affects the skin of the temples, sides of the forehead, and upper part of the cheeks *Infraorbital:* affects the skin of the lower eyelids and sides of the nose, upper lip, and mouth *Auriculotemporal:* affects the external ear and the skin from above the temples to the top of the skull *Mental:* affects the skin of the lower lip and chin		
Sixth	Abducent	Motor	Motion of the eye
Seventh	Facial	Sensory-motor	Motion of the face, scalp, neck, ear, and sections of the palate and tongue
Chief motor nerve of the face	*Posterior auricular:* affects muscles behind the ears at the base of the skull *Temporal:* affects the muscles of the temples, sides of the forehead, eyebrows, eyelids, and upper part of the cheeks *Zygomatic:* affects the muscles of the upper part of the cheeks *Buccal:* affects the muscles of the mouth *Mandibular:* affects the muscles of the chin and lower lip *Cervical:* affects the sides of the neck		
Eighth	Acoustic	Sensory	Sense of hearing
Ninth	Glossopharyngeal	Sensory-motor	Sense of taste
Tenth	Vagus	Sensory-motor	Motion and sensations of the ear, pharynx, larynx, heart, lungs, and esophagus
Eleventh	Accessory	Motor	Motion of the neck muscles
	Spinal branch: affects the muscles of the neck and back		
Twelfth	Hypoglossal	Motor	Motion of the tongue

Spinal or cervical nerves can also be affected by facial massage. The cervical nerves originate at the spinal cord and their branches supply the muscles and scalp at the back of the head and neck, as shown in **Table 13-3**.

> ### TABLE **13-3** Cervical Nerves Affected by Facial Massage

NERVE	LOCATION	FUNCTION
Greater occipital	Back of the head	Affects the scalp as far up as the top of the head
Lesser occipital	Base of the skull	Affects the scalp and muscles of this region
Greater auricular	Side of the neck	Affects the external ears and the areas in front and back of the ears
Cutaneous colli	Side of the neck	Affects the front and sides of the neck as far down as the breastbone

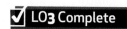 LO3 Complete

ARTERIES AFFECTED BY FACIAL MASSAGE

An artery is a tubular, thick-walled, elastic vessel that, like capillaries and veins, is part of the circulatory system that transports blood from the heart to all parts of the body. Blood returns to the heart through the veins. The primary arteries that are affected by facial massage are presented in **Figure 13-3** and **Table 13-4**.

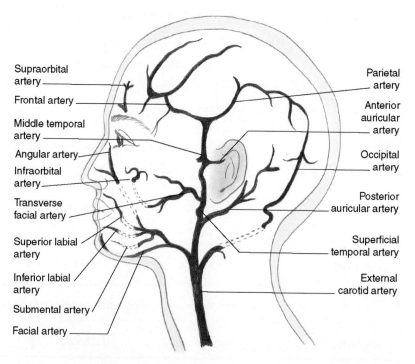

▶ **FIGURE 13-3**
Arteries of the head, face, and neck.

TABLE 13-4 Arteries Affected by Facial Massage

ARTERY	FUNCTION	ARTERIAL BRANCHES AND BLOOD SUPPLY AREAS
Common carotids	Main sources of blood supply to the head, face, and neck; located at the sides of the neck	*Internal division:* supplies the brain, eye sockets, eyelids, and forehead *External division:* supplies superficial parts of the head, face, and neck
External maxillary (facial artery)	Supplies the lower region of the face, mouth, and nose	*Submental:* supplies chin and lower lip *Inferior labial:* supplies lower lip *Angular:* supplies side of the nose *Superior labial:* supplies upper lip, septum, and wings of the nose
Superficial temporal	Continuation of external carotid: supplies muscles, skin, and scalp on the front, side, and top of the head	*Frontal:* supplies the forehead *Parietal:* supplies the crown and sides of the head *Transverse facial:* supplies the masseter *Middle temporal:* supplies the temples and eyelids *Anterior auricular:* supplies the anterior part of the ear
Occipital	Supplies the scalp and back of the head up to the crown	*Sternocleidomastoideus:* supplies the sternocleidomastoideus muscle
Posterior auricular	Supplies the scalp behind and above the ear	*Auricular:* supplies the skin in back of the ear

VEINS AFFECTED BY FACIAL MASSAGE

The deoxygenated blood returning to the heart from the head, face, and neck flows on each side of the neck in two principal veins: the internal jugular and the external jugular. The most important veins are parallel to the arteries and take the same names as the arteries. Both the internal and external jugular veins serve the head, face, neck, and chest.

Theory of Massage

Most clients enjoy a properly administered facial treatment for its stimulating or relaxing effects. Facial massage involves the manual or mechanical external manipulation of the face and requires a skillful touch. This is accomplished with the hands or with the aid of electrical appliances such as electric massagers or vibrators. Each massage movement is executed in such a way as to obtain a specific result.

The benefits of massage depend upon the type, intensity, and extent of the manipulations used. Massage must be performed systematically and never

in a casual or irregular manner. The condition of the skin and the general physical condition of the client should always be considered. Normal skin may receive soothing, mildly stimulating, or strongly stimulating massage treatments. Conversely, sensitive or slightly inflamed skin could be further damaged by massage and requires gentle, soothing manipulations with no pressure or friction. For this reason, it is crucial for the barber to perform a thorough client consultation and accurate skin analysis to determine the method and duration of massage manipulations to be used. Massage should always be performed in moderation and based on good judgment.

Massage should never be recommended or employed when the following conditions are present:

- Acute inflammation of the skin
- Severe skin lesions
- Pus-containing pimples
- High blood pressure
- Skin infections

MASSAGE MANIPULATIONS

When massaging any part of the head, face, or neck, any pressure employed should be applied in an upward direction. This rule should be followed in all massage manipulations, whether they are intended to stimulate, relax, or soothe the skin. When applying rotary manipulations, the same rule applies because the pressure should be applied on the upward swing of the movement.

An understanding of the motor points of the face is important in the performance of an effective facial massage. A **motor point** is a point on the skin over a muscle where pressure or stimulation will cause contraction of that muscle. A review of the motor points of the face (**Figure 13-4**) will assist you

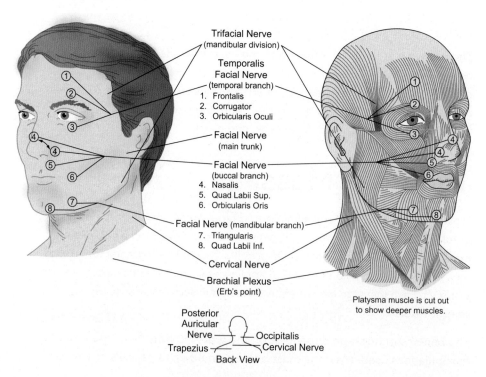

▶ FIGURE 13-4

Motor points of the face.

in learning the position and manipulation of the facial nerves that trigger facial muscles to contract during massage.

Effleurage (EF-loo-rahzh) is a stroking movement. It is a light, continuous movement that should be applied in a slow and rhythmic manner over the skin, with no pressure. The palms are used over large surfaces and the fingertips work the small surfaces, such as those around the eyes. Effleurage is frequently used on the forehead, face, and scalp for its soothing and relaxing effects and to apply lotions or creams.

To correctly position the fingers for the stroking movement, slightly curve the fingers with just the cushions of the fingertips touching the skin **(Figure 13-5)**. Do not use the ends of the fingertips for these massage movements since they are pointier than the cushions and the fingernails may scratch the client's skin.

To correctly position the palms for the stroking movement, keep your hands loose and your wrists and fingers flexible. Curve your fingers and palms to conform to the shape of the area being massaged **(Figure 13-6)**.

Pétrissage (PEH-treh-sahzh) is a kneading movement that is performed with light, firm pressure. In this movement, the skin and flesh are grasped between the thumb and fingers. As the tissues are lifted from their underlying structures they are gently squeezed, rolled, or pinched with a light, firm pressure. Pétrissage exerts an invigorating effect on the area being massaged. These kneading movements provide deeper stimulation to the muscles, nerves, and skin glands and also help to improve circulation.

Although kneading movements are usually used on large surfaces such as the shoulders and back, digital kneading can be used on the cheeks with light pinching movements **(Figure 13-7)**.

Friction is a deep rubbing movement in which pressure is applied on the skin while moving it over an underlying structure. The fingers or palms are employed to perform light circular friction on the face and neck. Friction has been proven beneficial to the circulation and glandular activity of the skin **(Figure 13-8)**.

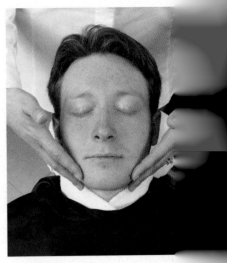

▲ **FIGURE 13-5**
Stroking movement with the fingertips.

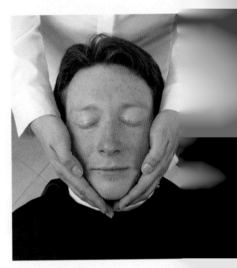

▲ **FIGURE 13-6**
Stroking movements with the palms.

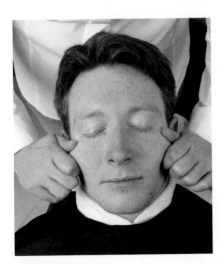

▲ **FIGURE 13-7**
Pétrissage.

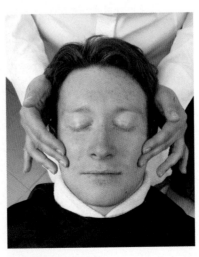

▲ **FIGURE 13-8**
Friction.

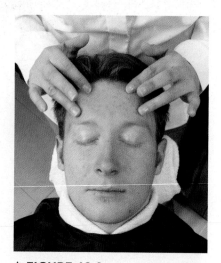

▲ FIGURE 13-9
Percussion.

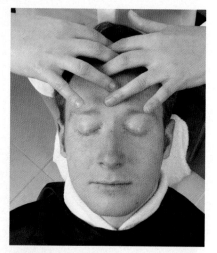

▲ FIGURE 13-10
Vibration.

Percussion or **tapotement** (tah-POHT-mant) consists of short, quick tapping, slapping, or hacking movements. This form of massage is the most stimulating and should be used with care and discretion. Tapping movements are the most gentle of the three and can be used in facial massage. Percussion movements stimulate the nerves to tone the muscles and impart a healthy glow to the part being massaged.

In tapping, the fingertips are brought down against the skin in rapid succession with even force **(Figure 13-9)**. In slapping movements, the palm is used to lightly strike the skin. One hand follows the other and slightly lifts the skin with each slapping stroke. Hacking movements employ the outer edges of the hands, which are struck against the skin in alternate succession, and are usually used on the back and shoulders.

Vibration is a rapid shaking movement that can be performed with the fingertips or an electric massager or vibrator. Both methods are used to transmit a trembling movement to the skin and its underlying structures. To prevent overstimulation, this movement should be used sparingly and should never exceed a few seconds' duration on any one area **(Figure 13-10)**.

PHYSIOLOGICAL EFFECTS OF MASSAGE

Skillfully applied massage influences the structures and functions of the body, either directly or indirectly. The immediate effect of massage is first noticed on the skin. The part being massaged reacts with an increase in its functional activities, such as more active circulation, secretion, nutrition, and excretion. There is scarcely an organ of the body that is not affected favorably by scientific massage treatments. Beneficial results that may be obtained by proper massage include:

- The skin and all its structures are nourished.
- Muscle fiber is stimulated and strengthened.
- Fat cells are reduced.
- Circulation of blood is increased.
- The activity of the skin and scalp glands is stimulated.
- The skin is rendered soft and pliable.
- The nerves are soothed and rested.
- Pain is sometimes relieved.

Facial Massage Manipulations

When performing facial massage manipulations, remember that an even tempo or rhythm induces relaxation. Once the manipulations have begun, one or both of the hands should remain on the skin at all times. When it becomes necessary to remove the hands, avoid abrupt motions and gently feather-off the hands from the skin.

Remember that massage movements are directed from the insertion toward the origin of a muscle to avoid damage to muscular tissues. Refer to Figure 13-4 and apply minimal pressure on the motor points when performing the massage manipulations listed below. Procedure 13-1 shows different massage movements that may be used on various parts of the face and neck. Your instructor may employ a different manipulation procedure that is equally correct. Use the following steps and illustrations to practice these techniques on a fellow student or model.

SUPPLIES

- Towels
- Massage cream
- Spatula
- Heading covering
- Drape

PREPARATION

1. Assemble supplies.

2. Wash your hands.

3. Drape model, recline chair, and cover hair with towel or plastic cap.

PROCEDURE

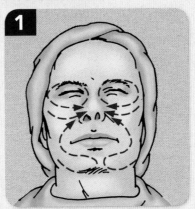

1 Remove massage cream from container with a clean spatula. Disperse the product over your hands and apply cream lightly over the face with stroking, spreading, and circulatory movements.

2 Stroke fingers across forehead with up-and-down movements.

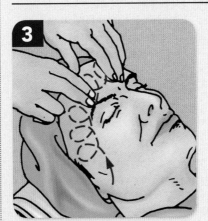

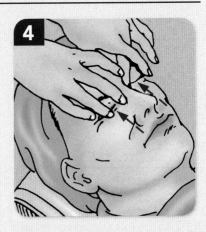

3 Manipulate fingers across the forehead with a circular movement.

4 Stroke fingers upward along the sides of nose.

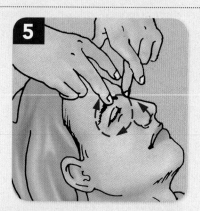

5 Apply a circular movement over the sides of nose and use a light, stroking movement around the eyes.

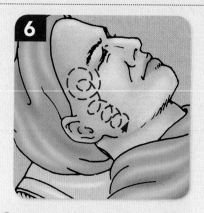

6 Manipulate the temples and then the front and back of the ears with a wide circular movement.

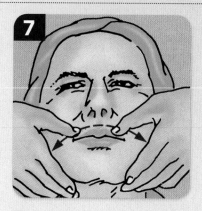

7 Gently stroke both thumbs across the upper lip.

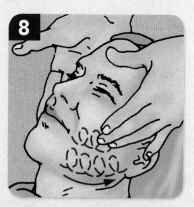

8 Manipulate fingers from the corners of the mouth to the cheeks and temples with a rotary (circular) movement. Manipulate fingers along the lower jaw from the tip of the chin to the ear using the same technique.

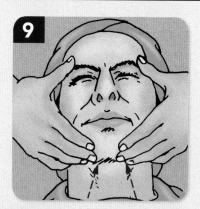

9 Stroke fingers above and below the lower jawbone from the chin to the ear. Manipulate fingers from under the chin and neck to the back of the ears and up to the temples.

10 Remove massage cream with a warm towel and pat dry.

CLEAN-UP AND DISINFECTION

1. Cleanse and disinfect all implements; store products and soiled towels appropriately.

2. Sanitize work area.

3. Wash your hands.

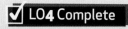

Facial Equipment and Applications

In addition to massage techniques performed with the hands, appliances such as massagers or vibrators, brush machines, electrical modalities, microdermabrasion, and light rays can be used to enhance the facial treatment service.

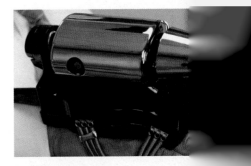

▲ FIGURE 13-11
Handheld massager.

The **electric massager** most often used in barbershops is a handheld unit that transmits vibrations through the barber's hand to the client's skin and muscles **(Figure 13-11)**. This type of massaging technique is used over heavy muscle tissue such as the scalp and shoulders to produce a succession of stimulating impulses. It has an invigorating effect on muscle tissue, increases the blood supply to the parts treated, is soothing to the nerves, increases glandular activity, and stimulates the skin and scalp. When used correctly, electric massagers can also be used to perform vibratory facials (See **Procedure 13-3:** Vibratory Facial).

CAUTION: Some hand massager appliances are heavy and cumbersome for smaller hands. Always "try one on for size" before purchasing.

The *brush machine* helps to stimulate, cleanse, and lightly exfoliate the skin. Many different models are available by a variety of manufacturers. Typically these units have two or three small brush attachments that can be rotated at different speeds **(Figure 13-12)**.

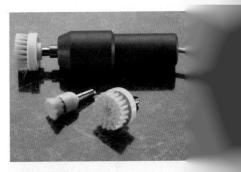

▲ FIGURE 13-12
The brush machine helps cleanse and lightly exfoliate the skin.

mini PROCEDURE

USING THE BRUSH MACHINE

Following proper set-up, draping, and hand sanitation, the procedure for using a rotary brush machine is as follows:

1 Perform a light cleansing on the skin.

2 Insert the appropriate size brush for the face into the handheld device.

3 Apply more cleansing cream to the skin.

CAUTION: Brush machines should never be used with products or drugs that thin or exfoliate the skin.

4 Dip the brush into water and begin the pattern of movement at the forehead.

5 Continue the rotation down the cheeks, nose, upper lip, chin, jaw, and neck areas. No pressure should be applied. Allow the brush to do the work with the bristles remaining straight **(Figure 13-13)**.

(Continued)

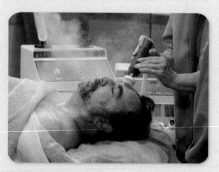

▲ FIGURE 13-13
To properly use the brush machine, a light touch is used, with no pressure on the skin.

6 Remoisten the brush as needed during the process. Dryer skin types require a slow, steady rotation. Thicker, oily skin types can tolerate a faster speed.

CAUTION: The rotary brush is *not* recommended for use on inflamed or acne-prone skin.

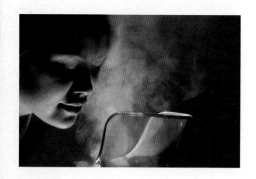

Steam towel or *hot towel cabinets* assure a ready supply of warm towels for facial services. To prepare steam towels, fold the towel lengthwise and then in half. Run hot water over the towel, wring out the excess water, and place the towel in the cabinet. Towels can also be prepared to facilitate a witch hazel steam by soaking dampened towels in a hot water witch hazel bath prior to wringing.

Steamers are electrical devices that produce and project moist, uniform steam that can be positioned over sections of the head or face for softening and cleansing purposes. The steam warms the skin, stimulates circulation, induces the flow of sebum and sweat, and has an antiseptic effect on problematic skin. Steam also helps to oxygenate the skin, which can be beneficial for sinus and congestion conditions.

Professional steamers are available in various sizes and models from tabletop units to facial machine components. Only distilled or filtered water should be used in a steamer because mineral and calcium deposits can damage the unit. Steamers may be used in place of hot towels for scalp and hair reconditioning treatments. When positioned over the scalp, the steam softens the skin, increases perspiration, and promotes the effectiveness of applied scalp tonics and lotions.

As you learned in Chapter 9, light rays are used to impart light therapy treatments to the skin. Infrared, ultraviolet, white, blue, and red rays are used to produce different effects through the use of therapeutic lamps. Review Table 9-3 for the types of light rays used in treatments and their beneficial effects.

Facial treatments performed with electronic facial machines are a form of electrotherapy. As you also learned in Chapter 9, there are several electrical

USING A FACIAL MACHINE STEAMER

Following proper set-up, draping, and hand sanitation, the procedure for using a facial machine steamer is as follows:

1 Pour distilled water into the steamer and allow the unit to preheat prior to the facial.

CAUTION: Do not let the water steam or boil for more than a minute with steamers that have glass components, as evaporation may cause glass breakage.

2 Position the steamer arm to the correct angle and height prior to the facial.

3 Have the client remove his shirt and recline on the facial bed. Drape with sheet or large towel and place a towel under the client's neck and over the shoulders to protect these areas from steam or dripping water.

4 Turn the machine away from the client and flip the switch on. Do not turn on the vaporizer switch until steam is visible.

5 When the water boils and steam is visible, flip on the vaporizer switch and slowly adjust the steam arm to a position about 15 inches from the client's face. The steamers can be moved father away if the steam becomes too hot or uncomfortable for the client.

CAUTION: Placing the steam to close to the skin can cause overheating and irritation.

6 Upon completion of the steam treatment, turn off the vaporizer switch first and then the on/off switch.

currents (modalities) used in electrotherapy: Tesla high-frequency, galvanic, faradic, and sinusoidal currents.

Each modality requires an *electrode* to apply and direct the current to the client's skin. The Tesla high-frequency modality requires only one electrode **(Figure 13-14)**, whereas galvanic, faradic, and sinusoidal modalities require two electrodes, one positive and one negative, to conduct the flow of electricity through the body. A positive electrode (anode) is red with a plus sign (+) and a negative electrode (cathode) is black with a minus sign (–) **(Figure 13-15)**.

The Tesla high-frequency and galvanic currents are the most common modalities used in the industry. Because the use of faradic or sinusoidal current by anyone other than a licensed physician is prohibited in some states, only facial treatments using the high-frequency or galvanic modalities are covered in this chapter.

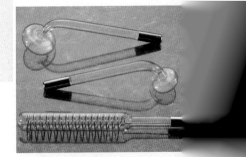

▲ **FIGURE 13-14**
Electrodes for the high-frequency machine.

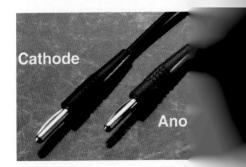

▲ **FIGURE 13-15**
Anode and cathode.

TESLA HIGH-FREQUENCY MACHINE

Tesla high-frequency current is characterized by a high rate of oscillation that is used for both scalp and facial treatments. Although it is sometimes called the violet ray because of its color, there are no ultraviolet rays in high-frequency current.

The primary actions of high-frequency current are thermal and antiseptic. Its rapid vibrations do not produce muscular contractions or chemical changes, so the physiological effects are either stimulating or soothing, depending on the method of application.

The electrodes for high-frequency machines are made of glass or metal. Their shapes vary from the flat facial electrode to the rake-shaped scalp electrode. As the current passes through the glass electrode, tiny violet sparks are emitted. All high-frequency treatments should be started with a mild current that is gradually increased to the required strength. The length of the treatment depends upon the condition to be treated. For general facial or scalp treatments, no more than 5 minutes should be allowed.

The high-frequency machine is a versatile tool that can benefit the client's skin in the following ways:

- Stimulates blood circulation
- Helps to oxygenate the skin
- Increases glandular activity
- Aids in elimination and absorption
- Increases cell metabolism
- Promotes antiseptic and germicidal action
- Generates a warm feeling that has a relaxing effect on the skin

CAUTION: Tesla high-frequency current should not be used on clients who are pregnant, suffer from seizures (epilepsy) or asthma, or who have high blood pressure, acne, a sinus blockage, a pacemaker, or metal implants.

APPLICATION OF HIGH-FREQUENCY CURRENT

Follow the manufacturer's directions for the proper use of Tesla high-frequency current. The two primary methods used in the barbershop are direct surface application and indirect application.

Direct surface application is performed with the mushroom or rake-shaped electrode for its calming and germicidal effect on the skin **(Figure 13-16)**. The heat that is generated has a sedative effect, and oily and acne-prone skin benefits from its germicidal action. The germicidal benefits of high-frequency current are produced only with the direct application method. This method can be used on clean, dry skin, over facial creams, or over gauze for a sparking effect.

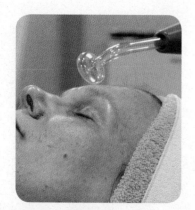

▲ FIGURE 13-16

Direct application method using high frequency.

DIRECT SURFACE APPLICATION

The procedure for direct surface application during a facial treatment is as follows:

1 Place the mushroom-shaped electrode into the handheld device.

2 Adjust the rheostat to the proper setting. If in doubt, start at a low setting and increase as needed.

3 Place an index finger on the glass electrode.

4 Apply the electrode directly onto the client's skin, beginning on the neck.

5 Glide the electrode over the skin in circular, upward movements on the neck toward the jaw, then the cheeks, chin, nose, and forehead areas.

NOTE: If the electrode tends to drag, place gauze between the skin and the electrode.

6 To remove the electrode from the skin, place an index finger over the glass and remove it. Turn the power switch off.

When applying high-frequency current to the face using the facial electrodes, movements are started on the neck and worked upward to the jaw, cheeks, chin, nose, and forehead.

Indirect application is performed with the client holding the wire glass electrode between both hands (**Figure 13-17**). To prevent shock, the power is turned on after the client is holding the electrode firmly and turned off before the electrode is removed from the client's hand. At no time is the electrode held by the barber or stylist. Indirect application of the current produces both a toning and stimulating effect on the skin that is ideal for aging and sallow skin.

Cleaning and Disinfection Procedures

After each use, clean the glass electrode by wiping it with a soap and water solution. Do not immerse the electrode directly in water. Next, place the end only of the electrode into a disinfectant solution for 20 minutes. Rinse with cool water, but do not get the metal parts wet. Dry with a clean towel and store in a covered container.

CAUTION: Do not place electrodes in an ultraviolet-ray cabinet sanitizer or autoclave.

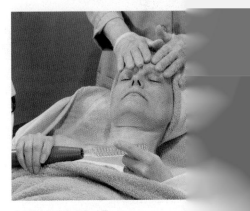

▲ **FIGURE 13-17**
Indirect application method using high frequency.

REMINDER

>>> When using high-frequency current, never use a skin or scalp lotion that contains alcohol prior to the electrical treatment.

mini PROCEDURE

INDIRECT APPLICATION

The procedure for indirect application during a facial treatment is as follows:

1 Apply cream to client's face.

2 Instruct the client to hold the wire glass electrode with both hands.

3 Place the fingers of one hand on the client's forehead.

4 With the opposite hand, turn the high-frequency machine on to a low setting.

5 Using both hands, perform tapping (tapotement) motions in a systematic manner over the client's face.

6 To discontinue the high-frequency service, remove one hand from the skin and turn the power off.

CAUTION: Do not lose contact with the client's skin during this procedure while the current is on.

GALVANIC MACHINE

The galvanic machine converts the oscillating current received from an outlet into a direct current **(Figure 13-18)**. The electrons then flow continuously in the same direction. This produces a relaxation response that can be regulated to target specific nerve endings in the epidermis. Galvanic current is used to produce chemical (desincrustation) and ionic (iontophoresis) reactions in the skin. This treatment is beneficial for oily skin problems and acne.

The galvanic machine has two poles, negative (–) and positive (+). Both are used for different effects. Several types of electrodes are available for the galvanic machine. The most popular are the desincrustator and the ionizing roller. To make proper contact, each electrode must be covered with cotton and the client must hold the opposite-polarity electrode.

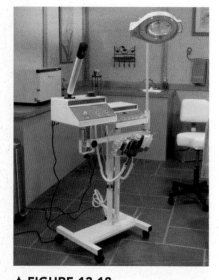

▲ FIGURE 13-18

"Five-in-one" machine, including galvanic electrodes.

Applications of Galvanic Current

Desincrustation is used to facilitate deep pore cleansing. During this process, the galvanic current is used to create a chemical reaction that helps to emulsify or liquefy sebum and waste. To perform desincrustation, an acid-based solution is placed on the skin's surface. When the current passes through certain solutions containing acids and salts, or passes through the tissues and fluids of the body, it produces chemical changes.

Iontophoresis means the introduction of ions. This process uses galvanic current to apply water-soluble solutions into the deeper layers of the skin. The current flows through conductive solutions by means of positive and negative polarities, or ionization. Once the charge of the solution is determined, the machine is set to the appropriate setting **(Table 13-5)**. The client holds

POSITIVE POLE (ANODE)	NEGATIVE POLE (CATHODE)
Cataphoresis	Anaphoresis
Causes an acid reaction	Causes an alkaline reaction
Calms and soothes nerve endings	Stimulates nerve endings
Decreases blood circulation	Increases blood circulation
Tightens the skin	Softens and relaxes tissue

mini PROCEDURE

APPLICATIONS OF GALVANIC CURRENT: DESINCRUSTATION

After preparing the client for the service, the desincrustation procedure is as follows:

1 Gently cleanse the skin prior to treatment.

2 Instruct the client to remove any jewelry from the hand that will be used to hold the electrode. Cover the electrode held by the client with a moistened sponge or piece of dampened cotton. This electrode is connected to the red wire (positive).

3 Prepare the desincrustator electrode (negative) by placing a dampened sponge or cotton pad into the black ring, then slide the ring back onto the electrode.

4 Dip the electrode into the desincrustation solution and apply the electrode to the client's forehead. Turn the switch to negative and set it at 0.05 micro-amperes. Gradually turn the rheostat clockwise to increase the intensity of the current. At this point the client will usually experience a metallic taste in the mouth and a slight prickling sensation, which indicate that the current is strong enough. Be sure to explain to the client the sensations he will experience and do *not* increase the current once these sensations are felt. The alkaline desincrustation solution will be attracted to the positive pole in the client's hand.

5 Gently glide and rotate the electrode over the facial areas that are oily. Before moving the electrode to another section of the face, the current is reduced back to zero and the process is repeated. The time spent doing the desincrustation part of the facial treatment will depend on the condition of the skin. Anywhere from 3 to 10 minutes may be required for normal to oily and acne-prone skin.

6 Upon completion, turn the machine off and remove the electrode. Use cotton pads or sponges to rinse the skin with warm water. Proceed with extraction of blackheads and pustules.

an electrode with the opposite charge **(Figure 13-19)**. Moistened sponges or cotton pads are also used in this process.

Phoresis is the process of forcing chemical solutions into unbroken skin by way of a galvanic current. The process of ionic penetration takes place in two forms: cataphoresis and anaphoresis.

Cataphoresis is the use of the positive pole (anode) to introduce an acid-pH product, such as an **astringent** solution, into the skin. Products that have a slightly acid pH are considered positive. The positive pole may also be used to close the follicles or pores after the treatment; decrease redness, as in mild acne; prevent inflammation after comedone and blemish treatment (by decreasing blood supply); soothe nerves; and harden tissues.

Anaphoresis is the use of the negative pole (cathode) to force an alkaline-pH product, such as desincrustation lotion, into the skin. Products with an alkaline pH are considered to be negative. The negative pole may be used to stimulate the circulation of blood to dry skin, stimulate nerves, and soften tissues. The procedure for ionization is the same as that used in the desincrustation process.

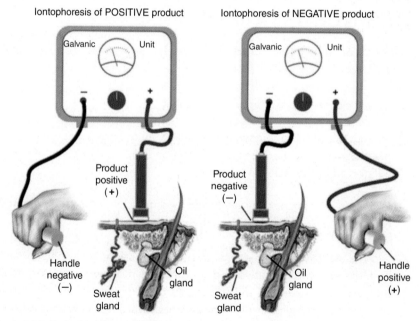

▲ **FIGURE 13-19**

Iontophoresis of positive and negative products.

Cleaning and Disinfection Procedures

Always follow the manufacturer's directions for cleaning and disinfecting facial machine components.

FACIAL MACHINES

Microdermabrasion

It is a relatively new form of mechanical exfoliation that entered the U.S. market around 1995. The microdermabrasion machine is an electronic vacuum that is used to spray micro-crystals across the skin's surface through a closed stainless steel or glass pressurized wand. If can be used to diminish sun damage, pigmentation, comedones, wrinkles, and coarse-textured skin. Although the machine and service are not standard features of most barbershops, they may be found in some high-end men's spas or grooming parlors.

CAUTION: Always check with your state regulatory agency about microdermabrasion rules in your state.

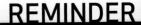

REMINDER

Always check with your state regulatory agency about microdermabrasion rules in your state.

Ultraviolet-Ray Lamps

Ultraviolet rays may be used to treat acne, tinea, seborrhea, and dandruff. Their germicidal effect helps to promote healing and may stimulate hair growth. Ultraviolet-ray lamps deliver these shortest light rays of the spectrum. The benefits of these shorter rays are obtained when the lamp is placed 30" to 36" from the skin.

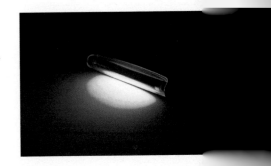

Average exposure to ultraviolet rays may produce redness of the skin, and overdoses may cause blistering. It is better to start with a 2 or 3 minute exposure and gradually increase the time to 7 or 8 minutes.

The barber must wear tinted safety goggles and the client opaque eye protectors to protect their eyes from the rays.

Infrared-Ray Lamps

Infrared rays generally produce a soothing and beneficial type of heat that extends for some distance into the tissues of the body. The effects of infrared rays on the exposed skin area include:

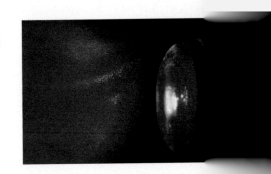

- Heating and relaxation of the skin without increasing the temperature of the body as a whole
- Dilation of blood vessels in the skin and increased blood flow
- Increased metabolism and chemical changes within skin tissues
- Increased production of perspiration and oil on the skin
- Relief of pain

The infrared-ray lamp is operated at an average distance of 30". It is placed closer at the start of the treatment and is then moved back gradually as the surface heat becomes more pronounced, in order to avoid burning the skin. Always protect the eyes of the client during exposure. Place pads saturated with dilute boric acid or witch hazel solution over the client's eyelids. See **Table 13-6** for a description of the effects of the different forms of light therapy.

TABLE **13-6** Effects of Light Therapy

TYPE OF LIGHT	BENEFICIAL EFFECTS
Ultraviolet	Increases the elimination of waste products Improves the flow of blood and lymph Has a germicidal and antibacterial effect Produces vitamin D in the skin Can be used to treat rickets, psoriasis, and acne Produces a tan
Infrared	Heats and relaxes the skin Dilates blood vessels and increases circulation Produces chemical changes Increases metabolism Increases production of perspiration and oil Deep penetration relieves pain in sore muscles Soothes nerves
White Light	Relieves pain in the back of the neck and shoulders Produces some chemical and germicidal effects Relaxes muscles
Blue Light	Soothes nerves Improves skin tone Provides some chemical and germicidal effects Used for mild cases of skin eruptions Produces little heat
Red Light	Improves dry, scaly wrinkled skin Relaxes muscles Penetrates the deepest Produces the most heat

SAFETY PRECAUTIONS FOR USING ELECTRICAL EQUIPMENT

- Disconnect any appliances when they are not being used.
- Study instructions before using any electrical equipment.
- Keep all wires, plugs, and equipment in a safe condition.
- Inspect all electrical equipment frequently.
- Avoid getting electric cords wet.
- Sanitize all electrodes properly.
- Protect the client at all times.
- Do not touch any metal while using electrical appliances.

- Do not handle electrical equipment with wet hands.

- Do not allow the client to touch metal surfaces when electrical treatments are being performed.

- Do not leave the room when the client is attached to any electrical device.

- Do not attempt to clean around an electric outlet when equipment is plugged in.

- Do not touch two metallic objects at the same time while connected to an electric current.

- Do not use any electrical equipment without first obtaining full instruction in its care and use.

The protection and safety of the client are the primary concern of the barber. All electrical equipment should be inspected regularly to determine whether it is in good working condition. Carelessness may result in shocks or burns. Barbers who practice safety precautions help to eliminate accidents, assuring greater comfort and satisfaction for their clients.

With a basic knowledge of the anatomical structure of the head, face, and neck and the primary subdermal systems, and the ability to perform massage manipulations manually or with electrical devices, you are now ready to engage in the analysis and performance of skin care.

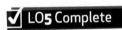
✓ LO5 Complete

Facial Treatments

The barber does not treat skin diseases but should be able to recognize various skin disorders so as to differentiate between those that can be serviced in the barbershop and those that should be referred to a physician. Facials performed in the barbershop are considered to be either preservative or corrective treatments.

Preservative treatments are intended to help maintain the health of facial skin. The performance of correct cleansing, massage, and electrical treatments can increase circulation, relax the nerves, activate skin glands, and increase cell metabolism.

Corrective treatments are used to correct skin conditions such as dryness, oiliness, blackheads, aging lines, and minor acne. In general, facial treatments are beneficial because they:

- cleanse the skin.
- increase circulation.
- activate glandular activity.
- relax tense nerves.
- maintain muscle tone.

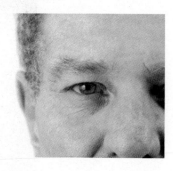

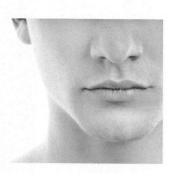

- strengthen weak muscle tissue.
- correct certain skin disorders.
- help prevent the formation of wrinkles and aging lines.
- improve skin texture and complexion.
- help to reduce fatty tissues.

To perform the full range of facial treatments presented in this text, the barber will require access to hot and cold water, soft terry cloth towels, therapeutic lamps, and a variety of preparations designed for facial treatments. These preparations include such items as facial creams, tonics, exfoliants, lotions, oils, packs, and masks.

SKIN TYPES

There are four basic skin types that the barber will need to recognize before the appropriate products can be chosen for a facial treatment. Skin type is primarily based on the amount of oil that is produced in the follicles from the sebaceous glands and the amount of lipids found between the cells. Skin types include dry, normal, combination, and oily. Any of these skin types can be sensitive to products, irritation, or the environment.

Dry skin does not produce enough oil, which is needed to protect the skin from environmental damage and aging. Dry skin needs extra care because it does not have this protection. The objective of a facial treatment for dry skin is stimulation of oil production and protection of the skin surface. In some cases, dry skin is also *dehydrated* skin that lacks water. In addition to drinking plenty of water, hydrating the skin with moisturizers and humectants can help minimize the negative effects of dryness and dehydration.

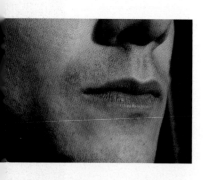

Normal skin has a good water/oil balance. The follicles are a normal size and the skin is free of blemishes. Maintenance and preservative care is the goal for this type of skin.

Combination skin can be both oily and dry in different areas of the face. The T-zone is the section of the face that incorporates the forehead, nose, and chin area. These areas tend to have more sebaceous glands and larger pores. The cheek and outer areas of the face tend to be dry. Water-based products work best for combination skin types.

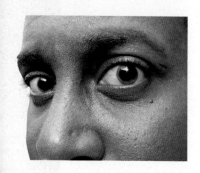

Oily skin is characterized by excess sebum (oil) production. The follicle size is larger and contains more oil. Oily skin requires more cleansing and exfoliation than other skin types, yet over-cleansing can strip and irritate the skin. If the skin is over-dried, it is not balanced and the body will try to produce additional oil to compensate for the dryness on the surface. Proper exfoliation and a water-based hydrator will help keep oily skin clean and balanced.

Wrinkles are depressions in the skin that have developed from repetitious muscle action moving in the same direction. Other factors that influence the formation of wrinkles include:

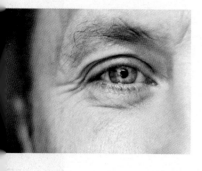

- Loosening of the elastic skin fibers due to abnormal tension or relaxation of the facial muscles

- Shrinking of the skin tissue as a result of aging
- Excessive dryness of the skin
- Improper facial care

SKIN ANALYSIS

A knowledge of skin types and conditions is necessary to performing an accurate skin analysis. It is preferable to analyze the skin with a magnifying lamp or light (Figure 13-20), but if one is not available, a close inspection of the skin will suffice. When analyzing the skin, it is important to note the client's skin type and condition and the skin's visible appearance and texture. Be sure to record this information on a client record card for future use (Figures 13-21 and 13-22). Follow these four guidelines when performing a skin analysis:

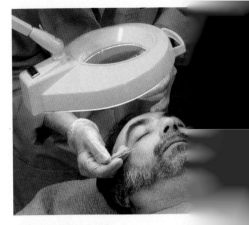

▲ **FIGURE 13-20**
Using a magnifying light to analyze the skin.

1. Observe the client's skin type, condition, and appearance; feel the texture.

2. Ask the client questions relating to the skin's appearance and home care routine.

3. Discuss the facial procedure and/or treatment plans as well as the products that will be used and why.

4. Encourage the client to ask questions and then determine a course of action together.

CONSULTATION CARD				
Name _____			Date of Consultation	
Address _____			D.O.B.	
City _____ State ____ Zip ____			Occupation	
Tel. (Home) _____ (Business) _____			Ref. by	
			Contraindications	
Medical History				
Current Medication				
Previous treatments				
Home Care Products used				
SKIN TYPE	Oily	Normal	Dry	Combination
SKIN CONDITION	Clogged pores	Sensitive	Dehydrated	Mature
Skin Abnormalities				
Remarks				

▲ **FIGURE 13-21**
Client consultation card (front).

FACIAL RECORD			
Date	Type of treatment	By	Products purchased
2/14	Cleansing, Peel - Relaxing Massage		Moisturizer with sunscreen
3/16	Cleansing, Peel Modelage Mask		Cleanser, Tonic Lotion
4/5	Cleansing, Peel High Frequency indirect		Moisturizer
4/26	Cleansing, Peel Massage	John	Dry skin cream
5/13	Cleansing, Peel Iontophoresis		
	Skin is showing marked improvement.		
6/1	Cleansing, Peel Relaxing Massage	Mary	

▲ **FIGURE 13-22**

Client consultation card (back).

SKIN CARE PRODUCTS

The type of facial treatment will determine the products needed to complete the procedure. Three essential skin care preparations, however, should be used before or after a shave service and during full facial treatments. These essential preparations are cleansers, toners, and moisturizers. Additional products such as exfoliating scrubs, masks, and treatment creams are used in conjunction with the essential preparations during the full facial treatment.

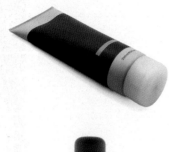

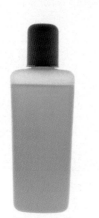

- *Cleansers* should be mild and easy to rinse from the skin. They are available as face washes, lotions, and creams for all types of skin and skin conditions. Face washes are usually water-based products with a neutral or slightly acidic pH effective on oily and combination skin types. Cleansing lotions are water-based emulsions for normal and combination skin that contain emollients or oils to soften the skin. Cleansing creams are oil-based emulsions that are used primarily to dissolve dirt and makeup. Because cleansing creams are heavier than cleansing lotions, performers use these products to remove heavy stage makeup.

- **Tonics,** which include *fresheners*, *toners*, and *astringents*, are used after cleansing and prior to the application of a moisturizer. These tonic lotions vary in strength and alcohol content and therefore vary in pH.

  Fresheners usually have the lowest alcohol content (0 to 4 percent) and are beneficial for dry, mature, and sensitive skin. *Toners* are designed to tone or tighten the skin and may be used on normal and combination skin types. The alcohol content range of toners is usually 4 to 15 percent. *Astringents* may contain up to 35 percent alcohol and are used for oily and acne-prone skin. Toners, fresheners, and astringents all help to remove cleanser residue and have a temporary tightening effect on the skin. Some restore the skin's natural pH after cleansing and others can help certain skin conditions.

- *Moisturizers* are the third essential product needed to perform a facial. Moisturizers are formulated to add moisture to the skin and are available for various skin types. They are also available in water-based and oil-based formulations.

NOTE: The use of cleansers, toners, and moisturizers following the shave service is discussed in Chapter 14.

There are other types of products for specific applications:

- *Exfoliating scrubs* are used to physically rub or remove dead cells from the skin surface. Granular scrubs for normal to dry skin may be used two times per week. Scrubs are available in cream, lotion, and gel forms for a variety of skin types. *Chemical exfoliants* consist of enzymes that digest dead skin cells at the skin surface or alphahydroxy acid that penetrates into the skin to dissolve intercellular adhesives. Alphahydroxy acid peels are much stronger than enzyme peels and require advanced training and certification to perform.

- *Masks* and *packs* draw impurities out of pores, tighten, tone, hydrate, soothe, and nourish the skin, depending on the ingredients. They are available in cream, gel, or clay forms and should be used according to skin type.

  Face packs and masks differ in their composition and usage. A mask is usually a setting product, which means that it dries after application, providing complete closure to the environment on top of the skin. Masks are most often applied directly to the skin and are known for their tightening and sebum-absorbing effects. Packs, also referred to as cream or gel masks, are usually applied to the skin over layers of gauze to hold the product in place over the skin. They are beneficial for sensitive skin and have excellent hydrating properties. Applied with a mask brush, they are allowed to set for about 10 minutes.

  High-quality packs and masks should feel comfortable while producing slight tingling and tightening sensations. Always follow the manufacturer's directions for preparation, application, and removal of the product from the skin.

  ▶ *Clay masks* are clay preparations used to stimulate circulation and temporarily contract the skin pores. They absorb sebum and are used on oily and combination skin types. Applied with a mask brush, they are allowed to set until dry, usually about 10 minutes **(Figure 13-23)**.

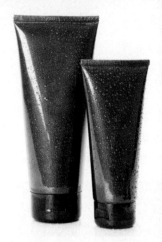

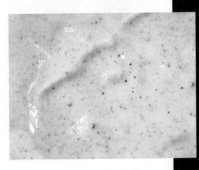

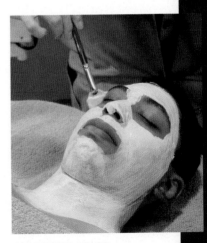

▲ FIGURE 13-23
Mask application.

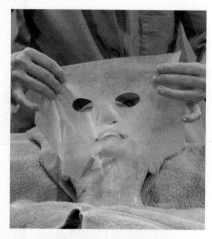

▲ FIGURE 13-24

Placing gauze on the client's face.

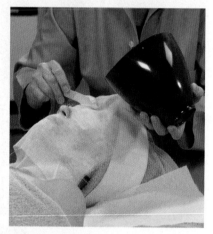

▲ FIGURE 13-25

Applying a mask over the gauze.

▶ *Paraffin wax masks* actually employ the pack application method. Specially prepared paraffin is melted at slightly more than body temperature before application. The client's skin is prepared by cleansing, followed by the application of a treatment cream. Eye pads are used and the paraffin is applied over gauze to prevent the facial hair from sticking to the wax **(Figures 13-24** and **13-25)**.

There are various facial masks and packs available for use in the barbershop. Hot-oil, milk and honey, egg white, and witch hazel packs have been around for many years. For proper use, the barber should always read the manufacturer's claims and directions. Judge the merits of the mask or pack before recommending it to a client.

• *Massage creams* are creams, lotions, or oils that provide slip during a massage while also nourishing and treating skin conditions.

• **Rolling cream** is a thick, smooth, non-granular exfoliating cream, usually pink, that has been used in barbershops for decades. It is applied in a thin layer over the skin, after which it is rolled off with a firm, stroking motion. As the rolling takes place, loose flaky skin and trapped impurities are lifted from the skin surface. The skin is left soft and smooth with increased circulation to the surface.

A general outline of the order in which skin care products will be used during facial treatments in this text is as follows:

1. Cleansing cream or lotion

2. Exfoliant (scrub or rolling cream)

3. Massage cream

4. Cleansing cream or lotion

5. Freshener (low alcohol content)

6. Mask or pack

7. Toner or astringent

8. Moisturizer

NOTE: Your instructor's recommended order of product application is equally correct.

Men's Skin Care Products

Several decades ago, men's personal care products consisted of basic items such as cologne, hair tonics or creams, deodorants, shaving creams, and aftershave lotions. The high-end versions of these basic items were often created as spin-off products from clothing designers. Even men's hair sprays were almost nonexistent before the 1960s. Today, however, products that have been developed specifically with males in mind are abundant on retail shelves and in shops and salons. The male consumer is finally getting the attention he deserves, and each year more men are experiencing the benefits of using skin care products on a regular basis.

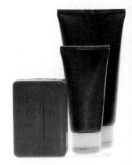

When choosing men's skin care products for use in the barbershop, it is important to think about the specific characteristics of a product that might appeal to men. For example, some men do not like highly fragranced or multi-step products. Creams should be simple, non-fragranced, and absorbent, with a matte finish rather than greasy or oily. Men also seem to prefer simpler routines and multi-purpose products. For example, a toner that serves as an aftershave may be chosen over the purchase and use of two separate products.

Although the quality of the product must be the barber's and the client's first consideration in product choices, packaging characteristics also need to be taken into consideration. Typically, tube packaging is preferred over jars, and size can also be a factor for the client who travels in his profession. One option is to stock barbershop retail shelves with larger containers for the client's home use and smaller, more convenient sizes for travel. As a general rule, use the products you retail for services performed within the shop. NOTE: Smaller packaged goods can also be used for promotions and marketing strategies in the barbershop (see Chapter 21).

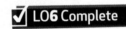

THE BASIC FACIAL

The basic facial, sometimes known as the *scientific rest facial*, is beneficial for its cleansing and stimulating action on the skin. It also exercises and relaxes the facial muscles. The procedural steps listed in **Procedure 13-2** represent one routine that is used to perform a basic facial at the barber's chair. It may be changed to conform to your instructor's method, different equipment, or new procedures in the industry.

VIBRATORY FACIAL

When using an electric massager on the face, avoid heavy contact with the client's skin. Delicate areas around the nose and upper cheek require a special technique using both of the barber's hands. The right-handed barber will attach the massager to his or her right hand. The left hand is placed on the client's skin. Next, the barber places his or her right hand on top of the left and the vibrations travel through this hand to the client's skin. Direct contact with the barber's right hand can be made to less delicate areas such as the forehead and jaw line, but pressure still needs to be avoided. **See Procedure 13-3.**

CAUTION

The vibrator should never be used when there is a known weakness of the heart or in cases of fever, abscesses, or skin inflammations.

Basic Facial Procedure

SUPPLIES AND EQUIPMENT

- Barber chair with headrest
- Steam towel cabinet
- Sink
- Container for soiled towels
- Container for paper and cotton products
- Terry cloth towels
- Headrest covering (paper or cloth towels)
- Nylon or vinyl drape
- Cotton pads or pledgets
- Spatulas
- Head covering
- Cleansing cream
- Exfoliating scrub
- Massage cream
- Tonics (toners, fresheners, astringents)
- Mask or pack
- Moisturizer
- Talc

PREPARATION

1. Arrange all necessary supplies in a convenient location.
2. Wash your hands.

PROCEDURE

1 Drape client and engage in consultation.

2 Perform skin analysis and make product selection.

3 Place a towel or paper barrier between the client's head and the headrest. Adjust the headrest and recline the hydraulic chair. Make sure the client is comfortable.

4 Protect the client's hair with a towel or cap.

NOTE: All products should be removed from their containers with a sanitized spatula to prevent contamination of the product. Do not dip your fingers into the containers!

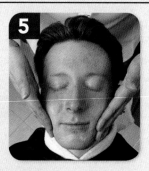

5 Apply cleansing cream over the face, using stroking and rotary movements.

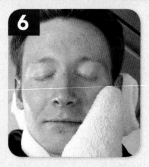

6 Remove the cleansing cream with a warm, damp towel.

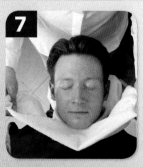

7 Apply two or three steam towels to open pores and loosen imbedded dirt and oils.

8 Reapply cleansing cream to the skin with the fingertips.

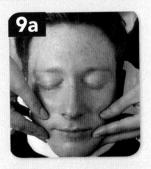

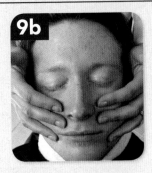

9 Gently massage the face with the hands or a brush machine, using continuous and rhythmic movements.

10 Wipe off excess cleansing cream with a warm towel.

11 Apply an exfoliating product and lightly massage over the skin.

12 Apply steam towel. Wipe off excess product until the skin is free of exfoliating residue.

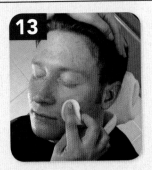

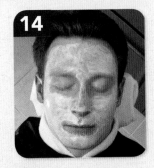

13 Gently wipe the selected tonic over the face and pat dry.

14 Apply mask or pack and allow to dry.

15 Apply tepid to warm towel to moisten mask or pack. Wipe off product until free of residue.

16 Again, gently wipe toner or astringent over the face and pat dry.

17 Apply a light coat of moisturizer using the effleurage movement.

18 Apply a light dusting of talc if the client desires it. Remove any excess.

19 Slowly raise the hydraulic chair and assist the client to a sitting position.

CLEAN-UP AND DISINFECTION

1. Discard all disposable supplies and materials.

2. Wipe containers and close tightly. Store in appropriate place.

3. Sanitize all non-disposable implements and tools.

4. Wash your hands.

POINTS TO REMEMBER

- Strive to have the client relax.
- Provide a quiet atmosphere.
- Organize and maintain supplies in a clean, orderly fashion.
- Follow a systematic procedure.
- Perform the facial massage properly.

CONDITIONS TO AVOID

- Harming or scratching the skin
- Excessive or rough massage
- Product in the client's eyes
- Towels that are too hot
- Breathing into the client's face
- Not being careful or sanitary
- Disinterest in the client's skin problems or conversation
- Leaving excess product on the skin
- Excessive talking that does not facilitate client relaxation
- Leaving the chair to obtain materials or supplies
- Heavy, rough, or cold hands

MASSAGE MOVEMENTS WITH AN ELECTRIC MASSAGER

The following steps outline massage movements to use with an electric massager:

1 Adjust the massager on the right hand and place the fingertips of the left hand on the client's left nostril. Place the vibrating right-hand fingers over the left-hand fingers to vibrate through the left hand.

2 Vibrate the skin with a few light up-and-down movements on the left side of the nose.

3 Gently slide the fingers along the upper cheek area and direct them toward the center of the forehead.

4 Place the vibrating right hand onto the skin and perform rotary movements toward the left temple. Pause for a moment.

5 Continue the rotary movements down along the jaw line toward the tip of the chin.

6 Vibrate from the chin back toward the cheek, using wider, firmer movements.

7 Continue with a slow, light stroke at the temple, around the left ear, over the jawbone, toward the center of the neck, and then below the chin.

8 Vibrate rotary movements over the neck, behind the ear, up to the temple, and then toward the center of the forehead.

9 Repeat steps 2 through 8 on the right side of the face.

10 Repeat steps 2 through 8 on both sides of the face again and proceed with step 5 of the vibratory facial procedure that follows.

Vibratory Facial

The procedure for a vibratory facial is similar to the basic facial with minor variations. Materials, implements, equipment, and preparation remain the same except for the addition of an electric massager. Again we emphasize that the following procedure may be changed to conform to your instructor's routine.

SUPPLIES

- Barber chair with headrest
- Steam towel cabinet
- Electric massager
- Sink
- Container for soiled towels
- Container for paper and cotton products
- Terry cloth towels
- Headrest covering (paper or cloth towels)
- Nylon or vinyl drape
- Cotton pads or pledgets
- Spatulas
- Head covering
- Cleansing cream
- Exfoliating scrub
- Massage cream
- Tonics (toners, fresheners, astringents)
- Mask or pack
- Moisturizer
- Talc

PREPARATION

1. Arrange all necessary supplies in a convenient location.

2. Wash your hands.

PROCEDURE

1 Drape the client and engage in consultation.

2 Perform skin analysis and make product selection.

3 Place a towel or paper barrier between the client's head and the headrest. Adjust the headrest and recline the hydraulic chair. Make sure the client is comfortable.

4 Protect the client's hair with a towel or cap.

5 Apply cleansing cream using stroking and rotary movements.

6 Remove the cleansing cream with a warm, damp towel.

7 Apply two or three steam towels to open pores and loosen imbedded dirt and oils.

8 Apply massage cream to the skin with the fingertips.

9 Administer the massage using the electric massager as described in the preceding section.

10 Wipe off excess massage cream with a warm towel.

11 Apply an exfoliating product and lightly massage over the skin.

12 Apply steam towel. Wipe off excess product until the skin is free of exfoliating residue.

13 Gently wipe the selected tonic over the face and pat dry.

14 Apply mask or pack and allow it to dry.

15 Apply tepid to warm towel to moisten mask or pack. Wipe off product until free of residue.

16 Again, gently wipe toner or astringent over the face and pat dry.

17 Apply a light coat of moisturizer using the effleurage movement.

18 Apply a light dusting of talc if the client desires it. Remove any excess.

19 Slowly raise the hydraulic chair and assist client to a sitting position.

CLEAN-UP AND DISINFECTION

1. Discard all disposable supplies and materials.

2. Wipe containers and close tightly. Store in appropriate place.

3. Sanitize all non-disposable implements and tools.

4. Wash your hands.

RULES FOR USING AN ELECTRIC MASSAGER

- Regulate the number of vibrations to avoid over-stimulation.

- Do not use the vibrator for too long in any one spot.

- Vary the amount of pressure in accordance with the results desired.

- Do not use a vibrator over the upper lip, as the vibrations may cause discomfort.

- For soothing and relaxing effects, give very slow, light vibrations for a very short time.

- For stimulating effects, give light vibrations of moderate speed and duration.

- To reduce fatty tissues, give moderately-timed, fast vibrations with firm pressure.

ROLLING CREAM FACIAL

The facial treatment once most often identified with the barbershop is the **rolling cream** facial. This is another facial treatment that is designed to cleanse and stimulate the skin. Due to the drying qualities of the rolling cream and the application process, this type of facial should be recommended only to clients with normal, oily, or thick skin. It should not be performed on skin that is dry, acne-prone, sensitive, or thin in texture. The rolling cream takes the place of the exfoliating product in the basic facial procedure, but has a different textural consistency that can be challenging to work with the first time around. Some tips for using rolling cream after the first cleansing and steaming processes of a basic facial follow.

mini PROCEDURE

PROCEDURE USING ROLLING CREAM

1 Apply dabs of rolling cream to the chin, cheeks, and forehead.

2 Dampen the fingertips of both hands with water and spread the cream evenly over the face and neck with smooth, stroking movements.

3 Massage the face and neck with uniform rotary, stroking, and rubbing movements with the cushion tips of the fingers in an upward direction until most of the cream has dried and rolled off.

4 Apply a small amount of cleansing cream to the face and neck, using lighter manipulations to remove residue.

5 Remove the cleansing cream with a warm towel.

6 Apply a witch hazel steam to the face and neck with one or more hot towels, following with one or two cool towels to close the pores (optional); or

7 Apply selected tonic. Dry and powder the face and neck.

8 Finish as for a basic facial.

FACIAL FOR DRY SKIN

Dry skin is caused by an insufficient flow of sebum from the sebaceous glands. The objective of a facial for dry skin is to help moisturize it. Dry-skin facials can be performed using infrared rays, galvanic current, or high-frequency current.

PROCEDURE WITH INFRARED RAYS

1 Prepare the client as for a basic facial.

2 Apply cleansing cream; remove cream with a warm, moist towel.

3 Sponge the face with a mild tonic for dry skin.

4 Apply massage cream to the face.

5 Apply lubricating oil or eye cream over and under the eyes.

6 Apply lubricating oil over the neck.

7 Cover the client's eyes with cotton pads moistened with witch hazel or a nonalcoholic freshener.

8 Expose the face and neck to infrared rays for not more than 5 minutes.

9 Perform massage manipulations three to five times.

10 Remove the massage cream and oil with pledgets or a warm, moist towel.

11 Apply tonic lotion suitable for dry skin. Blot the face dry with pledgets or a towel.

12 Apply moisturizer.

13 Complete and clean up as for a basic facial.

CAUTION

Do not permit infrared rays to remain on the body tissues for more than a few seconds at a time. Move your hand back and forth across the rays' path to break constant exposure on the client's skin. The total exposure time should not exceed 5 minutes.

PROCEDURE WITH GALVANIC CURRENT

The procedure for giving a dry-skin facial with galvanic current is similar to the procedure for giving a dry-skin facial with infrared rays, with a few changes:

1 Prepare the client as for a basic facial.

2 Apply cleansing cream; remove cream with a warm, moist towel.

3 Sponge the face with a mild tonic lotion for dry skin.

4 Apply a thick layer of ionized, oil-free gel to the face and neck.

5 Apply negative galvanic current for 5 to 7 minutes to open the pores.

6 Reapply gel to the face and neck.

(Continued)

7 Apply positive galvanic current for 4 to 6 minutes to close the pores.

8 Apply massage cream to the face.

9 Apply lubricating oil or eye cream around the eyes.

10 Apply lubricating oil over the neck.

11 Perform massage manipulations three to five times.

12 Remove the massage cream and oil with tissues or with a warm, moist towel.

13 Apply tonic lotion suitable for dry skin. Blot the face dry with pledgets or a towel.

14 Apply moisturizer.

15 Complete and clean up as for a basic facial.

PROCEDURE WITH INDIRECT HIGH-FREQUENCY CURRENT

1 Prepare the client as for a basic facial.

2 Apply cleansing cream; remove cream with a warm, moist towel.

3 Sponge the face with a mild tonic for dry skin.

4 Apply massage cream to the face.

5 Apply lubricating oil or eye cream over and under the eyes.

6 Apply lubricating oil over the neck.

7 Have client hold electrode in his right hand.

8 Perform manipulations, using the indirect method of applying high-frequency current, for 7 to 10 minutes. Do not use tapping movements and do not lift hands from the client's skin.

9 Apply two or three cool towels to the face and neck.

10 Remove the oil with tissues or a warm, moist towel.

11 Apply tonic lotion suitable for dry skin. Blot the face dry with pledgets or a towel.

12 Apply moisturizer.

13 Complete and clean up as for a basic facial.

FACIAL FOR OILY SKIN AND BLACKHEADS

Oily skin and/or blackheads (comedones) are caused by hardened masses of sebum formed inside a follicle. The sebaceous material in the follicle darkens when exposed to oxygen, thus forming a blackhead.

1 Prepare the client as for a basic facial.

2 Apply cleansing lotion and remove it with a warm, moist towel or facial sponges.

3 Place moistened eye pads on the client's eyes, then analyze the skin under a magnifying lamp.

4 Steam the face with three or four moist, warm towels or a facial steamer to open the pores.

5 Wear gloves and cover your fingertips with cotton and gently press out blackheads. Do not press so hard as to bruise the skin tissue.

6 Sponge the face with the appropriate astringent or toner.

7 Optional: Cover the client's eyes with pads moistened with a mild astringent. Apply ultraviolet light over the skin for 3 to 5 minutes.

8 Apply massage cream suitable for the skin condition and perform massage manipulations.

9 Remove cream with a warm, moist towel, cotton pads, or facial sponges.

10 Moisten a cotton pledget with an astringent lotion. Apply it to the face and neck with upward and outward movements to constrict the pores. Blot the excess moisture with tissues. For male clients with beards, use downward and outward movements in the same direction as the hair growth.

11 Apply moisturizer or protective lotion according to skin type.

12 Complete and clean up as for basic facial procedure.

CAUTION

Overexposure to ultraviolet rays can destroy skin tissue. Start with a 2 or 3 minute exposure time and gradually increase to 7 or 8 minutes.

FACIAL FOR ACNE

Acne is a disorder of the sebaceous glands and serious cases require medical direction. If the client is under medical care, the role of the barber is to perform facial treatments as prescribed by the client's physician and as indicated on the prescription. If in doubt, contact the physician directly. With a prescribed treatment plan, treatment of acne conditions by barbers should be limited to the following procedures:

1 Reduction of oily skin by local and topical applications

2 Removal of blackheads using proper procedures

3 Cleansing of the skin

4 Application of medicated and/or prescribed preparations

PROCEDURE

Because acne contains infectious matter, it is advisable to use vinyl or latex gloves and disposable materials, such as cotton cleansing pads.

1 Prepare the client as for a basic facial.

2 Cleanse the client's face as in a basic facial.

3 Place cotton eye pads over the client's eyes, then analyze the skin under the magnifying lamp.

4 Apply warm, moist towels to the face to open the pores for deep cleansing.

5 Extract comedones as in a facial for oily skin.

6 Cleanse the face with a cotton pad or sponge that has been sprinkled with astringent.

CAUTION: If high-frequency current is used in step 7, use a nonalcoholic toner in place of the astringent.

7 Optional: Apply high-frequency current with direct application over the affected area for up to 5 minutes, or cover the client's eyes with goggles and apply ultraviolet light over the skin for 3 to 5 minutes for its germicidal effects. Be guided by your instructor.

8 Apply prescribed acne treatment cream if available. Optional per physician's directions: Leave the eye pads in place and apply infrared lamp for 5 to 7 minutes to promote penetration of the treatment cream.

9 Leave the eye pads in place and apply a treatment mask that is suitable for the skin condition for 8 to 10 minutes.

10 Remove the mask with moist towels or sponges.

11 Apply astringent to the face with a wet cotton pad or sponge.

12 Apply protective fluid or special acne lotion.

13 Complete cleanup and sanitation procedures as for basic facial procedures.

> **REMINDER**
>
> >>> Make sure to ask the cl if they are sensitive to latex before using latex products.

HOT-OIL MASK

The hot-oil mask can be used for extremely dry, parched, and scaly skin that is prevalent during dry, hot, or windy weather. Although there are many commercially prepared products on the market, some older clients may request this service to soften, smooth, and stimulate skin tissues.

FORMULA FOR A HOT-OIL MASK

- 2 tablespoons of olive oil

- 1 tablespoon of castor oil (refined grade)

- $\frac{1}{4}$ teaspoon of glycerin

Mix the oils in a small container and warm.

PROCEDURE

1 Prepare the client as for a basic facial.

2 Prepare the mask. Saturate cotton pads (4" x 4") or an 18" square of gauze with the warm oil mixture.

3 Follow steps 1 through 11 as in basic facial.

4 After the manipulations, do not remove the massage cream. Place eye pads and gauze in position over the face.

5 Use red dermal light or an infrared lamp for 8 to 10 minutes.

6 Remove the mask and cream.

7 Finish as for a basic facial.

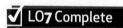 LO**7** Complete

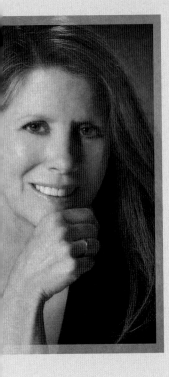

LEANIE KELLER

Leanie Keller is the Managing Director of men-u Grooming Products North America. She has been in the personal care industry for over 20 years, developing skin and haircare products distributed in over 110 countries. She is considered an expert in men's grooming products and is sought out by the media for her insights. Men-u Grooming Products are sold only through professionals. You can learn more about men-u shaving, skin, and hair products at http://www.men-uusa.com.

MEN'S SKIN CARE AND YOUR BUSINESS
WHAT EVERY BARBER SHOULD KNOW ABOUT HELPING CLIENTS AND INCREASING RETAIL SALES

You are in a unique position to be of tremendous help to your clients when it comes to the health of their skin, even if you do not offer skin care or shaving services. The fact that your clients are coming to you for their hair service indicates that they have a great deal of trust in you and your expertise. Moreover, during a hair service, you are able to get a 360-degree view of their face and neck, ask questions, and make suggestions in a non-threatening environment. Whether or not you choose to have the products you recommend to your clients available for purchase is up to you, but most successful barbers do.

MEN'S SKIN CARE TRENDS

There are several trends converging in the profession that should be of enormous benefit to your business. In 2007, the U.S. male grooming market reached $11 billion (just over a third the size of the female market) and continues to show robust growth without having yet attained its enormous potential. While men may not feel the high engagement and emotional connection women tend to feel about personal care and grooming products, they are increasingly embracing the attitude that the right products will make a difference in how they look and feel. This is largely being driven by increased education through the media, particularly men's magazines; greater numbers of men concerned with health, well being, and looking good; the aging population still competing in the workplace; and the younger guys having grown up with more product education overall.

And understanding men's needs, attitudes and behaviors towards skin care will open new avenues of opportunity for you and benefit your clients!

SHAVING AND SKIN CARE

To begin with, our studies indicate that over 80 percent of men shave and that many have never learned the correct way to perform this personal service. As a student of barbering, you know that improper shaving can lead to a host of skin issues such as razor burn, razor bumps, skin rash, and other irritations. Indeed, we can say the foundation to healthy male skin and the prevention of such skin irritations starts with the proper shaving techniques and products. This puts you, with your shaving training, in a unique position to help evaluate skin problems and offer solutions. For example, while your client is in the chair for a hair service, observe his skin. Casually, you might say "I notice you have some skin irritation on your neckline (or jaws, cheeks, etc.) and think it might be due to shaving." Ask questions such as "Do you shave after you shower?" or "How often do you change your blades?" or "What shaving cream do you use?" or "What products do you use after you shave?" and so forth. To get an idea of other kinds of questions to ask to help determine the things your client might be doing to cause razor burn or razor bumps, read *How to Prevent & Avoid Razor Burn: The 5 Key Shaving Mistakes and How to Avoid Them* at http://www.men-uusa.com/razor_burn_prevent.html. You will also see a link for a similar article on razor bumps, 99 percent of which are preventable with the correct shaving technique.

Although a great exfoliant, shaving removes up to two layers of the epidermis and places the skin in its most vulnerable condition. That is why your clients need to finish off their shave with two additional steps that will also promote excellent skin care. After shaving they should cleanse and tone with a product that contains a mild astringent (such as witch hazel) and natural anti-bacterial ingredients like tea tree oil. This will help prevent infections and blemishes associated with razor burn and razor bumps. Next, your clients should finish off with a moisturizer or aftershave balm (never aftershaves with alcohol!) to help balance the pH of the skin after the shaving process. Following these few simple steps should result in your clients having freshly shaved skin that is clean and moisturized and will help them look and feeling their best.

KEEP IT SIMPLE

The truth is, men want simple, straightforward products that work, do not cost a fortune, and are convenient to purchase from a trusted source such as their barbershop. Men are not usually interested in multiple lotions and potions, and if offered too many choices will become overwhelmed, get a glazed look in their eye, and back away. I've seen it happen! So if you believe they need to use a better shave cream, for instance, do not present them with multiple choices. Recommend one product. Ideally, the products you offer will have multiple uses, such as an aftershave balm that is also a general facial moisturizer. Your clients do not need a lot of different products, so be cautious of a manufacturer that has dozens of specialized skin care products for men—they obviously do not understand men and are simply applying the female market mentality to male grooming products.

MEN WANT INFORMATION AND RECOMMENDATIONS, NOT "SELLING"

Some barbers have an aversion to what they consider "selling," and men do not like to be "sold" to. But you do not have to sell. You are the expert and when you believe in a product this expertise and confidence shines through. Recommending a product that will benefit your client's skin becomes part of the general conversation during a service while he is in the chair. Just remember that men tend to respond to facts presented in a straightforward way: here's what it's for, here's how it works, here's what it will do, and this is why you need it.

PRODUCT SELECTION

When it comes to skin care, men are different from women and need solutions made specifically for them. Men tend to have thicker, oilier skin than women (due to the male hormone androgen) and therefore do not like the heaviness of typical female moisturizers. Our research shows they prefer moisturizers that go on lightly, dry quickly, and have a matte finish (never shiny). This is an important reason why you should look for products formulated specifically for men. A word of caution here, though: Some manufacturers of strong female brands simply label their female moisturizer formulas with "men's" on the bottle, so be careful in your selections and never purchase without trying the product yourself.

TRIAL IS THE KEY

As with hair care products, the best way to expose your clients to products that you believe in is by using the products in service. Ideally, the best way for your clients to try a moisturizer is to provide complimentary moisturizing treatments after every hair service. Simply apply a hot towel to the face and neck area for several minutes, then wipe the skin with the towel to remove any residual oils. Pat dry and apply the moisturizer to the face and neck areas using the effleurage massage movement. Not only will you introduce your client to the product, but you will have also given them a great experience they will remember and talk about.

Another inexpensive way to introduce clients to products is to provide them with a trial size of the product. Most manufacturers have smaller trial sizes you can use to promote services and retail sales. Yet another way is to simply demonstrate the products at your station by applying the product to the back of the client's hand or showing them how a shaving cream whips up, for example.

HOW TO MERCHANDISE YOUR PRODUCTS

There are three effective ways to sell retail products. We've already discussed problem evaluation and recommendations while the client is in the chair and the trial method through either service or sampling. The third way is through effective merchandising.

DISPLAY IT!

An effective way to retail your skin care products is to have a display in the waiting area on shelves that your clients can walk over and take a look at. Do not put products behind a glass display case. Many people, male or female, are reluctant to ask to see a product because they do not want to feel obligated to purchase it—so they will not ask in the first place. If they have access to a product off the shelf and are interested in learning more, they will ask you for more information.

Similarly, always have a special area or small shelf at each station to display the products. Your client is a captive audience during his hair service and will see the products. If interested, he will ask you about them. And, if you have identified a skin care need that you can help solve, it is helpful to have the products within reach to show him. One of each item is sufficient, and again, keep it simple!

In summary, although many men do not currently use skin care products, the market is growing each year. If you tie good skin care to the shaving process, they will respond. This is a proven way to help your clients get started on good skin care routines. You are the expert and they trust you, so keep it simple. Your clients benefit and you benefit by solidifying the service you provide your clients, which then translates into increased revenue for you.

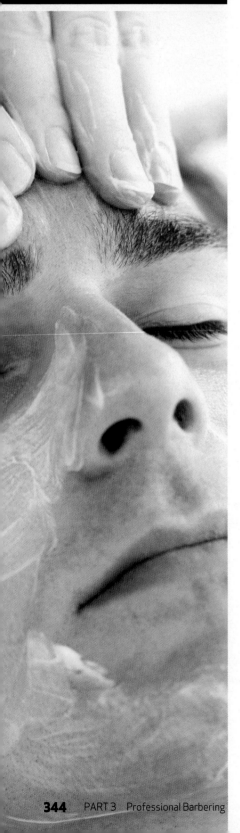

13 Review Questions

1. Identify three characteristics of the skin that may benefit from regularly scheduled facial services.

2. List important facial muscles associated with facial massage.

3. Explain what stimulation of the nerves achieves.

4. List the ways in which nerves may be stimulated.

5. Identify three cranial nerves that are important in massaging the head, face, and neck.

6. Identify the main arteries that supply blood to the entire head, face, and neck.

7. Identify the principal veins by which the blood from the head, face, and neck is returned to the heart.

8. List and describe the five basic massage movements and their effects on the skin.

9. List the benefits of facial massage.

10. List the electrical equipment that can be used in the performance of facial treatments.

11. List and describe the basic skin types.

12. List the steps involved in the performance of a basic facial.

13. Read and list the CAUTION and REMINDER boxes presented in this chapter.

Chapter
Glossary

astringent tonic lotions with an alcohol content of up to 35 percent; used to remove oil accumulation on oily and acne-prone skin

direct surface application high-frequency current performed with the mushroom- or rake-shaped electrodes for its calming and germicidal effect on the skin

effleurage light, continuous stroking movement applied with the fingers (digital) or the palms (palmar) in a slow, rhythmic manner

electric massager massaging unit that attaches to the barber's hand to impart vibrating massage movements to the skin surface

friction deep rubbing movement requiring pressure on the skin with the fingers or palm while moving the hand over an underlying structure

indirect application high-frequency current administered with the client holding the wire glass electrode between both hands

motor point a point on the skin, over a muscle, where pressure or stimulation will cause contraction of that muscle

muscles system that covers, shapes, and supports the skeleton; contracts and moves various parts of the body

percussion another name for tapotement

pétrissage kneading movement performed by lifting, squeezing, and pressing the tissue with a light, firm pressure

phoresis the process of forcing chemical solutions into unbroken skin by way of a galvanic current

rolling cream cleansing and exfoliating product used in facials to lift dead skin cells and dirt from the skin surface

tapotement most stimulating massage movement, consisting of short, quick tapping, slapping, and hacking movements

tonics include toners, fresheners, and astringents; are used after cleansing and prior to the application of a moisturizer

vibration in massage, the rapid shaking of the body part while the balls of the fingertips are pressed firmly on the point of application

14 Shaving and Facial Hair Design

☑ Learning Objectives

1 Discuss sanitation and safety precautions associated with straight razor shaving.

2 Demonstrate the ability to perform straight razor-holding positions and cutting strokes.

3 Identify the 14 shaving areas of the face.

4 Demonstrate a facial shave.

5 Demonstrate a neck shave.

6 Demonstrate a mustache and beard trim.

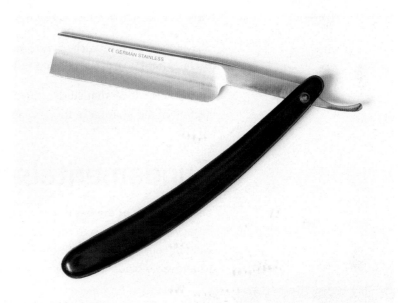

Key Terms

PAGE NUMBER INDICATES WHERE IN THE CHAPTER THE TERM IS USED.

backhand / 351	freehand / 351	reverse freehand / 351
close shaving / 371	neck shave / 373	second-time-over shave / 369
cutting stroke / 351	once-over shave / 371	styptic powder / 349
first-time-over-shave / 371	reverse backhand / 351	

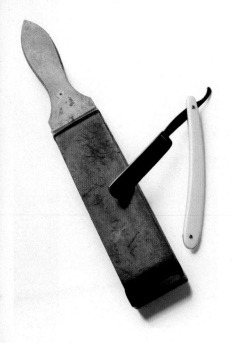

Although the advance of safety and electric razors over the past century has made it more convenient for men to shave at home, there will always be those clients who choose to indulge in a barbershop shave on an occasional, if not regular, basis. A full facial shave, complete with hot towels, lotions, and massage, is one of the most relaxing yet rejuvenating services that men can enjoy in the barbershop.

Admittedly, many traditional barbershops have felt the impact of new inventions, fashion trends, and the proliferation of unisex and franchise salons. Some have closed their doors forever and others are looking for younger barbers to replace 50-year veterans in the trade. Still others are part of the resurgence of barbers, barbershops, and barbering that is taking place nationwide as the male consumer seeks the ambience and services of a real barbershop once again. In essence, the cycle has gone full circle through technological advances, trends, and the mass-market approach. The barbershop has survived and today's barbers need to master traditional skills to ensure the longevity of the profession.

Shaving is an art. As such, it requires careful attention, skill, and practice to perfect. It rests with the student to learn the mechanics and perfect the art.

NOTE: It is critical that student barbers read and study the entire shaving section of this chapter before engaging in the performance of a facial shave.

Fundamentals of Shaving

Shaving is one of the basic services performed in the barbershop. The objective of shaving is to remove the visible part of facial and neck hair without causing irritation to the skin. Professional barbers use a straight razor (changeable blade or conventional) and warm lather when shaving a client.

There are certain general principles of shaving that apply to all men. Because each individual is different, there will also be exceptions to these principles that will require consideration. For example, the application of hot towels is a standard procedure in preparing the beard for shaving. Nevertheless, some clients may not be able to tolerate a hot towel on their skin. Other individual characteristics such as hair texture, hair growth pattern, and product sensitivity are variables that barbers must consider and make educated judgments about before proceeding with the shave service.

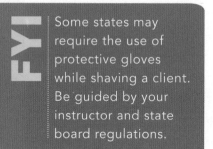

FYI Some states may require the use of protective gloves while shaving a client. Be guided by your instructor and state board regulations.

SANITATION AND SAFETY PRECAUTIONS ASSOCIATED WITH SHAVING

Some general rules to be observed when shaving include the following:

- Always disinfect razors before and after use. Disinfect replaceable or injector blades before use, then discard in a sharps container after use. Disinfect hones and strops before and after use when preparing a conventional straight razor.

- Always wash your hands before servicing a client.

- Always use clean linens, capes, and paper products.

- Always provide a cloth or paper barrier between the client's head and the headrest.

- Never proceed with the shave if the client has a skin infection or pustules. Doing so could spread the infection to other parts of the face or to the barber.

- If small cuts or nicks occur, wear gloves, pat cut dry with sterile cotton or tissue, and apply **styptic powder** or liquid with a cotton swab. Discard tissue and swab in a closeable plastic bag. Never use a styptic pencil or other astringent application that will come into contact with another person's skin.

- Lock the chair once the client is properly draped and in position for the shave.

- Always prepare facial hair for the shave with warm or hot towels and lather.

- Always use a light touch and a forward gliding motion that leads with the point of the blade.

- Always observe the hair growth pattern and shave with it, not against it.

- Do not use hot towels on skin that is chapped, blistered, thin, or sensitive.

- Lather against the grain *gently* to place the facial hair in a position to be shaved.

- Heavy beard growth requires more care in the lathering process and more steam towels than usual to effectively prepare it for the shave.

- Keep the fingers of the hand opposite the hand holding the razor dry to grasp, stretch, or hold the skin firmly during the shave service.

- Use the cushions of the fingertips to stretch skin in the opposite direction of the razor stroke.

- Apply lather neatly to the areas to be shaved and replace as necessary.

- Keep the skin moist while shaving.

- Follow through with shaving strokes from one shaving area to another; do not stop short.

- Use pH-balanced fresheners or toners when astringents are too harsh for sensitive skin.

- Curly facial hair requires special care as its growth characteristics may cause problems if the shave isn't performed correctly. Ingrown hairs are often the result of improper hair removal by a razor, tweezers, or trimmer. Curly hair has the tendency to grow in a

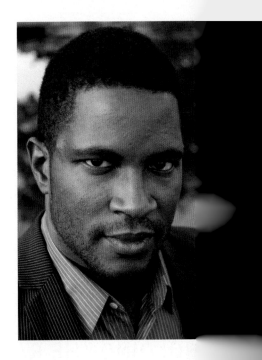

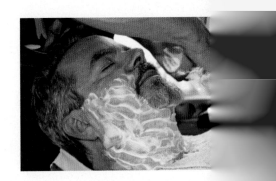

looped direction and as it grows out of the skin, it can bend back into the skin surface. Excessively close shaving, coupled with excessive pressure with clippers, trimmers, or razors, can damage skin to the point that new hair growth is trapped under the injured tissue. This can result in infected bumps on and under the skin surface (folliculitis) or scar tissue, or it may initiate a keloid condition.

- Be especially careful when shaving tender, sensitive areas beneath the lower lip, on lower part of the neck, and around the Adam's apple to avoid irritation or injury.

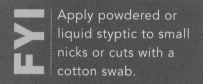
FYI Apply powdered or liquid styptic to small nicks or cuts with a cotton swab.

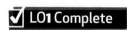
☑ **LO1 Complete**

RAZOR POSITIONS AND STROKES

mini PROCEDURE

HOLDING THE RAZOR

The first step in learning how to shave is to master the fundamentals of handling the razor. Review the parts of the razor, illustrated in **Figure 14-1**, so you can learn how to open and close the razor without injury.

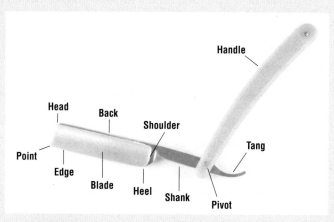
▲ **FIGURE 14-1**
Parts of the razor.

1 To open the razor, grasp the back of the razor's blade between the thumb and index finger of the dominant hand while holding the handle with the opposite thumb and index finger.

2 As the blade and handle separate by way of the pivot (**Figure 14-2a**), reposition the little finger of the dominant hand to rest on the tang as the handle is placed in an upward position (**Figure 14-2b**).

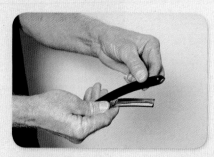
▲ **FIGURE 14-2a**
Opening the razor.

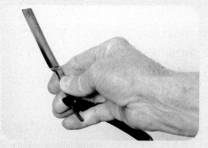
▲ **FIGURE 14-2b**
Positioning of the little finger.

(Continued)

3 The razor should be held between the thumb and index finger on the sides of the shank near the shoulder of the blade and rest across the second and third fingers, with the little finger bracing the razor (**Figure 14-2c**).

4 When closing the razor, release the little finger and bring the handle to the blade. Be careful the cutting edge does not strike the handle (**Figure 14-2d**).

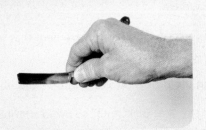

▲ **FIGURE 14-2c**

Positioning of the thumb and fingers.

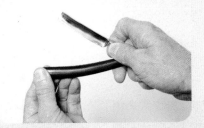

▲ **FIGURE 14-2d**

Close the razor carefully.

The term used to describe the correct angle of cutting with a razor is called the **cutting stroke.** To achieve a proper cutting stroke, the razor must glide over the skin surface at an angle with the point leading (**Figure 14-3**). This should be a light-handed forward gliding motion that is most often positioned to cut *with* the grain of the hair, not against it.

There are four razor positions and strokes used in the practice of barbering: **freehand, backhand, reverse freehand,** and **reverse backhand.** Position refers to the way the razor is held in the barber's hand to facilitate a technique or stroke movement. The actual movement of the razor while being held in one of the four positions is the stroke. Each of these techniques require consideration and diligent practice of the following:

▲ **FIGURE 14-3**

Angle of cutting stroke.

- **When to use a particular razor position and stroke** (see Practice Session 1)

- **How to hold the razor for each position and stroke**

  ▶ Position of the fingers, wrist, and elbow of the dominant hand in relation to the razor

  ▶ Position of the opposite hand on the client's skin in relation to the razor

  ▶ Position of your body in relation to the client to facilitate a razor position and stroke

- **How to hold or stretch the skin**

  ▶ Finding the balance between stretching the skin too much or too little

  ▶ Using the cushions of the finger tips to stretch the skin with the proper pressure

CAUTION

Always handle razors with extreme care. Warped or loose handles may cause the blade to pass through to the fingers when closing the razor.

REMINDER

 Be careful that the cuttir edge does not strike the handle when closing the razor.

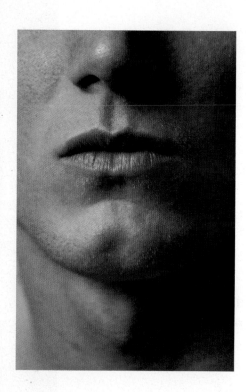

- ▶ Using the thumb and second finger as the primary digits for stretching the skin

- ▶ Stretching different areas of the skin in the opposite direction that the razor will travel

- **How to position and stroke the razor over the surface of the skin**

  - ▶ Positioning the razor at about a 30-degree angle relative to the skin surface

  - ▶ Using a forward gliding movement that leads with the point of the razor

  - ▶ Using the proper stroke length on different areas of the face

  - ▶ Using strokes of 1" to 3" to avoid shaving too far from the stretching point

  - ▶ Using shorter strokes around the mouth, over the ears, and on the sides of the neck

  - ▶ Developing a medium stroke speed to avoid very fast or very slow movements

  - ▶ Adjusting the rate of speed of the stroke according to the area being shaved

  - ▶ Using smooth strokes that carry through once started without stopping and starting

- **How to recognize growth patterns and the grain of the hair in different areas of the face**

  - ▶ Identifying areas where the direction of hair growth changes

  - ▶ Using the appropriate razor position and stroke for the area to be shaved

  - ▶ Adjusting stroke speed and pressure to accommodate the texture or density of the hair

  - ▶ Recognition and use of the terms *with the grain*, *against the grain*, and *across the grain*

- **How to work efficiently and effectively**

  - ▶ Making strokes so no lather is left behind

  - ▶ Keeping the non-dominant thumb and fingertips dry for stretching purposes

  - ▶ Starting strokes from a clean skin surface into the lathered surface

  - ▶ Wiping residual lather and hair from the razor in a safe and clean manner

  - ▶ Checking work for rough or missed patches

NOTE: If using a conventional straight razor, review honing and stropping procedures before learning each shaving stroke.

To shave the face with ease and efficiency, the barber employs three of the four positions and strokes:

- Freehand position and stroke

- Backhand position and stroke

- Reverse freehand position and stroke

The reverse backhand stroke is not used when shaving the face; however, it is employed at the sideburn and behind the ear areas during neck and outline shaves.

To master the correct hand and finger placement, razor control, and cutting strokes requires practice. Use the following exercises to become comfortable and proficient with a straight razor.

PRACTICE SESSION #1

Freehand Position and Stroke

1 How to hold the razor. The position of the right hand is as follows:

- Take the razor in the right hand. Hold the handle of the razor between the third and fourth fingers, with the tip of the small finger resting on the tip of the tang of the razor. The thumb should rest on the side of the shank near the shoulder of the blade. The third finger lies at the pivot of the shank and the handle with the first and second fingers in front of it on the back of the shank (**Figure 14-4**).

- Turn the hand slightly outward from the wrist with the elbow at a comfortable level.

The position of the left hand is as follows:

- Keep the fingers of the left hand dry in order to prevent them from slipping on the face.

- Use the left hand to stretch the skin in the opposite direction of the stroke under the razor (**Figure 14-5**).

2 How to perform the freehand stroke:

- Use a gliding stroke toward you.

- Lead with the point of the razor in a forward, gliding movement.

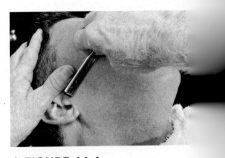

▲ **FIGURE 14-4**

Holding position of razor for freehand stroke.

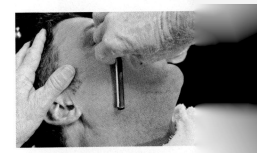

▲ **FIGURE 14-5**

Stretch the skin gently with the left hand.

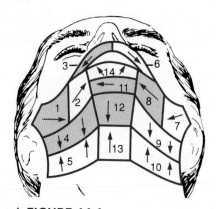

▲ FIGURE 14-6

Diagram of shaving areas of the face.

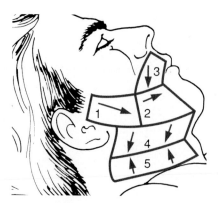

▲ FIGURE 14-7

Diagram of shaving areas on the right side of the face.

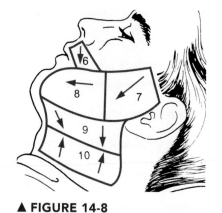

▲ FIGURE 14-8

Diagram of shaving areas on the left side of the face.

3 When to use the freehand stroke:

- The freehand position and stroke is used in 6 of the 14 shaving areas. See Nos. 1, 3, 4, 8, 11, and 12 in **Figures 14-6** through **14-8**.

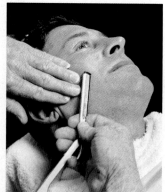

▲ FIGURE 14-9

Backhand holding position.

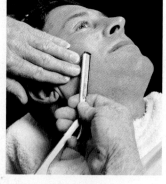

▲ FIGURE 14-10

Alternative backhand holding position.

Backhand Position and Stroke

1 How to hold the razor. The position of the right hand is as follows:

- The shank of the razor should be held firmly between the thumb and first two fingers at the pivot with the razor held in a relatively straight position.

- The underside of the handle rests on the third and fourth fingers **(Figure 14-9)**.

- An alternative method is to bend the handle slightly so the third finger barely rests at the end of the tang and the fourth finger is bent into the palm **(Figure 14-10)**.

- Turn the back of the hand away from you and bend the wrist slightly downward. Then raise the elbow so that you can move the arm freely. This is the position used for the backhand stroke with the arm movement. Some practitioners prefer to use a wrist movement, in which case the arm is not held as high.

The position of the left hand is as follows:

- Keep the fingers of the left hand dry in order to prevent them from slipping.

- Stretch the skin under the razor in the opposite direction of the stroke.

2 How to perform the backhand stroke:

- Use a gliding stroke away from you.
- Direct the stroke with the point of the razor leading in a forward, gliding movement.

3 When to use the backhand stroke:

- The backhand stroke is used in 4 of the 14 shaving areas and if preferred, in area 12. See Nos. 2, 6, 7, and 9 in Figures 14-6 through 14-8.

PRACTICE SESSION #3

Reverse Freehand Position and Stroke

The reverse freehand stroke hand and razor position is similar to the freehand stroke, but the stroke is performed in an upward rather than a downward direction, usually with the barber standing behind the client's head.

1 How to hold the razor. The position of the right hand is as follows:

- Hold the razor firmly in a freehand position.
- Turn the hand slightly toward you so that the razor edge is turned upward (**Figure 14-11**).

The position of the left hand is as follows:

- Keep the hand dry and use it to pull the skin taut under the razor.
- Position the fingers below or in back of the razor opposite the cutting edge and direction of the stroke.

2 How to perform the reverse freehand stroke:

- Use an upward, semi-arc stroke toward you with the point leading in a gliding movement.
- The movement is from the elbow to the hand with a slight twist of the wrist.

3 When to use the reverse freehand stroke:

- The reverse freehand stroke is used in 4 of the 14 shaving areas. See Nos. 5, 10, 13, and 14 in Figures 14-6 through 14-8.

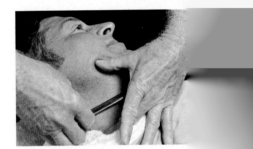

▲ **FIGURE 14-11**
Reverse freehand stroke.

Reverse Backhand Position and Stroke

The reverse backhand position and stroke require diligent practice to master. The holding position of the razor is the same as that for the backhand stroke except the elbow is positioned downward (closer to the barber's body) and the forearm in held upward. When using this stroke, employ a downward gliding stroke that follows along the natural hairline.

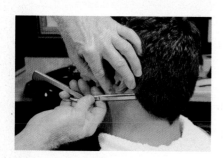

▲ FIGURE 14-12

Reverse backhand stroke.

1 How to hold the razor. The position of the right hand is as follows:

- Hold the razor firmly in the backhand position.

- Turn the palm of the hand to the right so that it faces upward.

- Drop the elbow close to the side.

The position of the left hand is as follows:

- Position the left hand so as to be able to draw the skin taut under the razor.

- The barber's hand will be positioned above the razor **(Figure 14-12)**.

2 How to perform the reverse backhand stroke:

- Use a smooth, gliding stroke, directed downward toward the point of the razor.

- Proceed with short cutting strokes directed downward and slightly outward.

3 When to use the reverse backhand stroke:

- The reverse backhand stroke is only used for making the left sideburn outline and for shaving the left side behind the ear during a neck shave while the client is sitting in an upright position.

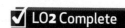
☑ **LO2** Complete

The cutting strokes described in the preceding section illustrate the holding and stroking positions that should be employed by the right-handed barber. The left-handed barber will need to reverse the starting position, as outlined in **Table 14-1**.

TABLE 14-1 Shaving Movements for Left-handed and Right-handed Barbers

MOVEMENT	AREA OF FACE FOR A LEFT-HANDED BARBER	POSITION	DIRECTION	AREA OF FACE FOR A RIGHT-HANDED BARBER
1	Left sideburn	Freehand	Down	Right sideburn
2	Left side of cheek	Backhand	Down	Right side of cheek
3	Left upper lip	Freehand	Down	Right upper lip
4	Left side below jaw	Freehand	Down	Right side below jaw
5	Left side of neck	Reverse freehand	Up	Right side of neck
6	Right upper lip	Backhand	Down	Left upper lip
7	Right sideburn	Backhand	Down	Left sideburn
8	Right side of cheek	Freehand	Down	Left side of cheek
9	Right side below jaw	Backhand	Down	Left side below jaw
10	Right side of neck	Reverse freehand	Up	Left side of neck
11	Across chin right to left	Freehand	Across	Across chin left to right
12	Below chin	Freehand or backhand	Down	Below chin
13	Middle of neck	Reverse freehand	Up	Middle of neck
14	Lower lip	Reverse freehand	Up	Lower lip

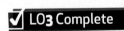

The Professional Shave

NOTE: During the shaving procedure, the right-handed barber stands at the client's right side, then moves in back of the client's head as required to execute the shaving strokes. The left-handed barber begins on the client's left side and moves behind the client's head in the same manner.

A professional shave consists of preparation, shaving, and finishing. The following procedure explain these steps in detail.

MATERIALS, IMPLEMENTS, AND EQUIPMENT

- Barber chair with headrest
- Sink
- Steam towel cabinet
- Sharps container
- Covered trash can
- Covered container for soiled towels
- Haircutting cape
- Terry cloth towels
- Barber's paper towels
- Headrest cover
- Straight razor and blades
- Shaving cream or gel
- Toner or astringent
- Moisturizing cream
- Comb and brush

PREPARATION

1. Assemble supplies.
2. Wash your hands.

PROCEDURE

A. PREPARING A CLIENT FOR A SHAVE

1 Seat the client comfortably in the chair.

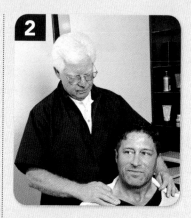

2 Ask the client to loosen his collar. Position a terry cloth towel from back to front, and lay the cape loosely over the client's shoulders from the front without it coming into contact with the client's neck.

3 Apply a fresh headrest cover and adjust the headrest to the proper height.

4 Recline the chair to a comfortable working angle.

5 Adjust and lock the chair to the proper height.

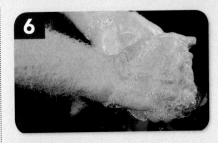

6 Wash your hands with soap and warm water, and dry them thoroughly.

7 Unfold a clean terry cloth towel, and lay it diagonally across the client's chest.

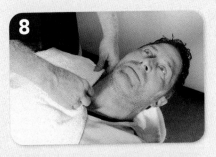

8 Tuck one corner of the towel along the right side of the client's neck, securing the edge tucked inside the neckband with a sliding movement of the forefinger of the left hand.

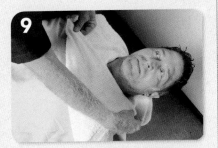

9 Cross the lower end of the towel to the other side of the client's neck and tuck under the neckband with a similar sliding motion.

10 Tuck a paper strip or paper towel into the neckband and lay it across the client's chest to use during the shave to wipe the razor clean of shaving cream and facial hair.

B. PREPARING A STEAM TOWEL

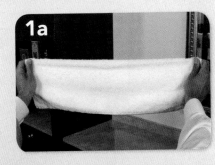

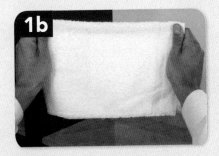

1 Fold a clean towel in half lengthwise. Then fold it in half again by bringing both ends of the towel together.

2 Place the folded towel under a stream of hot water, or wrap it around a disinfected faucet or hose spray, until it becomes thoroughly saturated and heated. Wring out the towel. Prepare 4-6 towels in the same manner and store in heated steam towel cabinet.

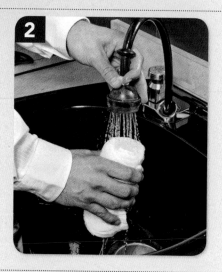

REMINDER

>>> Be sure to sanitize the hose, spray nozzle, and sink *prior* to preparing the steam towel.

CAUTION

Do not use a hot steam towel if the skin is sensitive, irritated, chapped, or blistered.

C. PREPARING THE FACE FOR SHAVING

Steaming and lathering the face are very important steps to preparing the skin for shaving. *Steaming* the face helps to soften the hair cuticle, provides lubrication by stimulating the action of the oil glands, and relaxes the client. *Lathering* serves to cleanse the skin, soften the hair, hold the hair in an upright position, and create a smooth surface over which the razor can glide more effectively. If the client has a mustache, trim and shape it prior to the shave service to prepare it for finish work with the razor.

The face is prepared for shaving as follows:

1 Test the temperature of the towel on your wrist. If it is too hot, hold the towel by the top corners and gently fan it back and forth for a few seconds. Test the towel again before applying it to the client's face.

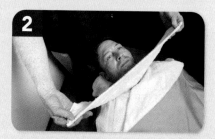

2 Standing behind the client's head, position the steam towel under and in front of the client's chin.

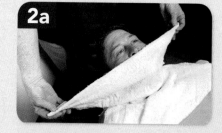

a. Fold the towel over the client's mouth and upper lip area to just under his nose.

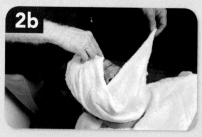

b. Cross the right hand section of the towel over to the client's left temple area.

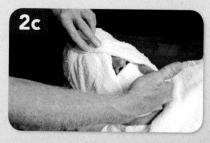

c. Bring the left hand section of the towel over toward the client's right side and smooth the fold.

3 Warm shaving lather is usually prepared in an electric latherizer.

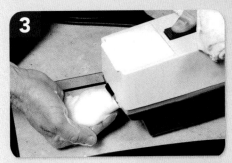

a. Transfer a quantity of lather into the hand, remove the steam towel, and spread lather evenly over the bearded areas of the face and neck to be shaved.

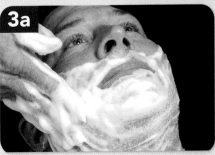

b. Use a rotary movement to briskly rub lather into the bearded area with the cushion tips of the fingers. Start at the neck and rub lather up to the right side of the face. Then gently turn the head with the left hand by lightly grasping the top of the head or the back of the head near the crown. Rub lather on the other side of the face and continue lathering until the bearded areas are covered. Rubbing time is from 1 to 2 minutes, depending on the stiffness and density of the beard.

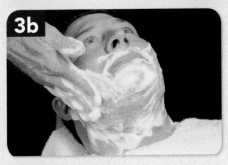

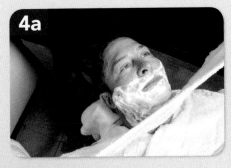

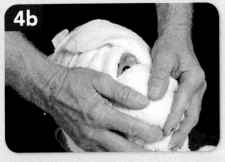

4 Test the temperature of a second steam towel and apply it over the lather. Mold or pat towel to conform to client's face. Repeat the steaming process if the beard is extremely coarse or dense.

5 Prepare the razor while the steam towel is on the client's face.

a. When using a conventional straight razor, strop the razor, immerse it in a disinfectant solution, rinse, and wipe dry.

b. When using a changeable-blade razor, disinfect the razor and new blade, rinse, wipe dry, and assemble.

> > > **REMINDER**

New blades for changeable-blade razors *do not* guarantee a sanitized blade. Clean and disinfect the razor and blades, rinse, wipe dry with a clean towel, and place in a clean, closed container until ready for use.

6 Remove the steam towel and wipe the lather off in one operation.

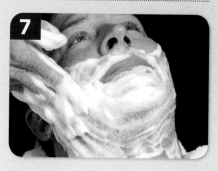

7 Re-lather the beard, then wipe the lather from your hands.

D. THE FACIAL SHAVE

Razor strokes should be correct and systematic. Proper coordination of both hands is necessary. While the right hand holds and strokes the razor, the fingers of the left hand gently stretch the skin area that is being shaved. Taut skin allows the beard hair to be cut more easily.

Loose skin tends to push out in front of the razor and can result in cuts or nicks. Stretching the skin too tightly, however, will cause irritation. The skin must be held firmly, neither too loosely nor too tightly, to create the correct shaving surface for the razor. To prevent slipping, remove lather with the thumb (e.g., at the sideburn hairline, area No. 1), or dry the skin to be touched (e.g., at the neck, below area No. 5). Keep the fingers of the non-dominant hand dry at all times.

CAUTION

Avoid sawing, scraping, pushing, or sideways movements with straight razors to avoid causing injury to the skin. Always employ a gentle gliding motion that leads with the point of the blade.

FIRST-TIME-OVER SHAVE

1 Shaving Area No. 1 – Freehand stroke

a. Standing at the right side of chair, gently turn the client's face to the left. Remove the lather from the hairline with the thumb of the left hand. Hold the razor in a freehand position.

b. Stretch the skin and begin at the hairline of the right sideburn. Use a gliding diagonal stroke that leads with the point of the razor and shave downward toward the corner of the mouth and jawbone.

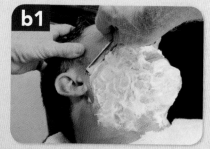

Beginning of stroke.

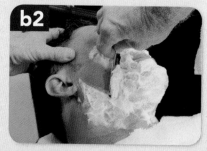

End of stroke.

2 Shaving Area No. 2 – Backhand stroke

a. Remain in the same position and wipe the razor clean on lather paper. Hold the razor in a backhand position.

b. Stretch the skin and use a diagonal stroke from point to heel to shave the right side from the angle of the mouth to the point of the chin.

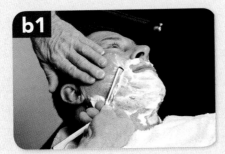

Beginning of stroke.

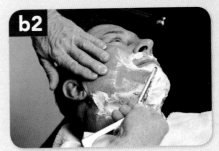

End of stroke.

3 Shaving Area No. 3 – Freehand stroke

a. Maintain the same body position and wipe the razor clean. Hold the razor in a freehand position.

b. To shave underneath the nostril, slightly lift the tip of the nose, taking care not to interfere with breathing. Stretch the upper lip by placing the fingers of the left hand against the nose while holding the thumb below the lower corner of the lip.

c. Shave underneath the nostrils and over the right side of the upper lip, using the fingers of the left hand to stretch the underlying skin. If the client has a mustache, shave the outline with the razor at this time.

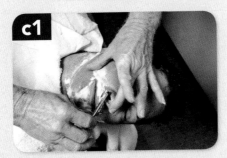

Beginning of stroke.

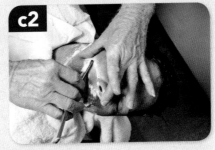

End of stroke.

REMINDER

>>> Shaving strokes on the upper lip are performed on a slight diagonal to follow the curves of the face; however, remember to shave *with the grain* in this area.

4 Shaving Area No. 4 – Freehand stroke

a. Shift your body position to face the front of the right side of the client's face.

b. Starting at chin level, stretch the skin, and shave that portion of the neck below the jawbone down to the change in the grain of the beard. Be sure to hold the skin taut between the thumb and fingers of left hand.

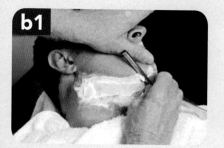
Beginning of stroke.

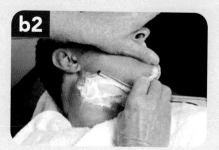
Mid-point of stroke.

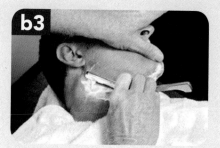
End of stroke.

REMINDER

>>> The beard should be shaved at an angle with the grain of the hair; therefore, the barber must determine when the reverse hand positions and strokes are the correct procedure for shaving the client's beard. For example: When the hair in shaving area No. 5 grows downward, the freehand stroke may be a better choice than the reverse freehand stroke.

5 Shaving Area No. 5 – Reverse freehand stroke

a. Move behind the chair. Hold the razor for a reverse freehand stroke.

b. Stretch the skin and shave the remainder of the beard upward with the grain. Do not expect to complete this shaving area in one stroke.

c. After completing the first stroke, reposition the razor just right of the previously shaved section until the entire area is shaved. This movement completes shaving of the right side of the face.

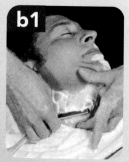
Beginning of stroke 1.

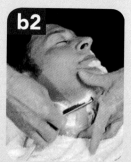
End of stroke 1.

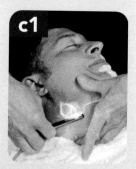
Beginning of stroke 2.

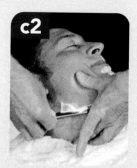
End of stroke 2.

6 Shaving Area No. 6 – Backhand stroke

a. Wipe the razor clean and strop if necessary. Stand to the right side of the client and turn the client's face upward so that you can shave the left upper lip. Re-lather if necessary. Hold the razor in the backhand position.

b. While gently pushing the tip of the nose to the right with the thumb and fingers of the left hand, stretch the skin and shave the left side of upper lip.

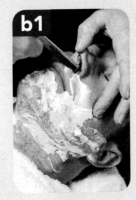 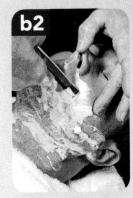

Beginning of stroke.   End of stroke.

7 Shaving Area No. 7 – Backhand stroke

a. Stand slightly back and at an angle from the client. Gently turn the face to the right. Re-lather the left side of the face.

b. Using the thumb, wipe lather from the hairline. Stretch the skin taut with the fingers of the left hand to prevent the razor from digging in along the ear. Stretch the skin and shave downward and slightly forward toward the corner of the mouth and jawbone.

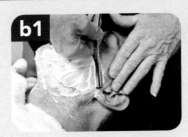 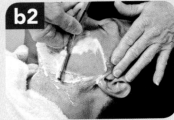

Beginning of stroke.   End of stroke.

8 Shaving Area No. 8 – Freehand stroke

a. Wipe off the razor. Stand to the client's right. Hold the razor in a freehand position.

b. Stretch the skin and shave downward on the left side from the angle of the mouth to the point of the chin.

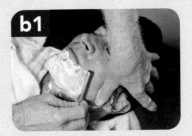 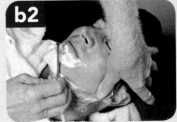

Beginning of stroke.   End of stroke.

9 Shaving Area No. 9 – Backhand stroke

a. Wipe off the razor. Maintaining the same body position, hold the razor for the backhand stroke.

b. With the fingers of the left hand stretching the skin, shave downward from the point of the chin to where the grain of the beard changes on the neck.

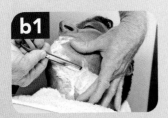 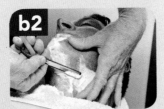 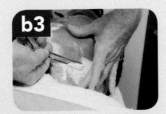 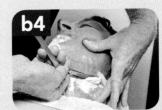

Beginning of stroke 1.   End of stroke 1.   Beginning of stroke 2.   End of stroke 2.

10 Shaving Area No. 10 – Reverse freehand stroke

a. Wipe off the razor. Stand behind the client. Hold the razor in the reverse freehand position.

b. Stretching the skin with the left hand, shave the left side of the lower neck area upward to where the grain of the beard changes.

c. Similar to area No. 5, after completing the first stroke, reposition the razor just left of the previously shaved section until the entire area is shaved. This completes the shaving of the left side of the face.

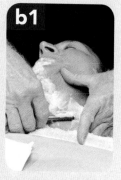

Beginning of stroke 1.

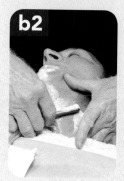

End of stroke 1.

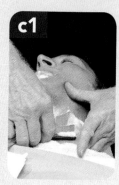

Beginning of stroke 2.

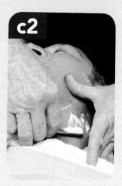

End of stroke 2.

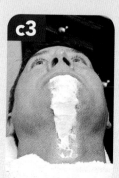

Completed right and left sides.

11 Shaving Area No. 11 – Freehand stroke

a. Stand at the client's side and turn the client's head so his face is pointing upward.

b. Holding the razor in a freehand position, stretch the skin, and shave across the upper part of the chin. Continue shaving until the entire chin area has been shaved to a point just below the jawbone.

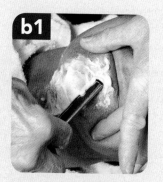

Beginning of stroke 1.

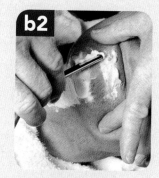

End of stroke 1.

Did **You** Know...

In shaving areas No. 11 and 14, the client can help to stretch the skin if he rolls his bottom lip slightly over his bottom teeth. This is sometimes called *balling-the-chin*.

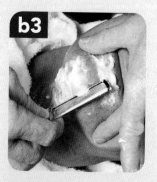

Beginning of stroke 2.

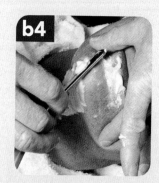

End of stroke 2.

12 Shaving Area No. 12 – Freehand or backhand stroke

   a. Using the freehand stroke, stretch the skin with the left hand and position the razor to arc downward just below the chin.

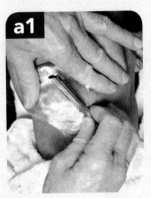

Position razor to arc downward.

   b. Continue this stroke until the grain of the beard (direction of hair growth) changes.

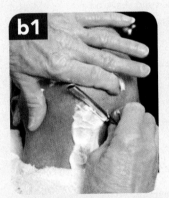
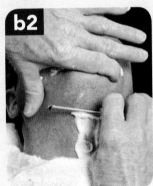
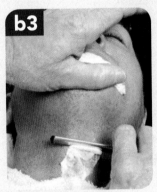

Beginning of stroke.   Mid-point of stroke.   End of stroke.

   c. Alternate method: Some barbers prefer to use the backhand stroke in shaving area No. 12.

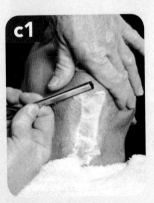
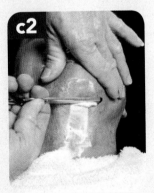
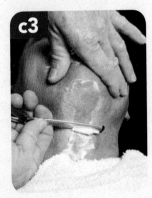

Beginning of stroke.   Mid-point of stroke.   End of stroke.

13 Shaving Area No. 13 – Reverse freehand stroke

a. Move behind the chair. Hold the razor for the reverse freehand stroke.

b. Stretch the skin below the chin and shave upward on the lower part of the neck. Stretch the skin away from the Adam's apple and shave on a slight diagonal to prevent nicks.

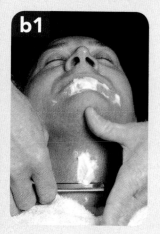 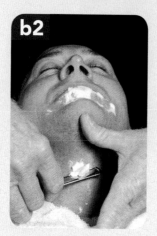 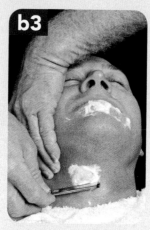 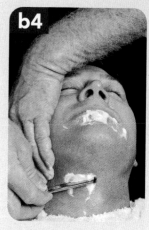

Beginning of stroke. End of stroke. Stretch skin and shave on a slight diagonal. Beginning of stroke. Stretch skin and shave on a slight diagonal. End of stroke.

14 Shaving Area No. 14 – Reverse freehand stroke

a. Remain behind the chair. Cup the client's chin and stretch the skin.

b. Using the reverse freehand stroke, use a few short scooping strokes to shave upward from the cleft of the chin toward the lower lip. You may also ask the client to ball his chin for this step.

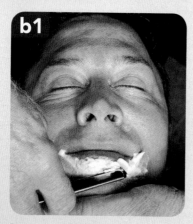 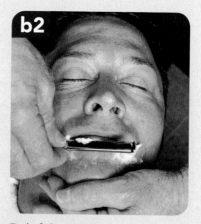

Beginning of short strokes. End of short strokes.

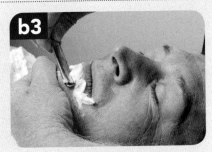

Beginning of short strokes—side view.

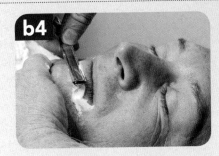

End of short strokes—side view.

c. Wipe off the razor and discard the towel or paper strip. This completes the first-time-over shave procedure.

15 **Second-Time-Over Shave**

The **second-time-over shave** follows a regular shave and serves to remove any rough or uneven spots. This technique may be considered a form of close shaving and care must be taken to avoid irritation or injury to the skin.

a. Dampen the client's face with water instead of lather.

b. Stretch the skin tightly and use the freehand stroke with a very light touch to shave with or across the grain to remove any residual facial hair.

E. FINAL STEPS OF THE FACIAL SHAVE

The final or finishing steps in shaving require attention to a number of important details.

1 Apply light facial cream or moisturizing lotion with an effleurage massage movement. Massage the cream into the skin using petrissage massage movements.

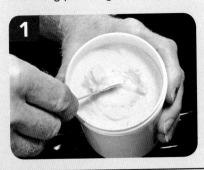

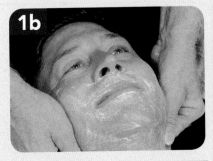

2 Prepare a moderately warm towel and apply it over the face.

CAUTION: Avoid excessively hot steam towels as the skin may be sensitive after the shave service.

A complete facial treatment may be performed at this time if the client desires the service; however, care should be taken not to irritate the skin with exfoliants, harsh scrubs, or high-pH astringents.

3 Remove the towel from the face.

4 Apply a toner or other mild astringent using cotton pledgets or a soft tissue to remove residual cream product. Pat gently; do not wipe or scrape against the skin.

5 Remove the towel from the client's chest and position yourself behind the chair.

6 Spread the towel over the client's face. Pat dry the lower part of the face, then the upper part. Remove the towel and fan the face dry.

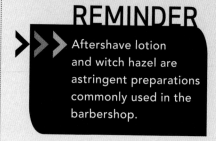

REMINDER

>>> Aftershave lotion and witch hazel are astringent preparations commonly used in the barbershop.

7 Move to the right side of the chair and wrap a clean dry towel around your hand. Sprinkle a small amount of talcum powder on the towel and apply evenly to the face.

8 Slowly raise the chair to an upright position.

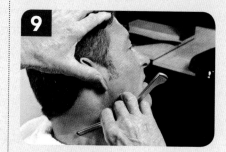

9 Offer to perform a neck shave (see Procedure 14-2).

10 Comb the hair neatly as desired.

11 Wipe off loose hair, lather, or powder from the client's face, neck, and clothing. Proceed with mustache trim, if not performed before shave service, or neck shave, as desired. Remove draping.

CLEAN-UP AND DISINFECTION

1. Cleanse and disinfect all implements; store soiled towels in appropriate container.

2. Sanitize work area.

3. Wash your hands.

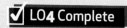
✔ LO**4** Complete

THE ONCE-OVER SHAVE

The **once-over shave** requires less time for a complete shave service and was popular when men patronized barbershops for their daily shaves. This shave should result in a smooth face without being a close shave. To perform an once-over shave, shave a few more strokes *across the grain* while completing each shaving movement. This will assure a complete and even shave with a single lathering. Remember to use a light hand to avoid causing irritation.

THE CLOSE SHAVE

Close shaving is the practice of shaving the beard *against the grain* of the hair during the second-time-over phase of the shave. This practice is undesirable because it may irritate the skin and lead to infection or ingrown hairs so barbers do not traditionally employ close-shaving methods. That said, barbers should be able to perform a close shave when the client's beard growth warrants it and he has requested the service.

mini PROCEDURE

1 Remove all traces of lather with a steam towel following the **first-time-over shave**. Turn the towel over and place it on the face.

2 Remove the steam towel and remoisten the bearded areas with water.

3 Using freehand and reverse freehand strokes as necessary to access the different shaving areas of the face, shave against the grain during the second-time-over shave.

4 When finished, wipe off the razor on lather paper, a neck strip, or a paper towel. Follow up with the final steps of the shave service, but do not offer to perform a deep cleansing facial at this time as doing so may irritate the skin. Discard all soiled papers in a closed container.

TIP: When employing the reverse freehand stroke, stand slightly behind the client. Stroke the grain of the beard sideways with your hand to help position the hair to be shaved in this manner.

TOWEL WRAPS

Properly trained barbers and stylists know how to wrap a towel around the hand with ease and skill for the following purposes:

- Cleansing and drying the face.
- Applying powder to the face.
- Removing all traces of powder, lather, and loose hair from the face, neck, and forehead.

Barbering students should practice the towel-wrapping methods illustrated in this procedure before beginning a facial shave service. **Figures 14-13a** to **14-13c** show one method of wrapping a cotton towel around the hand. **Figures 14-14a** to **14-14i** illustrate wrapping with a paper barber's towel. Either wrapping method can also be used with a flat-weave cotton towel.

PROCEDURE FOR CLOTH TOWEL WRAP

1 Grasp towel lengthwise (**Figure 14-13a**).

2 Holding your right hand in front of you, draw the upper edge of the towel across the palm of the right hand; then grasp the towel ends and twist (**Figure 14-13b**).

3 Wrap the twisted ends of the towel around the back of the hand and bring over the inside of the wrist (**Figure 14-13c**).

4 Hold the ends of the towel while in use to prevent them from flapping in the client's face.

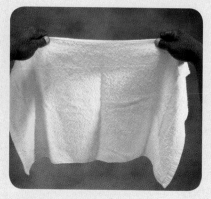

▲ **FIGURE 14-13a**
Grasp towel lengthwise.

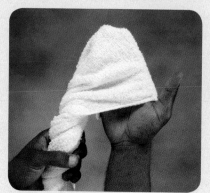

▲ **FIGURE 14-13b**
Draw towel over palm and twist the ends.

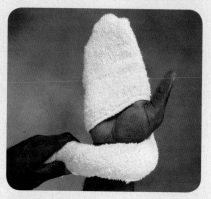

▲ **FIGURE 14-13c**
Wrap twisted towel ends around back of hand and across the wrist.

PROCEDURE FOR PAPER TOWEL WRAP

1 Grasp the towel lengthwise (**Figure 14-14a**).

2 Fold down the top third of the towel toward you (**Figure 14-14b**).

3 Holding the towel at one end, insert the two middle fingers into the fold (**Figure 14-14c**); maintain your grip on the towel with the thumb, index finger, and fourth finger.

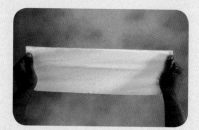

▲ **FIGURE 14-14a**
Grasp the towel lengthwise.

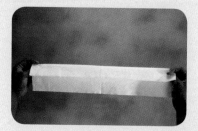

▲ **FIGURE 14-14b**
Fold down top third of towel.

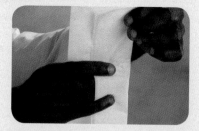

▲ **FIGURE 14-14c**
Insert two middle fingers into the fold.

(Continued)

4 Bring the top edge around the back of the hand and secure with the fourth finger (**Figures 14-14d** and **14-14e**).

5 Grasp the towel end and shift to a diagonal position (**Figure 14-14f**).

6 Wrap the remaining towel length around the back of the hand and insert thumb into the fold (**Figure 14-14g**).

7 Continue wrapping motion around the thumb (**Figure 14-14h**).

8 Tuck the towel end into wrap at the back of the hand (**Figure 14-14i**).

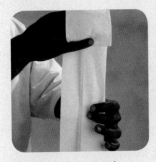

▲ **FIGURE 14-14d**

Bring top edge around hand and secure with fourth finger.

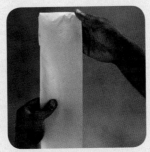

▲ **FIGURE 14-14e**

Figure 14-14d from barber's perspective.

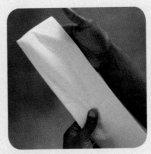

▲ **FIGURE 14-14f**

Reposition towel diagonally.

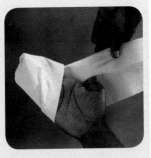

▲ **FIGURE 14-14g**

Wrap hand and insert thumb into fold.

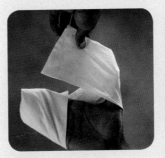

▲ **FIGURE 14-14h**

Wrap the thumb.

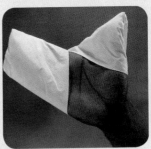

▲ **FIGURE 14-14i**

Tuck towel end into wrap at back of hand.

> **REMINDER**
> Neck dusters must never be used to remove hair from the face.

THE NECK SHAVE

A **neck shave** traditionally accompanies a facial shave and involves shaving the neckline on both sides of the neck behind the ears and across the nape if desired or necessary. Conversely, complete outline shaves that include the sideburn, around the ear, behind the ear areas, and sometimes the front hairline, typically follow a haircut.

> **REMINDER**
> Be sure to check the hairline and neck areas for moles, warts, or other hypertrophies before beginning the neck shave, and always follow the natural hairline.

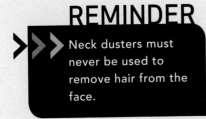

FYI A standard finishing service to a facial shave is a neck shave.

MATERIALS, IMPLEMENTS, AND EQUIPMENT

- Barber chair
- Sink
- Sharps container
- Covered trash can
- Covered container for soiled towels
- Haircutting cape
- Terry cloth towels
- Barber's paper towels
- Straight razor and blades
- Shaving cream or gel
- Witch hazel or antiseptic
- Comb and brush

PREPARATION

1. Assemble supplies.
2. Wash your hands.

PROCEDURE

A. PREPARING CLIENT FOR A NECK SHAVE

1 Following the facial shave, raise the chair slowly to an upright position.

2 Tuck the towel around the back of the neck. Leave the cape and towel loose enough to facilitate access to the sides and bottom of the neckline. Tuck a neck strip or paper towel into the neckline of the drape for wiping lather off the blade.

3 Check the neckline and behind-the-ear areas for moles, blemishes, or other conditions.

B. PERFORMING A NECK SHAVE

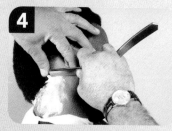

4 Apply lather. Stretch the skin behind the right ear with the thumb and shave along the natural hairline using a freehand stroke.

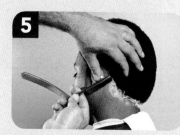

5 Repeat on the left side using a reverse backhand stroke.

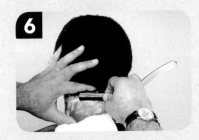

6 Use a freehand stroke to shave the nape area.

7 Clean the shaven part of the neckline with a towel or neck strip moistened with witch hazel, antiseptic, or warm water. Remove the towel from around the neck and dry thoroughly.

8 Position yourself behind the chair, place a clean dry towel around the client's neck, and comb or style the hair as desired by the client.

9 Take the towel from the back of the neck and fold it around the right hand. Remove all traces of powder and any loose hair.

10 Discard the towel and remove the chair cloth from the client. Make out the price check and thank the client as it is handed to him.

CLEAN-UP AND DISINFECTION

1. Cleanse and disinfect all implements.

2. Store soiled towels and papers in appropriate containers.

3. Sanitize work area.

4. Wash your hands.

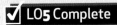

☑ **LO5 Complete**

While there are many reasons why a client may find fault with the shave procedure, the most common include:

- Dull or rough razors
- Unclean hands, towels, or drape
- Cold fingers
- Heavy touch
- Poorly heated towels
- Lather that is either too cold or too hot
- Glaring overhead lights
- Unshaven hair patches
- Scraping the skin and close shaving
- Offensive body odor or foul breath of the barber

Introduction to Facial Hair Design

In addition to cutting and styling hair, barbers and barber-stylists should be able to offer clients a full range of services for grooming facial hair. Unlike some decades of the past, men do not have to wait for fashion trends to decide to grow their mustaches or beards. Because today's style is one of individuality, barbering students should become proficient, or even specialize, in the design and trimming of men's facial hair. The client who wears a mustache and/or beard will frequent a shop that can provide both haircutting and facial hair design services.

The Mustache

The mustache is worn primarily for personal adornment rather than utility, and the wearer is usually very particular about how it is designed and maintained. Care, artistry, and sensitivity to the client's preferences are required for this service. Corrective shaping or redesign of the mustache by the barber helps clients with their daily maintenance and trimming at home until the next visit to the barbershop.

In addition to knowing how to trim and shape mustaches, barbers and barber-stylists should be able to understand and apply certain principles of mustache design.

MUSTACHE DESIGN

Choosing a suitable mustache design depends on the client's facial features, hair growth, and personal taste. As with hairstyling services, facial features are of primary importance in the selection process. The size of the mustache should correspond to the size of the features—such as a large design for heavy features and a smaller design for fine, small facial features.

Important facial characteristics that help to determine the choice of mustache design include width of the mouth; size of the nose; shape of upper lip area; width of the cheeks, jaw, and chin; and density of hair growth. As a general rule, be guided by the client's pattern of hair growth and avoid cutting into natural hairlines too deeply to minimize daily maintenance. Additional guidelines for mustache design and proportion are as follows:

- *Large, coarse facial features:* heavier-looking mustache

- *Prominent nose:* medium to large mustache

- *Long, narrow face:* narrow to medium mustache

- *Extra-large mouth:* pyramid-shaped mustache

- *Extra-small mouth:* medium, short mustache

- *Smallish, regular features:* smaller, triangular mustache

- *Wide mouth with prominent upper lip:* heavier handlebar or large, divided mustache

- *Round face with regular features:* semi-square mustache

- *Square face with prominent features:* heavier, linear mustache with ends slightly curving downwar

Additional mustache services that may be offered with a mustache trim include waxing mustache ends, penciling with temporary color, or coloring for overall color evenness or compatibility with scalp hair color.

Mustache Trim

MATERIALS, IMPLEMENTS, AND EQUIPMENT

- Barber chair with headrest
- Sink
- Sharps container
- Covered trash can
- Covered container for soiled towels
- Haircutting cape
- Terry cloth towels
- Barber's paper towels
- Headrest cover
- Haircutting shears
- Outliner or trimmer
- Straight razor and blades
- Shaving cream or gel
- Comb and brush

PREPARATION

1. Assemble supplies.
2. Wash your hands.

PROCEDURE

1 Drape the client as for a haircut service.

2 Consult with the client regarding shape preferences.

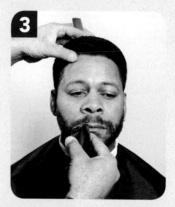

3 Trim the mustache to the desired length with an outliner. Check for evenness of length at the corners of the mouth.

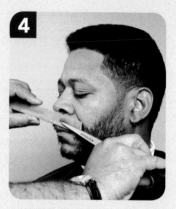

4 For safety, remove bulk from the mustache using the shear-over-comb technique.

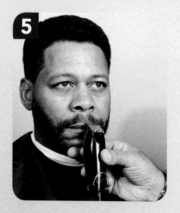

5 Shape the mustache with an outliner. If using a razor, apply shaving cream or gel, wipe off excess product with thumb or finger, and proceed with razor outlining.

CLEAN-UP AND DISINFECTION

1. Cleanse and disinfect all implements.
2. Store soiled towels and papers in appropriate containers.
3. Sanitize work area.
4. Wash your hands.

The Beard

The purpose of a beard or goatee is to balance the facial features and to correlate the proportions of face, head, and body. As with their mustaches, men are usually very particular about the design of their beards. Again, a careful approach, artistry, and sensitivity to the client's preferences are required for this service.

If the client is to receive a haircut service in addition to the beard trim, the decision must be made as to which service will be performed first. This is completely a matter of choice for the barber, as he or she will have his or her own reasons for doing so. Some barbers prefer to cut and style the hair prior to the beard trim so as to better balance the length and fullness of the beard with the hairstyle.

BEARD DESIGN

The correct shaping or design of the beard can emphasize pleasant facial features, minimize less desirable ones, and camouflage flaws. As with other hair design, it is important to develop a good eye for balance and proportion of the beard. Very few individuals have perfectly symmetrical face shapes, so barbers are usually challenged to create an illusion of symmetry. Use the natural hairline in the sideburn, cheek, and mustache areas as a guide. Also use the area under the chin, noting where the direction of hair growth changes, to help determine design options for outlines.

During the first trimming, it is advisable to leave the facial hair slightly longer than the desired end result. This helps to avoid cutting the hair too closely and leaves it long enough for re-trimming toward the end of the beard design service. Beard design and trimming is usually performed with a combination of the shears, comb, outliner and/or clippers, and razor.

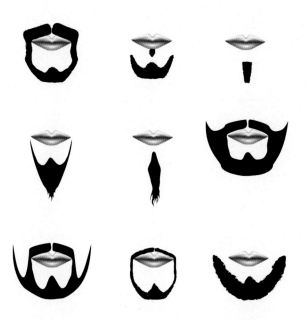

Beard Trim

MATERIALS, IMPLEMENTS, AND EQUIPMENT

- Barber chair with headrest
- Sink
- Sharps container
- Covered trash can
- Covered container for soiled towels
- Haircutting cape
- Terry cloth towels
- Barber's paper towels
- Headrest cover
- Haircutting shears
- Clippers
- Outliner or trimmer
- Straight razor and blades
- Shaving cream or gel
- Comb and brush

PREPARATION

1. Assemble supplies.
2. Wash your hands.

PROCEDURE

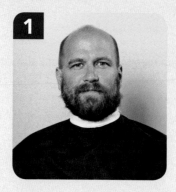

1 Drape the client as for a haircut service.

2 Consult with the client as to his desired design of the beard. Determine any preferences regarding length, density (thickness), and shape.

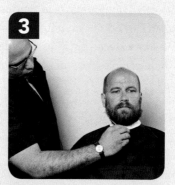

3 With the client in an upright sitting position, gently comb through his beard and check for hidden moles or growths. Study the client's facial features and offer design options. Discuss the client's preferences and reach a final decision about the design.

4 Apply fresh headrest cover. Adjust the headrest so the client's neck is supported while leaning his head back. The chair back may also be reclined at a slight angle, depending on your preference for reaching areas under the chin.

5 Place a towel underneath the chin to protect the client's neck from stray hairs (optional).

6 Trim excess hair using shear-over-comb or clipper-over-comb technique.

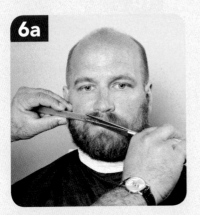

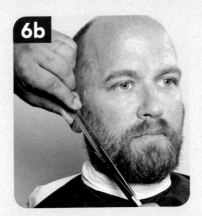

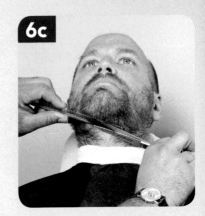

7 There are several approaches that can be used to create a design line with the outliner; all three methods are correct and depend only on personal preference and the characteristics of the beard you are working with.

a. Start in the center directly under the chin and outline the under part of the beard. Work to your left (client's right side) toward the back of the jaw and then from center to your right (client's left side). Move to the client's right side and cut in the design from the sideburn down to the guide created at the back of the jaw. Repeat on the left side.

b. Start at the right or left side in the sideburn area and angle the design line from the earlobe, working down to the jaw area. Continue cutting in the design line under the chin and around to the opposite sideburn.

c. Start at the right or left side in the sideburn area and angle the design line from the earlobe, working down to the back of the jaw. Repeat on the opposite side. Next, establish a guide in the center under the chin. Cut in the design line from the center to one side and connect with the guide at the back of the jaw. Repeat on the other side.

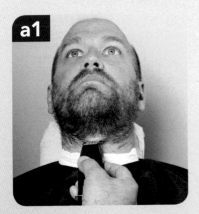

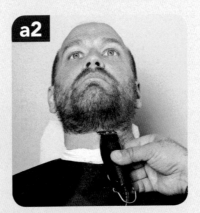

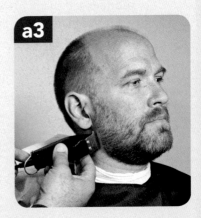

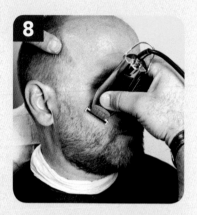

8 Outline the cheek and upper areas of the beard, blending with the sideburn area. Note: This procedure may be performed prior step 7 if desired.

9 Using the shear-over-comb or clipper-over-comb technique, taper and blend the beard from the outlined areas up to just under the bottom lip, mustache, and cheek areas.

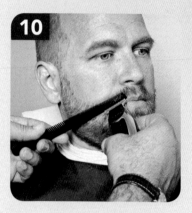

10 Trim and blend the mustache into the beard using shear, clipper, or outliner-over-comb technique.

11 Recline client, apply steam towel, lather areas to be shaved, shave carefully at the outline, and wipe clean.

12 Return client to sitting position.

13 Wipe off any remaining lather with a warm towel. Apply aftershave or tonic lotion.

14 Remember to check the proportion and shape of the beard in the mirror when the client is returned to a sitting position. Retouch the beard design with shears or outliner wherever necessary.

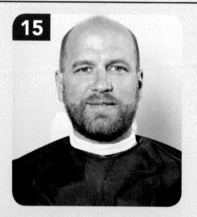

15 Style or cut the hair as needed for a finished look.

CLEAN-UP AND DISINFECTION

1. Cleanse and disinfect all implements.

2. Store soiled towels and papers in appropriate containers.

3. Sanitize work area.

4. Wash your hands.

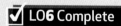
LO**6** Complete

MUSTACHE AND BEARD DESIGNING

In some cases, your client may desire more than a beard trim—he may desire
a whole new look! Such a request requires the barber to create a new beard
design that will complement and balance the structure of the client's face.

DESIGN ON STRAIGHT HAIR TEXTURE

Figures 14-15 to **14-25** show the process of creating a new mustache and
beard design from the design in Procedure 14-4.

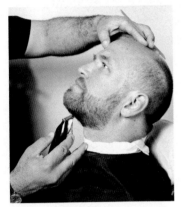

▲ FIGURE 14-15

Establish new design line from center.

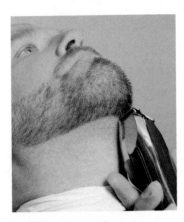

▲ FIGURE 14-16

New design line - front view.

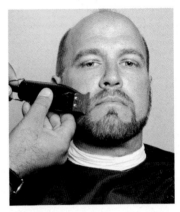

▲ FIGURE 14-17

Re-design chin and mustache areas.

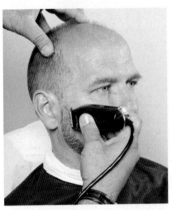

▲ FIGURE 14-18

Cut in new design line in cheek areas.

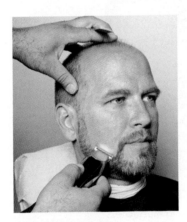

▲ FIGURE 14-19

Remove excess hair in cheek areas.

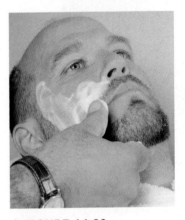

▲ FIGURE 14-20

Application of shaving cream.

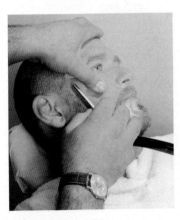

▲ FIGURE 14-21

Shaving sideburn outline.

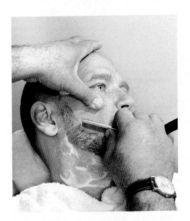

▲ FIGURE 14-22

Shaving cheek area.

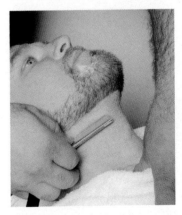

▲ FIGURE 14-23

Completion of shaving area No. 5.

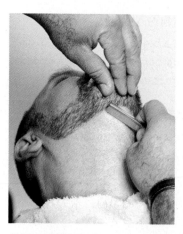

▲ FIGURE 14-24
Shaving area No. 12.

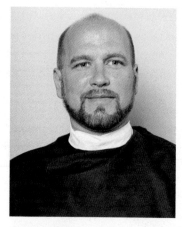

▲ FIGURE 14-25
Finished design.

DESIGN ON CURLY HAIR TEXTURE

Figures 14-26 to **14-36** start with a mustache and beard trim on curly hair and progress through to a mustache and goatee design. Note the three different design options that are shown in this progression.

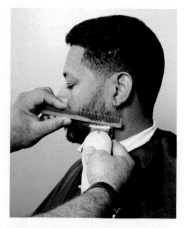

▲ FIGURE 14-26
Trimming excess hair using clipper-over-comb techinque.

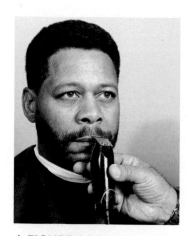

▲ FIGURE 14-27
Trimming mustache.

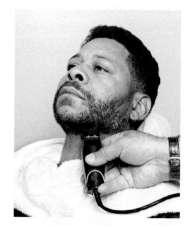

▲ FIGURE 14-28
Establishing design line under chin.

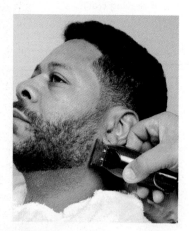

▲ FIGURE 14-29
Establishing design line at jaw and sideburn areas.

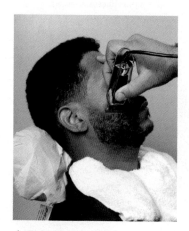

▲ FIGURE 14-30
Establishing design line in cheek areas.

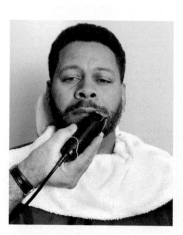

▲ FIGURE 14-31
Contouring mustache design line. End of Design No. 1.

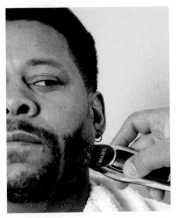

▲ FIGURE 14-32
Removing side hair to create a full goatee.

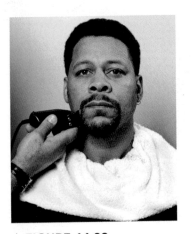

▲ FIGURE 14-33
Fine-tuning full goatee design line. End of Design No. 2.

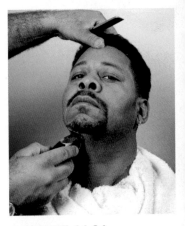

▲ FIGURE 14-34
Removing hair to create a chin goatee and patch.

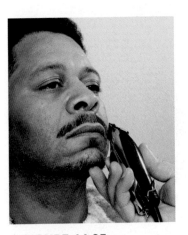

▲ FIGURE 14-35
Fine-tuning corners of mustache.

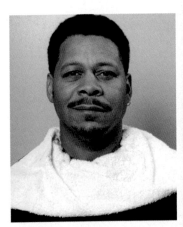

▲ FIGURE 14-36
Finished Design No. 3.

DESIGN ON COARSE, WIRY HAIR

Figures 14-37 to **14-44** show the basic steps for a mustache and beard design on coarse, wiry hair.

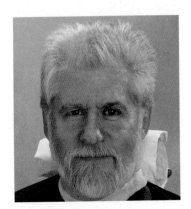

▲ FIGURE 14-37
Client before beard trim.

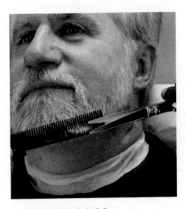

▲ FIGURE 14-38
Trim excess hair.

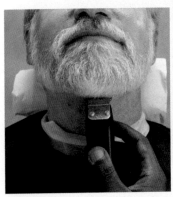

▲ FIGURE 14-39
Create a design line with outliner.

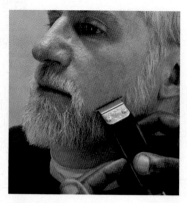

▲ FIGURE 14-40

Outline the cheek areas of the beard.

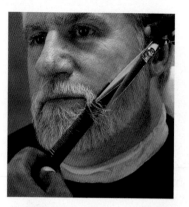

▲ FIGURE 14-41

Blend from outlined areas to mustache.

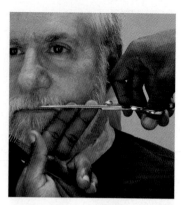

▲ FIGURE 14-42

Trim mustache.

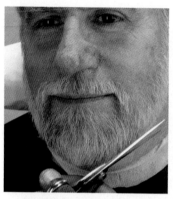

▲ FIGURE 14-43

Complete detail finish work on beard with shears.

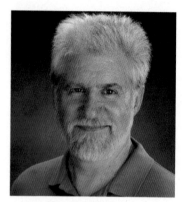

▲ FIGURE 14-44

Completed beard trim.

DESIGN ON MEDIUM TEXTURED HAIR

Figures 14-45 to 14-52 show the basic steps for a mustache and beard design on medium textured hair.

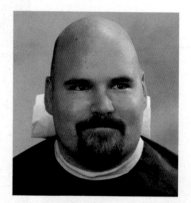

▲ FIGURE 14-45

Client before beard design.

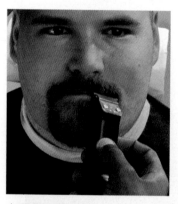

▲ FIGURE 14-46

Establish mustache length.

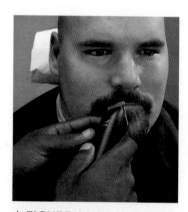

▲ FIGURE 14-47

Shape mustache from center to corner.

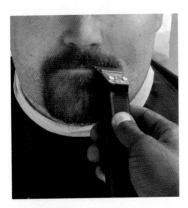

▲ FIGURE 14-48
Shape corner and ends of mustache.

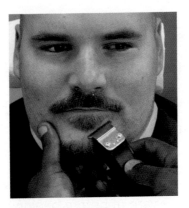

▲ FIGURE 14-49
Shape patch area under bottom lip (optional).

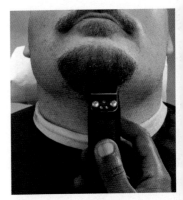

▲ FIGURE 14-50
Establish goatee design line.

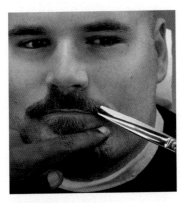

▲ FIGURE 14-51
Complete detail finish work on mustache, patch, and goatee with shears.

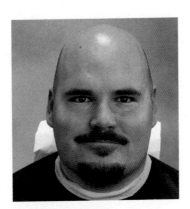

▲ FIGURE 14-52
Finished mustache and goatee design.

CLIPPERS, COMB, AND OUTLINER METHOD

Clippers may also be used for beard trimming, especially if one overall length is desired. Clipper-cut beard trims are most successful on clients whose beards are of an even density and texture. This is important to note because sometimes all-over-even cutting may produce whorls or patches, especially in wavy hair.

Some beard designs may require the use of a detachable-blade clipper to create uniform length throughout the beard. Follow steps 1 through 8 in Procedure 14-4. Then choose a blade size that leaves the hair close to the length of the client's beard. If more than a light trim is required, select the next size blade that will cut the hair to a shorter length. Repeat as required until the desired length is achieved. Always follow up with shears, outliner, and/or razor for final trimming and detail work.

The tremendous variety of mustache and beard designs is limited only by the creativity and expertise of the barber. Perfecting these skills will help you to meet the service requests of your clients while providing you with an additional outlet for creative design.

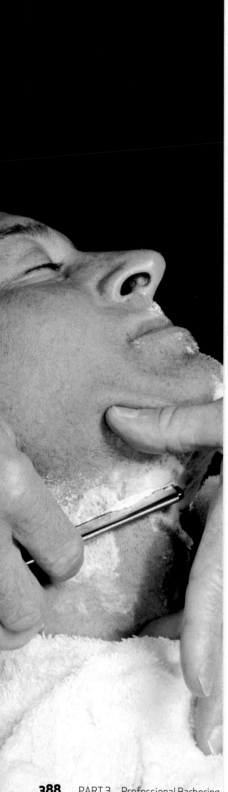

14 Review
Questions

1. Identify three client characteristics that barbers should be aware of before beginning the shave service.

2. List the steps to prepare the client for a shave.

3. What effect does shaving cream have on facial hair?

4. Describe the most effective way to rub lather into the beard.

5. What effect do hot towels have on facial hair?

6. Identify several skin conditions that may prohibit the application of hot steam towels.

7. Identify the four razor-holding positions.

8. What three razor-holding strokes are used in facial shaving?

9. Shaving strokes should be performed in what relation to the grain of the hair?

10. Identify the number of shaving areas on the face.

11. Explain the difference between a standard shave and a once-over shave.

12. List the finishing steps of a facial shave.

13. Identify at what step of the shave a facial might be suggested to the client.

14. Explain how a close shave differs from a standard shave and why it may be undesirable.

15. List important characteristics used to determine a mustache design.

16. Explain why some barbers prefer to cut and style the hair before performing a beard trim service.

Chapter
Glossary

backhand razor position and stroke used in 4 of the 14 basic shaving areas: Nos. 2, 6, 7, and 9

close shaving the procedure of shaving facial hair against the grain during the second-time-over shave

cutting stroke the correct angle of cutting the beard with a straight razor

first-time-over-shave first part of the standard shave consisting of shaving 14 areas of the face; followed by the second-time-over shave to remove residual missed or rough spots

freehand razor position and stroke used in 6 of the 14 shaving areas: Nos. 1, 3, 4, 8, 11, and 12

neck shave shaving the areas behind the ears, down the sides of the neck, and at the back neckline

once-over shave single-lather shave in which the shaving strokes are made across the grain of the hair

reverse backhand razor position and stroke used for making the left sideburn outline and shaving the left side behind the ear during a neck shave

reverse freehand razor position and stroke used in 4 of the 14 basic shaving areas: Nos. 5, 10, 13, and 14

second-time-over shave follows a regular shave to remove any rough or uneven spots using water instead of lather; may be considered a form of close shaving

styptic powder alum powder used to stop bleeding of nicks and cuts

15 Men's
HAIRCUTTING AND STYLING

CHAPTER OUTLINE

- ▶ The Client Consultation
- ▶ Basic Principles of Haircutting and Styling
- ▶ Fundamentals of Haircutting
- ▶ Haircutting Techniques
- ▶ Practice Sessions 1–10
- ▶ Procedures 15-1 to 15-10
- ▶ Introduction to Men's Hairstyling
- ▶ Safety Precautions for Haircutting and Styling

✓ Learning Objectives

AFTER COMPLETING THIS CHAPTER, YOU SHOULD BE ABLE TO:

1 Discuss the art and science of men's haircutting and styling.

2 Discuss the term *envisioning* and the importance of the client consultation.

3 Discuss facial shapes and anatomical features.

4 Identify and name the sections of the head as applied to haircutting.

5 Understand the fundamental terms used in haircutting.

6 Demonstrate basic cutting techniques: fingers-and-shear, shear-over-comb, freehand shear cutting, freehand clipper cutting, clipper-over-comb, and razor cutting.

7 Demonstrate shaving the outline areas.

8 Demonstrate disinfection procedures.

9 Demonstrate basic hairstyling techniques.

10 Discuss safety precautions used in haircutting and styling.

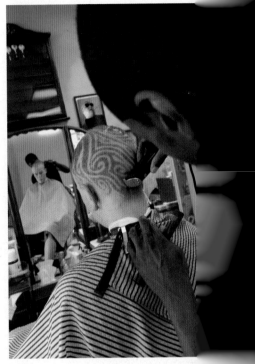

Key Terms

PAGE NUMBER INDICATES WHERE IN THE CHAPTER THE TERM IS USED.

angle / 398

arching technique / 410

blow-dry styling / 471

clipper-over-comb / 412

crest / 396

cutting above the fingers / 403

cutting below the fingers / 403

cutting line / 400

design line / 401

diagonal / 398

elevation / 399

envisioning / 393

facial shape / 393

fingers-and-shear / 403

freehand clipper cutting / 412

freehand shear cutting / 410

freehand slicing / 424

guide / 401

hair-locking / 477

horizontal / 398

layers / 401

outlining / 402

over-direction / 402

parietal ridge / 396

part / 400

parting / 400

projection / 399

razor-over-comb / 424

razor rotation / 425

reference points / 396

rolling the comb out / 409

shear-over-comb / 407

shear-point tapering / 410

stationary guide / 401

tapered / 401

tension / 402

texturizing / 402

thinning / 402

traveling guide / 401

vertical / 398

weight line / 402

The art of haircutting involves individualized and precise designing, cutting, and shaping of the hair. Mastering this art requires the competent use of a variety of tools, implements, techniques, and methods to achieve the desired result.

A good haircut is the foundation of a good hairstyle. The importance of this simple truth cannot be overstressed. Thorough instruction in the proper way to cut, blend, and taper the hair using clippers, shears, and razors provides the basics of this skill. Practice and application under an instructor's guidance are necessary for the achievement and refinement of those basic skills while in school. Later, when working in the barbershop, each client will present new challenges and learning opportunities that form the basis for future success.

The hairstyle, and therefore the haircut, should accentuate the client's best features and minimize the weakest ones. Hairstyle design requires the barber to consider the client's head shape, facial contour, neckline, and hair texture. The barber also needs to be guided by the client's preferences, personality, and lifestyle as well.

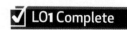

The Client Consultation

A thorough client consultation helps to eliminate any guesswork about the haircut or style to be performed and provides the perfect opportunity to perform the scalp and hair analysis. This is the time when the barber must determine just what it is the client is asking for in the way of a haircut or style. Phrases such as "a little off the top" or "over the ears" are not specific enough for haircutting purposes. How is "a little" measured? Is it a quarter inch or one inch? Does "over the ears" mean covering the ears or cutting around the ears? These interpretations are just two examples of why the consultation is so important to both the client and the barber.

Once the client has been seated and draped, the barber should be analyzing the client's hair and scalp during the conversation that leads to knowing what the client desires in the way of a service. This is the time to discover scalp conditions that may prohibit moving forward with the service, hair conditions that may require special conditioning or treatment, or hair texture and density issues that limit or enhance cutting and styling options. With this information the barber can make a professional judgment about what can or cannot be done in terms of services and the client's expectations.

Some basic questions that can be asked before the actual cutting begins that will assist the barber in envisioning the desired results include:

- *How long has it been since your last haircut?*

  Knowing that the average hair growth is about $\frac{1}{2}$" per month allows the barber to envision the preferred length of the hair before it grew out and needed to be cut again.

- *Do you prefer a similar style or are you looking for something new?*

  The answer to this question can lead the barber directly to the cutting stage or to further discussion with the client about appropriate styles and options.

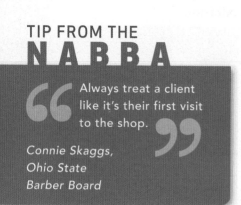

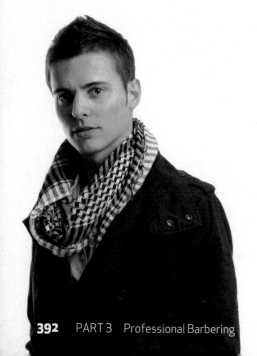

- *What is your usual morning routine (shampoo, blow-dry, etc.)?*

  The answer will indicate how much time the client is willing to spend on hair care.

- *Are you having any particular problems with your previous cut or style?*

  This question provides an opportunity to open dialogue about specific hair-related issues such as problem areas, length, fullness, growth and wave patterns, hair texture, density, and color.

Additional consultation questions should lead to answers that help the barber to determine the length of the sideburns, the shape of the neckline, and whether or not the client desires a neck shave, eyebrow trim, or other services. With practice and experience, barbers learn to ask specific questions that help to provide a clearer picture of the haircut or style the client desires.

Envisioning is the process of picturing or visualizing in your mind the finished cut and style based on what the client has told you. With the information gained through the consultation, the barber is better able to visualize the client's expectations of the haircutting service. It is essential to achieve this understanding *before* beginning the haircut.

Basic Principles of Haircutting and Styling

Each haircut is a representation and advertisement of the barber's work. Remember, a good haircut is the foundation of a good hairstyle!

Hairstyling has been defined as the artistic cutting and dressing of hair to best fit the client's physical needs and personality. Pay attention to details such as client comfort, sideburn length, outlines, balance, and proportion. The consultation should provide sufficient information about the client's lifestyle and personality to suggest a suitable style, but a study of facial shapes assists the barber in determining the *best* style for a client's features.

☑ **LO2 Complete**

FACIAL SHAPES

The **facial shape** of each individual is determined by the position and prominence of the facial bones. There are seven general facial shapes: oval, round, inverted triangular, square, pear-shaped, oblong, and diamond. In order to recognize each facial shape and then be able to give correct advice, barbers should be acquainted with the outstanding characteristics of each type. With this information, the barber can suggest a haircut and style that complements the facial shape, similar to the way that certain clothes flatter the body.

The following facial shapes should constitute a guide for choosing an appropriate style.

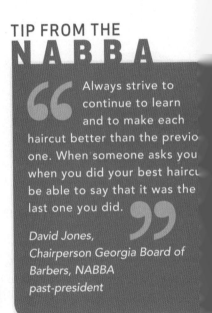

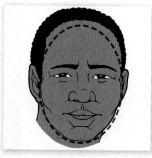

▲ FIGURE 15-1

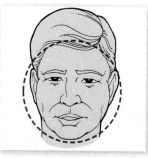

▲ FIGURE 15-2

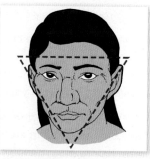

▲ FIGURE 15-3

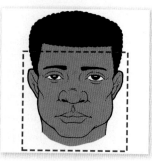

▲ FIGURE 15-4

Oval: The oval-shaped face is generally recognized as the ideal shape. Any hairstyle that maintains the oval shape is usually suitable (Figure 15-1). Try changing the part. Experiment, but keep in mind elements such as the client's lifestyle, comfort, and ease of maintenance.

Round: The aim here is to slim the face. Hair that is too short will emphasize fullness, so create some height on the top to lengthen the look of the face (Figure 15-2). An off-center part and some waves at eye level will also help lessen the full appearance of the face. Beards should be styled to make the face appear oval.

Inverted triangular: The potential problems with this facial shape are over-wide cheekbones and a narrow jaw line (Figure 15-3). Keep the hair close at the crown and temples and longer in back, or try changing the part and the direction of the hair. A full beard helps to fill out the narrow jaw.

Square: To minimize the angular features at the forehead, use wavy bangs that blend into the temples. This softens the square forehead and draws attention to a strong jaw (Figure 15-4). If a beard is worn, it should be styled to slenderize the face.

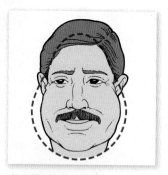

▲ FIGURE 15-5

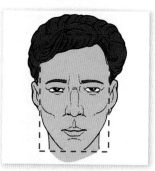

▲ FIGURE 15-6

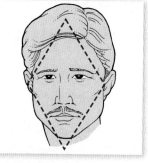

▲ FIGURE 15-7

Pear-shaped: This shape is narrow at the top and wide on the bottom (Figure 15-5). Create width and fullness at the top, temples, and sides to produce balance. Short, full styles are best, ending just above the jaw line where it joins the ear area. A body wave or medium-size curl perm is another way to achieve width at the top. If a beard is worn, it should be styled to slenderize the lower jaw.

Oblong: The long face needs to be visually shortened and the angularity hidden (Figure 15-6). Layered bangs brushed to the sides over the temples can camouflage or hide the front hairline, giving the illusion of a short facial shape. Wearing a mustache also helps to shorten the look of a longer face shape.

Diamond: The aim here is to fill out the face at the temples and chin and keep hair close to the head at the widest points (Figure 15-7). Deep, full bangs give a broad appearance to the forehead and a fuller back section adds width. A full, square, or rounded beard is also appropriate.

PROFILES

Always be aware of the client's profile since it can influence the appropriateness of a haircut or style for that particular individual.

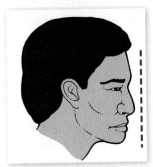

▲ FIGURE 15-8

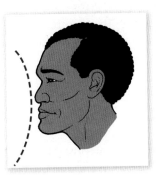

▲ FIGURE 15-9

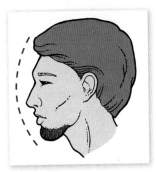

▲ FIGURE 15-10

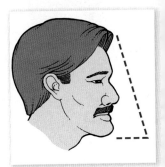

▲ FIGURE 15-11

Straight profiles tend to be the most balanced and can usually wear most hairstyles successfully (Figure 15-8).

Concave profiles require a close hair arrangement over the forehead to minimize the bulge of the forehead (Figure 15-9).

Convex profiles require some balance, so arrange the top front hair over the forehead to conceal a short, receding forehead (Figure 15-10). A beard or goatee minimizes a receding chin.

Angular profiles also have receding foreheads, but the chin tends to jut forward (Figure 15-11). Arrange the top front hair over the forehead to create more balance. A short beard and mustache help to minimize the protruding chin.

NOSE SHAPE

The shape of the nose influences the profile and should be studied both in profile and from a full-face view.

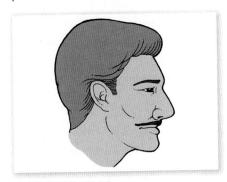

▲ FIGURE 15-12

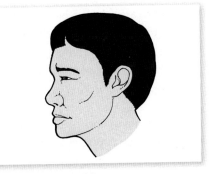

▲ FIGURE 15-13

Prominent nose shapes include a hooked nose, large nose, or pointed nose (Figure 15-12). Bring the hair forward at the forehead and back at the sides to minimize the prominence of the nose.

Turned-up nose shapes can usually wear shorter haircut styles because the size or heavy features associated with prominent nose shapes are not an issue (Figure 15-13). Experiment with combing the hair from different part lines, or comb the hair back on the sides.

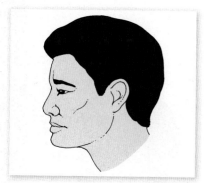

▲ FIGURE 15-14

Long neck.

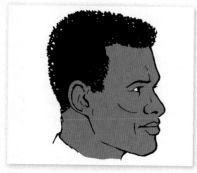

▲ FIGURE 15-15

Short neck.

NECK LENGTHS

The length of the neck is also a factor in determining the overall shape of the haircut and style. In most cases it is advisable to follow the client's natural hairline when designing a style; however, sometimes an overly long or very short neck limits the options. The length, density, growth pattern, and natural partings of the hair should be considered when deciding on a style that best complements the client's neck length.

Long necks are minimized when the hair is left fuller or longer at the nape **(Figure 15-14)**.

Short necks are best served by leaving the neck exposed to create an appearance of length **(Figure 15-15)**. Work with the natural hairline and perform a tapered cut that creates the illusion of a longer nape and neck area.

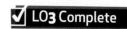

Fundamentals of Haircutting

The fundamental principles of haircutting should be thoroughly understood. The same general techniques are used in cutting, shaping, tapering, and blending men and women's hair. The differences between the two are usually evident in the overall design line, the contour or shape (which includes volume), and the finished style. The fundamental principles of haircutting pertain to the head form, basic haircutting terms, and different haircutting techniques.

THE HEAD FORM

In order to create consistent and successful results in haircutting, it is necessary to understand the shape of the head. Hair responds differently in different areas of the head because of the curves and changes from one section to the next. The ability to visualize these sections will assist student barbers in the development of individual cutting patterns, help to eliminate technical mistakes, reduce confusion during the haircutting process, and facilitate easier checking of the final result.

When designing and cutting hair, the barber should envision the sections of the head as depicted in **Figures 15-16** through **15-18**. These sections include the front, top (apex), temporal (crest), crown, sides, sideburns, back, and nape.

Reference points are points on the head that mark areas where the surface of the head changes or the behavior of the hair changes as a result of the surface changes. These points are used to establish proportionate design lines and contours.

- The **parietal ridge** is also known as the **crest**, *temporal*, *horseshoe*, or *hatband* area of the head. It is the widest section of the head, starting at the temples and ending just below the crown. When a comb is placed flat against the head at the sides,

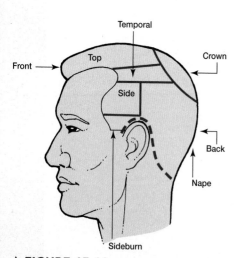

▲ FIGURE 15-16

Diagram of sections of head, side view.

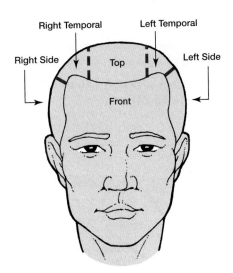

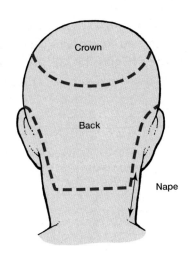

▲ FIGURE 15-17

Diagram of sections of head, front view.

▲ FIGURE 15-18

Diagram of sections of head, back view.

the parietal ridge begins where the head starts to curve away from the comb (**Figure 15-19**). The parietal ridge is one of the most important sections of the head when cutting hair because it serves as a transition area from the top to the front, sides, and back sections.

- The occipital bone protrudes at the base of the skull. When a comb is placed flat against the nape area, the occipital begins where the head curves away from the comb (**Figure 15-20**).

- The apex is the highest point on the top of the head (**Figure 15-21**).

- The four corners are located by crossing two diagonal lines at the apex (**Figure 15-22**). The lines will point to the front and back corners of the head.

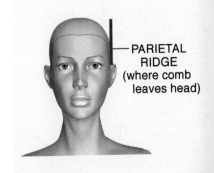

▲ FIGURE 15-19

The parietal ridge.

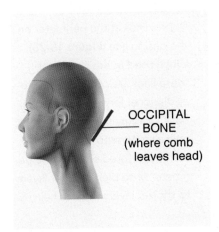

▲ FIGURE 15-20

The occipital bone.

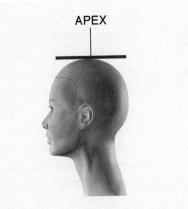

▲ FIGURE 15-21

The apex.

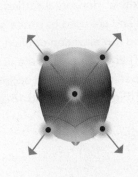

▲ FIGURE 15-22

The four corners.

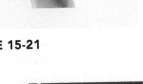

BASIC TERMS USED IN HAIRCUTTING

A *line* is simply a series of connected dots that result in a continuous mark. Straight and curved lines are used in haircutting to create design, shape, and direction (**Figure 15-23**). The three types of straight lines used in haircutting are horizontal, vertical, and diagonal lines (**Figure 15-24**).

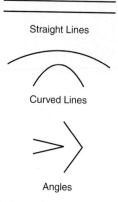

Straight Lines

Curved Lines

Angles

▲ FIGURE 15-23

Lines and angles.

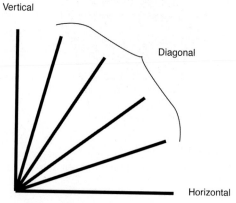

Vertical

Diagonal

Horizontal

▲ FIGURE 15-24

Horizontal, vertical, and diagonal lines.

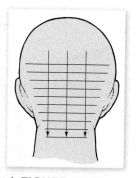

▲ FIGURE 15-25

Weight line at perimeter.

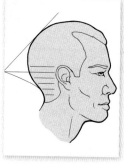

▲ FIGURE 15-26

Weight line at occipital.

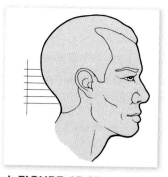

▲ FIGURE 15-27

Vertical partings facilitate layering.

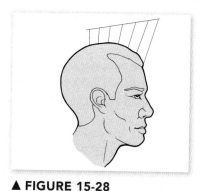

▲ FIGURE 15-28

Diagonal line within top front sections.

Horizontal lines are parallel to the horizon or floor and direct the eye from one side to the other. Horizontal cutting lines build weight and are used to create a one-length look and low elevation or blunt haircut designs. These *weight lines* are usually created at the perimeter or at the occipital area of a haircut (**Figures 15-25** and **15-26**).

Vertical lines are perpendicular to the floor and are described in terms of up and down. Vertical partings facilitate the projection of the hair at higher elevations while cutting. Vertical cutting lines remove weight within the cut and create layers that may be used to cut from short to long, long to short, or uniformly depending on finger placement (**Figure 15-27**).

Diagonal lines have a slanted direction and are used to create sloped lines at the perimeter on the design line (**Figure 15-28**). When used at the perimeter, these lines are often referred to as diagonal forward or diagonal back. Diagonal finger placement may also be used to create a stacked, layered effect at the perimeter or to blend longer layers to shorter layers within a haircut.

An **angle** is the space between two lines or surfaces that intersect at a given point. Angles help to create strong, consistent foundations in haircutting and are used in two different ways. Angles can refer to the degree of elevation at which the hair is held for cutting—for example, "angle the hair section at a 45-degree projection from the head"; or it can refer to the position of the fingers when cutting a section of hair (cutting line), as in "using a vertical parting, angle the fingers 45 degrees from the hairline to the occipital" (see Figure 15-32).

Elevation is the angle or degree at which a section of hair is held from the head for cutting, *relative from where it grows.* Elevation, also known as **projection,** is the result of lifting the hair section above 0 elevation, or natural fall. This projection of the hair while cutting produces graduation or layers and is usually described in terms of degrees **(Figure 15-29)**.

- *Zero elevation* is the lowest elevation and produces weight, bulk, and maximum length at the perimeter of a hair design.

- To perform a 0- elevation cut, a parting is made in the section to be cut **(Figure 15-30)**. After combing the hair straight down from where it grows, it is cut either against the skin (as in the nape or around-the-ear areas) or as it is held straight down between the fingers. Both stationary and horizontal traveling guides are used to create the design or perimeter line. The design line then serves as a guide for all subsequent partings that will be brought to the design (perimeter) line for cutting. This technique creates crisp, clean lines around the hairline on shorter hairstyles and achieves the standard "blunt cut" on longer hair.

- Holding the hair at *45 degrees* from where it grows is considered to be a medium elevation. Medium elevation or graduation creates layered ends or "stacking" within the parting of hair from the 0-degree distance to the 45-degree position. Movement and texture are created within the distance between the two degrees, depending on the length of the hair and the position of the angle in relation to the head form.

- Both stationary and horizontal traveling guides are used to achieve the graduated or stacked effect **(Figure 15-31)**. Use of a vertical parting projected at 45 degrees, with the fingers holding the parting angled at a 45-degree diagonal, will create a tapered effect **(Figure 15-32)**.

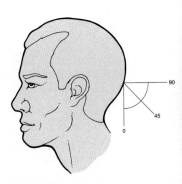

▲ FIGURE 15-29
Elevations relative to the head form.

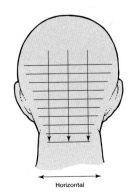

▲ FIGURE 15-30
Horizontal, zero elevation.

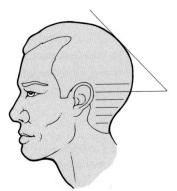

▲ FIGURE 15-31
Horizontal, 45-degree elevation.

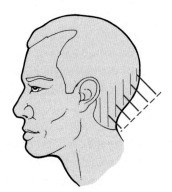

▲ FIGURE 15-32
Vertical parting with 45-degree finger placement.

- A *90-degree* elevation is the most common projection used in men's haircutting. It produces layering, tapering, and blended effects. When using a 90-degree elevation, the hair is held straight out from the head from where it grows. This requires a traveling guide in order to move around and over the curves of the entire head. Lengths in various sections of the head can vary, but the hair will still be blended overall. This is considered to be a high-elevation cut. A 90-degree elevation is used to create uniform layers as depicted in **Figure 15-33a**, where the each section of hair is the same length, or a tapered cut where hair is shorter at the nape and increasingly longer toward the top.

- To create a tapered effect like the one shown in **Figure 15-33b**, the hair is held from a vertical parting and cut closer to the head form in the nape and around-the-ear areas at a 90-degree projection. This requires positioning the fingers at a 45-degree angle from the hairline to hold the hair to be cut and then gradually repositioning the fingers in increments from perpendicular (to the floor) to beyond perpendicular to follow the curve of the head as the hair is blended into the crest and top sections.

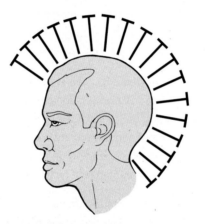

▲ FIGURE 15-33a
Uniform 90-degree layers.

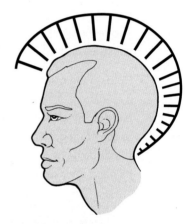

▲ FIGURE 15-33b
90-degree taper.

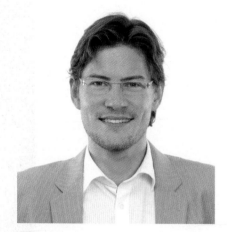

A **part** is a line that divides the hair at the scalp, separating one section of the hair from another. Parts or partings are used to create subsections to gain control of the hair while cutting. The position and direction of a *natural part* is determined by the direction or slant the hair takes as it leaves the follicle.

A **parting** is a smaller section of hair, usually $\frac{1}{4}$" to $\frac{1}{2}$" thick, parted off from a larger section of hair. The use of partings is essential to maintain control of the hair in manageable proportions and to perform precision cutting. Partings may be held horizontally, vertically, or diagonally, with a usual projection range of 0 to 180 degrees. The way that a parting is sectioned off from a subsection and held depends on the desired effect to be achieved.

The **cutting line** is the position of the fingers when cutting a section of hair. Because the shears follow the position and angle of the fingers when cutting, finger placement should be checked before cutting to avoid cutting in an unwanted line design (such as diagonal rather than horizontal), losing the guide, or cutting off too much hair.

The **design line** is the outer perimeter line of the haircut. It may act as a guide depending on the overall design of the haircut and the method the barber uses to achieve it. A design line can be reflected in the hanging length of a blunt or long-layered cut, along the hairline of a short cut, or along any haircut perimeter (**Figures 15-34a** and **15-34b**).

A **guide**, also known as a guideline or guide strand, is a cut that is made by which subsequent partings or sections of hair will be measured and cut. Guides are classified as being either stationary or traveling. Both types may originate at the outer perimeter (design line) of the hair or at an interior section, usually the crown area. Most haircuts are achieved by using a combination of the two types of guides.

- A **stationary guide** is used for overall one-length-looking designs at the perimeter, such as a solid-form blunt cut, or for maintaining the length of one section while subsequent partings are brought from other sections to meet it for cutting, producing either an overall long layered effect or extra length within a section (**Figure 15-35**).

- A **traveling guide** moves along a section of hair as each cut is made. Once the length of the initial guide has been cut, a parting is taken from in front of it or near it, combed with the original guide, and cut. Then a new parting is taken, combed with the second parting of hair, and cut against that guide. It is this use of the previous guide to cut a subsequent parting of hair that makes it a traveling guide. Care must be taken not to re-cut the original or subsequent guides as the barber moves along the section to cut a new parting. When performed properly, the traveling guide ensures even layering and blending of the hair from one section to another. Refer to Figures 15-33a and 15-33b.

Traveling guides are used internally within the cut to create blended layers; they are also used to finish perimeter designs after the hair is cut to the desired length from one section to another. For example, although a stationary guide is used when establishing the length at the perimeter, it becomes a traveling guide when subsequent cuts are made from left to right or right to left around the head form.

Layers are produced by cutting interior sections of the hair and can originate from the front, top (apex), crown, or perimeter (usually the design line). Layering can be angled (shorter on top and longer at the perimeter), uniform (even throughout), or fully tapered (longer on top and shorter at the perimeter) to blend or create fullness and/or a feathered effect.

Tapered, or tapering, means that the hair conforms to the shape of the head and is shorter at the nape and longer in the crown and top areas. Most men's haircut styles require some form of tapering, and blending of all of the hair lengths is extremely important (see Figure 15-33b).

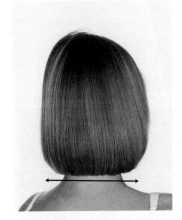

▲ **FIGURE 15-34a**
Horizontal blunt cut design line.

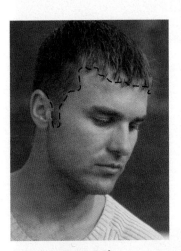

▲ **FIGURE 15-34b**
Short haircut design line.

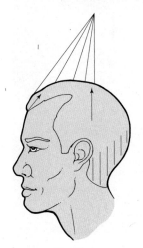

▲ **FIGURE 15-35**
Stationary guide.

A **weight line** refers to the heaviest perimeter area of a 0-elevation or 45-degree cut. It is achieved by using a stationary guide at the perimeter and may be cut in at a variety of levels on the head, depending on the style. In men's haircutting, weight lines may be used in combination with a tapered nape area or for longer hairstyles that *look* to be one length.

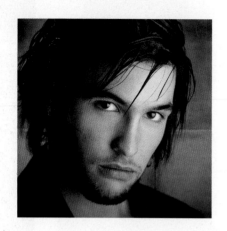

Texturizing is performed after the overall cut has been completed. Thinning or notching shears or razors can be used to create wispy or spiky effects within the haircut or along the perimeter.

Tension is the amount of pressure applied while combing and holding a section of hair for cutting. Tension ranges from minimum to maximum as a result of the amount of stretching employed when holding the hair between the fingers and the spacing between the teeth of the comb. For example, fine-toothed combs facilitate more tension while combing than wide-toothed combs.

- Use maximum tension on straight hair to create precise lines.
- Use minimal to moderate tension on curly and wavy hair as the hair may dry shorter than intended if maximum tension is used.

Thinning refers to removing excess bulk from the hair.

Outlining means marking the outer perimeter of the haircut in the front (optional, depending on hair texture), in front of and over the ears, and at the sides and nape of the neck.

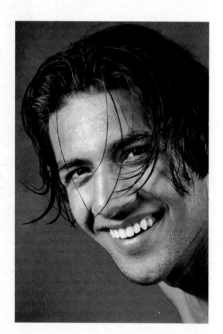

Over-direction creates a length increase in the design and occurs when the hair is combed away from its natural fall position rather than straight out from the head toward a guide. For example, in Figure 15-35, the front section of hair is over-directed back to the stationary guide at the top of the head.

Hairstyling is the art of arranging the hair in a particular style that is appropriately suited to the cut. Hairstyling may involve the use of styling aids such as hair spray, gel, tonic, oil sheen, pomade, or mousse; appliances in the form of blow-dryers or irons; and implements that include brushes, combs, clips, and so forth.

During the course of your barbering career, you will be introduced to a variety of haircutting terms. Terminology for the most part depends on who is presenting the information or technique and whether or not new terms have replaced former terminology. The same holds true for different style names. The important things to remember are that there are only so many angles and elevations used in haircutting; specific effects are created by using specific angles and elevations; and cut and style trends tend to be cyclical in nature. Variations of design will inevitably occur because history has a way of repeating itself in our industry. For example, crew cuts and boxed fades can be traced back to the years of World War II, finger waves were a hit in the 1920s, and braiding has probably been around since humans first walked the earth.

These examples simply reinforce the fact that barbers must become proficient in the basic skills in order to adapt those skills and techniques to whatever the current trend may be.

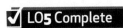

HAIRCUTTING TECHNIQUES

In Chapter 6, you were introduced to the correct holding positions for the comb, shears, clippers, and razor. The terms used to describe how we use these basic tools are *fingers-and-shear, shear-over-comb, freehand shear cutting, freehand clipper cutting, clipper-over-comb, razor-over-comb,* and *razor rotation.* It is important to note that almost every haircutting procedure requires a combination of techniques and tools. The most important factors that determine the tools used to achieve the haircut are the client's desired outcome, the texture and density of the hair, and the barber's personal preference. As a professional barber you should be comfortable and skillful with using all the tools of the trade.

Now it is time to begin your practical training in haircutting. Practice the following techniques and procedures to become familiar with different methods of using your tools.

FINGERS-AND-SHEAR TECHNIQUES

A **fingers-and-shear** technique may be used on many hair types from straight to curly. The three basic methods for using fingers-and-shear techniques are cutting on top of the fingers, cutting below the fingers, and cutting palm-to-palm.

NOTE: The blades of the shears should rest flat and flush to the fingers for these positions. Angling the shear blades may cause injury.

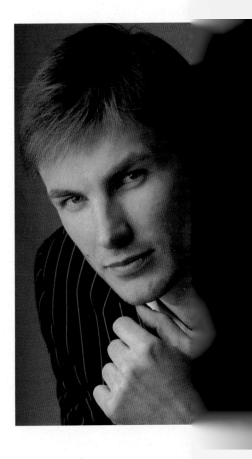

- **Cutting above the fingers** is frequently used in men's haircutting to cut and blend layers in the top, crown, and horseshoe areas (See Figure 15-36). It is also used when cutting hair that is held out at a 90-degree elevation from a vertical parting, such as at the sides and back of the head form (See Figure 15-37). Whether the barber's finger position is perpendicular to the floor or angled at 45 degrees in these sections, the cutting should be performed on the outside (on top of) the fingers.

- **Cutting below the fingers** is most often used to create design lines at the perimeter of the haircut (See Figure 15-38a).

- **Cutting palm-to-palm** may be preferred by some practitioners. Care must be taken not to bend the hair or to project it higher than intended from the head form when using this technique. Also remember that the shears follow finger placement, so avoid curling the fingers inward when cutting unless you want a curved cutting line (Figure 15-38b).

OBJECTIVE:

The objective of this practice session is to introduce you to three forms of finger-and-shear cutting. Only one parting from each of three primary sections of the head will be cut.

Fingers-and-Shear Technique with Mirror

1 Set up a freshly shampooed, conditioned, and combed mannequin in front of the mirror. Pick up the shears and comb in your dominant hand and face the mirror.

2 Palm the shears, comb through the top section of the hair, and create a part on the left side of the mannequin. Comb the hair over the top to the right. At the front part of the crown, position the comb at about a 45-degree angle relative to the surface of the head. Use the first few teeth of the comb to part off a $\frac{1}{4}$" thick parting. Comb the hair in front of the parting forward and away from you. With the teeth of the comb facing you, comb through the parting with the first two fingers of the opposite hand underneath the comb as you position the parting just below eye level at a 90-degree elevation. Leave about an inch of hair extending beyond your fingers. The fingers and comb should be in a horizontal position parallel to the floor (**Figure 15-36**).

3 Palm the comb in the opposite hand while simultaneously positioning the shears at the tip of the fingers holding the hair section. Check the position of your fingers and shears for parallel placement. Cut the hair projecting from between your fingers from the tips no further than the second knuckle. Be conscious of how you open and close the shears along your fingers as you cut the hair that extends beyond them. This fingers-and-shear placement will be used to cut 90-degree layers within the sections of the head form.

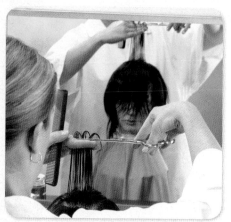

▲ FIGURE 15-36

Cutting above the fingers using a horizontal parting.

Fingers-and-Shear Technique with Mirror: Cutting Above the Fingers Vertically on the Right Side

1 Set up a freshly shampooed, conditioned, and combed mannequin in front of the mirror. Pick up the shears and comb in your dominant hand and face the mirror.

2 Palm the shears, comb through the hair, and make a part at the top of the crest on the right side of the mannequin. Comb the hair over the top to the left. Comb down through the hair on the right side and part off a $\frac{1}{4}$" thick vertical parting. With the teeth of comb facing you in a vertical position, comb through the vertical section of hair with the fingers of the opposite hand following underneath the teeth of the comb to position the hair at just below eye level at a vertical 90-degree elevation. Leave about an inch of hair extending beyond your fingers. The tips of the fingers holding the hair should be pointing downward. Both the fingers and comb should be in a vertical position, perpendicular to the floor.

3 Palm the comb in the opposite hand while simultaneously positioning the tips of the shears on top of the tips of the fingers holding the hair section. Your fingers and shears should be vertical and parallel to each other as the cutting begins **(Figure 15-37)**. Cut the hair projecting from between your fingers from the tips no further than the second knuckle. Be conscious of how you open and close the shears along your fingers as you cut. This fingers-and-shear placement will be used to cut 90-degree vertical layers within sections of the head form, using the perimeter for a guide.

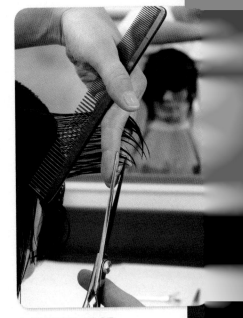

▲ **FIGURE 15-37**
Cutting above the fingers using a vertical parting.

Fingers-and-Shear Technique with Mirror: Cutting Below the Fingers at the Nape

1 Set up a freshly shampooed, conditioned, and combed mannequin in front of the mirror. Pick up the shears and comb in your dominant hand and face the mirror.

2 Palm the shears and part off the hair into four sections from ear to ear and from front to nape. Use a clip to secure the hair at the sides. Part off a $\frac{1}{4}$" to $\frac{1}{2}$" horizontal parting along the hairline from each back section. Secure the hair remaining above the partings in the back sections with clips. With the teeth of the comb facing downward at a slight angle relative to the hair and the fingers of the opposite hand placed on top of the comb, comb through the partings at the nape with no elevation. Leave about an inch of hair extending beyond your fingers. The fingers and comb should be in a horizontal position.

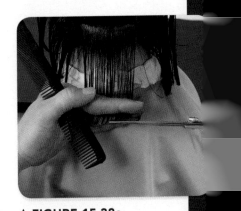

▲ **FIGURE 15-38a**
Cutting below the fingers at the perimeter.

3 Palm the comb in the opposite hand while simultaneously positioning the tips of the shears just below the fingertips holding the hair section. The fingers and shears should be horizontal and parallel to each other as the cutting begins **(Figure 15-38a** and **b)**. Cut the hair projecting from between your fingers from the tips no further than the second knuckle. Be conscious of how you open and close the shears along your fingers. This fingers-and-shear placement will be used to cut 0-elevation cuts along the perimeter, as the first cutting step in creating a design line, or to create weight lines within sections of the head form.

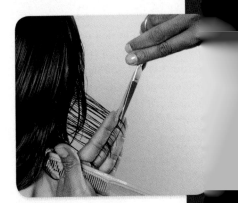

▲ **FIGURE 15-38b**
Cutting palm-to-palm.

OBJECTIVE:

The objective of this session is to practice different fingers-and-shear cutting techniques on a mannequin.

Fingers-And-Shear Technique on Mannequin

Drape the mannequin and proceed as follows:

1 **Top section.** This practice session begins with learning how to perfect the *cutting above the fingers* technique. Set up a freshly shampooed, conditioned, and combed mannequin in front of the mirror. Drape the mannequin and refer to Figure 15-36. Proceed as follows:

Palm the shears, comb through the top section of the hair, and create a part on the left side of the mannequin. Comb the hair over the top to the right. Start at the front part of the crown and make a horizontal $\frac{1}{4}$" parting across the top of the head. Using the dominant hand, comb the parting of hair straight up at 90 degrees from where it grows. Use the first and second fingers of the other hand to secure the 90-degree parting in a position for cutting. Palm the comb and position the fingers and shears parallel to the horizontal parting. Cut the hair to the desired length (be guided by your instructor) along the top of your fingers.

Comb through the parting of hair to check for evenness and fine-tune as needed. When held between the fingers at 90 degrees, the cut hair section should represent a clean horizontal line. You have just created a 90-degree guide for the top section.

NOTE: Make sure to palm the shears when using the comb, and palm the comb when cutting with the shears.

2 Part off a second parting, comb through it while picking up some of the previous parting, and comb it into a 90-degree position. Remember that the hair you are going to cut should be held at 90 degrees. When holding two partings of hair, the first parting will be very slightly over-directed to facilitate using it for a guide for the subsequent parting, which should be at a true 90-degree elevation. The second parting should be thin enough to see the guide from the first parting. Cut the second parting along your fingers and the horizontal line created with the first parting. Comb through, check, and fine-tune. You have just used the first parting as a traveling guide. Cut the entire top section in this manner.

3 **Back section.** Next, practice *cutting below the fingers* as in Figures 15-38 a and b. Start at the center of the nape. Create a $\frac{1}{4}$" to $\frac{1}{2}$" thick parting at the hairline. Use a clip to secure excess hair out of the way. Comb the parting straight down with no elevation, follow the comb with your fingers, and secure the parting for cutting. Cut below your fingers to the desired length. Comb, check, and fine-tune the cut parting. You have just cut below the fingers and established a guide

Here's a **Tip:**

To assist you in developing a rhythm for using a traveling guide, say the following to yourself as you go through the procedure in step 1: part on 1; comb forward on 2; pick up on 3; and cut on 4.

for the perimeter. Continue cutting the perimeter through the back section and around to the sides. Check to make sure the sides are even in length. This perimeter cut becomes the design line. Use the design line as a guide to cut subsequent partings in each section at the perimeter.

4 **Side sections.** To practice cutting *above the fingers* on a *vertical parting*, start on the right side. Section off a $\frac{1}{4}$" thick vertical parting from the crest to the perimeter. Comb the parting into a 90-degree projection, holding it straight out from the head form. Finger position should be vertical and perpendicular to the floor as in Figure 15-37. Using the perimeter as a guide, cut the hair that extends beyond the fingers. Repeat this step using vertical partings around the head until all the hair is layered from the design line to the top section. Note the layering that took place during this exercise. You have just created layers by cutting above the fingers using the design line as a guide and vertical partings held at 90 degrees.

NOTE: The tips of the fingers should be positioned at the end of the perimeter guide as it is held out at 90 degrees from a vertical parting. When the perimeter length is used as a guide at 90 degrees, the hair cut above it should not influence the overall hanging length of the hairstyle.

When both horizontal and vertical fingers-and-shear cutting techniques have been practiced, refer to Procedure 15-1 to perform a complete haircut using these techniques. See Procedure 15-2 for a variation of this method. Be guided by your instructor in learning other techniques.

The fingers-and-shear cutting method used in Procedure 15-1 produces a well-balanced, evenly blended precision cut that is adaptable to almost any hair type. Some exceptions are excessively thick, bristly hair and very short, overly curly hair. The rule to follow is this: *If a parting can be made in the hair and picked up between the fingers to put into a position for cutting, precision layering can be performed.* The hair should be clean and uniformly moist to maintain control of the hair and to produce the most precise cut.

FYI

Traditionally, men's h___ is not sectioned off ___ with a hair clip unles___ the length of the hai___ warrants it. When working with long ha___ there are three areas where a hair clip ma___ necessary to hold so___ of the hair out the w___ while cutting: the to___ section, at the sides, at the nape when cu___ in a design line.

THE SHEAR-OVER-COMB TECHNIQUE

The **shear-over-comb** technique is used to cut the ends of the hair and is an important method used in tapering and clipper cutting. The comb is used to position the hair to be cut and acts similarly to holding a section of hair between the fingers. Most shear-over-comb cutting is performed in the nape, behind the ears, around the ears, and in the sideburn areas of a cut. An entire haircut, however, may also be accomplished using this method. Use vertical working panels to cut in the nape and sideburn areas. Cutting the areas behind and around the ears usually requires some diagonal positioning of the comb for safety and easier access to the section. To learn the shear-over-comb technique, practice the following exercises in front of a mirror.

OBJECTIVE:

The objective of this session is to learn how to manipulate the shears and comb in tandem to perform shear-over-comb cutting.

Shear-Over-Comb Technique with Mirror

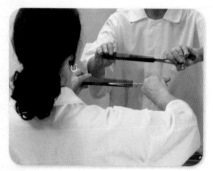

▲ FIGURE 15-39

Positioning of comb and shears.

1 Pick up the shears firmly with the right hand and insert the thumb into the thumb grip. Place the third finger into the finger grip and leave the little finger on the finger-brace of the shears. Practice using the thumb to open and close the shears.

2 Pick up the comb with the left hand and place the fingers on top of the teeth with the thumb on the backbone of the comb **(Figure 15-39)**.

NOTE: Students should start with the coarse teeth of the comb until competent at rolling the comb out and positioning the hair to be cut. After sufficient skill has been developed, use the fine teeth of the comb.

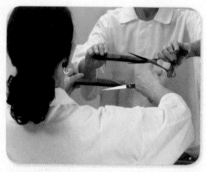

▲ FIGURE 15-40

Open and close the shears in tandem with the upward movement of the comb.

3 Practice aligning the still blade of the shears with the comb at the level where the teeth join the back as in Figure 15-39. The shears and comb should be parallel to each other. Next, move the comb upward, opening and closing the shears in tandem with the movement of the comb **(Figure 15-40)**. After several cutting movements, roll the teeth of the comb away from you (as if you were combing a client's hair) by using the thumb and the first two fingers in a key-turning motion **(Figure 15-41)**. Master these techniques before attempting to do an actual haircut.

NOTE: The preceding procedures may be changed to conform to your instructor's technique.

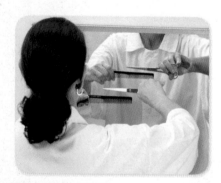

▲ FIGURE 15-41

Roll the comb using a key-turning motion.

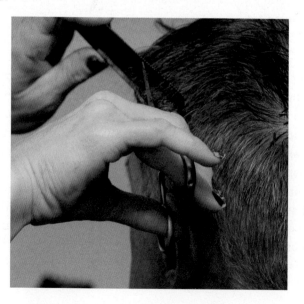

OBJECTIVE:

The objective of this session is to practice manipulating the shears, comb, and hair using the shear-over-comb technique on a mannequin.

Shear-Over-Comb Technique on Mannequin

Drape the mannequin and proceed as follows:

1 Start at the hairline in the center of the nape area.

2 With the teeth of the comb pointing upward, comb into a section of hair at the hairline, rolling the comb out toward you (**Figure 15-42**). When performed correctly, the hair should protrude from the teeth of the comb and be in a position for cutting. This is called **rolling the comb out.**

3 Hold the comb parallel with the still blade of the shears, as shown in Figure 15-39, and control the movement of the cutting blade with the thumb.

4 While manipulating the shears, move both the shears and the comb slowly upward at the same time, cutting the hair in the process. Stop at the occipital area.

5 Turn the teeth of the comb down when combing the hair down toward the hairline, as shown in Figure 15-41.

6 Begin the next working panel by including some hair from the center section with the hair to the right or left of center. There should now be two lengths of hair in the comb: shorter hair from the center section and longer hair from the second section. The shorter hair from the center section becomes the guide for the second panel (**Figure 15-43**). Finish one vertical strip at a time before proceeding with the next section.

7 To practice cutting along the sides of the neck, position the comb diagonally behind the ear parallel to the hairline. Proceed to trim the hair as described for the nape area.

8 Continue to practice the shear-over-comb technique in front of and around the ear. Make sure to blend the hair from the nape section to the sides of the neck and the around-the-ear areas.

Be guided by your instructor to learn other variations of this method, such as beginning on the right or left sides.

Once the shear-over-comb technique has been practiced on the mannequin, refer to Procedure 15-2 to perform a haircut using this method.

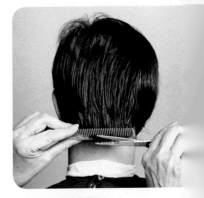

▲ **FIGURE 15-42**
Position the hair to be cut by rolling the comb out.

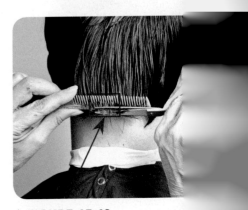

▲ **FIGURE 15-43**
Center point, cut to guide.

FREEHAND SHEAR CUTTING TECHNIQUE

Freehand shear cutting is a technique that does not require the use of the fingers or a comb to control the hair while the actual cutting is performed. Instead, the hair is combed or picked out to reveal stray hairs. The shears are then employed with a consistent open-and-close motion that skims over the surface of the hair to cut any stray hairs protruding from the design. These comb-and-cut steps are repeated as often as necessary in the final stages of a haircut, beard trim, or other procedure to fine-tune the work and are especially effective for trimming very curly hair textures (see Procedure 15-4, step 13 for example).

SHEAR-POINT TAPERING

Shear-point tapering is a useful technique for thinning out difficult areas of the hair caused by hollows, wrinkles, whorls, and creases in the scalp. Dark and ragged hair patches on the scalp can be minimized by this special technique. The shear-point taper is performed with the cutting points of the shears (**Figures 15-44** and **15-45**). Only a few strands of hair are cut at a time and then combed out. Continue cutting around the objectionable spot until it becomes less noticeable and blends in with the surrounding hair or hairline.

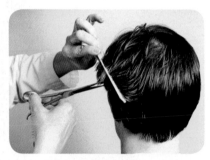

▲ **FIGURE 15-44**
Shear-point taper in back left section.

ARCHING TECHNIQUE

The **arching technique** is the method used to mark or outline the haircut along the hairline at the bottom of the sideburns, in front of the ears, over the ears, and down the sides of the neck. This portion of outlining the haircut is accomplished with the points of the shears, an outliner, and/or a razor and is part of the finish work of most haircuts.

As with the other techniques in this text, the following practice session is simply one method of performing the procedure. Be guided by your instructor for variations in the method.

▲ **FIGURE 15-45**
Shear-point taper in nape area.

PRACTICE SESSION #5

OBJECTIVE:

The objective of this session is to learn to manipulate the shears in the tighter, smaller areas around ears and to become comfortable in performing the arching technique with this tool.

Arching Technique

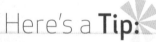

Here's a Tip:

Before beginning the arching procedure, check to determine if one sideburn is longer than the other. Start on the side with the shortest sideburn to avoid unnecessary repetition of the procedure.

1 Hold the shears with the right hand.

    a. Pick up the shears and insert the thumb in the thumb grip. Place the third finger into the finger grip and the little finger on the brace of the shears.

    b. Gently tug the client's ear down.

2 Arch the right side.

    a. Start the outline as close to the natural hairline as possible **(Figure 15-46)**.

    b. Start in front of the ear and cut a continuous outline around the ear and down the side of the neck **(Figures 15-47a** and **15-47b)**.

    c. Reverse the direction of arching back to the starting point **(Figure 15-48)**.

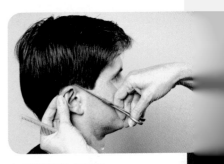

▲ **FIGURE 15-46**
Start outline at hairline.

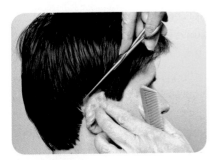

▲ **FIGURE 15-47a**
Arching around the ear in a continuous line.

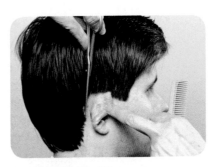

▲ **FIGURE 15-47b**
Continuing line in back of the ear.

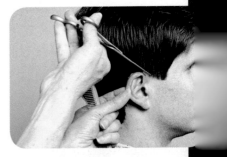

▲ **FIGURE 15-48**
Reverse the direction of arching.

    d. Continue arching around the ear until a definite outline is formed.

    e. Square off and establish the length of the right sideburn **(Figure 15-49)**.

3 Arch the left side.

    a. Start in front of the left ear and cut a continuous outline with the shears over the left ear and down the side of the neck **(Figures 15-50a** and **15-50b)**.

    b. Reverse the direction of the shears and return to the starting point. Continue arching around the ear until a definite outline is formed.

    c. Square off of the left sideburn to match the right sideburn **(Figure 15-51)**.

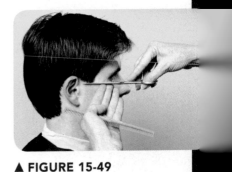

▲ **FIGURE 15-49**
Establish length of right sideburn.

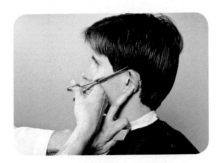

▲ **FIGURE 15-50a**
Beginning of arching on left side.

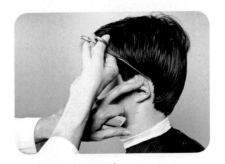

▲ **FIGURE 15-50b**
Arch over the ear and continue to back of the ear.

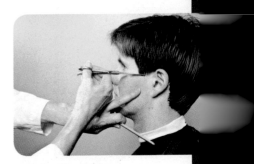

▲ **FIGURE 15-51**
Cut left sideburn to match the right sideburn.

CLIPPER CUTTING

Clippers are versatile tools that can be used in several ways to cut a variety of hair textures and styles. The standard techniques are **freehand clipper cutting** and **clipper-over-comb** cutting. As a general rule, clipper cutting is followed up with shear and comb work to fine-tune the haircut and/or to perform the arching technique.

DIRECTIONAL TERMS USED IN CLIPPER CUTTING

Cutting and tapering the hair with clippers can be accomplished in the following ways:

- Cutting *against the grain* is accomplished by cutting the hair in the opposite direction from which it grows (**Figures 15-52** and **15-53**). Taper the hair by gradually tilting the clipper until it rides on its heel.

- Cutting *with the grain* means the cutting is performed in the same direction in which the hair grows (**Figures 15-54** and **15-55**). When using a clipper on hair that has a tight curl formation, try to cut with the grain or growth pattern. Cutting tight, curly hair against the grain clogs up the clipper blades and may leave patches or spots in the haircut.

- When cutting *across the grain* with clippers, the hair is cut neither with nor against the grain. This direction in cutting is usually performed on transition areas in the crest or side regions. (**Figures 15-56** and **15-57**).

- In whorl areas, or in places where the hair does not grow in a uniform manner (**Figure 15-58**), cutting the hair in a *circular motion* using clippers is advisable.

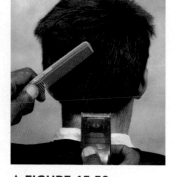

▲ **FIGURE 15-52**

Cutting against the grain on straight hair.

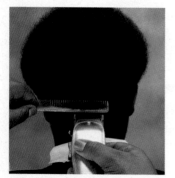

▲ **FIGURE 15-53**

Cutting against the grain on curly hair.

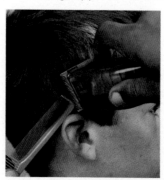

▲ **FIGURE 15-54**

Cutting with the grain on straight hair.

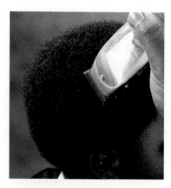

▲ **FIGURE 15-55**

Cutting with the grain on curly hair.

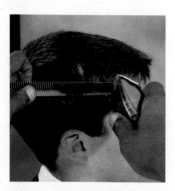

▲ **FIGURE 15-56**

Cutting across the grain on straight hair.

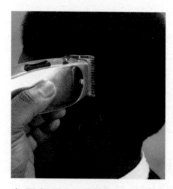

▲ **FIGURE 15-57**

Cutting across the grain on curly hair.

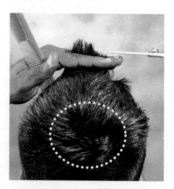

▲ **FIGURE 15-58**

Whorl in crown area in straight hair.

ARCHING WITH A CLIPPER OR TRIMMER

Many barbers prefer to use an outliner or trimmer with a fine cutting edge to square off sideburns and perfect the outline around the ears and down the sides of neck. This method of arching is efficient and precise due to the maneuverability of the smaller cutting head of the tool. If the desired result can be accomplished with the standard clipper, that method is equally acceptable (**Figures 15-59a** to **15-59c**).

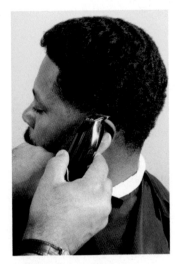

▲ FIGURE 15-59a
Arching with outliner front of the ear.

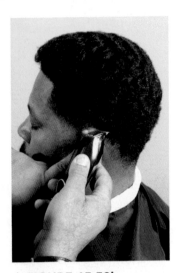

▲ FIGURE 15-59b
Arching with outliner around ear.

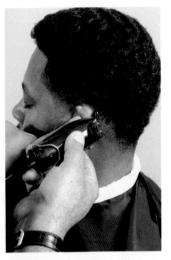

▲ FIGURE 15-59c
Arching with outliner behind the ear.

FREEHAND AND CLIPPER-OVER-COMB CUTTING

Freehand clipper cutting requires a steady hand and consistent use of the comb or hair pick while cutting. The use of the comb or pick is important for two reasons: First, both implements put the hair into a position to be cut, and second, both implements help to remove the excess hair cut from the previous section. This provides the barber with a clearer view of the cutting results and any areas that may need re-blending.

True freehand clipper cutting technique tend to be used on two extremes of hair length: (1) very short straight, wavy, and curly lengths in which little clipper-over-comb work is performed (**Figure 15-60**), and (2) longer, very curly hair lengths that require more sculpting (**Figure 15-61**). The freehand method

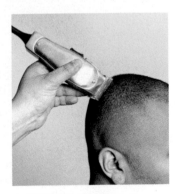

▲ FIGURE 15-60
Freehand clipper cutting on wavy hair texture.

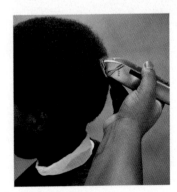

▲ FIGURE 15-61
Freehand clipper cutting on curly hair texture.

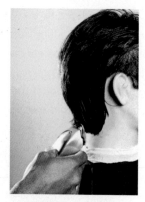

▲ **FIGURE 15-62a**
Freehand clipper cutting on straight hair texture.

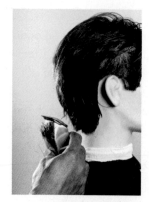

▲ **FIGURE 15-62b**
Freehand clipper cutting on straight hair texture.

Did **You** Know...

The use of guards is not considered to be a form of freehand clipper cutting; nor is this technique usually acceptable for state board practical examinations.

can also be used to cut in the nape, back, and sides of medium-length straight hair textures (**Figures 15-62a** and **15-62b**).

For short hair styles, clippers with detachable blades range from size 0000 (close to shaving) to size $3\frac{1}{2}$, which leaves the hair approximately $\frac{3}{8}$" inch long. Detachable blades should not be confused with clipper attachment combs, most commonly known as guards. Guards are placed on top of a clipper blade, allowing for more hair length to remain while cutting.

Freehand clipper cutting is also used for tightly curled hair when a natural look is the desired result. Because most tightly curled hair grows up and out of the scalp, rather than falling to one side or another as with straighter hair types, this hair texture lends itself to being picked out and put into position for free-hand clipper cutting. Cutting this type of hairstyle requires a keen eye for balance, shape, and proportion as the hair is sculpted into the desired form.

Clipper-over-comb cutting can be used for the entire haircut or to blend the hair from shorter tapered areas to longer areas at the top, crest, or occipital. Much like the shear-over-comb technique, the comb places the hair in a position to be cut and utilizes the same blending principles (**Figure 15-63a** to **15-64**). Freehand clipper cutting, clipper-over-comb, and fingers-and-shear work are techniques that are frequently combined to perform a single haircut.

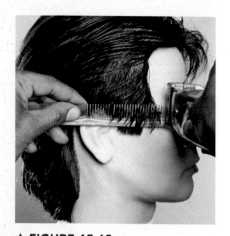

▲ **FIGURE 15-63a**
Horizontal Clipper-over-comb on straight hair.

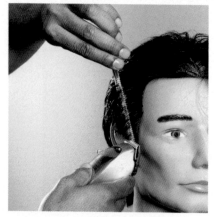

▲ **FIGURE 15-63b**
Vertical clipper-over-comb on straight hair.

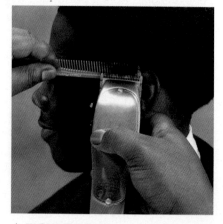

▲ **FIGURE 15-64**
Clipper over comb on curly hair.

OBJECTIVE:

The objective of this session is to practice the clipper-over-comb and freehand clipper cutting methods on straight hair textures.

Clipper Cutting on Straight-Haired Mannequin

This practice session will involve clipper-over-comb cutting and standard freehand clipper cutting using an all-purpose comb.

1 How to hold the clipper and comb for *clipper-over-comb cutting:*

   a. Pick up the clipper with the dominant hand.

   b. Place the thumb on the top left side and fingers underneath along the right side of the clipper. Hold it firmly but lightly to permit freedom of wrist movement.

   c. Use the largest numbered detachable clipper blade or fully open the adjustable blade clipper.

   d. Begin in the center of the nape area and comb the hair down with the opposite hand **(Figure 15-65a)**.

   e. With the teeth of the comb pointing upward, comb into a section of hair at the hairline, rolling the comb out toward you as in **Figure 15-65b**.

   f. Use the clipper to cut the hair section to the desired length. Comb through, check, and begin the next section to the right or left of center.

2 Clipper-over-comb: cutting the nape area

   a. For a gradual, even taper from shorter to longer in each section of hair, keep rolling the comb out to put the hair in a position to be cut.

   b. Gradually taper the hair from the hairline to an inch or two above the hairline. Do not taper higher than the occipital for this exercise, or cut into the hair along the sides of the neck at this point **(Figure 15-66)**.

3 Clipper-over-comb: cutting the sides

There are two comb positions that can be used to cut the sides depending on the hair texture, density, and the desired result: horizontal and vertical.

   a. *Horizontal:* Begin in the front of the ear and position the comb parallel to the hairline. Roll the comb out at about a 45-degree

REMINDER

▲ >>> When using the clipper-over-comb technique to taper, be sure to tilt the comb away from the head to create a blended taper from shorter to longer sections.

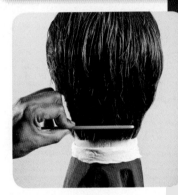

▲ FIGURE 15-65a
Comb the hair down.

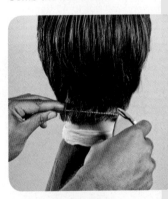

▲ FIGURE 15-65b
Roll the comb out to put the hair in position to be cut.

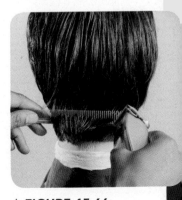

▲ FIGURE 15-66
Cut to the occipital area.

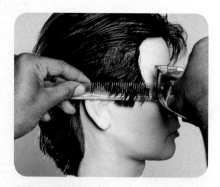

▲ FIGURE 15-67

Position the comb horizontally and parallel to the hairline.

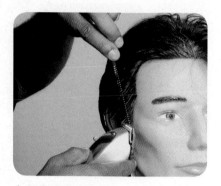

▲ FIGURE 15-68

Position comb vertically at the hairline and roll out to 45 degrees.

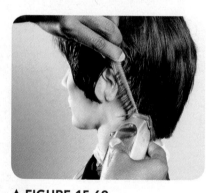

▲ FIGURE 15-69

Position the comb at the hairline behind the ear.

projection and cut (**Figure 15-67**). Follow the forward curve of the hairline around the ear.

b. *Vertical:* Position the comb on an angle from the bottom of the sideburn and roll the comb out about 45 degrees (**Figure 15-68**). Cut hair extending beyond the teeth of the comb.

4 Clipper-over-comb: cutting behind the ears

a. The guide around the ears and at the corner of the neck should be visible.

b. Place the comb parallel to the hairline on a diagonal, roll the comb out, and blend from the guide at the back of the ear to the nape corner (**Figure 15-69**). The hair in the tapered areas should blend from the nape to the side of the neck and around the ear.

5 How to hold the clipper for freehand clipper cutting:

a. Pick up the clipper with the dominant hand.

b. Place the thumb on the top left side and fingers underneath along the right side of the clipper. Hold it firmly but lightly to permit freedom of wrist movement. Depending on the section of the head form being cut, the holding position will change for comfort and access to the area.

c. Use the largest-numbered detachable clipper blade or fully open the adjustable blade clipper.

d. Begin in the center of the nape area and comb the hair down with the opposite hand.

e. Palm the comb and steady the clipper with the tip of the index finger of the opposite hand.

6 Freehand clipper cutting: the nape area

a. Begin with the clipper blades open. With the teeth of the bottom blade placed flat against the skin at the center of the nape hairline, gradually tilt the blade away from the head so that the clipper rides on the heel of the bottom blade. Lightly guide the clipper upward into the hair to about an inch above the hairline (**Figures 15-70a** and **15-70b**). Remember, this is just a practice session to become familiar with the clippers, so avoid removing too much hair.

b. Continue to work the center section, stopping just below the occipital. This will set the guide length for left and right of the center panel. Maintain the gradual taper from shorter to longer hair and do not taper higher than the occipital for this exercise (**Figure 15-70c**).

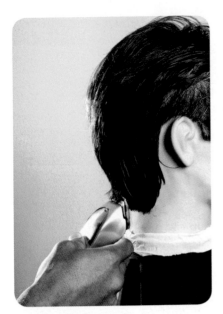

▲ FIGURE 15-70a

Lightly guide the clipper upward from the hairline into the hair about an inch above the hairline.

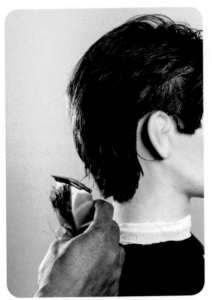

▲ FIGURE 15-70b

Removal of hair at lower nape area.

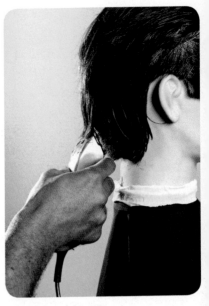

▲ FIGURE 15-70c

Guide the blades through the ends of the hair.

   c. Do not move the clipper into the hair too fast as it may have a tendency to jam the clipper blades and pull the hair.

   d. After tapering one panel of hair, comb it down, check the results, and start tapering the section to the right or left of center. Be guided by your instructor.

7 Freehand clipper cutting: the sides

   a. Begin at the front of the ear at the hairline and comb the hair down. Tilt the clipper at about a 45-degree angle so that the first few teeth of the blades will be used for cutting the curve around the ear.

   b. Bend the ear forward and continue cutting along the hairline, meeting the top of the hairline at the side of the neck.

8 Freehand clipper cutting: behind the ears

   a. The guide around the ears and at the corner of the neck should be visible.

   b. Comb the hair down and blend from the nape corner to the guide at the back of the ear. The hair in the tapered areas should blend from the nape to the side of the neck and around the ear.

When the clipper-over-comb and freehand techniques have been practiced on the mannequin, refer to Procedure 15-3 to perform a medium-length haircut using these methods. Be guided by your instructor to learn other variations, such as beginning on the right or left sides.

FYI

The style will determi[ne] the point on the head [at] which the tapered area[s] blended into longer ha[ir.] Short styles, such as bu[zz] cuts, crew cuts, and fa[des] have a high taper and are blended in the cre[st] areas; longer styles ma[y] blended at or just bel[ow] the occipital. There ar[e] many variations as the[re] are heads of hair to cu[t.]

OBJECTIVE:

The objective of this session is to practice the freehand clipper cutting method on tightly curled hair textures.

Clipper Cutting on Mannequin with Tightly Curled Hair

1 Hold the clipper as for freehand clipper cutting.

2 Use a pick or Afro comb to comb the hair up and outward from the scalp.

3 If the hair is too thick or too tightly curled to use an all-purpose comb while cutting, use a wide-tooth comb to practice the clipper-over-comb technique as performed on the model in Figure 15-64.

4 When the clipper-over-comb technique has been completed, practice the freehand clipper cutting method in Figure 15-61.

Be guided by your instructor as to where to begin the clipper cut and the order of the subsequent sections. Some barbers prefer to start in the center of the nape area, while others work from right to left or left to right. As long as the hair is tapered evenly, all methods are equally correct.

Once the clipper-over-comb and freehand clipper cutting techniques have been practiced on the mannequin, refer to Procedure 15-4 to perform a medium-length haircut on tightly curled hair using these methods. Be guided by your instructor to learn other variations of this method.

CLIPPER CUT STYLES

Variations of basic clipper cut styles have been around since the hand clipper was invented (**Figure 15-71**). Flat tops, crew cuts, and the Quo Vadis are three of the most popular styles that have stood the test of time and cyclical haircut trends.

Flat tops are very short on the sides and in the back areas, as are crew cuts. Flat tops are traditionally slightly longer in the front and crest sections and flat across the top of the head form. The top of the crest area should look squared off when viewed from the front. Variations of the style and length of the top section will be determined by the client's preference, hair texture, and hair density. Clippers and shears are usually used to cut a flat top (**Figure 15-72a**).

Some general guidelines for cutting the flat top style are as follows:

1. Stand behind the client. The hair at the crown is cut flat to about $\frac{1}{4}$" to $\frac{1}{2}$" in length and about 2" to 3" in width.

2. Stand in front of the client. Position the comb flat across the front center area, cutting the hair to a length of 1" to $1\frac{1}{2}$", depending on the

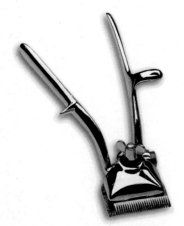

▲ FIGURE 15-71

Hand clipper.

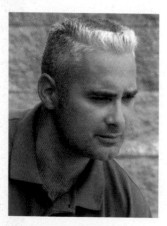

▲ FIGURE 15-72a

Flat-top style.

client's preference. This cutting area will span the width of the client's top section. Cut straight across from side to side.

3. Ask the client if the front hair is at the desired length. If not, re-cut the front section.

4. Complete all finish work such as arching and the neck shave. Refer to Haircutting Procedure 15-8.

Crew cuts are also referred to as the *short pomp* or *brush cut*. The length of hair on the sides and back of the head usually determines the crew cut style, as described in the following list.

- Short sides and back: short crew cut.
- Semi-short sides and back: medium crew cut.
- Medium sides and back: long crew cut.

Generally, the back and sides are cut first and relatively high to the bottom of the crest area. The hair on top is then combed from front to back to make it stand up, followed by blending the tapered area to the crest and top sections. Since the top section should be smooth and almost flat, use a wide-toothed comb to provide a level guide. Begin cutting in the front to the desired length and cut back toward the crown. This section should be graduated in length from the front hairline to the back part of the crown. Repeat the procedure until the top section has been cut. When viewed from the front, the top section should blend with the top of the crest, with a slight curvature to conform to the contours of the head. Use the shears and comb to smooth out any uneven spots left by the clipper work (**Figure 15-72b**). Refer to Procedure 15-8.

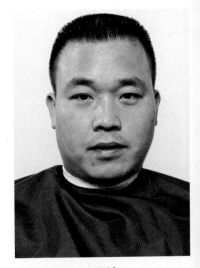

▲ **FIGURE 15-72b**
Crew cut style.

The brush cut is a variation of the crew cut and is popular with young men, as it requires the least attention. The sides and back areas are cut as for a short crew cut, but the hair on top is cut the same length all over, about $\frac{1}{4}$″ to $\frac{1}{2}$″, and follows the contours of the head.

The *Quo Vadis* is a popular haircut style that is suitable for very curly hair. The main objective with this haircut is to achieve an even and smooth cut over the entire head. Since the hair is cut close to the scalp, clipper lines and patches are readily noticeable. Be guided by the natural hair growth pattern and cut with the grain to avoid gaps. Outline and taper the nape area with a #000 clipper blade and then use a #1 clipper blade over the rest of the head (**Figure 15-73**).

BASIC TAPERING AND BLENDING AREAS

To simplify the clipper or shear cutting procedures, the primary tapering and blending areas of haircut styles may be identified as belonging to one of four basic classifications: long cuts and trims, medium lengths, semi-short lengths, and short cuts. A variety of hairstyles, such as the fade and bi-level, can be created from these basic classifications to suit the client's tastes and desires.

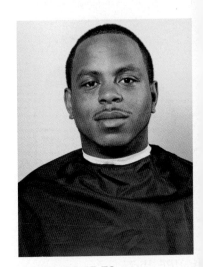

▲ **FIGURE 15-73**
Quo Vadis style.

Long haircut styles and trims usually require the least amount of clipper tapering. Tapering is performed from the nape hairline to just above the bottom of the ear and below the occipital using the fingers-and-shear, shear-over-comb,

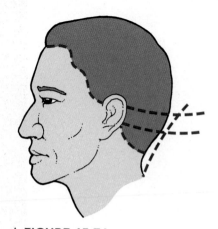

▲ FIGURE 15-74

Taper area for longer hair style.

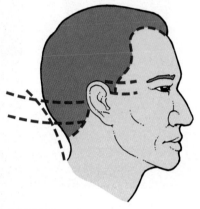

▲ FIGURE 15-75

Taper area for medium-length style.

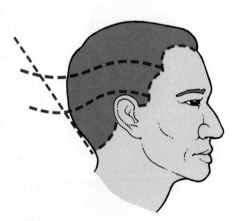

▲ FIGURE 15-76

Taper area for semi- short style.

or clipper-over-comb techniques **(Figure 15-74)**. An outliner or trimmer is used to remove fine hair at the nape and along the sides of the neck. Sideburns and over-the-ear areas are shortened using the shear-over-comb method along the natural hairline and then outlined with trimmers and/or a razor.

Medium-length styles do not usually have a scalped appearance, although the hair is cut closer to the head than in longer styles **(Figure 15-75)**. Clipper cutting in the nape should be performed with the clipper tilted on its heel until it reaches a point about midway to the ears. In the sideburn areas, the taper should end no higher than the tops of the ears. An outliner or razor is used at the nape hairline.

Semi-short styles usually require tilting the clipper back off the hair as the top of the ear areas are viewed from the back section. The hair in the back may be left slightly longer than on the sides. In the sideburn areas, the clipper tapers out at about the top of the ears. When cutting around the ears, remove about $\frac{1}{2}$" from the hairline, then use an outliner to trim the sideburns and around the ear areas **(Figure 15-76)**.

Short haircut styles usually require cutting up to the crest area and then gradually tilting the heel of the clipper back as the clipper is brought up until it runs off the curve of the head. This movement is repeated all the way around the head form. An outliner is used to taper the sideburns and nape **(Figure 15-77)**.

The *fade style* derives its name from the fact that the hair at the nape and sides is cut extremely close, becoming gradually longer in the crest and lower crown areas and longest at the top. Hence, it fades to nothing at the hairline.

This cut requires close cutting from the nape to the bottom of the crest or horseshoe area. The sides are cut to the temporal region using the next-longer clipper blade, or one that will taper in the crest area to the top section. The top section is cut and blended to the crest **(Figure 15-78)**. To gradually blend the fine clipper taper with the longer clipper taper, tilt the heel of the clippers, moving with and across the grain as necessary.

A *bi-level style* is most often achieved with clippers and shears. The clipper is used to cut the nape and sides to the desired length **(Figure 15-79)**. The top is either layered and texturized or cut to one length using a weight line. The weight line may vary in style lengths.

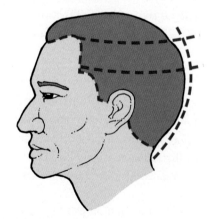

▲ FIGURE 15-77

Taper area for short styles.

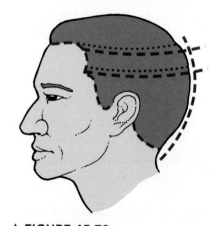

▲ FIGURE 15-78

Taper area for a fade style.

For a medium-length style, the top, crown, and crest area hair is sectioned off and secured with a hair clip. Clipper cutting is performed up to the occipital area in the back and on the sides to the bottom of the crest. A horizontal parting is taken from the secured hair to establish a design/guide line. The hair is cut at 0 elevation until all the partings are cut. Using the design line as a guide, the hair is projected at 45 or 90 degrees to produce layers if desired. Using clipper cutting for a shorter length, bi-level style usually requires cutting higher into the temporal region with slight blending to the top section.

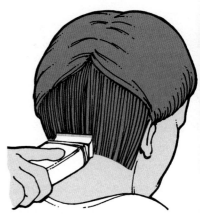

▲ **FIGURE 15-79**
Taper area for a bilevel style.

POPULAR SIDEBURN LENGTHS

When trimming or redesigning the length of sideburns, every effort should be made to make sure that the sideburns appear even in length. When seen in profile, the client's ear, eye, or other anatomical feature may be used as a general guide for trimming the sideburns. However, *always check the length of both sideburns by facing the client toward the mirror*. No one's face is truly symmetrical, and differences will be noticed when viewing the client from the front. In addition, check to see that the thickness (density) of the sideburns complements the facial shape and hairstyle (**Figures 15-80** through **15-84**).

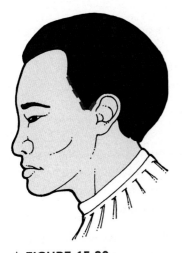

▲ **FIGURE 15-80**
Short sideburn.

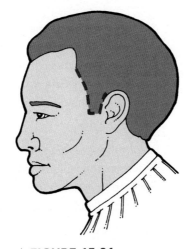

▲ **FIGURE 15-81**
Medium sideburn.

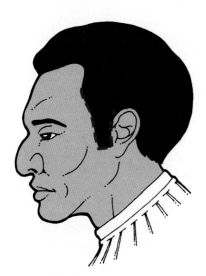

▲ **FIGURE 15-82**
Long sideburn.

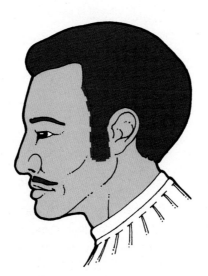

▲ **FIGURE 15-83**
Extra-long sideburn.

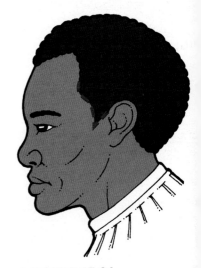

▲ **FIGURE 15-84**
Pointed sideburn.

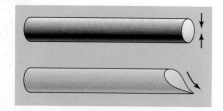

▲ FIGURE 15-85

Shear cut and razor cut strands.

RAZOR CUTTING

Razor cutting provides an opportunity for the barber to create a variety of different effects in the hair (**Figure 15-85**). It is especially suitable for thinning, shortening, tapering, blending, or feathering specific areas and can help make resistant hair textures more manageable. For client comfort and a precise cut, the hair should always be clean and damp. As always, the barber must consider the client's styling wishes, features, head shape, facial contour, and hair texture. The technique of handling a razor should be mastered completely before attempting to use it to cut a client's hair.

CAUTION: The use of a razor with a safety guard is recommended for the beginner. Once the student barber is proficient in the techniques, the razor may be used without a safety guard.

RAZOR STROKING AND COMBING

Proper stroking of the razor and combing during the tapering process are of utmost importance in razor cutting. It is better to taper a little at a time than to taper too much.

- *Arm and hand movements:* Some barbers prefer the arm movement, in which the razor stroking and combing is done with stiff arms, using the elbows as a hinge. Others use both wrist and arm movements. This is a matter of preference. The barber should develop a technique best suited to the individual and that gives the desired results.

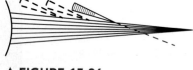

▲ FIGURE 15-86

Light taper-blending.

- *Razor taper-blending:* Razor cutting is thought by some barbers to be the best technique to use for tapering and blending the hair. The cutting action of the razor permits a smoother blend than that usually accomplished with shears and/or clippers.

  ▶ *Light taper-blending* requires that the razor is held almost flat against the surface of the hair. Note the small amount of hair that is cut when the blade is only slightly tilted and very little pressure is used (**Figure 15-86**).

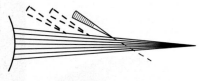

▲ FIGURE 15-87

Heavier taper-blending.

  ▶ *Heavier taper-blending* is performed with the razor held up to 45 degrees from the surface of the hair strand. As the razor is tilted higher and a little more pressure is used, the depth of the cut increases (**Figure 15-87**).

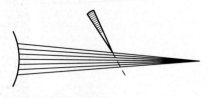

▲ FIGURE 15-88

Terminal blending.

  ▶ *Terminal blending* means that the angle of the razor blade is increased to almost 90 degrees. Short sawing strokes are used. Other terms used for terminal blending are *hair-end tapering* and *blunt cutting* (**Figure 15-88**).

- *Razor and comb coordination:* Razor stroking and combing are done in a continuous movement. The razor tapers while the comb removes the cut hair and re-combs the section for the next stroke or strokes (**Figures 15-89** to **15-91**).

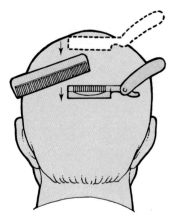

▲ FIGURE 15-89

Crown area: razor and comb coordination.

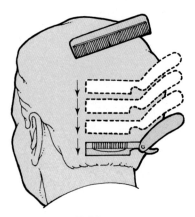

▲ FIGURE 15-90

Nape area: razor and comb coordination.

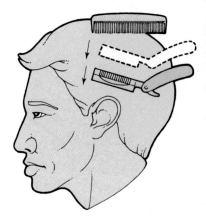

▲ FIGURE 15-91

Side areas: razor and comb coordination.

HAIR TEXTURES AND RAZOR CUTTING

- *Coarse, thick hair* requires more strokes and heavier tapering than other textures. The first strip of hair is combed, followed by three razor strokes, and followed again with the comb. The comb removes the cut hair and re-combs the hair, allowing the barber to see how much hair has been cut. It also helps to keep the guide in view for use in tapering the next strip **(Figures 15-92 to 15-94)**.

- *Medium-textured hair* requires fewer razor strokes and lighter pressure than coarse, thick hair as pictured in **Figures 15-95 to 15-98**.

- *Fine hair* typically does not have any bulk to remove; however, the razor may be used to blend hair ends to achieve a particular hairstyle. Stroking of the razor is usually lighter than that used for medium-textured hair.

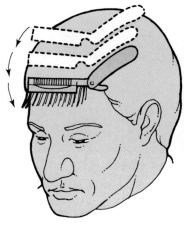

▲ FIGURE 15-92

Top area. Consideration must be given to the hairstyle to be created. The stroking and the pressure of the razor largely depend upon the amount of hair to be removed to achieve the finished hairstyle.

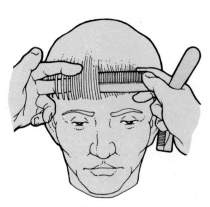

▲ FIGURE 15-93

Front hair. To equalize the length of long and uneven front hair, pick up the hair with the comb in the right hand. Hold the hair straight out between the middle and index fingers of the left hand.

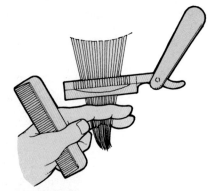

▲ FIGURE 15-94

Palm the comb to the left hand. Hold the razor at an angle, and with short, sawing strokes cut the hair to the desired length.

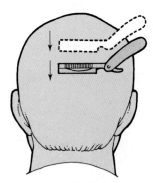

▲ FIGURE 15-95

Crown area: two long strokes are used.

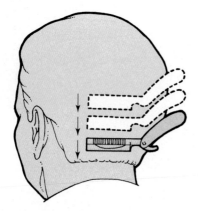

▲ FIGURE 15-96

Nape area: three short strokes are used.

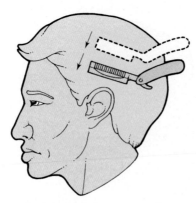

▲ FIGURE 15-97

Left and right sides of the head: two short strokes may be used.

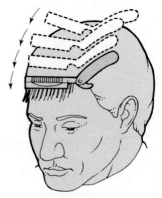

▲ FIGURE 15-98

Top area: the stroking and pressure of the razor in this area are the same as for the sides and back area.

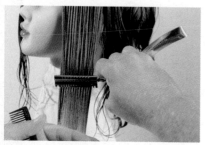

▲ FIGURE 15-99

Removing weight with freehand slicing.

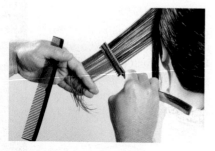

▲ FIGURE 15-100

Releasing weight from a subsection.

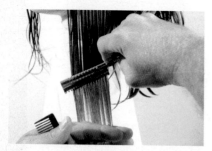

▲ FIGURE 15-101

Establishing a design line at the perimeter.

TERMS ASSOCIATED WITH RAZOR CUTTING

Removing weight can be accomplished by holding a parting of damp hair out from the head with the fingers positioned at the end of the section. Place the razor flat to the hair and gently stroke the razor to remove a thin sheet of hair from the section. This technique tapers the ends of the hair (**Figure 15-99**).

Freehand slicing can be used in the mid-shaft of a section or at the ends of the hair. The hair is combed out from the head and held between the fingers where the tip of the razor is used to slice out pieces of hair. This technique releases weight from the subsection and allows for more movement within the hairstyle. When used to cut the design line, freehand slicing the ends helps to create soft perimeters (**Figures 15-100** and **15-101**).

Razor-over-comb cutting is slightly different from shear- or clipper-over-comb techniques in which the comb is used to project the hair into a position for cutting. In razor-over-comb cutting, the razor is held in the freehand position and situated just above the comb as it follows the comb's downward direction through the hair (**Figure 15-102**). Short, precise strokes with medium

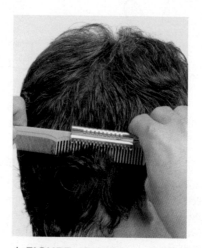

▲ FIGURE 15-102

Razor-over-comb technique.

pressure are applied to the surface of the hair. This technique is often used to taper nape areas or to soften weight lines.

Razor rotation is performed by using a rotating motion with the comb and razor as the hair is being cut. In the first movement, the razor follows the comb through the hair. Then the comb follows the razor and so on (**Figure 15-103**).

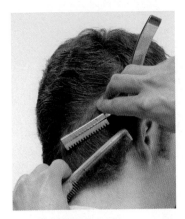

▲ **FIGURE 15-103**
Razor rotation.

HAIR SECTIONING FOR RAZOR HAIRCUTTING

There are several effective ways to section the hair for razor cutting. These include the two-section, three-section, four-section, and five-section methods. All methods begin by combing the hair into the umbrella effect, which is created by combing the hair into natural directions from the crown (**Figure 15-104**). Be guided by your instructor.

- *Two sections:* First, part the hair from ear to ear across the crown. All hair in front of the part is combed forward. All hair behind or below the part is combed down (**Figure 15-105**).

- *Three sections:* First, part the hair from ear to ear across the crown. All top and side hair is combed forward. Then make a vertical part from the crown to the nape. Each of these subsections is combed toward the sides. In the nape area where there is no part, comb the hair down (**Figure 15-106**).

- *Four sections:* Add one more section to the previous three sections. Make a top center part and comb each side down (**Figure 15-107**).

- *Four sections, alternate method:* First, part the hair from ear to ear across the crown. Second, section the right side from the center of the right eyebrow to the crown and comb down. Make another section on the left side from the center of the left eyebrow to the crown and comb down. Comb all back hair down (**Figure 15-108**).

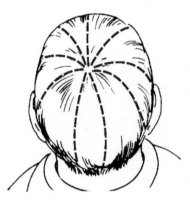

▲ **FIGURE 15-104**
Umbrella effect.

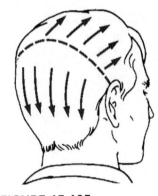

▲ **FIGURE 15-105**
Two sections.

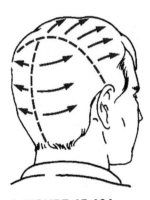

▲ **FIGURE 15-106**
Three sections.

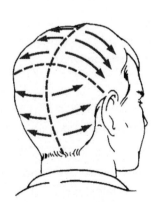

▲ **FIGURE 15-107**
Four sections.

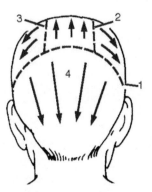

▲ **FIGURE 15-108**
Four sections (alternate method).

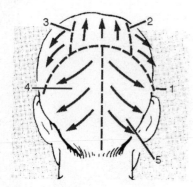

▲ FIGURE 15-109
Five sections.

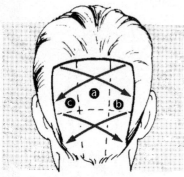

▲ FIGURE 15-110
Back.

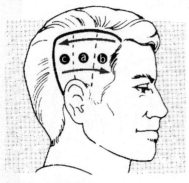

▲ FIGURE 15-111
Sides.

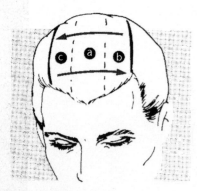

▲ FIGURE 15-112
Top.

• *Five sections:* Sectioning is the same as the alternate four-section except that the back section is divided in two and combed as indicated by the arrows in **Figure 15-109**.

A pattern for cutting needs to be established by the barber so that there is a plan to follow. In this text, one basic plan is followed. Other procedures may be different but equally correct. Be guided by your instructor.

- Back part of head (**Figure 15-110**)
  ▶ Downward
  ▶ Top right to left, downward
  ▶ Top left to right, downward

- Right side of head (**Figure 15-111**)
  ▶ Downward
  ▶ Toward the back
  ▶ Toward the face

- Left side of head
  ▶ Downward
  ▶ Toward the back
  ▶ Toward the face

- Top hair (**Figure 15-112**)
  ▶ Crown to forehead
  ▶ Top left side
  ▶ Top right side

RAZOR-CUTTING TIPS

- The hair must be clean and damp for best results and to avoid client discomfort. Maintain moisture content throughout the cut.

- Avoid tapering too close to the hair part or the scalp. Tapering the hair too closely to the hair part will cause the hair to stand up, making the part look ragged. Coarse hair that is cut too closely to the scalp will have short, stubby hair ends that will protrude through the top layer.

- Avoid over-tapering as it is difficult to correct a haircut after too much hair has been removed.

RAZOR-CUTTING SAFETY PRECAUTIONS

- Handle the razor properly, keeping it closed whenever not in use.

- Be aware of the people around you when working with any sharp tool or implement. A careless motion can cause injury to yourself or others. Do not annoy or distract anyone who is in the process of performing a service.

- Purchase and use only good-quality haircutting implements.
- Use changeable-blade razors and dispose of used blades in a sharps container.
- Replace dull razor blades, during a cut if necessary, as a dull blade will pull the hair and cause pain or discomfort to the client. Dull blades will also influence the quality of the haircut.

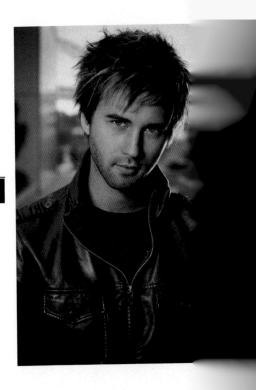

PRACTICE SESSION **#8**

OBJECTIVE:

The objective of this session is to become familiar with manipulating the razor using freehand slicing, razor-over-comb, and razor rotation cutting techniques.

Razor Cutting on a Mannequin

1 Pick up the razor (with guard) with the dominant hand.

2 Comb hair into the umbrella effect.

3 Position yourself behind the mannequin.

4 Hold the razor in a freehand position.

5 Use the freehand slicing technique to create a design line in the nape area.

6 Use the razor-over-comb technique to taper the nape area.

7 Use the razor rotation method to blend the hair at the occipital with the nape area.

Once the razor-cutting techniques have been practiced on the mannequin, refer to Haircutting Procedure 15-6 to perform a haircut using these methods. Be guided by your instructor to learn other variations of this method.

☑ **LO6 Complete**

HAIR THINNING AND TEXTURIZING

Hair thinning is used to reduce the bulk or weight of the hair. The barber can use thinning (serrated) shears, regular shears, clippers, or a razor for this purpose. Regardless of the tool used to perform the procedure, some general rules to follow when removing bulk from the hair are as follows:

- Make a careful observation of the hair to determine the sections that require some reduction in bulk or weight and cut accordingly.
- Avoid cutting top surfaces of the hair where visible cutting lines can be seen.
- Part off and elevate the hair to be cut to avoid cutting too deeply into the section.
- Avoid cutting too closely to the scalp or part lines.

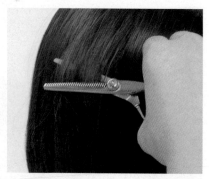

▲ **FIGURE 15-113**

Removing bulk midshaft with thinning shears.

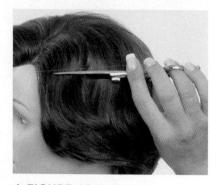

▲ **FIGURE 15-114**

Slicing on hair surface to remove bulk.

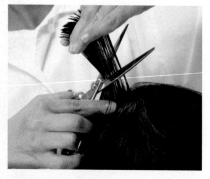

▲ **FIGURE 15-115**

Carving with shears to remove bulk.

REMOVING BULK

- *Thinning*: When thinning with serrated shears, the hair parting is combed and held between the index and middle finger. The shears are placed about mid-shaft on the strands and a cut is made (**Figure 15-113**). If another cut is necessary it should be made about 1" from the first cut. Do not cut twice in the same place.

- *Slicing and carving*: There are two slicing methods that can be used to remove bulk with regular shears. **Figure 15-114** shows the slicing technique performed on the surface of the hair. The second method requires parting off a vertical section of hair and elevating it between 45 and 90 degrees. Standing from the side of the hair projection, open the shears and position the parting close to the pivot. Carve through the partings with a curving motion that removes hair from the under portion of the parting as the motion is continued to the hair ends (**Figure 15-115**).

- *Slithering*: Yet another method used to remove bulk with regular shears is slithering. In this procedure a thin parting of hair is held between the fingers. The shears are positioned for cutting, and an up-and-down sliding motion along the parting is combined with a slight closing of the shears each time they are moved toward the scalp (**Figure 15-116**).

REMOVING WEIGHT FROM THE ENDS

Removing weight from the ends helps to taper the perimeter of graduated and blunt haircuts. This can be accomplished using thinning shears by elevating the section and placing the shears at an angle as the cuts are made or by using the comb to put the hair into position for cutting (**Figure 15-117**).

To remove weight with regular shears, *point cutting* or *notching* can be used to reduce weight in the ends of the hair. For either technique, a parting is held between the fingers, and the tips of the shears are used on a vertical angle to create points or notches in the hair (**Figure 15-118**).

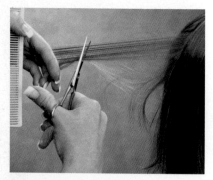

▲ **FIGURE 15-116**

Slithering.

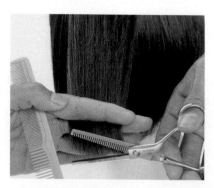

▲ **FIGURE 15-117**

Removing weight from the ends.

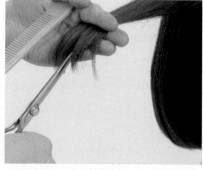

▲ **FIGURE 15-118**

Notching.

Both clippers and razors can be used to remove weight from the ends of the hair. Use a clipper-over-comb technique to put the hair ends in a position to be cut and position the clipper blades under the ends of the hair. Use a *reverse* rotation technique with the clipper to comb through and cut the ends from one section to another. The razor-over-comb technique should be used when lightening hair ends with a razor.

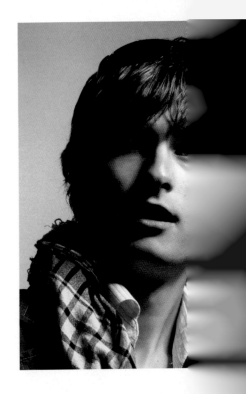

SHAVING THE OUTLINE AREAS

The performance of a neck shave and the shaving of the outline areas as a feature of the haircut service contribute to the appearance of the finished cut and provide the client with a true barbershop experience. This standard operating procedure in finishing a haircut follows the outlining or trimmer work.

The traditional *neck shave* consists of shaving the sides of the neck and across the nape with a razor. The *outline shave* includes the sideburn areas and around the ears and nape area. In African American styles, the front hairline is often included (Refer to **Figures 15-120** to **15-128**). The following preparation steps should be used in the performance of these shaving services:

1. Remove all cut hair from around the head and neck with a clean towel, tissues, or hair vacuum.

2. Loosen the cape and remove the neck strip used during the haircut. Be careful that loose clippings do not fall down the client's neck or shirt.

3. Pick up the cape at the lower edge, fold it upward to the top edge, and gather the four corners together. Remove the cape carefully so that cut hair does not fall on the client. Turn away from the chair and drop the lower edge of the cape, giving a slight shake to dislodge all cut hair.

4. Replace the cape, resting it a few inches away from the neck so that it does not touch the client's skin.

5. Spread a terry cloth or paper towel straight across the shoulders and tuck it loosely around the client's neck. Secure the cape and fold the towel over the neckband. The drape should be loose enough to permit easy access to the neck area. Tuck a towel or neck strip into the neckband of the drape for wiping the razor **(Figure 15-119)**.

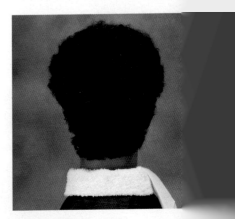

▲ FIGURE 15-119
Draping for outline shave.

OBJECTIVE:

The objective of this session is to practice the finger placement on the head form in relation to the razor and razor strokes used in performing an outline shave.

Shaving the Outline Areas on a Mannequin

Preparation: To avoid ruining the mannequin, apply a thin band of colored glue around the hairline and allow to dry thoroughly before shaving, or practice without a blade in the razor to master the position of the shaving strokes.

1 Apply a light coating of lather at the hairline of the sideburns, around and over the ears, the front hairline, down the sides of the neck, and across the nape. *Apply lather to the back of the neck and/or the front hairline of the client only if these areas are to be shaved.* Rub the lather in lightly with the balls of the fingers or thumb.

2 Shave the right side.

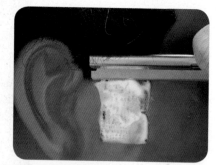

▲ **FIGURE 15-120**
Shave sideburn to desired length.

   a. Hold the razor for a freehand stroke.

   b. Place the left thumb on the scalp above the point of the razor and pretend to stretch the skin under the razor.

   c. Shave the sideburn to the desired length (**Figure 15-120**).

   d. Shave around the ear at the hairline and straight down the side of the neck, using the freehand stroke with the point of the razor. Be careful not to shave into the hairline at the nape of the neck (**Figures 15-121** through **15-123**).

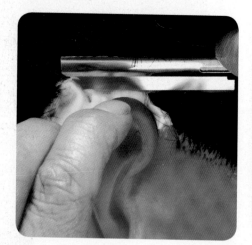

▲ **FIGURE 15-121**
Shaving around the ear.

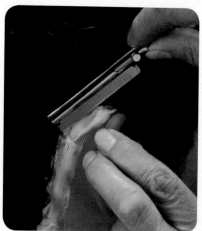

▲ **FIGURE 15-122**
Shaving in back of the ear.

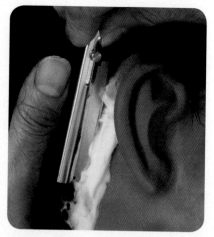

▲ **FIGURE 15-123**
Shaving behind the ear to the nape corner.

3 Shave the left side.

   a. Hold the razor for the backhand stroke.

   b. Place the left thumb on the scalp above the razor point, and pretend to stretch the skin under the razor.

   c. Shave the sideburn to the proper length using the backhand stroke (**Figure 15-124**).

   d. Shave around the ear at the hairline, using the freehand stroke.

   e. Shave the side of the neck below the ear, using the reverse backhand stroke with the point of the razor (**Figure 15-125**). Hold the ear away with the fingers of the left hand. If the stroke is done with one continuous movement, a straight line will be formed down the side of the neck.

   f. Shave the nape area with a freehand stroke (**Figure 15-126**).

4 Shave the front hairline.

   a. Start in the center of the front hairline and work toward the corners using a freehand stroke to the client's right side and a backhand stroke to the client's left side (**Figure 15-127**).

   b. Follow the natural hairline, shaving the outline through the temporal area to the front corner of the sideburns (**Figure 15-128**).

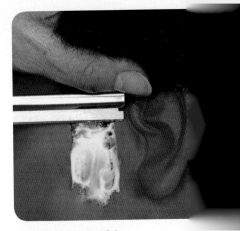

▲ **FIGURE 15-124**
Shave the left sideburn using reverse backhand stroke.

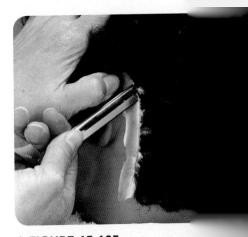

▲ **FIGURE 15-125**
Shave left side of neck to nape using the backhand stroke.

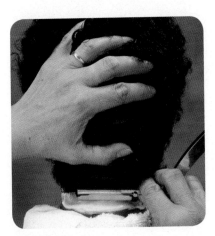

▲ **FIGURE 15-126**
Use the freehand stroke to shave the nape area.

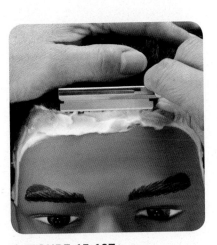

▲ **FIGURE 15-127**
Start at center of front hairline and shave toward corners.

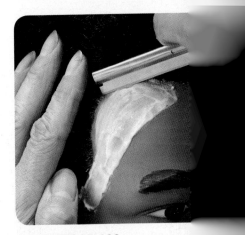

▲ **FIGURE 15-128**
Follow the natural hairline to the sideburn

Be guided by your instructor to learn other variations of this method.

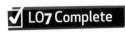

✔ **LO7 Complete**

Fingers-and-Shear Precision Cut on Model

MATERIALS, IMPLEMENTS, AND EQUIPMENT

- shampoo and haircutting cape
- terry cloth towels
- neck strips
- disposable barber towels
- clipper disinfectant and coolant
- shampoo and conditioner
- shaving cream or gel
- styling products
- talc
- spray bottle with water
- all-purpose, taper, and flat-top combs, picks, etc.
- styling brushes
- shears and blending shears
- clippers and outliners
- straight razor and blades
- hair clips
- blow dryer
- hand mirror

PREPARATION

1. Wash your hands.

2. Conduct model consultation.

3. Drape the model for wet service.

4. Shampoo and towel dry hair.

5. Remove waterproof cape; replace with a neckstrip and haircutting cape.

6. Face the model toward the mirror and lock the chair.

REMINDER

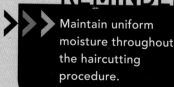

>>> Maintain uniform moisture throughout the haircutting procedure.

PROCEDURE

A. STEP 1

1 Comb the hair down in the front, sides, and back. Standing behind the model, take a $\frac{1}{4}$" to $\frac{1}{2}$" parting (depending on the density of the hair) at the forward-most part of the crown.

2 Comb the parting straight up at 90 degrees and hold it between the fingers of the left hand.

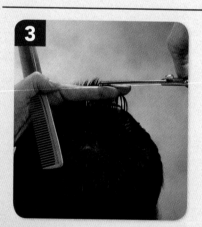

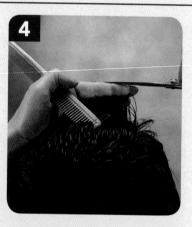

3 Bend the parting from right to left to determine at what length the hair will bend (bending point) to lie down smoothly (usually between 2" and 3"). When this length has been determined, re-comb the parting and, using the fingers of the left hand as a level, cut the hair that extends beyond the fingers. This cut establishes the traveling guide for the top section.

4 Pick up a second parting, retaining the guideline, comb, and cut. (The guideline should be visible and parallel to the top of the fingers.) A rhythm will soon develop: part hair for parting (1); comb hair in front of parting forward so it does not interfere with first parting (2); comb parting, retaining previous guide (3); and cut hair that extends past the guideline (4).

5 Complete the top section of hair, moving forward toward the front with each parting and cut. Remember to hold each parting that is to be cut at a 90-degree elevation from where it grows.

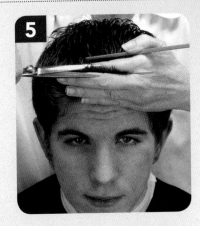

B. STEP 2

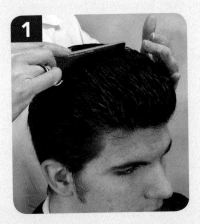

1 Comb the top section back. Move to the model's left side. Starting at the forehead, part off the top section of hair, front to back, with the thumb and middle finger.

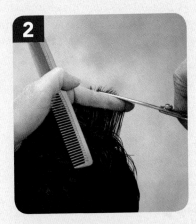

2 Hold the original guideline and a $\frac{1}{2}$" parting at the crown at 90 degrees and cut. This establishes the guide for the crown and back sections.

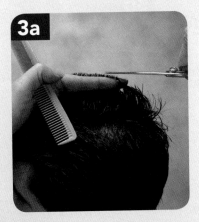

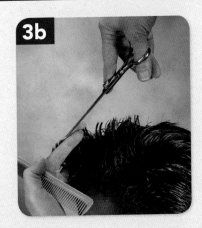

3 Work forward, still maintaining a side-standing position. Following the arc and contour of the head, even off any length that does not blend with the traveling guide. If Step 1 was performed correctly, no more than $\frac{1}{4}$" of hair should need to be evened or blended. Step 2 is a checkpoint for your work in the top section.

C. STEP 3

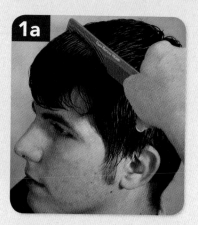 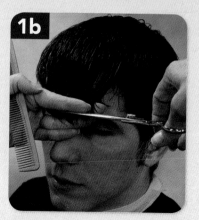

1 Comb the hair forward and move in front of the model. Holding the front hair section between the fingers of the left hand at 0 elevation, begin in the center and cut to the desired length to establish the front design line. Cut right and then left of the center to the ends of the width of the eyebrows, or to include the temporal area. The front and temporal design line has just been completed and will act as a traveling guide for the temporal area.

D. STEP 4

1 Move behind the model.

2 Beginning on the right side, pick up the front hair of the temporal/crest region. A small amount of the previously cut top hair should be visible.

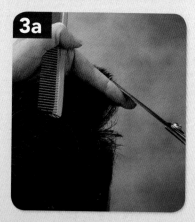 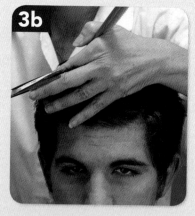

3 a. Hold the hair at 90 degrees and cut to the top guide.

    b. Front view of cutting right temporal section.

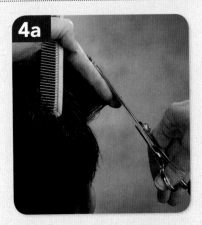

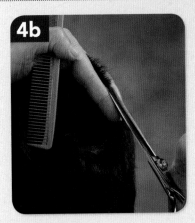

4 Continue cutting the crest area, working back to the center of the crown area. Cut hair only from the temporal region; do not pick up side hair. When approaching the crown area, reposition yourself so as to move toward the model's left, but not as far as the side of the model.

E. STEP 5

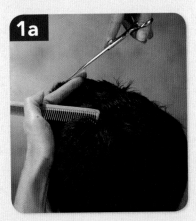

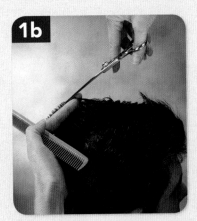

1 Repeat Step 4 on the left side of the model's hair. Cuts will be made *from* the top guide through the temporal region, rather than *to* the top guide. If the front design line was cut correctly, the excess hair in the front temporal region should not exceed 1″ to $1\frac{1}{2}$″. The crown hair from the right and left sides should meet upon completion of Step 5.

2 The top, temporal, and crown areas are now cut.

3 Comb the hair for Step 6.

F. STEP 6

1 Moving to the right of the model, comb the hair straight down on the sides.

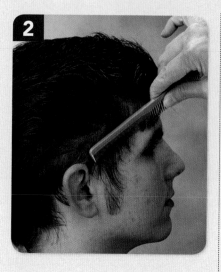

2 Take a $\frac{1}{4}$" to $\frac{1}{2}$" horizontal parting at the hairline, from the top of the ear to the sideburn area, and a diagonal parting of the same thickness from the right temple to the sideburn.

3 Comb the remaining hair back or secure it with a hair clip.

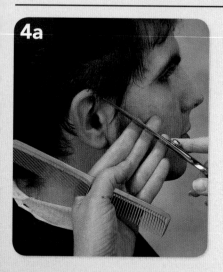

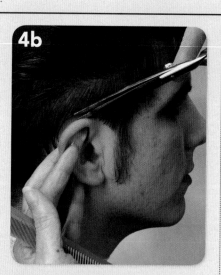

5 Move toward the front of the model facing the temporal and side areas.

4 Cut the design line either around the ears or to cover part of the ears at the desired length. If cutting around the ear, gently bend or slightly tug the ear down out of the way.

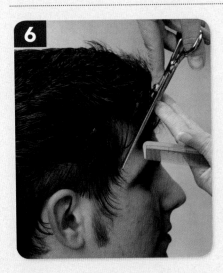

6 Using the front and side design lines (which are acting as guides), cut the hair between these two points against the skin, cutting along the natural hairline.

7 Holding the hair between the fingers at the lowest elevation possible, check the design line cut.

8 Proceed cutting the remaining side hair section, repeating the partings as the density of the hair requires.

9 Repeat this procedure on the left side, then check the length of the sides in the mirror for evenness.

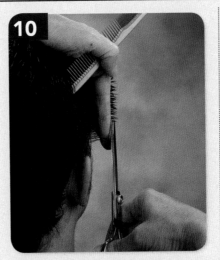

10 Move behind the model. Pick up the hair in vertical partings, holding it straight out to the side at 90 degrees. The design/guide line should be visible at the tips of the fingers when working on the right side of the model's head.

11 Make a straight, vertical cut from the design/guide line, cutting off any hair that extends past the guide.

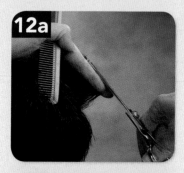

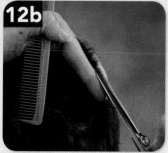

12 Continue cutting partings of hair while following the contour of the head until reaching the temporal/crest region. The hair lengths should meet and blend. Check the procedure by checking the blend of hair from the side design/guide line to the top section guide.

13 Proceed until all the side hair is cut. Stop at the topmost point behind the ear. Repeat for the left side. You may be positioned facing the client in order to work from the design/guide line up when blending the hair, or you may prefer to remain behind the model.

14 The front, top, temporal, crown, and side areas are now cut.

G. STEP 7

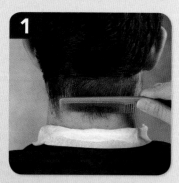

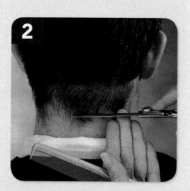

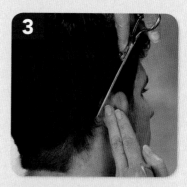

1 Move behind the model. Section off a $\frac{1}{4}$" to $\frac{1}{2}$" horizontal parting at the nape of the neck. Secure excess hair with a clip if necessary.

2 Starting in the center of the nape, cut the hair to the desired length; cut left and then right to the corners of the nape area. Check the design line cut.

3 Move to the model's right side. Part off a $\frac{1}{4}$" to $\frac{1}{2}$" section along the hairline. Cut hair in a downward direction from the side design line guide to right nape corner.

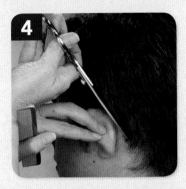

4 Comb and check the cut. Repeat for the left side. A backhand shear cutting position is required to cut downward on the model's left side.

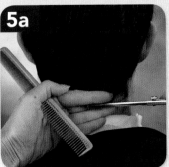

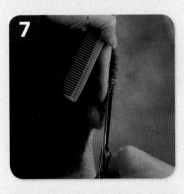

5 Part off a subsequent parting and comb hair down. Holding the design/guide line and parting between the fingers, cut hair at a low elevation or against the skin. Continue to take partings as the density requires, cutting the nape and behind-the-ear areas against the skin.

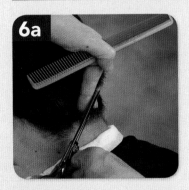

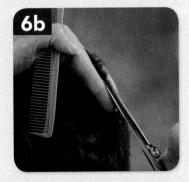

6 Pick up the hair in vertical partings at 90 degrees; blend through the back section up to meet the guides in the crown and crest areas.

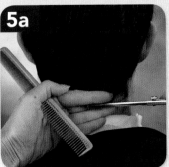

7 Proceed until the entire back section is cut and sides are blended to the back.

8 Check the entire haircut by combing the hair up in 90-degree sections, making sure that the hair blends from one section to another.

9 Perform a neck shave and shave outline areas as desired.

H. STEP 8

1 Dry the model's hair in a free-form style. This method requires the barber to move the dryer briskly from side to side while drying the hair. Begin at the nape, using a brush or comb in the left hand to hold midsection hair out of the way while drying the underneath hair first. The nozzle of the dryer should be pointing downward, 6" to 10" away from the hair. As the hair dries, check the cut for blending qualities. Proceed to dry the sides and top.

2 Brush the hair into place using a directional nozzle, if needed.

FYI

Cross-checking is the process of parting off subsections opposite from the elevation or direction at which they were cut to check for precision of line or blending. For example, a vertical subsection cut at a 90-degree projection can be cross-checked by parting off the subsections horizontally at 90 degrees.

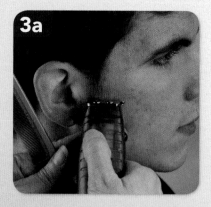

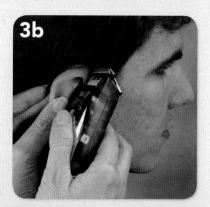

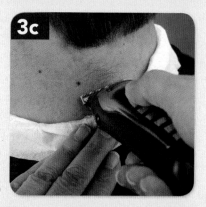

3 Use a trimmer (outliner) to clean up sideburns, sides (in around-the-ear styles), and nape. Check the behind-the-ear area for any difference in hair length or design. Complete finish work by performing a neck shave after outlining the bottom of the sideburn and around-the-ear areas with a razor.

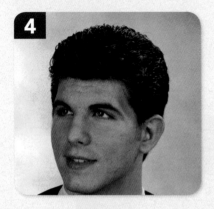

4 Re-comb the hair into the finished style.

5 Consult with the client regarding the use of a styling aid.

6 The haircut and style are now complete. Dust or vacuum stray hairs, making sure none remain on the client's face or neck.

CLEAN-UP AND DISINFECTION

1. Wash and disinfect tools and implements.

2. Clean surfaces and chair.

3. Sweep up hair and deposit in closed receptacle.

4. Deposit used blades in a sharps container.

5. Dispose of paper goods and/or linens.

6. Wash your hands.

I. ALTERNATIVE FINGERS-AND-SHEAR TECHNIQUE

Some barbers prefer to begin fingers-and-shear cutting in the front section or with a side part established in the hair. Be guided by the following steps and your instructor.

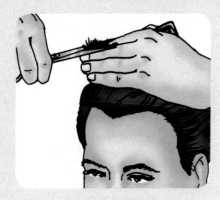

1 Comb model's hair into desired style with a side part. Start at the front hairline and project a parting of hair to 90 degrees. Cut to desired length and use as a traveling guide to cut back toward the crown.

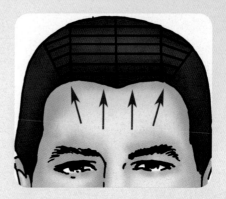

2 Pick up hair from the front temporal/crest area using the same procedure as in Step 1 to cut back toward the crown. Continue cutting all around the crest area through to the left side; or stop at the center of the crown and repeat procedure on the left side, working from the front to the crown. Continue with Steps 6–8 of Procedure 15-1, Fingers-and-shear precision cut on model.

Shear-Over-Comb Technique on Model

MATERIALS, IMPLEMENTS, AND EQUIPMENT

- shampoo and haircutting cape
- terry cloth towels
- neck strips
- disposable barber towels
- clipper disinfectant and coolant
- shampoo and conditioner
- shaving cream or gel
- styling products
- talc
- spray bottle with water
- all-purpose, taper, and flat-top combs, picks, etc.
- styling brushes
- shears and blending shears
- clippers and outliners
- straight razor and blades
- hair clips
- blow dryer
- hand mirror

PREPARATION

1. Wash your hands.
2. Conduct model consultation.
3. Drape the model for wet service.
4. Shampoo and towel dry hair. Blow-dry hair if dry cutting is preferred.
5. Remove waterproof cape; replace with a neckstrip and haircutting cape.
6. Face model toward the mirror and lock the chair.

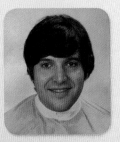

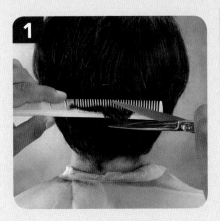

1 Comb the hair. Start cutting in the nape area, trimming hair to the desired length and thickness up to the occipital.

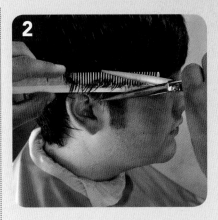

2 Move to right side and begin shear-over-comb cutting from the sideburn hairline into the side section.

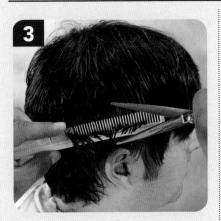

3 Continue technique over and behind the right ear.

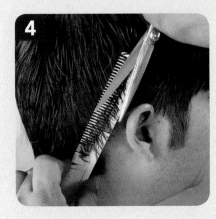

4 Using a diagonal comb position, blend the hair behind the ear to the hair at the right corner of the nape along the hairline.

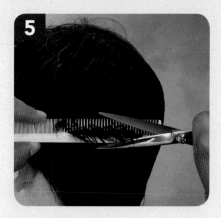

5 Blend hair at the side of the neck into the back section.

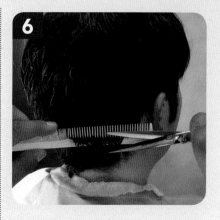

6 Move to left side and repeat shear-over-comb cutting from the sideburn hairline into the side section.

7 Continue technique over and in back of the left ear.

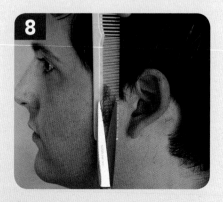

8 Using a diagonal comb position, blend the hair behind the ear to the hair at the left corner of the nape along the hairline.

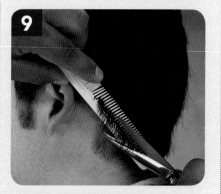

9 Blend hair at the side of the neck into the back section.

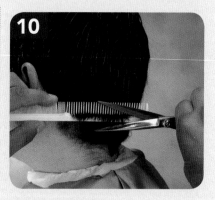

10 Blend hair from the occipital to the crown.

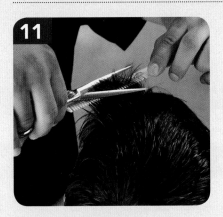

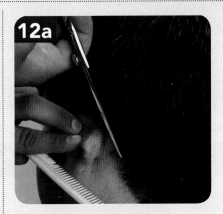

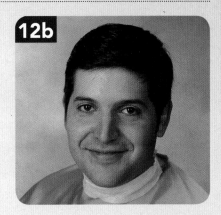

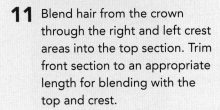

11 Blend hair from the crown through the right and left crest areas into the top section. Trim front section to an appropriate length for blending with the top and crest.

12 Outline sideburns, around the ear, and behind-the-ear areas with shears, followed by the trimmer. Finish the haircut with a neck and/or outline shave as the client desires. Also consult with the client regarding the use of a styling aid. Style the hair as desired. The haircut and style are now complete. Dust or vacuum any stray hairs on the client's face or neck.

CLEAN-UP AND DISINFECTION

1. Wash and disinfect tools and implements.

2. Clean surfaces and chair.

3. Sweep up hair and deposit in closed receptacle.

4. Deposit used blades in a sharps container.

5. Dispose of paper goods and/or linens.

6. Wash your hands.

Freehand and Clipper-Over-Comb Technique on Model with Straight Hair

PREPARATION

1. Wash your hands.

2. Conduct model consultation.

3. Drape the model for wet service.

4. Shampoo and towel dry hair. Blow-dry hair if dry cutting is preferred.

5. Remove waterproof cape; replace with a neckstrip and haircutting cape.

6. Face model toward the mirror and lock the chair.

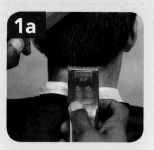

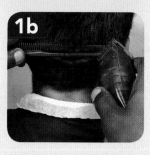

1 Comb the hair. Start in nape area and freehand taper the first inch or so of hair. Proceed with clipper-over-comb cutting to the occipital and lower crown areas.

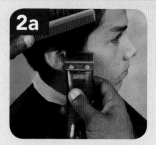

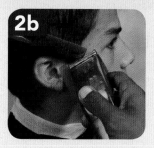

2 Move to right side and establish the length of the sideburn. Begin clipper-over-comb cutting from the sideburn hairline into the side section.

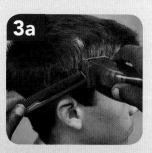

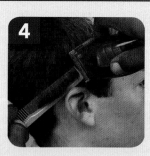

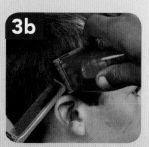

3 Continue technique above and in back of the right ear.

4 Using a diagonal comb position, blend the hair behind the ear to the hair at the right corner of the nape along the hairline.

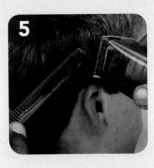

5 Blend hair on the right side of the neck into the back section.

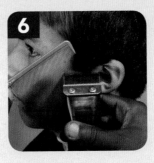

6 Move to left side and establish sideburn length. Begin clipper-over-comb cutting into the side section.

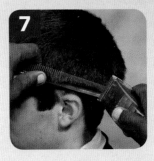

7 Continue technique above and in back of the left ear.

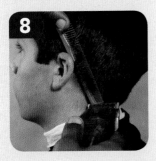

8 Using a diagonal comb position, blend the hair behind the ear to the hair at the left corner of the nape along the hairline.

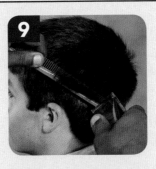

9 Blend hair at the side of the neck into the back section.

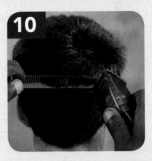

10 Blend hair from the occipital to the crown.

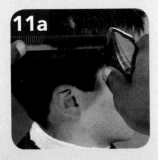

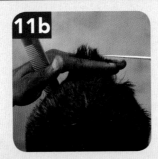

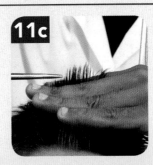

11 Blend hair from the crown through the right and left crest areas to meet the side sections. Trim top section using fingers-and-shear method to achieve the desired length. Check blending and fine-tune using fingers-and-shear method.

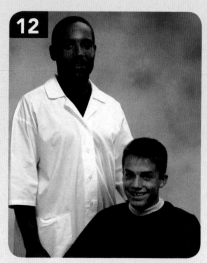

12 Outline sideburns, around the ear, behind-the-ear areas, and nape with shears and then trimmer. Complete finish work by performing a neck shave after outlining the bottom of the sideburn and around-the-ear areas with a razor. Consult with the client regarding the use of a styling aid, then style the hair as desired. The haircut and style are now complete . Dust or vacuum any stray hairs from the client's face or neck.

CLEAN-UP AND DISINFECTION

1. Wash and disinfect tools and implements.

2. Clean surfaces and chair.

3. Sweep up hair and deposit in closed receptacle.

4. Deposit used blades in a sharps container.

5. Dispose of paper goods and/or linens.

6. Wash your hands.

Freehand and Clipper-Over-Comb Techniques on Model with Tightly Curled Hair

MATERIALS, IMPLEMENTS, AND EQUIPMENT

- shampoo and haircutting cape
- terry cloth towels
- neck strips
- disposable barber towels
- clipper disinfectant and coolant
- shampoo and conditioner
- shaving cream or gel
- styling products
- talc
- spray bottle with water
- all-purpose, taper, and flat-top combs, picks, etc.
- styling brushes
- shears and blending shears
- clippers and outliners
- straight razor and blades
- hair clips
- blow dryer
- hand mirror

PREPARATION

1. Wash your hands.
2. Conduct model consultation.
3. Drape the model for wet service.
4. Shampoo and towel dry hair. Blow-dry hair if dry cutting is preferred.
5. Remove waterproof cape; replace with a neckstrip and haircutting cape.
6. Face model toward the mirror and lock the chair.

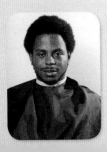

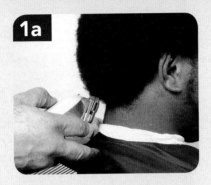

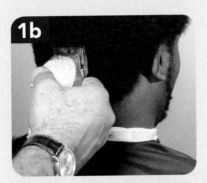

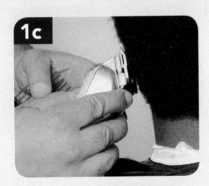

1 Comb or pick the hair out. Start in nape area and freehand taper or clipper-over-comb taper the first inch or so of hair. If hair density allows, proceed with clipper-over-comb cutting to the occipital area. If the hair is thick, freehand clipper cut to the occipital area. Continue cutting back section until nape to occipital is completed.

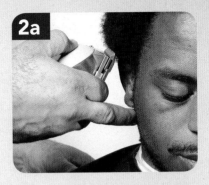

2 Move to right side to cut and blend from the sideburn hairline up to the crest.

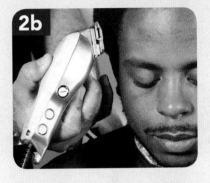

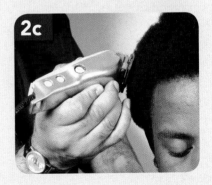

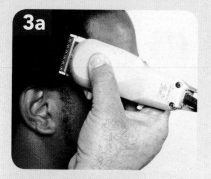

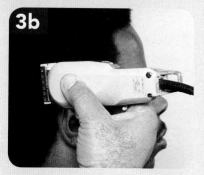

3 Blend sides toward back section.

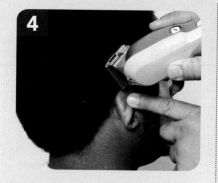

4 Blend the hair behind the ear to the right corner of the nape.

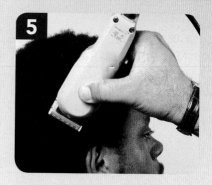

5 Blend the hair behind the ear to nape in the back section.

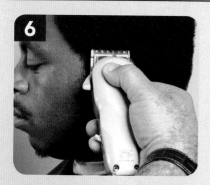

6 Move to left side and repeat cutting steps from sideburn hairline to the crest.

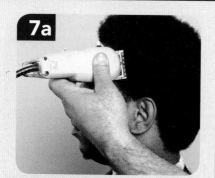

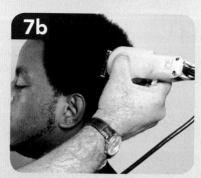

7 Continue blending on left side above ear.

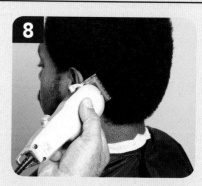

8 Blend the hair behind the ear to the corner of the nape along the hairline.

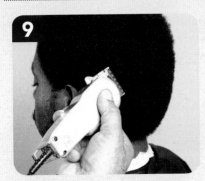

9 Blend the hair at the side of the neck into the back section.

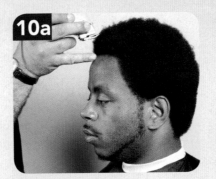

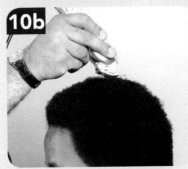

10 Establish guide in front center of top section and cut back to crown area.

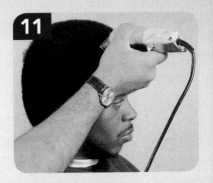

11 Blend crest to top guide around the entire head.

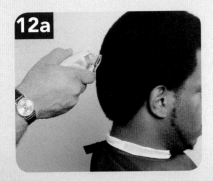

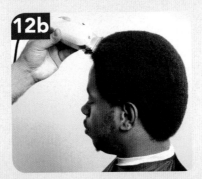

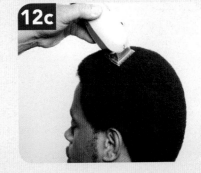

12 Blend occipital area to crest and check the blend to the top section.

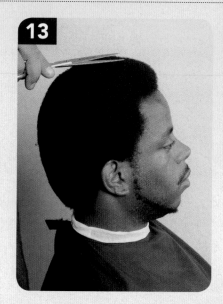

13 Comb or pick hair out. Fine-tune with shears.

14 Outline sideburns, around the ear, and behind-the-ear areas with clippers or trimmers. Consult with the client regarding the use of a styling aid and style the hair as desired. The haircut and style portion of the service is now complete. Finish with the neck and outline shaving procedure shown in Procedure 15-5. Dust or vacuum stray hairs from the model's face and neck.

CLEAN-UP AND DISINFECTION

1. Wash and disinfect tools and implements.

2. Clean surfaces and chair.

3. Sweep up hair and deposit in closed receptacle.

4. Dispose of paper goods and/or linens.

5. Wash your hands.

Shaving Outline on Model with Tightly Curled Hair

MATERIALS, IMPLEMENTS, AND EQUIPMENT

- shampoo and haircutting cape
- terry cloth towels
- neck strips
- disposable barber towels
- clipper disinfectant and coolant
- shampoo and conditioner
- shaving cream or gel
- styling products
- talc
- spray bottle with water
- all-purpose, taper, and flat-top combs, picks, etc.
- styling brushes
- shears and blending shears
- clippers and outliners
- straight razor and blades
- hair clips
- blow dryer
- hand mirror

PREPARATION

1. Model should still be draped from the haircut service.

2. Disinfect razor and blades.

3. Wash your hands.

4. Loosen cape and apply towel to neckline, leaving it loose enough for access when securing the drape.

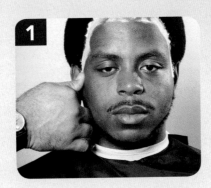

1 Apply a light coating of lather at the front hairline and rub the lather in lightly with the balls of the fingers or thumb.

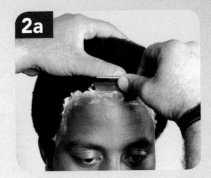

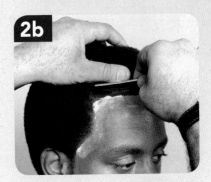

2 Stand at a slight diagonal to the model's forehead on his right side. Stretch the skin in the forehead area. Using a freehand stroke, shave along the front hairline into the temple area.

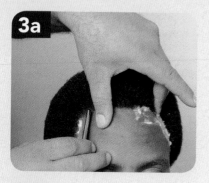

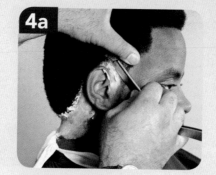

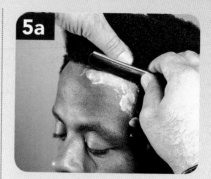

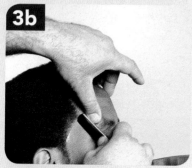

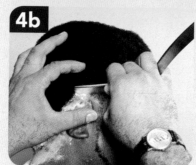

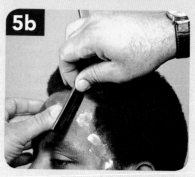

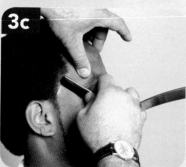

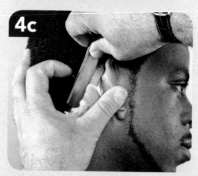

5 Move to the model's left side. Reapply lather at forehead as necessary. Stretch the skin in the forehead area and repeat freehand strokes to the temple.

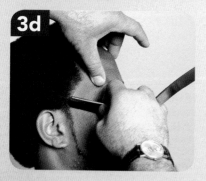

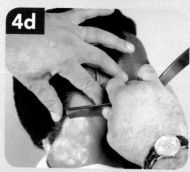

3 Next, shave from the temple along the hairline to the front of the sideburn.

4 Apply lather around and behind the ear. Shave around the ear and down the side of the neck, using the freehand stroke with the point of the razor. Hold the ear away with the fingers of the left hand as necessary for safety. Be careful not to shave into the hairline at the nape of the neck.

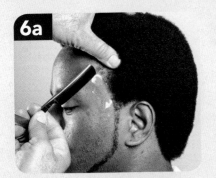

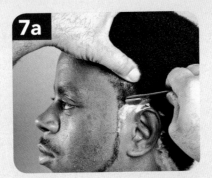

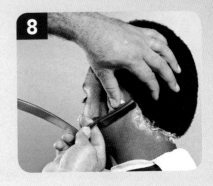

8 Employ the reverse backhand stroke to shave down the side of the neck with the point of the razor. Be careful not to shave into the hairline at the nape of the neck.

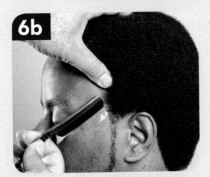

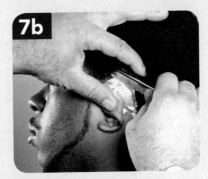

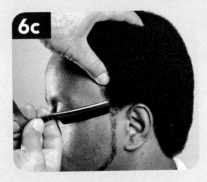

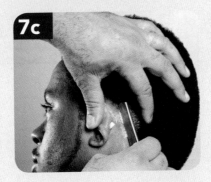

6 Use the backhand stroke to shave from the temple to the front sideburn area.

7 Apply lather around and behind the ear. Use the freehand stroke to shave in front of and around the ear at the hairline, holding the ear away with the fingers of the left hand as necessary for safety.

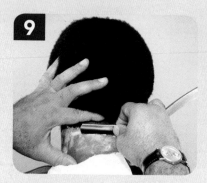

9 Shave the nape area with a freehand stroke. Clean up model's hairline with a warm, moist towel.

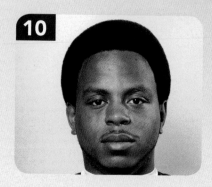

10 Apply astringent, moisturizing cream, talc, or after-shave lotion as desired. Figure 10 shows a finished outline shave.

CLEAN-UP AND DISINFECTION

1. Wash and disinfect tools and implements.

2. Clean surfaces and chair.

3. Sweep up hair and deposit in closed receptacle.

4. Deposit used blades in a sharps container.

5. Dispose of paper goods and/or linens.

6. Wash your hands.

Razor Cutting on Model

MATERIALS, IMPLEMENTS, AND EQUIPMENT

- shampoo and haircutting cape
- terry cloth towels
- neck strips
- disposable barber towels
- clipper disinfectant and coolant
- shampoo and conditioner
- shaving cream or gel
- styling products
- talc
- spray bottle with water
- all-purpose, taper, and flat-top combs, picks, etc.
- styling brushes
- shears and blending shears
- clippers and outliners
- straight razor, blades, and guard
- hair clips
- blow dryer
- hand mirror

PREPARATION

1. Wash your hands.
2. Conduct model consultation.
3. Drape the model for wet service.
4. Shampoo and towel dry hair.
5. Remove waterproof cape; replace with a neckstrip and haircutting cape.
6. Face model toward the mirror and lock the chair.

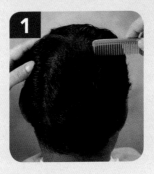

1 Section the hair into four sections from crown to nape, crown to front, and crest to sides. Subdivide the back section into three subsections.

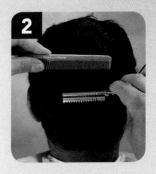

2 Begin in the center section just below the crown. Taper the hair using the razor rotation technique, one strip at a time in a downward direction to the hairline. Blend each new cut with the hair previously trimmed. Use short, even razor strokes to avoid ridges, lines, or any appearance of unevenness.

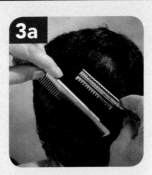
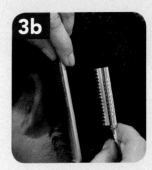

3 Comb the hair downward from the top right side toward the left midsection in the back. Lightly taper from right to left in the top section. Taper the lower section to blend with the nape hair.

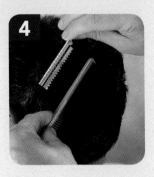
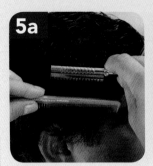
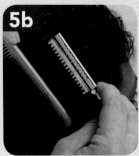
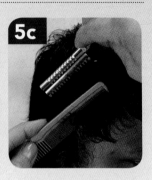

4 Comb the hair downward from the top left side toward the right. Repeat the procedure used in Step 3.

5 Comb side hair downward and subdivide it into three vertical partings. Begin tapering about $\frac{3}{4}''$ from the crest. Taper downward through the three sections to the hairline. Comb the hair toward the back and taper lightly in that direction, then blend with the back section. Comb the hair forward and taper lightly toward the face, trimming the perimeter (design) line as needed.

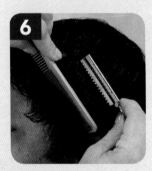
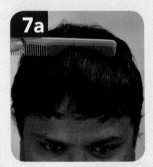
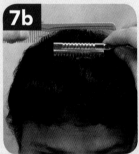
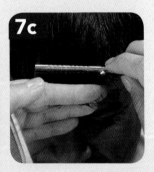

6 Repeat Step 5 procedures on left side of head.

7 Comb top hair forward with even distribution over the head form. Start tapering just forward of the crown in the top section. Work toward the forehead on the right side. Repeat on the left side, then taper the center section. Make sure to blend all three sections. Hold the front section at a low elevation and trim using the freehand slicing technique.

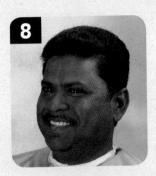

8 Comb through the cut, redistributing the sections in a variety of directions to check for blending and evenness. Consult with the client regarding a neck shave, outline shaving, and the use of styling aids. Style the hair as desired. The haircut and style are now complete. Dust or vacuum stray hairs, making sure none remain on the client's face or neck.

CLEAN-UP AND DISINFECTION

1. Wash and disinfect tools and implements.

2. Clean surfaces and chair.

3. Sweep up hair and deposit in closed receptacle.

4. Deposit used blades in a sharps container.

5. Dispose of paper goods and/or linens.

6. Wash your hands.

Clipper Cutting—Close Fade Cut on Model

The standard characteristics that apply to the many variations of fade cuts today include a close, tight cut at the sides and back; blending at the occipital and crest areas; and a customized design at the temples and front sections. To facilitate blending, the clipper blades are opened or closed, based on the hair's density and curl pattern.

MATERIALS, IMPLEMENTS, AND EQUIPMENT

- shampoo and haircutting cape
- terry cloth towels
- neck strips
- disposable barber towels
- clipper disinfectant and coolant
- shampoo and conditioner
- shaving cream or gel
- styling products
- talc
- spray bottle with water
- all-purpose, taper, and flat-top combs, picks, etc.
- styling brushes
- shears and blending shears
- clippers and outliners
- straight razor and blades
- hair clips
- blow dryer
- hand mirror

PREPARATION

1. Wash your hands.
2. Conduct model consultation.
3. Drape the model for wet service.
4. Shampoo and towel dry hair.
5. Remove waterproof cape; replace with a neckstrip and haircutting cape.
6. Face model toward the mirror and lock the chair.

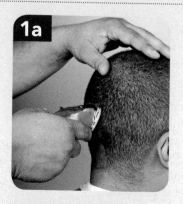

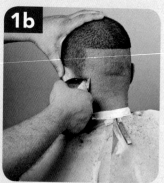

1 Set the clipper blade in the closed position to achieve a close cut. Start at the center of the nape, cutting to the bottom of the parietal ridge. Cut the sections right and left of center through the back section.

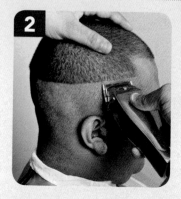

2 Move to the right side (or left, depending on preference) and cut from the hairline to the top, middle, or bottom of the crest area as desired by the client. Cut around the ear and into the previously cut back section, cutting up and/or across as the growth pattern allows. Complete cutting the opposite side in the same manner.

REMINDER

>>> Cutting against the grain achieves a closer cut than cutting with the grain. Procedure 15-7 shows one method to achieve a close fade cut. Be guided by your instructor for different techniques and fade style variations.

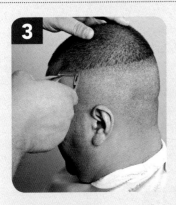

3 When the back and sides are completed, open the clipper blades (one-quarter of the way for fine hair; almost one-half for thick hair) and cut a $\frac{1}{4}''$ to $\frac{3}{4}''$ thick section at the point where you previously stopped cutting at the crest. Note the difference in hair length through the parietal ridge in Figure 3. Continue cutting only in this section from the right side, across the back, and into the left side area. Option: You may choose to stop at the center back and cut *from* the left side to the center back.

4 Open the blades another quarter and repeat the procedure in Step 3, cutting another $\frac{1}{4}''$ thick section above the one previously cut. Repeat as necessary.

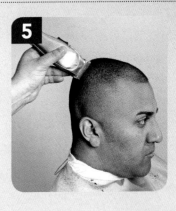

5 Open the blades completely. Starting in the crown area, blend the hair with the grain through the top, then on a slight diagonal into the shorter hair at the crest. Complete this step around the entire head.

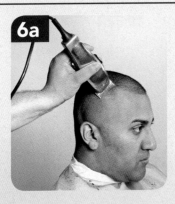 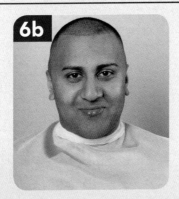

6 Close the blades slightly and blend from the bottom of the top section into the top of the crest area. Continue to close the blades slightly as you work through the crest, fading it into the side sections. Finish with the trimmer and/or outline shave to define the hairline. The haircut is now complete. Dust or vacuum stray hairs, making sure none remain on the client's face or neck.

CLEAN-UP AND DISINFECTION

1. Wash and disinfect tools and implements.
2. Clean surfaces and chair.
3. Sweep up hair and deposit in closed receptacle.
4. Deposit used blades in a sharps container.
5. Dispose of paper goods and/or linens.
6. Wash your hands.

MATERIALS, IMPLEMENTS, AND EQUIPMENT

- shampoo and haircutting cape
- terry cloth towels
- neck strips
- disposable barber towels
- clipper disinfectant and coolant
- shampoo and conditioner
- shaving cream or gel
- styling products
- talc
- spray bottle with water
- all-purpose, taper, and flat-top combs, picks, etc.
- styling brushes
- shears and blending shears
- clippers and outliners
- straight razor and blades
- hair clips
- blow dryer
- hand mirror

PREPARATION

1. Wash your hands.
2. Conduct model consultation.
3. Drape the model for wet service.
4. Shampoo and towel dry hair.
5. Remove waterproof cape; replace with a neckstrip and haircutting cape.
6. Face model toward the mirror and lock the chair.

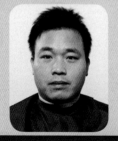

A. FLAT TOP

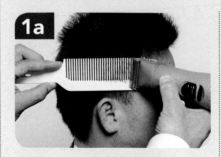

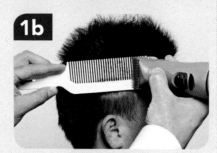

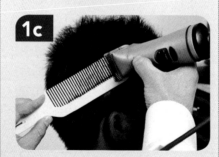

1 Start on preferred side using a clipper-over-comb technique with a flat top comb and a #1$\frac{1}{2}$ blade. Cut from the hairline to the crest. Cut through to back section and repeat on opposite side.

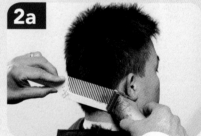

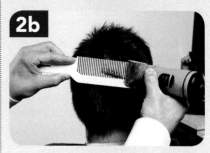

2 Move to back and use a #1 blade to taper the hairline. Taper and blend through the back section.

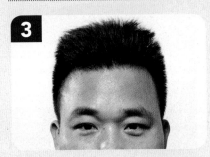

3 Work medium-hold gel through the hair in top section and blow-dry the hair up and back from the scalp. The goal is to position the hair to stand straight up from the scalp.

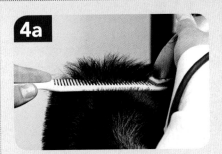

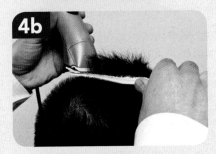

4 Stand in back of the model and use a #1 blade to blend and round the corners of the crown area, then establish a guide in the top section. Continue cutting over the top section toward the front using a horizontal comb placement.

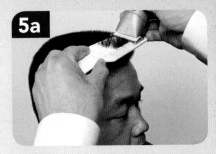

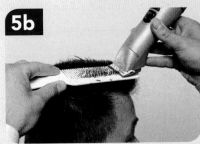

5 Working from in front of the model, cut and blend the front section from the top section to the top of the crest. The comb placement in this section should be slightly angled (or elevated) from shorter to longer hair. This means the comb will rest closer to the head in the shorter crest areas and farther away from the head in the front section. Use the length of the front guide and the shorter length guide at the crest to determine the angle of comb placement. Repeat on opposite side.

6 Re-comb and blow-dry as necessary. Finish with neck or outline shave. The haircut and style are now complete. Dust or vacuum stray hairs, making sure none remain on the client's face or neck. Figures 6a and 6b show the finished cut.

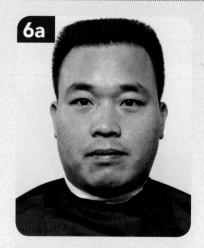

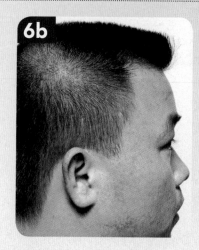

B. CREW CUT

The crew cut is a shorter and more rounded style than the flat top.

1 Using a # $1\frac{1}{2}$ blade, cut with the grain and angle the comb from the crown to the front. The hair should be cut closer at the crown and gradually longer toward the front. Use the top section as a guide to round out the crest areas.

2 Use a $\frac{3}{8}$" blade to cut and blend against the grain through the sides and back areas up to the crest.

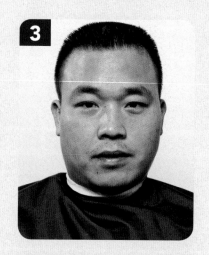

3 Re-comb and finish with neck or outline shave. The haircut and style are now complete. Dust or vacuum stray hairs, making sure none remain on the client's face or neck.

CLEAN-UP AND DISINFECTION

1. Wash and disinfect tools and implements.
2. Clean surfaces and chair.
3. Sweep up hair and deposit in closed receptacle.
4. Deposit used blades in a sharps container.
5. Dispose of paper goods and/or linens.
6. Wash your hands.

Taper Cut on Curly Hair Texture

MATERIALS, IMPLEMENTS, AND EQUIPMENT

- shampoo and haircutting cape
- terry cloth towels
- neck strips
- disposable barber towels
- clipper disinfectant and coolant
- shampoo and conditioner
- shaving cream or gel
- styling products
- talc
- spray bottle with water
- all-purpose, taper, and flat-top combs, picks, etc.
- styling brushes
- shears and blending shears
- clippers and outliners
- straight razor and blades
- hair clips
- blow dryer
- hand mirror

PREPARATION

1. Wash your hands.

2. Conduct model consultation.

3. Drape the model for wet service.

4. Shampoo and towel dry hair. Blow-dry hair if dry cutting is preferred.

5. Remove waterproof cape; replace with a neckstrip and haircutting cape.

6. Face model toward the mirror and lock the chair.

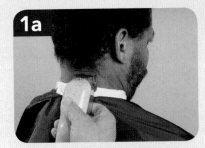

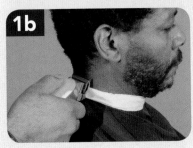

1 Comb or pick the hair out. Open the clipper blades and freehand clipper cut the nape area from the hairline.

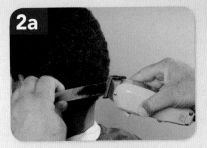

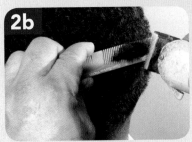

2 Use the clipper-over-comb technique to cut and blend through the back section. Depending on the length and density of the hair, do not remove too much hair from the occipital area. Taper cuts are shorter at the perimeter and gradually increase in length to the top section.

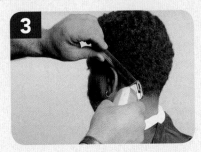

3 Move to the model's left side and blend the hair behind the ear using a diagonal comb placement.

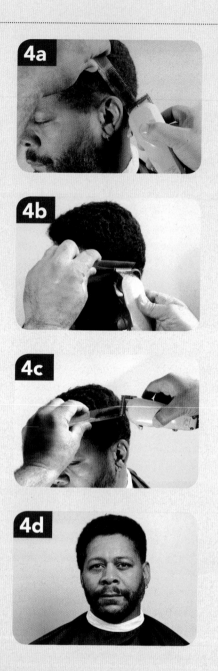

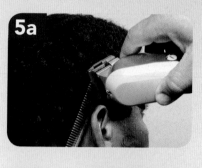

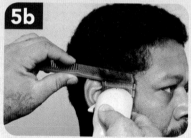

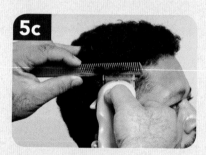

5 Repeat tapering and blending steps on the opposite side.

4 Continue tapering around the ear and into the side section. Taper and blend toward crest area. Compare the rounded uncut shape of the model's hair on his right side with the tapered shape of his left side in Figure 4d.

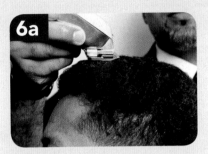

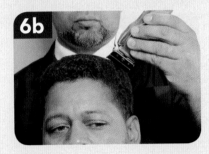

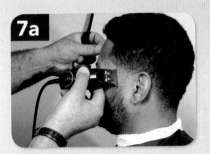

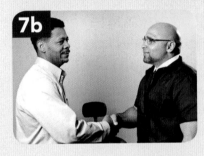

6 Pick out or comb through the top section. Blend hair through the top and crest areas. Check work.

7 Finish with outliner to clean up hairline. Note tapered nape area in Figure 7a. The taper cut is now complete. Finish with the neck and outline shaving if requested. Dust or vacuum stray hairs from the model's face and neck.

CLEAN-UP AND DISINFECTION

1. Wash and disinfect tools and implements.

2. Clean surfaces and chair.

3. Sweep up hair and deposit in closed receptacle.

4. Dispose of paper goods and/or linens.

5. Wash your hands.

Head Shaving

The shaved head is one of today's current fashion trends that many men choose regardless of the density or growth pattern of their hair. A head shave should be performed with a changeable-blade or conventional straight razor.

CAUTION: Do not adjust outliner blades flush with each other to accomplish this service as doing so may cause serious injury to the client's skin. Excess hair can be removed with clippers using #0000 or balding blades. The following is one method used to perform a head shave.

MATERIALS, IMPLEMENTS AND EQUIPMENT

- shampoo and haircutting cape
- terry cloth towels
- neck strips
- disposable barber towels
- clipper disinfectant and coolant
- shampoo and conditioner
- shaving cream or gel
- talc
- spray bottle with water
- all-purpose, taper, and flat-top combs, picks, etc.
- clippers and outliners
- straight razor and blades
- hand mirror

PREPARATION

1. Wash your hands.
2. Conduct model consultation.
3. Drape the model for wet service.
4. Shampoo and towel dry hair.
5. Remove waterproof cape; replace with a neckstrip and haircutting cape.
6. Face model toward the mirror and lock the chair.

1 Examine the scalp for any abrasions, primary or secondary lesions, or scalp disorders.

3 Apply shaving cream or gel and lather. Next, apply two or three steam towel treatments to soften the remaining hair.

2 Remove excess hair length with the clippers. Use a balding clipper blade if available. Shampoo the remaining hair and reexamine the scalp.

4 Start at the back and use a freehand stroke to shave with the grain of the hair from the crown to the nape. Use the opposite hand to stretch the skin taut as needed for each area to be shaved. Follow the curve of the head, taking short strokes with the first half of the blade from its point to midsection.

5 Move in front of the client and tip his head forward slightly. Continue shaving from the crown to the front hairline, reapplying lathering agent as needed.

NOTE: Keep the skin moist to facilitate shaving.

6 When the top section is completed, work down the sides. Just below the crest, hold the ear out of the way with the left hand, finish shaving the side, and carefully shave in front of and around the ears.

7 Upon completion of the head shave, check for any missed areas. Remove remaining lather with a warm towel, apply witch hazel or toner, and follow with a cool towel application for 2 to 3 minutes.

CLEAN-UP AND DISINFECTION

1. Wash and disinfect tools and implements.
2. Clean surfaces and chair.
3. Sweep up hair and deposit in closed receptacle.
4. Deposit used blades in a sharps container.
5. Dispose of paper goods and/or linens.
6. Wash your hands.

✓ LO8 Complete

HAIRCUT FINISH WORK

In addition to neck and outline shaves, two other finishing services traditionally performed in the barbershop include trimming the eyebrows and trimming excess hair from the nostrils and ears. Barbers should always ask their clients if they would like one or all of these finishing services.

TRIMMING THE EYEBROWS

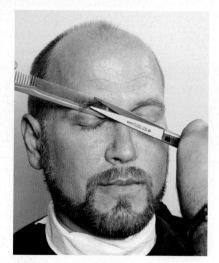

▲ **FIGURE 15-129a**

Using shear-over-comb technique to trim eyebrows.

Eyebrow trimming may require a combination of techniques, depending on the length and density of the brow hair. Shear-over-comb is the most popular but an outliner-over-comb technique can be used as well. Freehand shear cutting is sometimes required to cut individual stray hairs that extend beyond the natural arch of the brow and should be done carefully. Safety and protection of the client's eyes should always be the first consideration when using any technique (**Figures 15-129a** to **15-129c**).

TRIMMING EXCESS NOSTRIL AND EAR HAIR

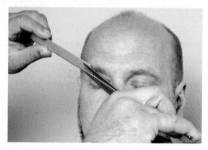

▲ **FIGURE 15-129b**

Mid-point of eyebrow trim.

Outliners with T-shaped blades or nose hair trimmers are the safest tools to use for trimming excess hair from the nostrils. If using a T-bladed trimmer, simply grasp the tip of the nose between your thumb and index finger and gently tilt it up or to the side and position the first few teeth of the blades on a slight diagonal to trim the hairs. Follow the manufacturer's directions for using nose hair trimmers, as there are several different styles available on the market.

Trimming excess hair in or around the ears is also performed with an outliner or trimmer. Some barbers prefer a T-bladed tool because it is easier to maneuver the blades in small tight areas like the ears. Always dust off residual hair in and around the ears after trimming.

Introduction to Men's Hairstyling

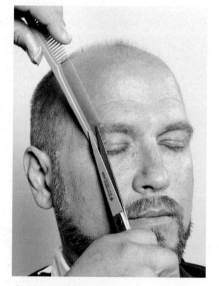

▲ **FIGURE 15-129c**

End point of eyebrow trim.

Hairstyling is the art of arranging the hair into an appropriate style following a haircut or shampoo. Today, many haircuts require minimal hairstyling techniques due to the quality of the cuts, current styles, and the availability of effective styling aids such as gels, mousses, and styling sprays. Other haircuts require more styling attention, such as blow-drying or picking the style into place. In this section, the methods discussed for styling men's hair include natural drying, finger styling, scrunch styling, blow-drying, and blow-waving.

NATURAL DRYING

As the name implies, natural drying is the term used when the hair is left to air-dry naturally. Typically the hair is combed into place or arranged with the fingers and allowed to dry in place. Some men prefer to apply gels, pomades, or other styling products to aid in holding the hair in place while it dries, while others prefer to apply products after the hair is dry. Since it is never a good idea to let a client leave the barbershop with wet hair, the use of a heat lamp or blow-dryer with a diffuser can speed up the drying process for this natural style.

FINGER-STYLING

Finger-styling may or may not utilize the blow dryer to style the hair. Sometimes the hair is simply styled with the fingers and allowed to dry naturally, much like many clients do at home. When a blow dryer is used, the technique involves lifting, raking, or directing the hair to give it direction as it dries and produces a more textured appearance than brush styling. Diffuser attachments and styling products can also be used with this technique, depending on the texture and density of the hair and the desired outcome (**Figure 15-130**).

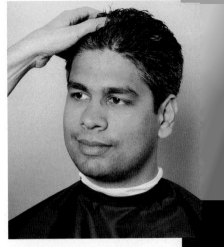

▲ **FIGURE 15-130**
Finger styling.

SCRUNCH-STYLING

Scrunch-styling is actually a form of finger styling that is typically used on wavy to curly hair patterns with some length to create a tousled look. A diffuser attachment can be used while lifting and squeezing the hair between the fingers. Wavy and curly hair may require the application of a spray gel or a light pomade to reduce the frizzy hair ends that sometimes accompany these hair textures (**Figures 15-131a** and **b**).

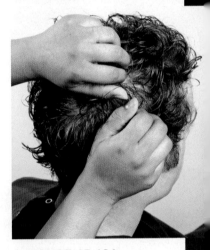

▲ **FIGURE 15-131a**
Scrunch styling technique.

BLOW-DRY STYLING

Blow-dry styling is the technique of drying and styling damp hair in one operation and has revolutionized the hair care industry. While some men may not wish to do more than comb their hair into place and let it dry, the use of a blow-dryer offers some options for speed-drying and special-effects styling, such as blow waving.

The implements most often used to style men's hair with a blow dryer are combs, picks, and a variety of brushes. Some barbers prefer a narrow brush with wire or hard plastic bristles. Others prefer vent or grooming brushes. In most cases, the texture of the hair and the desired effect will dictate the type of implement to use (**Figures 15-132** and **15-133**).

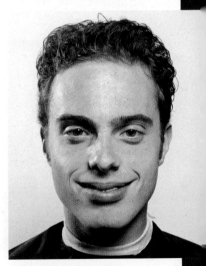

▲ **FIGURE 15-131b**
Finished scrunch styling.

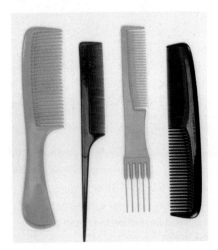

▲ **FIGURE 15-132**
Combs.

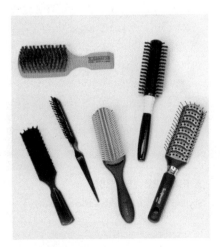

▲ **FIGURE 15-133**
Brushes.

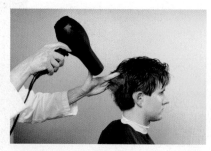

▲ FIGURE 15-134a
Freeform blowdrying using the fingers.

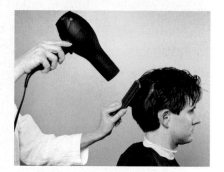

▲ FIGURE 15-134b
Freeform blowdrying using a brush to release hair while drying.

F◉CUS ON...

Keep the air and the hair moving when blow-dry styling to prevent burning the client's scalp.

The blow-drying techniques used in men's hairstyling are freeform, stylized or blow waving, and diffused.

BLOW-DRYING TECHNIQUES

Freeform blow-drying is a quick, easy method of drying the client's hair that is probably most like the techniques men use at home (**Figure 15-134a**). This technique can build fullness into the style while allowing the hair to fall into the natural lines of the cut (**Figure 15-134b**). Some barbers choose this method for the following reasons:

- It shows the client the ease with which the style can be duplicated.

- It demonstrates the quality of the haircut as the hair falls into place.

- The blow-drying service is accelerated.

- It allows the barber to check the accuracy of the work as the hair falls into place.

Stylized blow-drying creates a more finished appearance because each section is dried in a definite direction with the aid of a comb or brush followed by the dryer. Heat makes physical changes in the hair when using the blow dryer in this fashion. The hair will look smoother and more precisely directed overall; this look may be achieved with or without styling products, depending on the texture of the hair (**Figures 15-135a** to **15-135c**). When a comb or brush and the blow-dryer are used to create wave patterns and

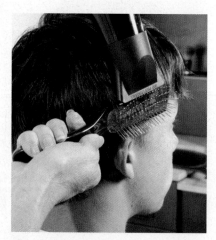

▲ FIGURE 15-135a
Styling the side section with blow dryer and brush.

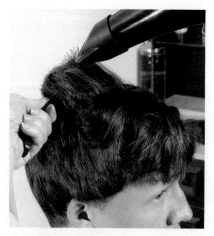

▲ FIGURE 15-135b
Styling and drying the top section.

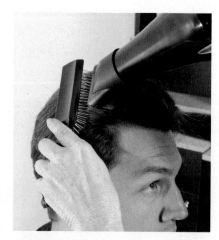

▲ FIGURE 15-135c
Finish work over the surface of the hairstyle. Follow the brush with the dryer.

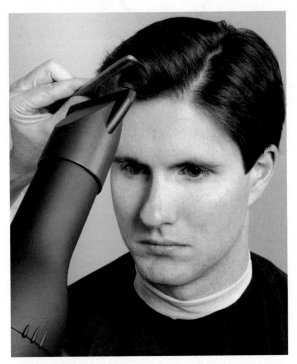

▲ **FIGURE 15-136a**
Create a ridge or bend in the hair near the scalp with the comb.

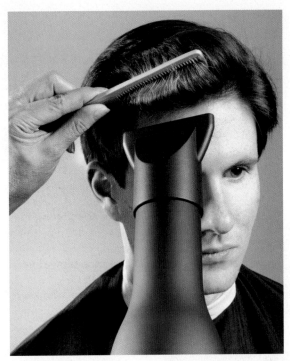

▲ **FIGURE 15-136b**
Set the ridge with heat from the blow dryer.

direction in the hair, the technique is called *blow waving* (**Figures 15-136a** and **15-136b**).

Diffused drying is used when the client desires to maintain the natural wave pattern of the hair, as opposed to temporarily straightening it with the blow-dryer and brush. Diffused drying is an effective option to use when arranging or picking out very curly hair textures, manipulating sculpting and styling products, or employing scrunching.

BUILDING VOLUME

Occasionally extra volume is needed in the crown, crest, or top (apex) areas of a style to create a more proportionate look. To build volume and/or to create an even contour throughout the hairstyle, use the blow-dryer and brush in the following manner:

1. Lift the hair with the brush, bending the section as the blow dryer is directed at the base of the section and followed through to the ends (Refer to Figure 15-135b). Avoid burning the scalp.

2. Follow the same procedure to build fullness on the sides. Use horizontal partings if the hair is to be styled down on the sides and vertical or diagonal partings if the hair will be brushed back.

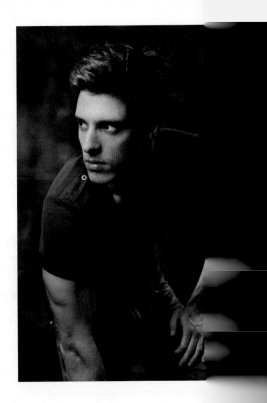

OBJECTIVE:

The objective of this session is to learn to manipulate the hair, brush, and blow-dryer for styling purposes.

Blow Dry Styling on a Mannequin

FREE-FORM BLOW-DRYING

1 After completing the mannequin haircut performed in Practice Session #4, moisten and comb the hair into the basic style.

2 Hold the blow-dryer in the dominant hand. The dryer should be held 6" to 10" from the area being dried at an angle with the nozzle pointing downward on the hair and should be moved briskly from side to side as it dries the hair.

3 Beginning at the nape area, hold the hair above the hairline out of the way with a brush or comb in the opposite hand (**Figure 15-137**). As the hair underneath is dried, the brush or comb releases the next layered section for drying. Comb or brush the hair down after each section is dried.

4 Dry the sides in the same manner (**Figure 15-138**).

5 The top should be dried loosely and then brushed in to the desired style, followed by the blow-dryer (**Figure 15-139**).

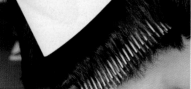

▲ **FIGURE 15-137**

Freeform blow-drying nape and back sections.

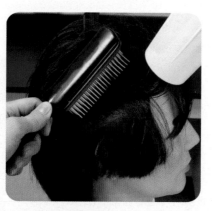

▲ **FIGURE 15-138**

Drying the side section.

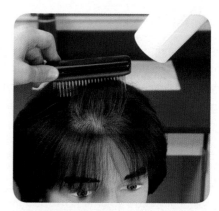

▲ **FIGURE 15-139**

Drying the front section.

6 Apply different styling aids such as mousses, gels, and hairsprays to compare and contrast the effects.

STYLIZED BLOW-DRYING

1 Remoisten the mannequin hair. Begin in the back section and lift a section of hair with the comb or brush. While combing or brushing through the parting, follow the movement with the dryer to apply a concentrated stream of heated air to the section. Repeat the process until the hair is dry in that section and continue the process with subsequent partings or sections of hair (**Figure 15-140**).

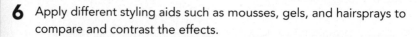

▲ **FIGURE 15-140**

Follow the brush with concentrated heat from the dryer.

2 Dry the sides in the same manner.

3 To create lift or direction in the top section, work from the natural part, parting off a section with the comb or brush. Elevate for desired fullness and follow with the blow dryer. This is actually a form of blow waving because the dryer heat is used to set or give direction to the hair.

4 To create a definite direction in the front section, the comb or brush can be used on top of a section of hair along the hairline. Insert the comb/brush about $1\frac{1}{2}$" from the hairline, first drawing the comb/brush a little to the back and then toward the hairline in one motion. This will create a ridge or bend in the hair that will set it in a different direction (**Figure 15-141**). Lift the hair for volume (**Figure 15-142**). Adjust the blow-dryer to hot and direct the hot air back and forth until a soft ridge has been formed. Repeat, following these instructions, for subsequent sections in the top and crest areas.

5 Apply a suitable styling aid to finish the styling service.

DIFFUSED BLOW-DRY STYLING

1 Use a curly-haired mannequin to practice drying with a diffuser attachment. Moisten the hair in preparation for combing or detangling.

2 Pick the hair out into the basic shape of the desired style (**Figure 15-143a**).

3 Begin drying in the back section working toward the crown and sides. Gently pick the hair out as the dryer is moved from section to section (**Figure 15-143b**).

4 Dry the sides in the same manner.

5 Dry the top section forward from the crown, picking the hair out as each area is dried (**Figure 15-143c**).

6 Apply a suitable styling aid to complete the styling service.

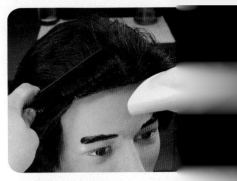

▲ **FIGURE 15-141**
Create a ridge or bend in the hair with the comb.

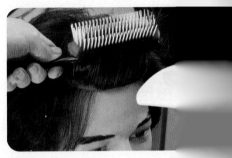

▲ **FIGURE 15-142**
Lift the hair for volume.

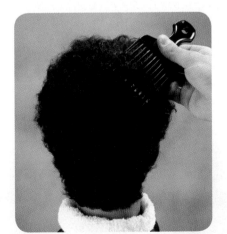

▲ **FIGURE 15-143a**
Pick out the hair.

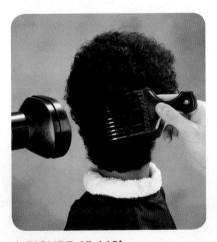

▲ **FIGURE 15-143b**
Begin drying in the back section.

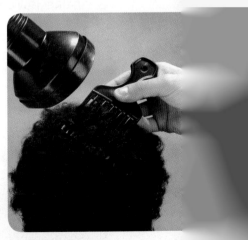

▲ **FIGURE 15-143c**
Dry top section.

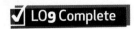

✓ **LO9 Complete**

BRAIDS AND LOCKS

The techniques associated with styling the hair into braids and locks is a form of natural hair care that originated in Africa thousands of years ago. Natural hair care has gained such popularity that an entirely new division of the hair care industry has developed. As a recognized professional segment of our industry, natural hair care is an active and exciting division that is currently involved in education, licensing, and legislative changes to meet the needs of its educators, practitioners, and clients.

BRAIDS

While there are many variations of braids and braiding styles, *on-the-scalp cornrows* are one of the most popular styles chosen by men today **(Figure 15-144)**. If the client has very short hair, you will be working close to the scalp across the curves of the head. The braid may begin at the nape, top, or sides depending on the desired finished result.

Figures 15-146 to 15-150 illustrate the underhand braiding method used to create cornrows.

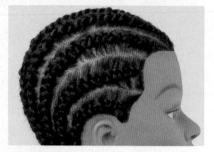

▲ **FIGURE 15-144**
Cornrows.

mini PROCEDURE

CORNROW BRAIDING

1 Apply and massage essential oil to the scalp **(Figure 15-145)**. Determine the correct size and direction of the cornrow base. Create two parallel partings to form a neat row for the cornrow base **(Figure 15-146)**.

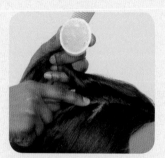

▲ **FIGURE 15-145**
Massage essential oil through hair.

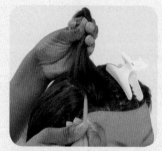

▲ **FIGURE 15-146**
Part out a panel.

2 Divide the parting into three strands. Place fingers close to the base and cross the left strand under the center strand **(Figure 15-147)**.

3 Cross the right strand under the center strand **(Figure 15-148)**.

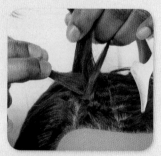

▲ **FIGURE 15-147**
Pass left strand of hair under center strand.

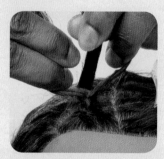

▲ **FIGURE 15-148**
Pass right strand under center strand.

(Continued)

4 With each crossing under, pick up hair from the base of the panel and add it to the outer strand before crossing it under the center strand (**Figures 15-149** and **15-150**).

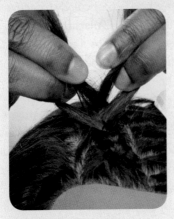

▲ **FIGURE 15-149**

Add hair to left outer strand.

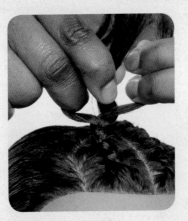

▲ **FIGURE 15-150**

Add hair to right outer strand.

5 Braid subsequent panels in the same manner. Finish with oil sheen or an appropriate styling aid for a finished look.

LOCKS

Locks, also known as dreadlocks, are created from natural-textured hair that is intertwined together to form a single network of hair. **Hair-locking** is the process that occurs when coiled hair is allowed to develop in its natural state without the use of combs, heat, or chemicals. The more coil revolutions within a single strand, the faster the hair will coil and lock.

Cultivated locks are those that are intentionally guided through the natural process of locking. There are several ways to cultivate locks such as twisting, braiding, and wrapping. The preferred and most effective technique is palm- or finger-rolling, depending on the length of the hair.

When consulting with the client who is considering locks, it is important to stress the following:

- Once locked, the locks can be removed only by cutting them off.

- The hair locks in progressive stages that can take from six months to a year to complete.

- General maintenance includes regular shop visits for cleaning, conditioning, and re-rolling. Once the hair locks into compacted coils, it may be shampooed regularly and managed with a non-petroleum-based oil. Heavy oils should be avoided.

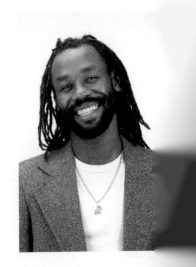

Two basic methods for locking men's hair, which is traditionally shorter at the beginning of the locking process, are the comb technique and the palm- or finger-rolling method. The procedures are as follows:

- *Comb technique:* This method is particularly effective during the early stages of locking and involves placing the comb at the base of the scalp and spiraling the hair into a curl with a rotating motion. With each revolution, the comb moves down along the strand until it reaches the end of the hair shaft.

- *Palm- or finger-rolling:* This method takes advantage of the hair's natural tendency and ability to coil. Rolling begins with shampooed and conditioned hair. Next, part the hair in horizontal rows from the nape to the front hairline and divide the rows into equal subsections. Apply gel to the first subsection to be rolled. Begin rolling at the nape by using the index finger and thumb to pinch the hair near the scalp, then twist the strands in one full clockwise revolution. Use the fingers or palms to repeat the clockwise revolutions down the entire strand (**Figure 15-151**). Maintain a constant degree of moisture by spraying with water as needed. Once all the hair has been rolled, place the client under a hood dryer set on low heat. When the hair is completely dry, apply a light oil to add sheen to the hair.

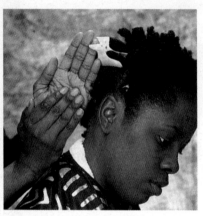

▲ **FIGURE 15-151**
Palm rolling.

Safety Precautions for Haircutting and Styling

- Use all tools and implements in a safe manner.

- Use the right tool for the job.

- Always use a neck strip or towel as a barrier between the cape and the client's neck.

- Use smooth movements when raising or lowering chairs and seat backs.

- Properly sanitize, disinfect, and store tools and implements.

- Avoid applying dryer heat in one place on the head for too long.

- Keep metal combs away from the scalp when using heat.

- Keep work area clean and sanitized.

- Sweep the floor after every client and dispose of hair clippings appropriately.

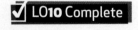

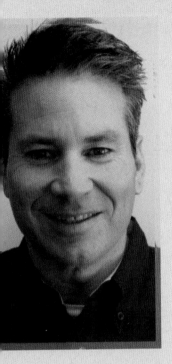

DAVE ALBERS, NATIONAL SALES MANAGER
GRAHAM PROFESSIONAL BEAUTY PRODUCTS

Dave Albers has been in the industry since 1982 and is currently the national sales manager for Graham Professional Beauty Products. Dave has represented Graham Professional as a committed industry partner at NABBA and professional conferences for many years and is a valued associate of the barbering and beauty industries.

Graham Professional Beauty Products, founded in 1955, is a division of Little Rapids Corporation (LRC), a privately held specialty paper company in Green Bay, Wisconsin. It is one of four divisions that also service the medical, dental, and OEM industries with 550 employees and annual sales of 250 million.

Graham Beauty's major product lines are Sanek Neck Strips, Barbee Towels, Handsdown Ultra products, Cellucotton, Salon Fit Vinyl Gloves, Spa Essentials, and Wrapit styling products. With over 65 product stock-keeping units, Graham Beauty is dedicated to providing stylist and barbers with a wide range of high-quality, high-performance professional products.

THE POWER OF PEACE OF MIND
CONFIDENT CLIENTS ARE LOYAL CLIENTS

Clients trust you to give them the look they want, but they also trust you with their health and safety. Let them know the lengths you go to meet sanitation standards. It'll do wonders for their peace of mind—and your client retention rate.

The safety and sanitation of barbershop and salon procedures have been getting a lot of media attention lately, and clients are beginning to wonder what measures their stylist takes to ensure a clean salon environment. Taking the time to let your clients know your procedures and precautions makes a big difference, not only in their comfort level but also in their trust in you—and in the barbershop they choose for their next visit.

From haircutting to shaving, sanitation standards affect just about everything that is done in your barbershop. Take advantage of these opportunities to share important safety and sanitation information with your clients.

THE ISSUE OF LATEX ALLERGIES

An increasing number of people are allergic to natural rubber latex, and the beauty industry has responded by developing disposable synthetic gloves that give you the peace of mind of knowing your client will not have an allergic reaction during a barber treatment.

Let your clients know they have no need to worry about a latex reaction, and assure them that because the gloves you are using are disposable, there is literally no chance of cross-contamination because they are not re-used. If you do happen to use synthetic rubber gloves that can be re-used, explain how you clean and disinfect them after every use to guard against cross-contamination.

SANITIZING VS. DISINFECTING VS. STERILIZING

Some clients may question you about how you "sterilize" your tools because they may not realize that there are important differences between sanitizing, disinfecting, and sterilizing. You can explain that sterilizing requires dry or steam heat, which is impractical in the shop, but that all your tools and implements are first washed (sanitized) and then disinfected before and after use.

THE COMFORT OF SINGLE-USE PRODUCTS

Disposable products offer the highest level of cleaning—and peace of mind—by greatly reducing the likelihood of cross-contamination, simply because they are used only once. When you use them, let your clients know the added safety benefits.

For example, point out that disposable neck strips not only protect skin from being irritated by capes but also act as a germ barrier. Mention to clients how disposable towels protect their skin and hair from irritants and contaminants.

SHOW OFF YOUR LICENSE

Display your up-to-date license proudly where it is easily visible to your clients. Not only do the barber laws in most states require this, but displaying your credentials are always a good way of building client confidence and loyalty.

Your clients expect the highest standards of safety and sanitation from your salon. That is the promise of a professional barber. By going the extra mile to ensure that your safety practices are communicated to your clients, you reinforce this promise. At the same time, you achieve a barber stylist's ultimate goal—an amazing barbershop experience for your clients.

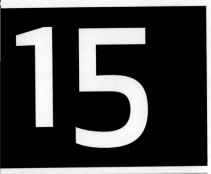

Review
Questions

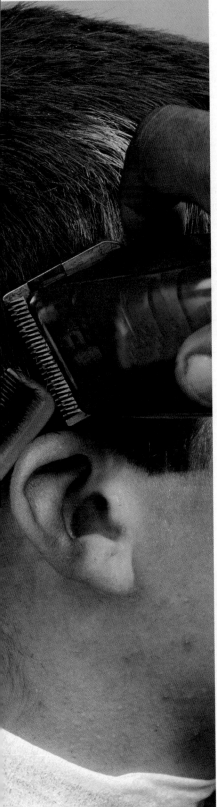

1. List the characteristics of the art of haircutting.

2. Explain what a good hairstyle should accomplish.

3. List the physical considerations that help to determine the best haircut and style for an individual.

4. Explain the process of envisioning.

5. List the haircutting areas of the head used in men's haircutting.

6. List and define the basic haircutting terms.

7. List the cutting techniques used in men's haircutting.

8. What is the difference between a neck shave and an outline shave?

9. Does an outline shave *always* include shaving the hairline at the forehead? Why or why not?

10. Explain why the hair should be in a damp condition for razor cutting.

11. Describe the razor rotation technique.

12. Explain the differences between freeform blow-drying and stylized blow-drying techniques.

13. Explain the braiding techniques used to create cornrows.

14. Define hair-locking.

15. Why do state barber boards most often require a licensure candidate to perform a taper cut during the practical exams?

Chapter
Glossary

angle the space between two lines or surfaces that intersect at a given point; in haircutting, the hair is held away from the head to create an angle of elevation

arching technique method used to cut around the ears and down the sides of the neck

blow-dry styling the drying and styling of the hair with a blow-dryer and implements or fingers.

clipper-over-comb cutting over a comb with the clippers

crest the widest area of the head, also known as the parietal ridge, temporal region, hatband, or horseshoe

cutting above the fingers method of holding the hair section between the fingers so that cutting can be performed on the outside of the fingers; used with horizontal or vertical 90-degree projections of hair

cutting below the fingers method of holding the hair section between the fingers so that cutting can be performed on the inside of the fingers; used in 0- and 45-degree elevation cutting

cutting line the position of the fingers when cutting a section of hair

design line usually the perimeter line of a haircut

diagonal lines positioned between horizontal and vertical lines

elevation angle or degree at which a subsection of hair is held, or elevated, from the head when cutting; also referred to as projection

envisioning the process of visualizing a procedure or finished haircut style

facial shape oval, round, inverted triangular, square, oblong, diamond, and pear-shaped

fingers-and-shear technique used to cut hair by holding the hair into a position to be cut

freehand clipper cutting generally interpreted to mean that guards are not used in the cutting process

freehand shear cutting cutting with shears without the use of fingers or a comb to control the hair

freehand slicing method of removing bulk from a hair section with the shears

guide section of hair, located at either the perimeter or the interior of the cut, that determines the length the hair will be cut; also referred to as a guideline; usually the first section that is cut to create a shape

hair-locking the process that occurs when coily hair is allowed to develop in its natural state without the use of combs, heat, or chemicals

horizontal lines parallel to the horizon

layers graduated effect achieved by cutting the hair with elevation or over-direction; the hair is cut at higher elevations, usually 90 degrees or above, which removes weight

outlining finish work of a haircut with shears, trimmers, or razor

over-direction combing a section away from its natural falling position, rather than straight out from the head, toward a guideline; used to create increasing lengths in the interior or perimeter

parietal ridge widest area of the head, also known as the crest, hatband, horseshoe, or temporal region

part a line that divides the hair at the scalp.

parting a line dividing the hair of the scalp that separates one section of hair from another or creates subsections from a larger section of hair

projection angle or elevation that hair is held from head for cutting

razor-over-comb texturizing technique in which the comb and the razor are used on the surface of the hair

razor rotation texturizing technique similar to razor-over-comb, done with small circular motions

reference points points on the head that mark where the surface of the head changes or the behavior of the hair changes, such as ears, jaw line, occipital bone, apex, etc.; used to establish design lines that are proportionate

rolling the comb out a method used to put the hair into position for cutting by combing into the hair with the teeth of the comb in an upward direction

shear-over-comb haircutting technique in which the hair is held in place with the comb while the shears are used to remove length

shear-point tapering haircutting technique used to thin out difficult areas in the haircut, such as dips and hollows

stationary guide guideline that does not move, but all other hair is brought to it for cutting

tapered haircuts in which there is an even blend from very short at the hairline to longer lengths as you move up the head; *to taper* is to narrow progressively at one end

tension amount of pressure applied when combing and holding a section, created by stretching or pulling the section

texturizing removing excess bulk without shortening the length; changing the appearance or behavior of hair through specific haircutting techniques using shears, thinning shears, clippers, or a razor

thinning removing bulk from the hair

traveling guide guideline that moves as the haircutting progresses; used when creating layers or graduation; also referred to as moving or movable guidelines

vertical lines that are straight up and down

weight line a visual line in the haircut, where the ends of the hair hang together; the line of maximum length within the weight area: heaviest perimeter area of a 0-degree (one-length) or 45-degree (graduated) cut

16 Men's
HAIR REPLACEMENT

CHAPTER OUTLINE

- ▶ Hair Replacement Systems
- ▶ Measuring for Hair Replacement Systems
- ▶ Procedures 16-1 to 16-4
- ▶ Cleaning and Styling Hair Replacement Systems
- ▶ Procedures 16-5 to 16-6
- ▶ Selling Hair Replacement Systems
- ▶ Alternative Hair Replacement Methods

☑ Learning Objectives

AFTER COMPLETING THIS CHAPTER, YOU SHOULD BE ABLE TO:

1 Discuss reasons why men may purchase a hair replacement system.

2 Recognize supplies needed to service hair replacement systems.

3 Demonstrate how to measure a client for a hair replacement system.

4 Explain how to create a hair replacement template.

5 Explain how to apply and remove a hair replacement system.

6 Describe how to fit and cut in a hair replacement system.

7 Describe how to clean and service a hair replacement system.

8 Discuss selling hair replacement systems.

9 Discuss alternative hair replacement methods.

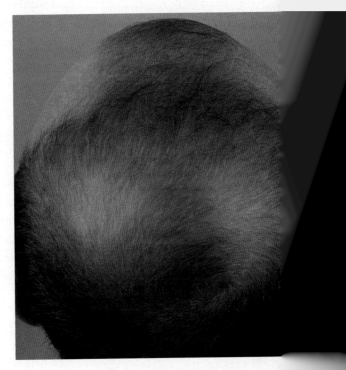

Key Terms

PAGE NUMBER INDICATES WHERE IN THE CHAPTER THE TERM IS USED.

finasteride / 515

flap surgery / 516

full head bonding / 502

hackling / 487

hair replacement system / 486

hair solution / 486

hair transplantation / 516

lace-front / 501

minoxidil / 515

root-turning / 488

scalp reduction / 516

styling or wig
block / 490

toupee / 486

From early Assyrian, Egyptian, and Roman times, hairpieces and wigs have been worn in an attempt to cover balding pates, as a part of ceremonial ritual, or in conformance with the prevailing fashion. False beards and mustaches, dreadlocks, full-bottom wigs, partial wigs, periwigs, side rolls, bobbed wigs, clubs, and queues all played a role in this history from ancient times to the present. During the eighteenth century, the word **toupee** was used to describe the front section of hair, also known as the foretop. This section of hair was grown long enough to cover the front part of the wig, which was placed farther back on the head in order to blend the natural hair with the artificial wig hair. Over time, the foretop was combed higher and extended back toward the crown until it became one long tail of hair. Over the years, the term *toupee* evolved to mean a small wig for men that covered the top or crown of the head, and still later the term *hairpiece* was adopted. Today the industry uses the terms **hair replacement system** or **hair solution.** These changes in terminology are the result of new bonding technologies and continued improvements in the base designs of hair replacement products. The days of your father's toupees or "rugs" are over. No longer is the hairpiece placed on the wig stand at night, to be applied to the scalp in a morning ritual. In keeping with these industry changes, the terms *hair replacement system* and *hair solution* will be used interchangeably throughout this chapter.

For centuries, barbers were involved with the making and styling of wigs. Today, the care and fitting of men's hair replacement systems in the barbershop continues the traditions established so long ago. Although not all barbers choose to specialize in these services, the professional who can design, fit, and custom-cut a hair replacement system can open the door to increased clientele and financial gain.

Men wear hair replacement systems for a variety of personal reasons. Some men choose to cover their thinning or bald areas because they feel it makes them look younger. Others just might prefer how they look with more hair. Regardless of the motivation, men have several options when it comes to deciding how to achieve the "look" they want (**Figures 16-1** and **16-2**).

Hair replacement options range from topical applications of drugs such as minoxidil to hair replacement systems to surgical hair transplantation and scalp reduction. This chapter focuses primarily on men's hair replacement systems with a brief discussion of other alternatives available to men with hair loss conditions.

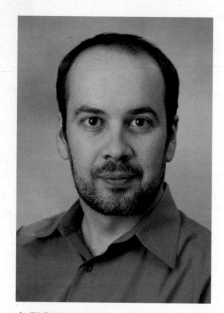

▲ **FIGURE 16-1**

Before hairpiece.

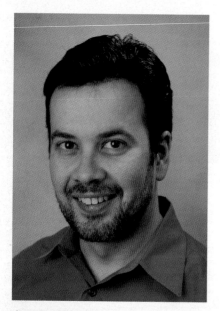

▲ **FIGURE 16-2**

After hairpiece.

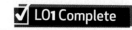

Hair Replacement Systems

The quality of a hair replacement system varies with the kind of hair used in its manufacture and the way in which it is constructed. The barber is often the one to measure, fit, cut, and style the system once it has been received from the supplier.

HUMAN HAIR

Human hair is a desirable choice for a quality hair solution, although synthetic fibers can simulate the look and feel of human hair as well. The advantages of human hair include a more natural look and texture, durability, and the ability to tolerate chemical process such as permanent waving or hair coloring. Some of the disadvantages associated with a human hair solution is that it reacts to climate changes, fades with exposure to light, requires styling maintenance, and can become damaged just as natural hair can.

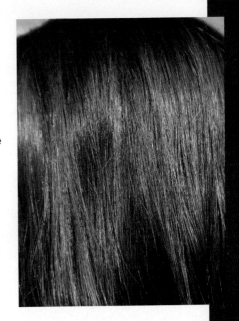

Human hair solutions are usually cleaned with shampoo and conditioner formulated for hair replacement systems. Always follow the manufacturer's directions. In today's market, human hair has become the most popular choice when it comes to hair replacement. The combination of human hair and new base designs results in a natural-looking hair replacement that is virtually undetectable.

Most of the human hair used in hair solutions is imported and must be prepared for use. The process usually includes chemical cleaning with an acid solution, sorting, and **hackling** (the process used to comb through the hair strands to separate them). However, most of the cuticle is removed in the processing of the hair. This means the hair becomes more like a fabric, so it should be treated as such. No harsh solvents or acetones should be used to clean the hair.

SYNTHETIC HAIR

Synthetic hair is used in the production of full wigs and some hair solutions. It is challenging to make synthetic hair that matches the texture of human hair, which makes it difficult to blend the piece with the client's natural hair. Synthetic fibers also possess a high gloss that makes them more noticeable, and they tend to mat and tangle easily when blended with human or animal hair. Overall, synthetic hair replacement systems can usually be cleaned with cleaner solutions, are less costly than human hair, and do not oxidize or lose their style.

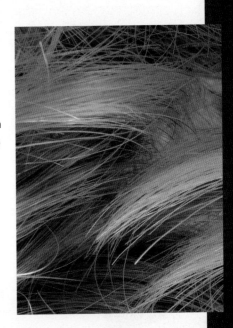

MIXED HAIR

Mixed-hair products, such as human hair blended with synthetic or animal hair, are often used in the manufacture of theatrical or fashion wigs. Horse and yak hair, as well as angora and sheep's wool, are some of the materials used in the manufacture of wigs and hair solutions. Angora has a finer texture than yak and may be used at the front hairline to create a softer and more natural look.

BASES AND CONSTRUCTION

Hair replacement systems may be machine-made, hand-made, or made by a combination of both methods. They are typically available with hard, soft, mesh, net, polyurethane, or combination bases. The materials used in base construction include silk, nylon, or plastic mesh; lace; thin (onion)

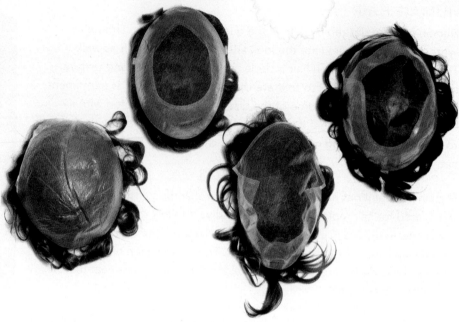

▲ FIGURE 16-3

Base Constructions - L to R: full skin base; thin skin & french lace; bio-lace, french lace, & skin; polyurethane & monofiliment.

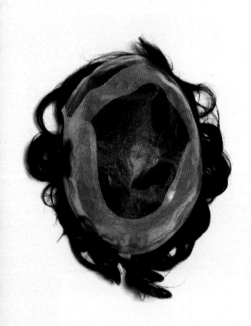

skin; or a combination of materials. Some professionals prefer a doubled base material for increased strength and a more exact fit **(Figure 16-3)**.

Knotting refers to the way the hair is attached to the base of the hair solution. Knotting methods include single knotting, V-looping, and single hair injection into the base. The single-knot method is frequently used and, although durable, may come untied during the cleaning process. Double-knotted hair helps the hair to remain intact through use and cleaning, but may not produce as natural a look as other knotting methods. Plastic or nylon-mesh bases resist shrinkage and wrinkling when cleaned in water-based solutions or shampoos.

Root-turning refers to sorting the hair strands so that the cuticle points toward the hair ends in its natural direction of growth. When a manufacturer states that a hair solution is root-turned, it means that the hair has been attached to the base with the cuticle of the hair strands in this natural position. Hair that has been root-turned minimizes tangling and matting because the cuticle scales are flowing in the correct direction.

New construction techniques with more natural-looking materials are constantly evolving in the manufacture of hair replacement systems. The new generation of manufacturing techniques has completely changed the industry, resulting in hair replacement systems that can look and feel quite natural.

STOCK AND CUSTOM HAIR REPLACEMENT SYSTEMS

Hair replacement systems are available from manufacturers and distributors in stock sizes and colors, which allows the barber to maintain an inventory of these products. Stock systems, or *pre-custom systems* as the industry now

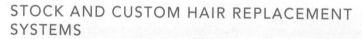

refs to them, can be used as samples to show prospective hair replacement clients what a replacement system might look like or may be customized to fit the client if one happens to be the correct color.

Custom hair solutions are tailored to the client's head shape and hair replacement needs. This customization requires the barber to create a template or pattern and a color matching sample for the supplier to use as a guide in the production of the hair solution.

A template or contour analysis should be done prior to fitting any hair solution. This analysis will help to determine whether the client has the option of purchasing a stock product or requires a custom-made hair solution.

OBTAINING THE HAIR REPLACEMENT SYSTEM

It is advisable for the barber who is interested in servicing or supplying hair replacement systems to study this area of the industry in detail. Decisions will have to be made about manufacturers, supplies, products, and equipment; naturally, this should be done with as much knowledge as possible.

The selection of a hair replacement manufacturer to work with is an important decision that should be based on the manufacturer's ability to meet the barber's needs in terms of cost, time, and product quality. The following sample questions may help to guide the selection of a manufacturer to provide hair replacement goods to the barbershop.

- What hair materials are used in the construction of the hair solution: human, synthetic, or mixed?

- What chemical treatments have been applied?

- If the hair is human hair, is it graded in terms of strength, elasticity, and porosity?

- Will the manufacturer stand behind their product?

- What is the life expectancy of the hair solution?

- Does the manufacturer have the ability to create custom colors?

- Is technical training offered about the manufacturer's products?

SUPPLIES FOR HAIR REPLACEMENT SERVICES

Most barbershops will already have many of the tools and implements required for hair solution services **(Figure 16-4)**. The few supplies that are not standard items, like special adhesives or solvents, can be obtained from a barber or hair replacement supply company. Be guided by the following checklist when purchasing hair solution service supplies.

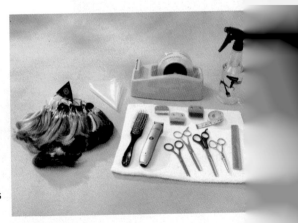

▲ FIGURE 16-4
Supplies for hairpiece services.

- Adhesive remover
- Alcohol
- Blow-dryer
- Client record cards
- Clippers
- Comb
- Double-sided adhesive tape
- Envelopes
- Grease pencil
- Hair density chart
- Hair net
- Haircutting shears
- Manufacturer's color ring
- Measuring tape
- Plastic wrap
- Razor
- Scissors (for cutting pattern)
- Small brush
- Spirit gum/adhesive
- **Styling or wig block**
- Thinning shears
- T-pins
- Transparent tape
- Wig cleaner

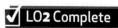
✓ **LO2 Complete**

Measuring for Hair Replacement Systems

Once the client consultation has been performed and an understanding has been reached about the type of hair solution to be purchased, a preliminary haircut should be performed.

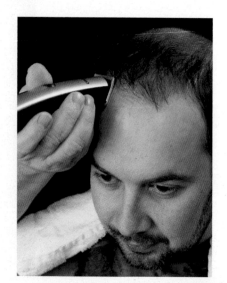

▲ FIGURE 16-5
Trim the front section.

To achieve a natural look, the client's hair should be allowed to grow fairly long to make it easier to blend it with that of the hair solution. When performing the preliminary cut, the hair should be lightly trimmed, leaving a long neckline and length close to the ears at the sides. Make sure to trim the front section as well **(Figure 16-5)**. After the preliminary cut is finished, the longest cuttings are gathered and put into an envelope for use as a texture and color guide for the manufacturer.

The sizes of men's hair solutions are commonly measured in inches. For example, a 6"–by–4" piece would be 6" long from front to back and 4" wide. In the manufacturer's code, the larger number refers to the length unless otherwise indicated. Tape measurements alone can be used for ordering stock hair solutions. Custom pieces, however, require a pattern or template of the client's head form in the area of hair loss.

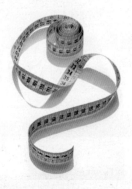

PLASTER MOLD FORM

Today, some manufacturers prefer plaster of Paris models. These models are made after creating the pattern but, instead of tape, plaster is applied while the client holds the plastic wrap in place. The plaster forms a hard mold that allows the manufacturer to create a perfect fit when creating the base. The manufacturer then pours a foam mold into the cast to create a permanent mold for the client to use again and again.

Making A Template

SUPPLIES

- Grease pencil
- Tape measure
- Plastic wrap
- 12 strips of $\frac{3}{4}''$ transparent tape (preferably the dull-finish type for easy writing)
- Permanent marker

PREPARATION

1. Perform client consultation.

2. Perform preliminary haircut.

3. After the preliminary cut is finished, the longest cuttings are gathered and put into an envelope for use as a texture and color guide for the manufacturer.

PROCEDURE

Measuring

For a front hairline to look natural, it should not be too low on the forehead. The original, natural hairline should be followed as closely as possible. The following procedure is a standard method of measuring for a hair solution.

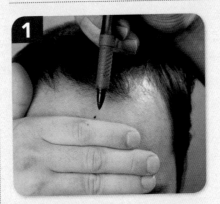

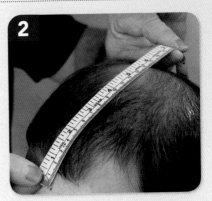

1 Place four fingers above the eyebrow with the last finger resting on the bridge of the nose. Make a dot with a grease pencil on the forehead directly in line with the center of the nose to indicate where the hair solution is to begin.

2 Place the tape measure on the dot. Measure the length to where the back hair begins and mark the tape measure. Be sure to measure back to where substantial growth begins and disregard sparse hair between the forehead and bald crown areas.

3 The next measurement is across the top, directly over the sideburns. This is the place where the front hairline of the hair solution blends in with the client's own hair at the sides of the head. Measure across the crown area if it is noticeably different from the front width. These measurements can be used to order a stock hair solution.

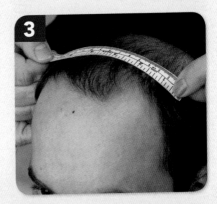

✓ **LO3** Complete

Creating a Template

To create a template for a custom hair solution, assemble the measuring tape, plastic wrap, 12 strips of $\frac{3}{4}''$ transparent tape (preferably the dull-finish type for easy writing), and grease pencil or permanent marker.

1 Trim excess or stray hairs.

2 Place approximately 2 feet of plastic wrap on top of the client's head and twist the sides until they conform to the contour of the head.

3 Place four fingers above the eyebrows and make a dot on the pattern to indicate the new hairline. Place additional dots as follows:

- Two dots on each side where the front hairline is to meet the client's own hairline
- Two dots in back of the head on each side of the balding spot
- One dot at the center back edge of the bald spot to determine the length of the area to be covered

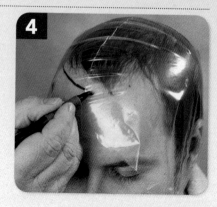

4 Connect the dots with a pencil to outline the balding area. Ignore minor irregularities and sparse areas.

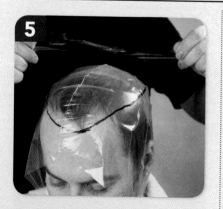

5 While the client holds the plastic wrap, place each precut strip of tape across the bald area to stiffen the template so it holds its shape.

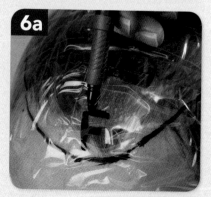

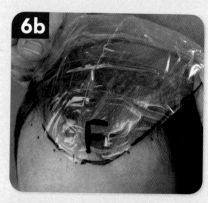

6 Mark the front part of the template *F* and the back *B* as in Figure 6a. Then remove the template and cut around the edge with scissors. After cutting the outline, replace the template over the balding area. Make sure this area is covered exactly. Although it is better to have a foundation that is slightly smaller than one that is too large, accuracy is very important.

7 Attach samples of the client's hair to the template or client card for color matching by the manufacturer.

8

1. Hairpiece without lace front

   a) Without side part ☐

   b) With left side part ☐

   c) With right side part ☐

2. Hairpiece with lace front

   a) With side part ☐

   b) With left side part ☐

   c) With right side part ☐

3. Hair color variations:

a) Front:	Natural ☐	Percentage of gray ☐
	Streaked ☐	Front and top lighter ☐
b) Temples:	Natural ☐	Percentage of gray ☐
c) Back:	Natural ☐	Percentage of gray ☐

4. Complexion:

   a)   Ruddy: ☐

   b)   Dark: ☐

   c)   Light: ☐

5. Details:

   a)   Partials ☐   Patches ☐   Fill-ins ☐

6. Photograph (may or may not be required by manufacturer).

8 Create a client record card, which can also serve as an information sheet when ordering stock and custom hair solutions. Send the measurements, template, and hair samples to the manufacturer with any special instructions.

CLEAN-UP AND DISINFECTION

1. Wash and disinfect tools and implements.

2. Clean surfaces and chair.

3. Sweep up hair and deposit in closed receptacle.

4. Dispose of paper goods and/or linens.

5. Wash your hands.

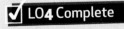
✓ **LO4 Complete**

Making a Plaster Mold Form

SUPPLIES

- Waterproof cape
- Towels
- Plastic bowl for mixing
- Plaster gauze strips
- Scissors or shears
- Black and white eyeliner pencils
- Permanent marker
- Tape

PREPARATION

1. Drape client.

2. Cut six plaster gauze strips at 9" or 10" and eight plaster gauze strips at 4".

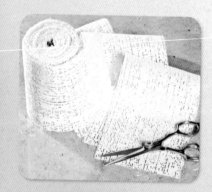

PROCEDURE

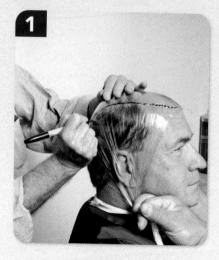

1 Stretch plastic wrap over client's head, twist the sides, and have the client hold the ends so the wrap conforms to his head.

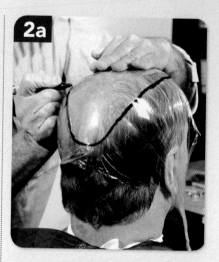

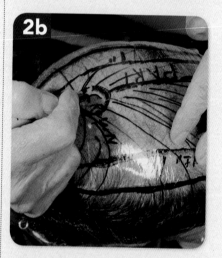

2 Mark the pattern and add details.

3 Apply towel around client's neck.

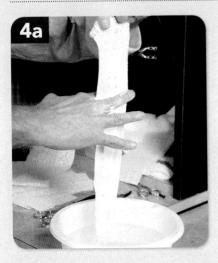

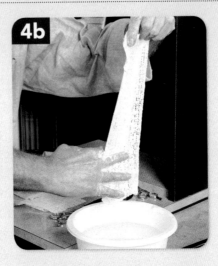

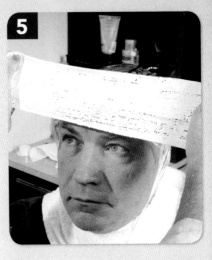

4 Mix plaster and water. Dip a gauze strip into the plaster bath and use two fingers to gently squeeze excess water from the strip from top to bottom.

5 Apply the first strip from front to back.

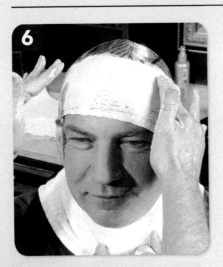

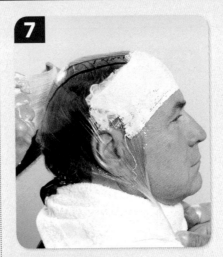

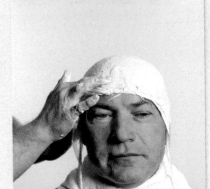

6 Smooth out the strip following the contour of the head from the front around to the temple areas.

7 Apply the second strip from back to front, making sure to smooth the strip to the contour of the head.

8 Apply shorter strips across the top of the head.

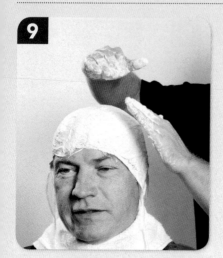

9 Repeat the process to create second and third layers of the gauze strips.

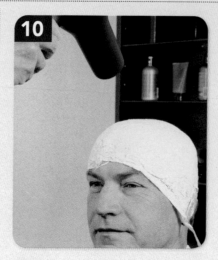

10 Blow-dry to set the plaster until completely dry.

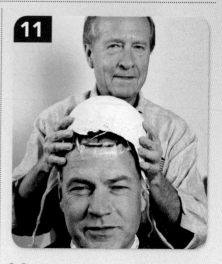

11 When the mold is dry, gently remove it by lifting it off the client's head. If any hair sticks to the plaster, mist the area with water to remove.

FYI It is extremely important to smooth out the gauze strips to fit the contour of the head.

12 Trim excess plaster from mold.

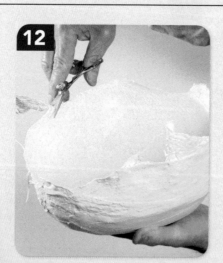

12

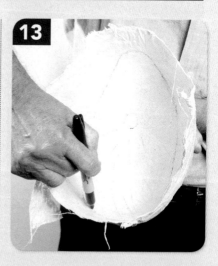

13

REMINDER

>> Do not use good haircutting shears to cut anything other than hair. Use an old pair of shears or scissors to cut gauze strips, plastic wrap, bases, and so forth.

13 The inside of the mold should have a faint outline of the pattern. Trace over the outline with a permanent marker. Write the client's name and date on the outside of the plaster mold.

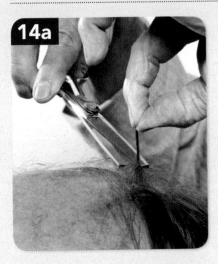

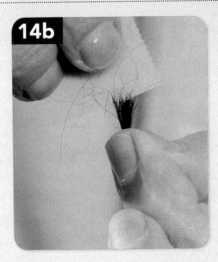

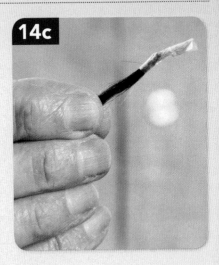

14 Gently twist a small section of hair from the client's crown and cut with thinning shears to create a sample. This color will be used in the front, top, and crown areas of the hair replacement. Wrap scotch tape around the base of the hair sample to keep it in place. Take separate hair samples from the temple, side, and back areas, as they tend to have more gray.

15 Shampoo and condition the client's hair.
Important: The plaster mold will need to cure for 24 hours before shipping it to the manufacturer.

CLEAN-UP AND DISINFECTION

1. Wash and disinfect tools and implements.

2. Clean surfaces and chair.

3. Sweep up hair and deposit in closed receptacle.

4. Dispose of paper goods and/or linens.

5. Dispose of leftover plaster mixture; use paper towels to wipe mixture from bowl before washing and deposit in trash.

6. Wash your hands.

Customizing a Stock (Pre-Custom) Hair Replacement System

SUPPLIES

- Plastic and tape template
- Scissors
- Canvas block and stand
- T-pins or tipped straight pins
- Shampoo and conditioner
- Towels
- Razor blade

PREPARATION

1. Drape client.
2. Perform client consultation.

PROCEDURE

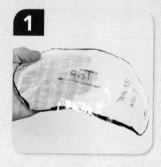

1 To customize a stock hair replacement, use the plastic and tape template.

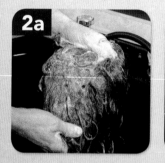 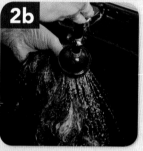 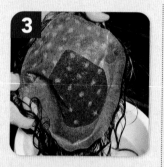 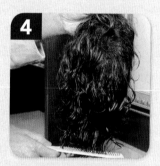

2 Shampoo the hair replacement system and rinse thoroughly.

3 Condition the replacement and rinse lightly, leaving a small amount of conditioner in the system.

4 After swishing the system through the water a few times, remove it and comb gently.

5 Towel-blot the hair replacement system and invert it.

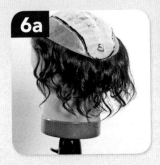 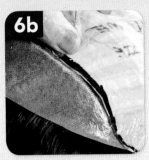

6 Drag the system over the back of the canvas block, making sure all the hair is behind the front edge of the hair replacement. Invert the template and place it on the hair replacement, making sure to use as much of the natural hairline of the replacement as possible. Secure the template and system to the block with pins.

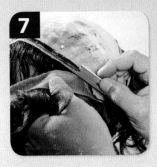

7 Use the tip of the razor blade to carefully cut the base, using the template as a guide. Cut all the way around the base, but do not cut the hair.

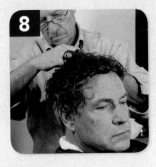

8 After the base has been cut, remove the pins from the canvas block and check for fit.

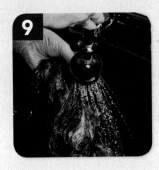

9 Rinse out excess conditioner and lay the replacement system to the side.

CLEAN-UP AND DISINFECTION

1. Wash and disinfect tools and implements.

2. Clean surfaces and chair.

3. Sweep up hair and deposit in closed receptacle.

4. Dispose of paper goods and/or linens.

5. Discard used razor blade in a sharps container.

6. Wash your hands.

Congratulations! You have just created a custom hair replacement system. You are now ready to apply the system.

APPLYING AND REMOVING HAIR REPLACEMENT SYSTEMS

Non–Lace Front System

1 Before adjusting a hair solution to the scalp, trim the front hairline and clean the entire bald area with a piece of cotton dampened with rubbing alcohol, or soap and water, then dry thoroughly.

2 Apply two-sided tape in a V shape on the front reinforced area of the foundation (**Figure 16-6**). This tape holds the hair solution close to the scalp. Place additional pieces of tape on the reinforced parts of the foundation at the sides and back of the hair solution.

3 Place four fingers above the eyebrow to locate the hairline. Position the hair solution at the hairline using the center of the nose as a guide. When the hair solution is in the proper position, press down firmly on the various taped areas (**Figure 16-7**).

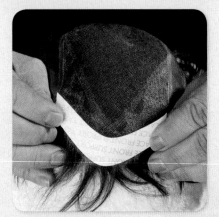

▲ **FIGURE 16-6**
Apply two-sided tape in V-shape.

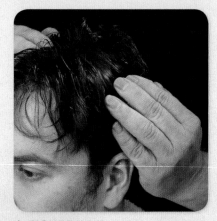

▲ **FIGURE 16-7**
Attach the hairpiece, press down firmly on taped areas.

Removing a Non–Lace Front System

Reach up under the hair solution with the fingertips at the front section and detach the tape from the scalp (**Figure 16-8**). Make sure the tape stays on the foundation so that it can be reactivated with spirit gum.

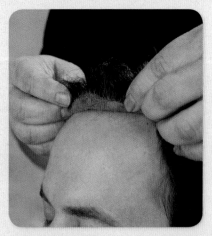

▲ **FIGURE 16-8**
Removing a hairpiece.

(Continued)

Lace-Front System

A **lace-front** hair solution is recommended when the hair is worn in an off-the-face style. It is scarcely visible from the front view and provides the required lightness for a natural-looking hairstyle.

1 Clean the bald area with rubbing alcohol or with soap and water.

2 Remove hair on the scalp where the tape or lace is to be attached (**Figure 16-9**).

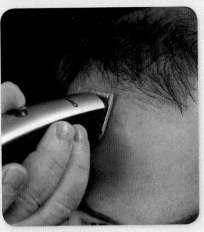

▲ **FIGURE 16-9**
Remove hair on scalp where hairpiece will attach.

3 Attach strips of two-sided tape to reinforced parts of the foundation, usually near the front, on the sides, and at the back of the hair solution. Note that reinforced areas vary with the design of the foundation and the manufacturer's specifications. Never apply tape directly to the lace.

4 Adjust the hair solution to the desired position using the four-finger method. Press it down into place with the back of a comb (**Figure 16-10**) to ensure that oils from the fingers do not stain the tape.

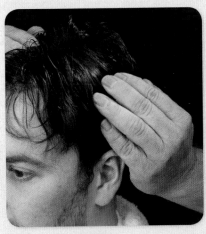

▲ **FIGURE 16-10**
Adjust the hairpiece.

REMINDER

>>> Reinforced areas of a lace-front hair solution vary with the design of the foundation and the manufacturer's specifications. Never apply tape directly to the lace.

(Continued)

Removing a Lace-Front Hair Solution

Before removing a lace-front hair solution, dampen the lace with acetone or solvent in order to loosen it from the scalp **(Figure 16-11)**. Do not pull or stretch the lace. To apply solvent, use a piece of cotton or a brush. After the lace becomes loosened, use the fingertips to remove the tape from the scalp **(Figure 16-12)**. Do not pull off the hair solution by tugging on the hair. Clean the reinforced areas with a small brush dipped in acetone or other solvent.

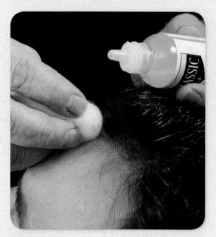

▲ **FIGURE 16-11**
Dampen lace with solvent to remove hairpiece.

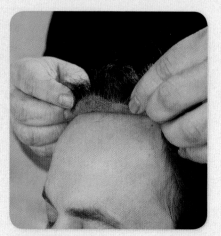

▲ **FIGURE 16-12**
Remove hairpiece gently.

FULL HEAD BONDING

Full head bonding is the process of attaching a hair replacement system to the head with an adhesive bonding agent. This allows the replacement system to adhere to all areas of the head rather than just being held in place with double-sided tape. Barbers can ask their suppliers about which copolymer should be used for full head bonding. The adhesives used with hair replacement systems are water-soluble. Be sure to remind clients to always allow the adhesive to dry for a few minutes after shampooing and before styling.

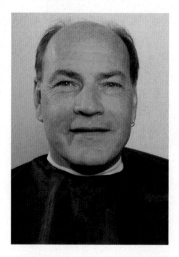

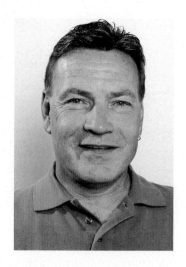

Full Head Bonding

SUPPLIES

- Waterproof cape
- Towels
- Material Safety Data Sheet (MSDS) for adhesive
- Razor blades
- Canvas block
- Soft-bond adhesives
- Eyeliner pencil
- Make-up sponges
- Plastic wrap
- Transparent tape
- Permanent marker or pen

PREPARATION

When preparing to do a full head bond, follow *all* the manufacturer's directions for using the adhesive.

1. Perform a patch test with any adhesive 24 hours before applying.

2. Wash your hands.

3. Drape the client and shampoo hair and scalp with a pH-balanced shampoo.

4. Towel dry and change drape to a haircutting cape.

5. Always make sure the base of the hair replacement is dry before applying.

PROCEDURE

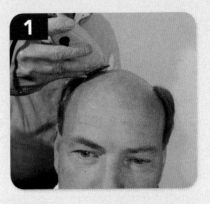

1 Trim the client's scalp with edgers.

---

2 Rinse excess hair from the scalp.

3 Dry the hair again after the client's scalp is rinsed. Do not touch the client's scalp with your hands after this step.

4 Select the correct adhesive for the hair replacement system.

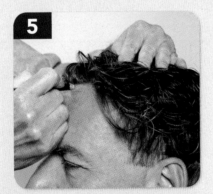

5 Place the hair system on the client's head. With an eyeliner pencil, mark exactly where the system needs to be placed. Remember to never bond on a client's wrinkle or too far back on the client's scalp.

6 Shake the adhesive product well before applying.

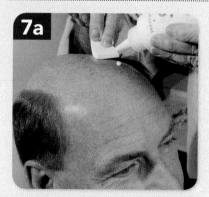

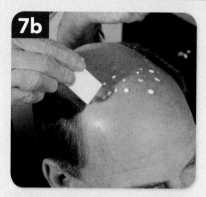

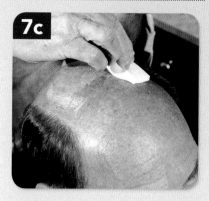

7 Apply a small amount of adhesive in a circular motion onto the client's clean scalp. Use a cosmetic sponge to distribute the adhesive evenly over the scalp. The adhesive will appear white until it dries completely to clear state.

8 When the first coat is dry, apply a second coat and let it dry. Repeat these steps for a total of four times, remembering to use small amounts of adhesive.

9 Once the adhesive is completely dry, it is time to apply the hair solution.

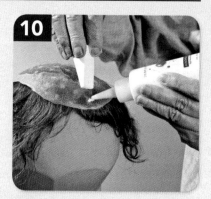

10 Apply one coat of adhesive to the base of the hair replacement system. Do not apply adhesive to any lace present in the system.

11 Stand behind the client and hold the solution in both hands. Place the system at the front hairline and start rolling the hair solution back, applying pressure without stretching the solution. Make sure not to wrinkle the base of the solution.

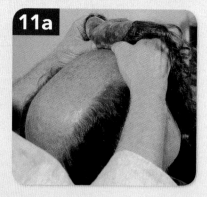

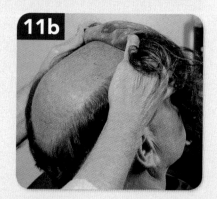

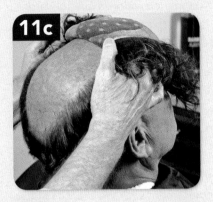

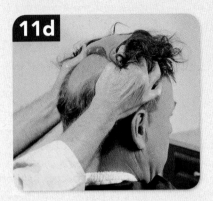

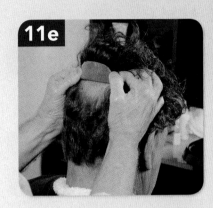

12 Once the system is fully on, use the back of a comb to check around the perimeter of the replacement for wrinkles. Smooth out any minor inconsistencies.

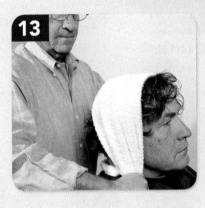

13 Take a towel and place it over the system. Stretch both ends of the towel and pull down tightly to ensure an even fit.

CLEAN-UP AND DISINFECTION

1. Wash and disinfect tools and implements.

2. Clean surfaces and chair.

3. Sweep up hair and deposit in closed receptacle.

4. Dispose of paper goods, sponges, and/or linens.

5. Wash your hands.

The hair system is now ready to be cut. After cutting and blending, remember to tell the client to allow 24 to 48 hours before shampooing.

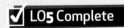
☑ **LO5** Complete

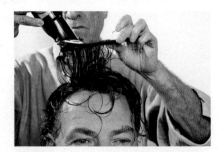

▲ FIGURE 16-13a

Remove excess hair from top section.

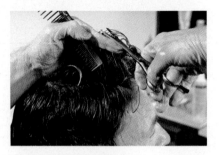

▲ FIGURE 16-13b

Blending top section.

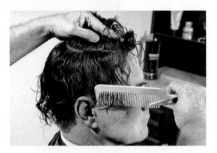

▲ FIGURE 16-14

Comb sides down and blend to hairline.

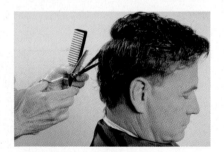

▲ FIGURE 16-15

Blend back section with thinning shears.

CUTTING, TAPERING, AND BLENDING HAIR REPLACEMENT SYSTEMS

- *Top section*: Remove excess length using the clipper-over-comb or fingers-and-shear method at a 90-degree elevation. Work forward from front of crown to forehead. Repeat this step using shears to blend top section (**Figures 16-13a** and **16-13b**).

- *Sides*: Comb the side hair down and blend with the natural hairline from temple to sideburn to the ear (**Figure 16-14**). Taper and blend from side hairline to crest. Taper gradually so replacement system will be undetectable when blended with the client's natural hair.

- *Back*: Cut any excess hair length from the replacement. Use thinning shears to blend the ends of the replacement with the client's natural hair (**Figure 16-15**).

Important: After cutting and blending, remember to tell the client to allow 24 to 48 hours before shampooing.

Congratulations! You have just completed cutting and customizing a hair replacement system (**Figures 16-16a** and **16-16b**).

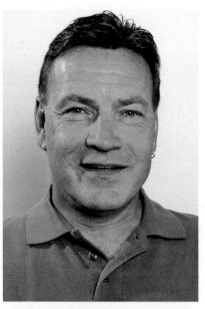

▲ FIGURE 16-16a

Hair replacement system – front view.

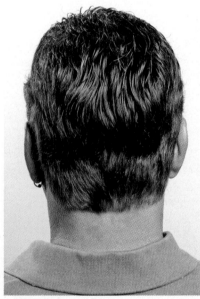

▲ FIGURE 16-16b

Hair replacement system – back view.

NOTE: If the front hairline appears heavy, use a razor or thinning shears to remove weight. Be sure to make very narrow partings in order to form a natural-looking front hairline and blend with the crest hair. Do not over-cut!

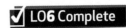
✓ LO6 Complete

PARTIAL HAIR REPLACEMENT SYSTEMS

For a small degree of hair loss, a partial lace fill-in may be all that is required. Partial hair solutions can be made for the front or crown areas of the head. The measuring, application, and cutting techniques are the same as those used for full hair solution styles. Be sure to shave the area to be covered so the spirit gum will adhere better to the scalp and the hair solution.

FACIAL HAIR REPLACEMENT SOLUTIONS

Facial hair solutions are attached with spirit gum. Mustaches, sideburns, and beards may all be attached in the same manner. Clean the facial area and apply spirit gum to the appropriate section. Wait until the gum is tacky, position the piece, and gently press down with a lint-free cloth. Trim the piece to the desired style.

FULL WIGS

While most men might not choose to wear a full wig, many women enjoy the coverage, convenience, and instant style changes they can achieve with wigs. Ready-to-wear wigs are usually made of the synthetic fiber Kanekalon.

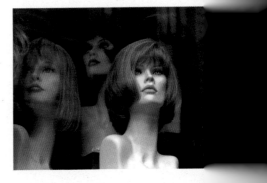

Full, ready-made wigs are constructed on a stretch cap made of lightweight elastic. The wig has permanent elastic bands at the sides designed to hold it in place. It should fit comfortably, but tightly enough to maintain its position without slipping, shifting, or lifting. Wigs come in a wide variety of colors and in many different styles.

Cleaning and Styling Hair Replacement Systems

The life of a hair replacement system depends on its construction and the overall treatment it receives. Manufacturers furnish instructions on the care of their hair solutions that both the barber and client should follow carefully. Clients should have at least two hair solutions to ensure that one will always be in good condition while the other one is being serviced and maintained.

Cleaning Wigs

Cleaning a ready-made wig is a fairly quick and easy process. Use the guidelines provided and the manufacturer's cleaning instructions for this process.

SUPPLIES

- Manufacturer's recommended cleaning solution
- Mixing bowl
- Towels
- Wig block
- Wide-toothed comb
- Brush
- T-pins

PROCEDURE

1 Brush the wig thoroughly to remove all surface dirt and residue.

2 Mix a solution of warm water and wig solution in a bowl.

3 Dip the entire wig into the solution; swish it around in the solution.

4 Rinse the wig in clean, cold water.

5 Blot it dry with a towel.

6 Turn the wig inside out and dry it with a towel.

7 Pin the wig to a head mold or wig block of the correct size.

8 Carefully brush the hair into place.

9 Permit the wig to dry naturally, pinned to the form.

10 If necessary, use cool air to dry the wig quickly.

11 When dry, brush into the proper style.

CLEAN-UP AND DISINFECTION

1. Wash and disinfect tools and implements.
2. Clean surfaces and chair.
3. Dispose of paper goods and/or linens.
4. Wash your hands.

Cleaning Human Hair Replacement Systems

Hair solutions must be kept clean just as natural hair must be kept clean. Cleaning should be performed carefully to help maintain the life of the hair solution. Use the following guidelines and the manufacturer's recommendations to clean a hair solution.

SUPPLIES

- Manufacturer's recommended cleaning solution
- Tape removal solvent
- Mixing bowl
- Towels
- Wig block
- Wide-toothed comb
- Brush
- T-pins

1 Remove all the old tape and clean any reinforced areas by lightly dabbing with recommended solvent.

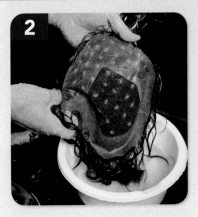

2 Put enough cleaner in a glass bowl so that the hair system can be submerged. Invert the hair replacement with the inside up and place into cleaning solution. Soak for 3 to 5 minutes. Swish the replacement back and forth (or dip it up and down) in cleaning solution until all residue is removed from the hair and foundation. If the cleaning solution darkens, replace it with fresh solution and repeat the swishing process.

4 Place a towel on a flat surface and place the hair replacement on the towel with the inside facing up. Gently press out the cleaner with the towel.

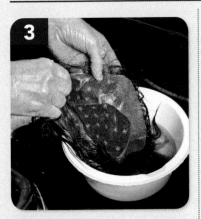

3 Gently tap the edge of the hair replacement with a small brush or your fingers until the adhesive has been removed. Do not rub or scrub.

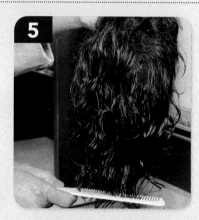

5 Hold the replacement by the front section and comb gently.

6 Fasten the replacement to the wig block with T-pins, style with blow-dryer, and store until client picks it up, or dry hair replacement and reattach to client's scalp.

CLEAN-UP AND DISINFECTION

1. Wash and disinfect tools and implements.

2. Clean surfaces and chair.

3. Dispose of paper goods and/or linens.

4. Dispose of used cleaning solution and solvents per manufacturer's recommendation.

5. Wash your hands.

CLEANING SYNTHETIC HAIR REPLACEMENT SYSTEMS

Synthetic hair solutions should always be cleaned with a solvent. Attach the hair solution to a plastic foam head mold with T-pins and immerse it in lukewarm water with the recommended solvent. Do not use hot water, which would cause the hair solution to shrink or become matted and tangled. Swish the hair solution around in the shampoo solution. Rinse with clean, lukewarm water. Permit the hair solution to dry naturally, pinned on the mold overnight; if time does not permit, place it under a dryer with cool air. Some hair solutions may be dry-cleaned, so always follow the manufacturer's instructions.

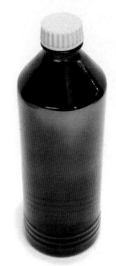

BASIC HAIR REPLACEMENT SYSTEM CARE

- Use the manufacturer's tape, antiseptic, cleaner, and softeners.

- When the hair solution is not being worn, it should be placed on an appropriate block.

- Some hair solutions should be removed for showering and swimming.

- Clean the hair solutions after the first week of wear, and then every three to four weeks or as needed.

- Never fold hair solutions.

- Always follow manufacturer's recommendations for removing hair solutions.

- Apply light hairdressings and spray sparingly and with even distribution.

- Set hair solutions with plain water.

RECONDITIONING HAIR REPLACEMENTS SYSTEMS

Reconditioning treatments should be given as often as necessary to prevent dryness or brittleness of the hair. Reconditioning treatments may also be used to liven up hair solutions that look dull and lifeless.

A small amount of reconditioner may be used, as directed by the manufacturer. If a slight color adjustment is necessary due to fading or yellowing, a suitable temporary color rinse is recommended. Select the rinse carefully so that the color matches that of the client's hair.

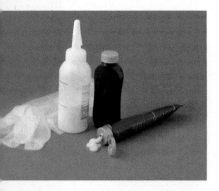

COLORING HAIR REPLACEMENT SYSTEMS

Permanent haircoloring products (aniline derivatives) can be used only on hair solutions made of 100 percent human hair. Use the following procedure and manufacturer's recommendations when coloring a hair solution with permanent haircoloring products.

1 The hair solution is first cleaned with a solvent.

2 Cover the head form block with plastic material to prevent staining from the coloring product.

3 Secure the hair solution firmly with T-pins or straight pins in the front, back, and sides.

4 Give a strand test on a small section of hair to determine the color desired. If using a tint with peroxide, apply it on a dry hair strand.

5 Mix the desired shade of haircoloring product.

6 Apply with a haircoloring brush.

7 Comb the color product through lightly, being careful not to saturate the foundation.

8 Test every 5 minutes until the desired shade is obtained.

9 After processing, rinse thoroughly with warm water. Shampoo and condition according to manufacturer's directions.

10 Comb and set into the desired style.

PERMANENT WAVING HAIR REPLACEMENT SYSTEMS

Permanent waving a hair solution requires time, creativity, and careful attention to detail. The objective is to create a natural look that blends the system with the client's natural hair. The hair system is attached to a wig or styling block with T-pins and should be custom wrapped according to the contours of the client's head.

The rod placement does not rest on the scalp of the hair system as it would in a perm procedure on natural hair. Instead,

(Continued)

the rods are *floated* to eliminate weight and rod marks on the base. Floating is accomplished by using T-pins to support the rod above the base of the hair system. The pins are inserted at both ends of the rod and are held in place by the rubber band of the perm rod. After the hair system has been rodded and secured with the T-pins, use the following guidelines to complete the process.

1 Select a mild permanent wave solution appropriate for bleached or damaged hair types. Hold the wig block upside down and rotate while applying the solution. Allow the excess solution to drip into the sink before setting the block back on the stand.

2 Take a test curl every minute until processing is complete.

3 Rinse the hair replacement system for 10 to 15 minutes. The system does not require the application of a neutralizing solution.

4 Thoroughly blot each rod with paper towels to absorb as much water as possible.

5 Remove the T-pins and hang the block upside down. Leave the rods in the hair solution and cover loosely with a plastic cap for 24 hours.

6 On day two, remove the cap and allow the system to dry for another day. Remove the rods only when the hair is completely dry.

GENERAL RECOMMENDATIONS AND REMINDERS

- Comb hair solutions carefully to avoid matting, loss of hair, or damage.

- Use a wide-tooth comb to avoid weakening or damaging the foundation.

- Never rub or wring cleaning fluids from the hair solution. Let it dry naturally.

- Be careful not to cut too much hair when cutting, tapering, and blending a hair solution.

- Take accurate measurements to assure a comfortable and secure fit.

- Recondition hair solutions as often as necessary to prevent dryness, brittleness, or dullness of the hair.

- Brush and comb hair solutions with a downward movement.

- To avoid damage to the foundation, never lighten or cold-wave a hair solution.

- If coloring is necessary, it must be done with care.

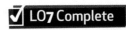

Selling Hair Replacement Systems

In order to sell men's hair solutions, it is important to know why men buy them. As discussed in the first part of this chapter, men wear hair replacements for a variety of personal reasons. When a man expresses an interest in wearing a hair solution to his barber, he won't appreciate a hard-sell approach. His interest has already been made evident, and he is simply looking for guidance and purchasing information at this stage. It is the barber's responsibility to educate the client about the possibilities and options available to him.

Just as a hard-sell approach should be avoided, the barber should never promise what cannot be delivered nor raise the client's expectations to an unreasonable level. For example, it is not professionally ethical to convince an elderly man that he can recapture the appearance of his 40s with a hair solution. It simply cannot be done. The color of the hair solution is also an important consideration. Dark, opaque colors are not recommended for any age group, especially older persons. It is better to recommend a salt-and-pepper blend or medium-brown shade. The more natural-looking the color, the less obvious the hair solution will appear.

MARKETING TECHNIQUES

- *Hair replacement system display*: One or two correctly styled hair solutions displayed in the shop will alert clients to the fact that hair solution services are performed there. Make certain that the sample is clean and nicely styled. It should be large enough to cover the average balding area of a man, since most clients will be men with an average amount of hair loss, and many may want to try it on.

  NOTE: Be sure to shampoo the hair replacement after each client.

- *Referrals and word-of-mouth*: These two methods may be a slower approach, and are not to be relied on exclusively for new business, but they are still very effective forms of advertising. Personal referrals are the best evidence of pleased and satisfied clients.

- *Window displays*: Window displays can add to increased hair replacement sales. Before-and-after illustrations in the shop window let the walk-by and drive-by traffic know that hair replacement systems can be obtained through the barbershop. These illustrations can also offer encouragement to those clients whom you feel cannot be approached directly with the idea of wearing a hair solution. As they become more comfortable with the idea of a hair replacement or see other men in the shop receiving these services, they may feel more inclined to explore their own options.

- *Personal approach*: The personal approach may certainly be used to suggest a hair replacement system to a client; however, it must be a tactful approach. Wait for an opening during the consultation or haircutting service when the client brings up his hair loss condition in the conversation, then offer him the opportunity to try on a hair solution. A quick demonstration may convince him of his improved appearance and lead to a sale.

- *Print ads*: Print ads include all printed advertising, from coupons to billboards. It is important to advertise hair replacement services because not all barbershops pursue this market. In many areas an extra line in the telephone book that mentions hair replacement systems will pay for itself. Your phone book also may contain a special listing for hair goods. This is another good classification in the phone directory in which to place an advertisement.

  In some communities, newspaper advertising is inexpensive and profitable. If a model is used, be sure to secure a model release for any photos that might be used in the ads. Even if the model is your best friend, do not assume that a release is unnecessary.

- *Web sites, online videos, and blogs*: Use today's technology to reach consumers. Hire a site developer or use your own creativity to establish your presence in cyberspace.

- *Personal experience*: If you wear a hair replacement yourself, you can develop an excellent promotional approach. Often, nothing is more convincing than your own before-and-after demonstration. The fact that you wear a hair solution with assurance and complete ease can make a very strong impression on prospective hair replacement clients.

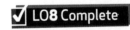 **✓ LO8 Complete**

Alternative Hair Replacement Methods

In addition to hair replacement systems and hair solutions, there are two other approaches to hair replacement available. The first are the drugs minoxidil and finasteride, which are known by different brand names depending on the manufacturer. The second is surgery, which includes procedures such as hair transplantation, scalp reduction, and flap surgery.

A 2 percent solution of **minoxidil** applied twice daily has been shown to be moderately effective for about 50 percent of the men using it. Clinical studies conducted by Pharmacia and Upjohn (the maker of Rogaine-brand minoxidil, recently acquired by Pfizer) revealed that 26 percent of the men reported average to dense hair growth, and 33 percent reported minimal hair growth, after four months of treatment with Rogaine. Minoxidil is available for both men and women in two different strengths: 2 percent (regular) and 5 percent (extra-strength formula).

Finasteride is an oral medication that is prescribed for men only to stimulate hair growth. Although it is considered more effective and convenient than minoxidil, its possible side effects include weight gain and loss of sexual function.

FYI

Low-light laser thera also known as laser hair enhancement, w approved by the FD 2007 for the promot of healthy hair growt Studies associated with this non-surgica procedure report ha growth as a result of cold-beam, red-light laser treatments that stimulate or increase blood circulation and cell regeneration in the hair follicles. Thi service can be offere in the barbershop by purchasing a low-ligh laser machine from a manufacturer, provid your clients with yet another option for h replacement.

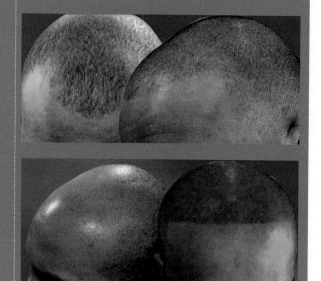

SURGICAL HAIR RESTORATION

The three types of surgical hair restoration available are hair transplants, scalp reduction, and flap surgery.

- **Hair transplantation** is strictly a medical procedure that should be performed only by licensed medical professionals. The process consists of removing hair from normal-growth areas of the scalp, such as the back and sides, and transplanting it into the bald areas under a local anesthetic. Small sections of hair ranging from single strands to larger plugs of 7 to 10 hairs are surgically removed, including the hair follicle, papilla, and hair bulb, and reset in the bald area. With today's technological advances in hair restoration, micrographs have replaced the larger plug sections of the past few decades. The transplanted hair usually grows normally in its new environment, while the area from which the hair was removed heals and shrinks in size to a very tiny scar.

  The surgeon must select the hair to be transplanted with care, taking into consideration color, texture, and type. Placement of the hair in the direction of natural growth to permit proper care and complimentary styling is also an important factor. Transplanted hair can last a lifetime if the service is performed properly. If the doctor is skilled and the individual cares for the hair as directed, hair transplants can be very successful as a method of permanently eliminating baldness.

- **Scalp reduction** is a process by which the bald area is removed from the scalp and surrounding scalp areas with hair growth are pulled together to fill in the spot.

- **Flap surgery**, like scalp reduction surgery, removes the bald scalp area. A flap of hair-bearing skin is then attached to what was the bald area.

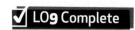

LO9 Complete

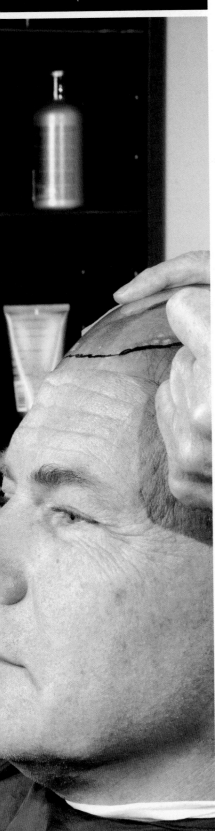

Review
Questions

1. Explain why some men might choose to wear a hair replacement system

2. What two types of hair are used to make men's hair replacement systems?

3. List the steps in measuring for a hair replacement system.

4. What important information should be labeled on a template?

5. List the steps for applying a hair replacement system with tape.

6. What type of product is used in a full head bonding application?

7. What type of product is used to clean hair replacement systems?

8. Name two medications that may be prescribed to encourage hair growth.

9. Name the oral medication that should not be prescribed for women.

10. List three surgical methods of hair replacement.

Chapter
Glossary

finasteride an oral medication prescribed for men only to stimulate hair growth

flap surgery a surgical technique that involves the removal of a bald scalp area and the attachment of a flap of hair-bearing skin

full head bonding the process of attaching a hair replacement system to all areas of the head with an adhesive bonding agent.

hackling process used to comb through the hair strands to separate them

hair replacement system formerly called a hairpiece; also known as a hair solution.

hair solution any small wig used to cover the top or crown of the head and integrated with the natural hair

hair transplantation any form of hair restoration that involves the surgical removal and relocation of hair, including scalp reduction and flap surgery

lace-front popular hair solution style used for off-the-face styles

Minoxidil topical medication used to promote hair growth or reduce hair loss

root-turning refers to sorting the hair strands so that the cuticle points toward the hair ends in its natural direction of growth.

scalp reduction the surgical removal of a bald area, followed by the pulling together of the scalp ends

styling or wig block head-shaped form made of plastic, foam, or other materials used as a stand for a wig or hair replacement system.

toupee outdated term used to describe a small hair replacement that covers the top or crown of the head

PART 4

ADVANCED BARBERING SERVICES

17 Women's
HAIRCUTTING AND STYLING

CHAPTER OUTLINE

☑ Learning Objectives

AFTER THE COMPLETION OF THIS CHAPTER, YOU SHOULD BE ABLE TO:

1 Perform four basic women's haircuts.

2 Demonstrate mastery of texturizing techniques.

3 Perform basic wet styling techniques.

4 Perform basic blow-dry styling techniques.

5 Perform thermal curling and straightening techniques.

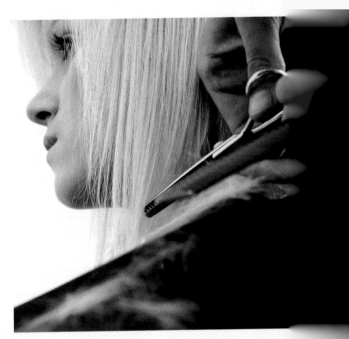

Key Terms

PAGE NUMBER INDICATES WHERE IN THE CHAPTER THE TERM IS USED.

base / 555

blow-dry styling / 549

blunt cut / 523

circle / 555

curl / 555

graduated cut / 528

hair molding / 549

hair pressing / 556

hair wrapping / 549

half off-base / 555

long layered cut / 537

off-base / 555

on-base / 555

stem / 555

thermal styling / 555

uniform layered cut / 533

In general, the concept of a barbershop implies a male domain. However, many women have been known to seek the haircutting services of a barber rather than visit the local beauty salon. It seems that no matter how traditional the atmosphere or the clientele of the barbershop, invariably a woman will walk in and request a service. Maybe she likes the way her husband or son's hair has been cut, or perhaps she wants a precisely blended short, tapered cut. In either scenario, the professional barber should be willing and able to accommodate the request.

Other types of shops, such as unisex salons, maintain a fairly equal ratio of male to female clientele. In this environment, barbers must be proficient in cutting and styling women's hair as well as men's. Should you choose to work in a shop or salon that provides services to both men and women, embrace it for the learning experience it is and the enhanced effect it can have on your professional future.

In Chapter 14, you learned the basic foundations of cutting and styling men's hair. This chapter will assist you in applying that knowledge to the performance of women's cuts and styles. For the most part, the same terminology will be used to accomplish the four basic haircuts in this chapter. These include the blunt cut, graduated cut, uniform layered cut, and long layered cut.

Since women's hairstyles do not usually end with the haircut, this chapter will also introduce some basic styling techniques for women's hair. Styling women's hair tends to be a more involved process than styling men's hair and includes techniques such as wet setting, finger waving, pin curls, hair wrapping, and thermal styling. This chapter addresses only those techniques that can be accomplished using a blow-dryer, thermal irons, or hair-wrapping methods. For information and procedures regarding wet setting, finger waving, and pin curls, refer to the *Milady's Standard Cosmetology* textbook.

Basic Haircutting

One of the main differences between cutting women's hair and cutting men's hair is that men's cuts usually appear more angular whereas women's cuts may be more rounded and soft looking. This is important to keep in mind, especially when sculpting short hairstyles for women. Just because the hair is short doesn't mean that it has to look masculine. Points and curves along the design line, rather than straight horizontal lines, will soften the look of a woman's short cut. Styling also plays an important role in the final look of a short haircut. A little wave, some soft feathering directed toward the face, height in the crown, or wisps at the neckline, all help to soften the look of a short haircut design. Remember to visualize the finished cut and style before beginning the service.

GENERAL HAIRCUTTING REMINDERS

- Start with clean, conditioned hair.

- Pay attention to the client's head position.

- Pay attention to your body position.

- Pay attention to your finger placement. Comb through and practice the finger placement you will use before actually cutting the hair.

- Take consistent, clean partings to produce more precise results.

- Keep the hair moist when cutting.

- Work with natural growth patterns.

- Use the appropriate amount of tension when combing and holding sections of hair.

- Comb through partings or subsections *from the scalp*, not halfway down the section.

- Always work with a guide or guideline. If you cannot see the guide, don't cut! Take a thinner parting or reverse back through the procedure until you find a visible guide.

- Use the mirror to check length and proportion. It is one of your most important tools.

- Plan for the shrinkage factor that results when the hair dries or when cutting wavy and curly hair textures.

- Always check and cross-check your work.

The art of haircutting is made up of variations and combinations of four basic haircuts: blunt, graduated, uniform layered, and long layered. As with men's haircutting, a variety of elevations **(Figure 17-1)** and hand positions are used to create these effects. Review Chapter 15 if necessary.

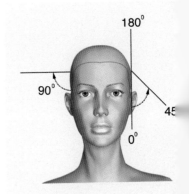

▲ FIGURE 17-1
Cutting elevations.

Blunt Cut (0 Elevation)

The **blunt cut** is also known as a *one-length cut* because all the hair ends at one hanging level to form a weight line at the perimeter. Blunt cuts *look* like all the hair is the same length, but the hair is actually shorter underneath, with each subsequent parting being longer as it travels over the curves of the head to reach the weight line. The head should be held in an upright position to avoid shifting the hair out of its natural fall position. If the head is positioned forward, graduation will be created within the cut. The design line at the perimeter may be cut to reflect horizontal, convex (rounded), diagonal forward, or diagonal back lines **(Figures 17-2 to 17-4)**. Figure 17-4 illustrates the technical pattern of a blunt cut with a diagonal forward design line.

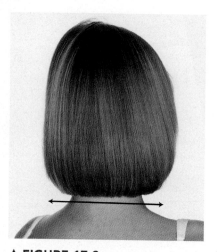

▲ FIGURE 17-2
Horizontal blunt cut.

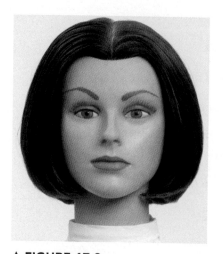

▲ FIGURE 17-3
Finished blunt cut.

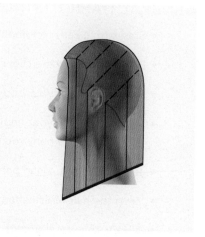

▲ FIGURE 17-4
Blunt cut technical with diagonal forward design line.

HAIRCUTTING TIPS FOR BLUNT CUTS

- Shampoo and condition the hair before cutting.

- Maintain uniform moisture while cutting.

- Work with the natural growth patterns of the hair.

- Keep the client's head upright and parallel to the floor.

- Take clean partings and subsections.

- Comb through the subsections twice from scalp to ends before cutting, and cut parallel to the part.

- Follow the comb with the fingers to maintain control of the hair parting.

- Cut with uniform minimal to moderate tension, depending on hair texture and elasticity.

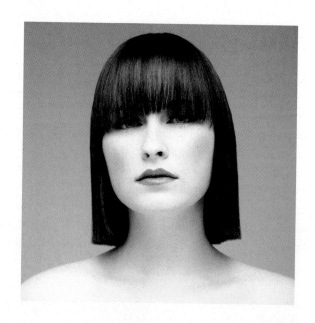

Blunt Cut

The method used to create the following blunt cut is somewhat different from other techniques you may be familiar with. Rather than working the four sections individually, this method provides a big-picture view of the haircutting areas and their relationship to each other throughout the entire haircut. Read through the procedure and discuss the steps before attempting the haircut. Remember to mist the hair as needed throughout the haircut. Be guided by your instructor for alternative methods of achieving a blunt cut.

SUPPLIES

- Towels
- Shampoo cape
- Shampoo and conditioner
- Chair cloth or cape
- Neckstrip
- Sectioning clips
- Brush
- All-purpose and tail combs
- Shears
- Blow-dryer
- Spray bottle with water

PREPARATION

1. Wash your hands.

2. Conduct the client consultation and hair analysis.

3. Drape the client and perform shampoo service.

4. Towel dry hair and drape for haircut.

PROCEDURE

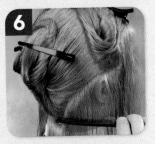

1 Comb the hair and part off into four sections from front to nape and from ear to ear over the top of the head form.

2 Secure sections with clips.

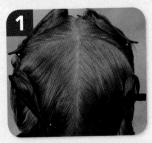

3 Beginning at the front right section, take a $\frac{1}{2}$" parting from the hairline. Secure remainder of hair in clip.

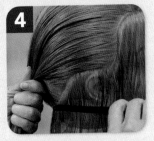

4 Move to the back right section and repeat the parting process, making sure to connect the parting lines from the side, to behind the ear, to the nape.

5 Repeat this process on the left side of the head.

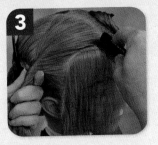

6 Comb through the $\frac{1}{2}$" partings all around the head.

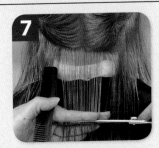

7 Move to the center back; comb through a section approximately 2" wide. Establish back guide at the desired length.

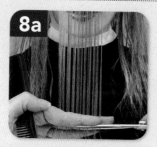
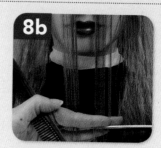

8 Move to the center front and establish a guide in the front section. Be sure that the length of the front guide will accommodate the intended design line. Example: for the horizontal design line, front guide length should be even with back guide length; for the diagonal forward design line, front guide length should be longer than back guide length; for the diagonal back design line, front guide length should be shorter than back guide length.

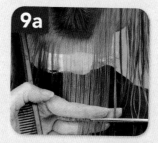
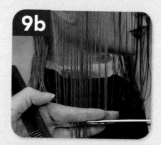

9 Move to the center back. Comb through the guide at a 0 elevation and, moving to the right, use the section as a guide to cut through to the corner of the back and into the side area. Continue cutting the design line until it meets with the front guide.

10 Repeat the process, working from the center back, to cut in the left side design line until it meets the front guide.

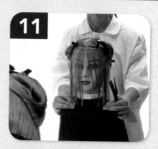

11 Comb through and check the design line; fine-tune as necessary. Check the sides for even length. Do not proceed until the design line is as precise as possible.

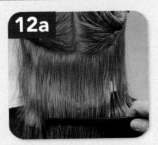
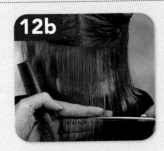
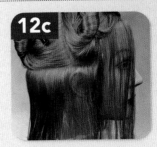

12 Move to the back and release another $\frac{1}{2}$″ parting from both back sections. Comb through the first and second partings at 0 elevation and cut the second parting using the design line as a guide. Continue cutting the back section in this manner until the parting meets the first side partings created in Step 9, usually around occipital height.

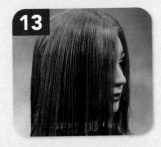

13 All subsequent partings will be parted off from the four sections to create one parting all the way around the head.

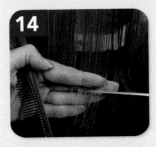

14 With the design line clearly established, cutting the subsequent partings can be performed from back to sides to front or from front to sides to back. Cut subsequent partings to the design line until all the hair is cut.

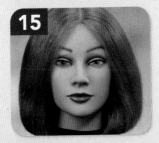

15 Cross-check your work by using vertical partings to view any excess hair strands. Fine-tune the entire cut as necessary, style the hair, and check again.

CLEAN-UP AND DISINFECTION

1. Clean and disinfect tools and implements.

2. Sanitize chair and workstation.

3. Dispose of towels and paper goods.

4. Sweep the floor.

5. Wash your hands.

Graduated Cut (45 Degrees)

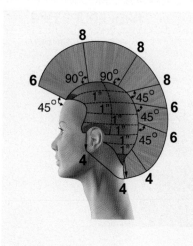

▲ FIGURE 17-5

Graduated cut technical.

A **graduated cut** has a wedge or stacked shape that is created by cutting with tension at low to medium elevations. The most common elevation for a graduated cut is 45 degrees, which creates layers within the hair between 0 and 45 degrees. These layers build weight and volume along the perimeter of the hairstyle. See **Figure 17-5** for a technical illustration of a graduated cut.

The graduated haircut can be accomplished with either horizontal or vertical partings. The horizontal method is described in the following procedure, with references to the vertical parting technique noted as applicable.

HAIRCUTTING TIPS FOR GRADUATED CUTS

- Coarse, curly, and thick hair appears to graduate more than straight hair textures.

- Graduation makes fine hair of average density appear thicker and fuller.

- Avoid weight lines and graduation on fine, low-density hair types.

- Maintain the same elevation around the perimeter when cutting in design lines.

- Maintain even, uniform tension and moisture throughout the haircut.

- Blend from one parting or subsection to another.

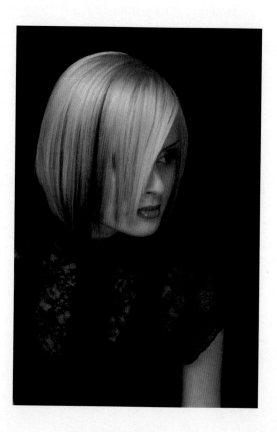

Graduated Cut

SUPPLIES

- Towels
- Shampoo cape
- Shampoo and conditioner
- Chair cloth or cape
- Neckstrip
- Sectioning clips
- Brush
- All-purpose and tail combs
- Shears
- Blow-dryer
- Spray bottle with water

PREPARATION

1. Wash your hands.

2. Conduct the client consultation and hair analysis.

3. Drape the client and perform shampoo service.

4. Towel dry hair and drape for haircut.

PROCEDURE

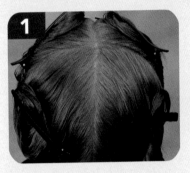

1 Comb the hair and part off into four sections from front to nape and from ear to ear as in Figure 1.

2 Secure sections with clips.

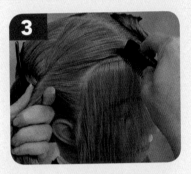

3 Beginning at the front right section, take a $\frac{1}{2}$" parting from the hairline as in Figure 3. Secure remainder of hair in a clip.

4 Move to the back right section and repeat the parting process, making sure to connect the parting lines from the side, to behind the ear, to the nape as performed in the blunt cut.

5 Repeat this process on the left side of the head.

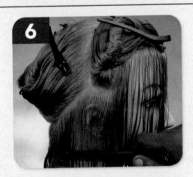

6 Comb through the $\frac{1}{2}$" partings all around the head.

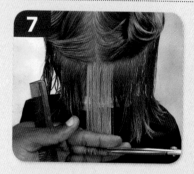

7 Move to the center back; comb through a section approximately 2" wide. Establish the back guide at a 45-degree elevation.

8 Move to the center front and establish a guide at a 0 or low elevation in the front section. Be sure that the length of the front guide will accommodate the intended design line.

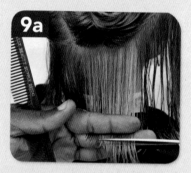

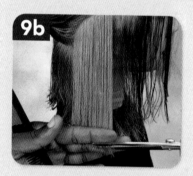

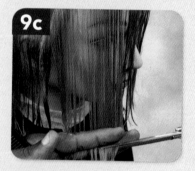

9 Move to the center back; comb through the guide horizontally at a 45-degree elevation. Cut to the right, using the guide to cut to the corner (9a). Use a portion of the back guide to begin the side guide/design line, using a horizontal traveling guide at the perimeter (9b). Continue cutting the design line until it meets with the front guide (9c).

10 Repeat the process, working from the center back to cut in the left side design line until it meets the front guide.

11 Comb through and check the design line; fine-tune as necessary. Check the sides for even length. Do not proceed until the design line is as precise as possible.

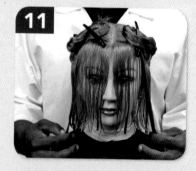

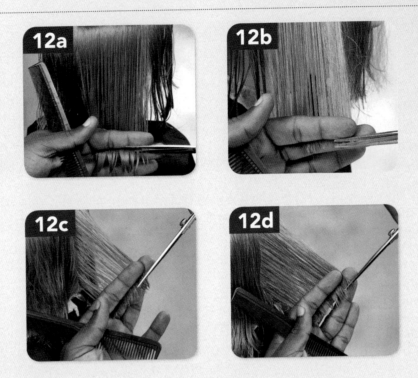

12 Move to the back and release another $\frac{1}{2}''$ parting from both back sections. Comb through the first and second horizontal partings while projecting to 45 degrees and cut the second parting using the design line as a guide. Continue cutting the back section in this manner until the partings meet the side and front partings created in Step 9.

Vertical Cutting Option: Using the design line as a guide, take a vertical parting and position the fingers at a 45-degree angle as shown in Figure 12c. Use this as a guide for cutting subsequent vertical partings around the head. Be careful to cut each section at the same elevation with the same angle of finger position. Also be sure that each section of hair blends from one vertical parting to another (Figure 12d).

13 All subsequent partings will be parted off from the four sections to create one parting all the way around the head.

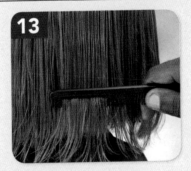

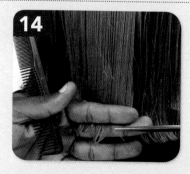

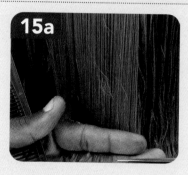

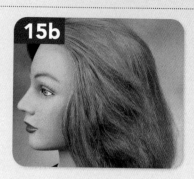

14 With the design line clearly established, cutting the subsequent partings can be performed from back to sides to front or from front to sides to back. Cut subsequent partings at the design line with a 45-degree elevation until the haircut is completed.

15 Check your work, fine-tune as necessary, style the hair, and check again.

CLEAN-UP AND DISINFECTION

1. Clean and disinfect tools and implements.

2. Sanitize chair and workstation.

3. Dispose of towels and paper goods.

4. Sweep the floor.

5. Wash your hands.

Uniform Layered Cut (90 Degrees)

In a **uniform layered cut,** all of the hair strands are cut to the same length at a 90-degree projection, straight out from the growth source. A traveling guide is used on the interior sections to create layers within the entire haircut. When finished, the cut will look soft and textured and conform to the head shape without weight lines or corners at the perimeter.

A uniform layered cut can be used to cut short or long layered styles. The main points to remember are to hold the hair that is being cut at a 90-degree projection from *where it grows* and to always use a guide from one section to the other. See **Figure 17-6** for a technical illustration of a uniform layered cut.

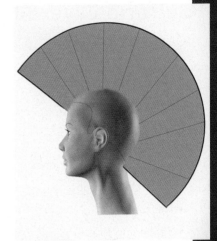

▲ **FIGURE 17-6**
Uniform layered cut technical.

HAIRCUTTING TIPS FOR UNIFORM LAYERED CUTS

- Establish an interior guide first, then set a guide at the perimeter to avoid cutting off too much hanging length in the style.

- The thinner the parting, the more volume will be created within the cut.

- Work with the natural growth pattern, wave formation, and density of the hair.

- Always make sure the hair is blending from one section to another.

- Always check design lines for blending on the perimeter of the cut.

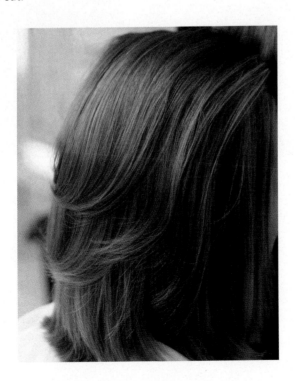

Uniform Layered Cut

SUPPLIES

- Towels
- Shampoo cape
- Shampoo and conditioner
- Chair cloth or cape
- Neckstrip
- Sectioning clips
- Brush
- All-purpose and tail combs
- Shears
- Blow-dryer
- Spray bottle with water

PREPARATION

1. Wash your hands.

2. Conduct the client consultation and hair analysis.

3. Drape the client and perform shampoo service.

4. Towel dry hair and drape for haircut.

PROCEDURE

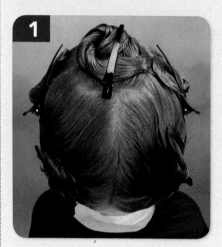

1 Comb the hair into a natural fall position. If the hair is long, part off into five sections: top, two sides, and two back panels. Secure sections with clips if necessary.

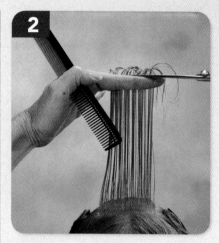

2 Stand behind the client and comb a horizontal parting from the high point of the head form into a 90-degree elevation. Establish guide.

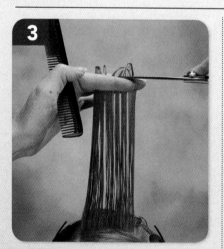

3 Use the first guide as a traveling guide to cut the top section toward the front area.

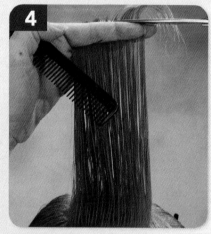

4 Comb the top section back. Move to the side. Starting at the forehead, part off the top section of hair, front to back, with the thumb and middle finger. Hold the original guide line and a $\frac{1}{2}$" parting at the crown at 90 degrees, and cut. This establishes the guide for the crown and back sections.

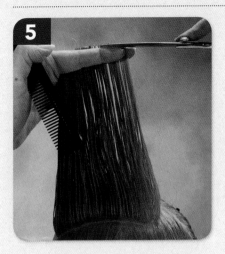

5 Work forward, still maintaining a side-standing position. Following the arc and contour of the head, even off any length that does not blend with the traveling guide. If the horizontal partings were cut correctly, no more than $\frac{1}{4}$" of hair should need to be evened.

6 Comb the hair into natural fall. Pick up the crown area guide and hold at a 90-degree elevation. Use a vertical parting to cut the hair from the crown to the nape.

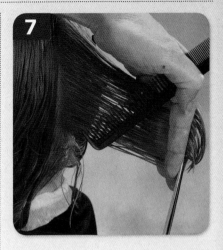

7 Once a vertical panel of hair has been cut to the appropriate length, use it as guide to cut the remainder of the back section. Vertical partings may be cut from the crown to the nape or from the nape to the crown (establish perimeter design line first), depending on preference.

8 Comb the back section into natural fall and establish a perimeter design line at 0 elevation.

9 Continue the design line into the sides and front areas. Check length on sides for evenness.

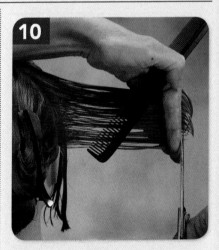

10 Move behind the client. Part off a vertical subsection from the hair on the right side. Hold the parting straight out to the side at 90 degrees. The design/guide line should be visible at the tips of the fingers when working on the right side of the client's head.

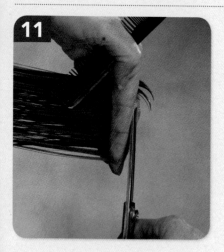

11 Make a straight, vertical cut from the design/guide line, cutting off any hair that extends past the guide. Maintain uniform moisture.

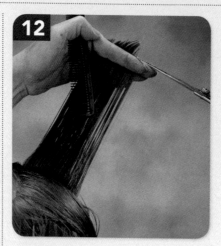

12 Continue cutting partings of hair while following the contour of the head until reaching the guide in the top section. The hair should meet. Check the procedure by checking the blend of hair from the side design/guide line to the top section guide.

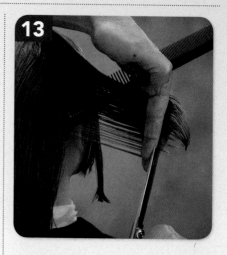

13 Proceed until all the side hair is cut. Use vertical partings to blend the side hair to the back hair. Repeat procedure on the left side. Option: Stand facing the client to facilitate working from the design/guide line up when blending the hair on the left side of the head.

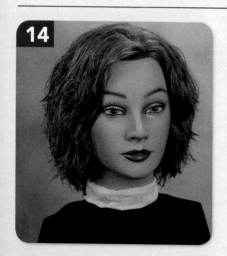

14 Comb and check the cut. Style as desired. The figure shows the uniform layered cut in a scrunched style.

CLEAN-UP AND DISINFECTION

1. Clean and disinfect tools and implements.

2. Sanitize chair and workstation.

3. Dispose of towels and paper goods.

4. Sweep the floor.

5. Wash your hands.

Long Layered Cut (180 Degrees)

A **long layered cut** consists of increased layering that is achieved by cutting the hair at a 180-degree elevation. This produces progressively longer layers from the top to the perimeter and begins with a stationary guide in the top section. **Figure 17-7** depicts the technical pattern of a long layered cut.

HAIRCUTTING TIPS FOR LONG LAYERED CUTS

- Comb through parting or subsections from scalp to ends with even tension.

- Work with only as much hair as is comfortable and controllable. Create thinner working panels of hair if the combination of length and density becomes unmanageable.

- If in doubt about what the remaining hanging length of the hair will be when it is cut to the top guide, cut in the design line at the perimeter first.

- Avoid steps and gaps between the layers. Blend sections from long to short or short to long.

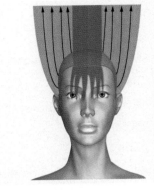

▲ **FIGURE 17-7**
180-degree long layered technical.

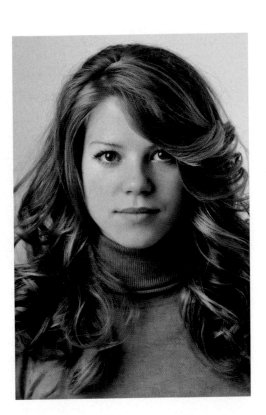

Long Layered Cut

SUPPLIES

- Towels
- Shampoo cape
- Shampoo and conditioner
- Chair cloth or cape
- Neckstrip
- Sectioning clips
- Brush
- All-purpose and tail combs
- Shears
- Blow-dryer
- Spray bottle with water

PREPARATION

1. Wash your hands.

2. Conduct the client consultation and hair analysis.

3. Drape the client and perform shampoo service.

4. Towel dry hair and drape for haircut.

PROCEDURE

1 Comb the hair into a natural fall position. Part off into five sections: top, two sides, and two back panels. Secure sections with clips.

2 Stand behind the client and comb a horizontal parting about an inch wide from the high point of the head into a 90-degree elevation. Establish a guide.

3 Use the first guide as a traveling guide to cut the top section toward the front area.

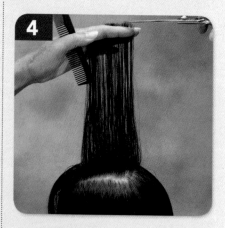

4 Comb the top section back. Move to the side. Starting at the forehead, part off the top section of hair, front to back, with the thumb and middle finger. Elevate the hair to 90 degrees and even off any length that does not blend with the traveling guide. Maintain uniform moisture.

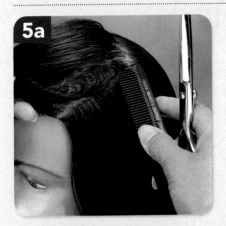

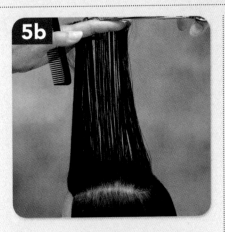

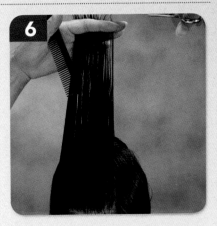

5 From a side-standing position, hold the top guide at 90 degrees and take a $\frac{1}{4}''$ to $\frac{1}{2}''$ horizontal parting from the top of the crest section on the side. Comb the side parting of hair up to the top guide and cut. Continue working down the side until all the hair has been cut at a 180-degree elevation to the top guide. Repeat on the other side.

6 Cut the back sections in the same manner as the sides. Continue until both back panels are cut.

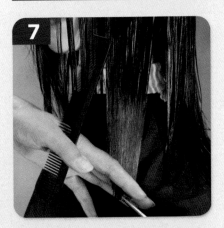

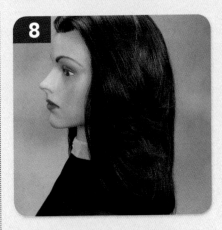

7 Comb the hair down into natural fall. Beginning at the center back, trim and fine-tune the perimeter design line. Check the sides for evenness. Check the layers for blending.

8 Style the hair as desired.

CLEAN-UP AND DISINFECTION

1. Clean and disinfect tools and implements.

2. Sanitize chair and workstation.

3. Dispose of towels and paper goods.

4. Sweep the floor.

5. Wash your hands.

Gallery of Cuts: Technicals and Finished Styles (Figures 17-8 to 17-31)

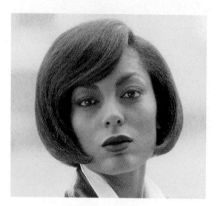

▲ **FIGURE 17-8**

Blunt cut.

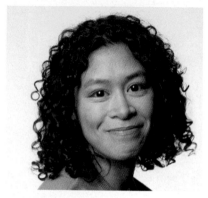

▲ **FIGURE 17-9**

Blunt cut on curly hair.

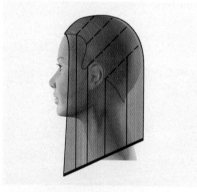

▲ **FIGURE 17-10**

Blunt cut technical with diagonal forward design.

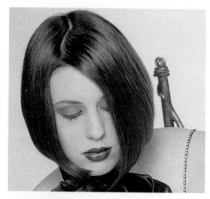

▲ **FIGURE 17-11**

Diagonal forward bob.

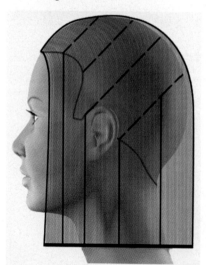

▲ **FIGURE 17-12**

Blunt cut technical.

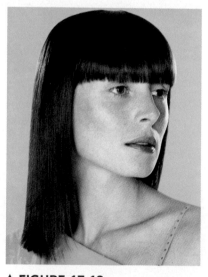

▲ **FIGURE 17-13**

Longer blunt cut with one-length bangs.

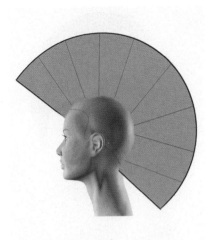

▲ FIGURE 17-14
Graduated cut technical.

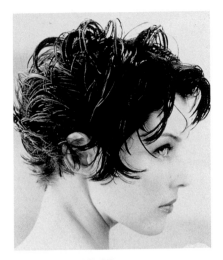

▲ FIGURE 17-15
Graduated cut on curly hair.

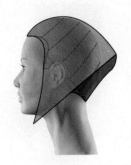

▲ FIGURE 17-16
Graduated bob technical.

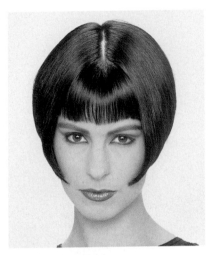

▲ FIGURE 17-17
Finished graduated bob.

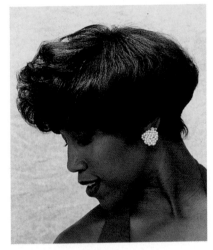

▲ FIGURE 17-18
Bob variation.

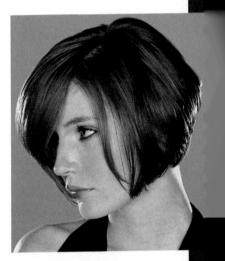

▲ FIGURE 17-19
Bob variation.

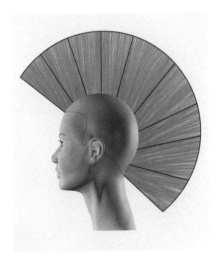

▲ FIGURE 17-20
Uniform layered cut technical.

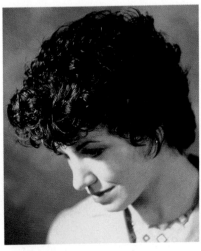

▲ FIGURE 17-21
Uniform layered cut on curly hair.

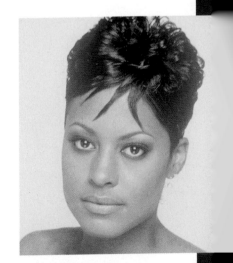

▲ FIGURE 17-22
Uniform layer with taper variation.

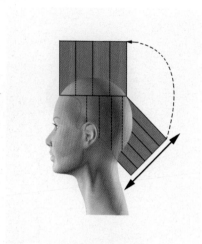

▲ **FIGURE 17-23**
Uniform layer with taper variation technical.

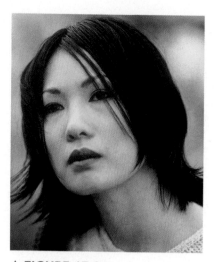

▲ **FIGURE 17-24**
Uniform layer variation.

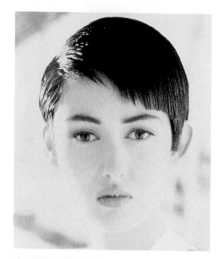

▲ **FIGURE 17-25**
Uniform layer with taper variation.

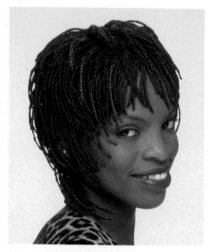

▲ **FIGURE 17-26**
Uniform layer braided style.

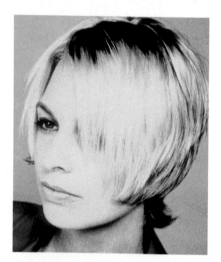

▲ **FIGURE 17-27**
Uniform layered cut variation.

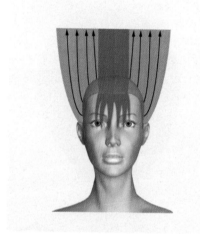

▲ **FIGURE 17-28**
180-degree long layered technical.

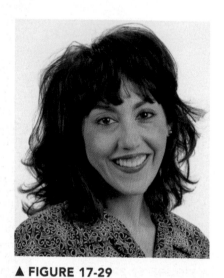

▲ **FIGURE 17-29**
Long layered cut.

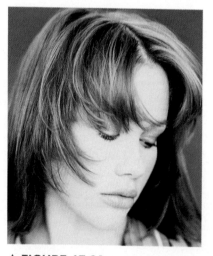

▲ **FIGURE 17-30**
Long layered cut.

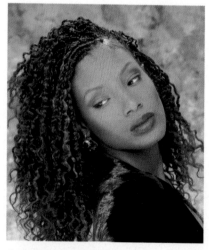

▲ **FIGURE 17-31**
Long layered braided style.

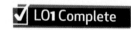
☑ **LO1 Complete**

Cutting Curly Hair Textures

Curly hair types range from large, loose curl patterns to tight, springy curls. Any of the four cutting elevations can be used on curly hair; however, the results will be different from those achieved on straighter hair types. For example, curly hair tends to graduate naturally due to the elasticity and curl pattern of the hair. Use less elevation if strong angles are the objective.

The trough and crest formation of the waves in curly hair textures needs to be taken into account when performing a haircut. Depending on the amount of curl, cutting the hair parting in the trough of the wave may cause the hair ends to flip out from the head form. Conversely, cutting just after the crest of the wave as it dips toward the trough may encourage the hair to fall inward toward the head form (**Figure 17-32**).

Knowing where to cut on the wave is helpful when cutting all lengths of curly hair and should be considered when analyzing the hair texture. It is most important when cutting shorter hairstyles, especially maintenance cuts on regular customers, because the amount of hair to be cut may have to be adjusted according to the wave pattern at any given time. For example, a client with wavy to curly hair has a standing appointment every four weeks. Assume that the hair grows at an average of $\frac{1}{2}$" per month. If the hair was cut at a point just after the crest of the wave during the previous haircut service, those hair ends may now be part of the subsequent trough that develops as the hair curls naturally. It would not be correct to automatically cut off $\frac{1}{2}$" of hair during the next visit because it may encourage the curl to wave out from the head form. Cutting a little less or a little more will place the cut line at the crest of the wave again and encourage the hair to curl toward the head form instead of away from it.

TECHNIQUES FOR CUTTING NATURAL CURLY STYLES

Depending on the overall length of the hair, short natural cuts on extremely curly hair can be created by using the freehand clipper or fingers-and-shear cutting technique. The hair is tapered at the perimeter and may be tapered, rounded, or wedged from the sides to the top section. When using clippers, the hair should be clean and dry. Fingers-and-shear cutting is usually performed on clean damp hair.

The decision to use clippers or shears will depend on the density and texture of the hair. Thick, coarse hair types are easier to cut with the clippers. Curly hair of medium density and a softer curl may lend itself to shear cutting. The rule for fingers-and-shear cutting on extremely curly hair is that if a parting can be made and held between the index and second finger, fingers-and-shear cutting can be performed.

HAIRCUTTING TIPS FOR CLIPPER CUTTING CURLY HAIR

- Observe the density and curl pattern closely. Sometimes extremely curly hair gives the illusion that the scalp won't be seen if the hair is cut close, but in reality, it may continue to curl in upon itself in small tufts, leaving partings throughout the hair and scalp exposed.

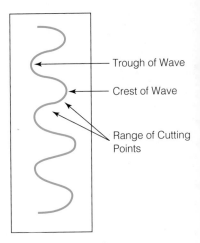

▲ FIGURE 17-32
Crest and trough formation of waves.

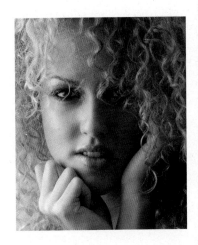

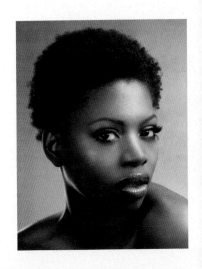

Clipper Cut Natural Style

SUPPLIES

- Towels
- Shampoo cape
- Shampoo and conditioner
- Chair cloth
- Neckstrip
- Clipper
- Comb and pick
- Shears
- Blow-dryer with diffuser attachment

PREPARATION

1. Wash your hands.

2. Conduct the client consultation and hair analysis.

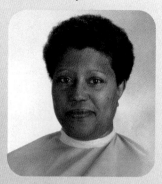

3. Drape the client and perform shampoo service.

4. Dry hair with diffuser attachment and drape for haircut.

PROCEDURE

1 Pick the hair out using a wide-toothed comb or pick.

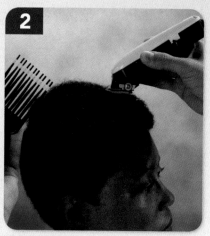

2 Set a guide in the top center section.

3 Move to the back and have the client bow her head forward slightly. Begin the taper at the nape using a clipper-over-comb technique. Allow the hair to gradually increase in length as you move up toward the occipital area.

4 Move to the next working panel in the back section using the first cut as a guide. Cut to the occipital.

5 Continue cutting the back section in this manner, working one panel at a time while following the head shape.

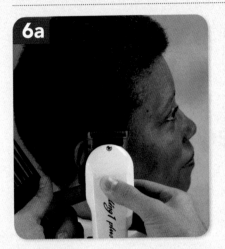

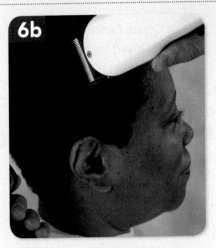

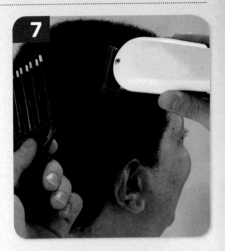

6 Move to the right side and cut from the hairline over the ears to the crest area, creating a tapered, rounded, or wedged shape as desired. Blend the sides to the back section behind the ear. Repeat the procedure on the left side.

7 Blend the hair from the crest to top section. Remember to lift the hair out at 90 degrees with the pick or comb.

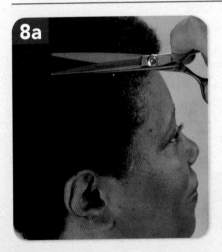

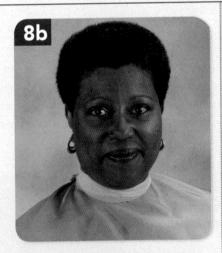

8 To complete the cut, comb through the hair in the direction that the client will be combing it. Check the cut and fine-tune with shears. Apply dressing to finished cut if desired.

CLEAN-UP AND DISINFECTION

1. Clean and disinfect tools and implements.

2. Sanitize chair and workstation.

3. Dispose of towels and paper goods.

4. Sweep the floor.

5. Wash your hands.

- Use your comb as a guard around the hairline to avoid cutting the hair too close to the head.

- After each cut with the clipper, comb or pick the hair to check the effect.

- Create flattering and proportionate design forms throughout the crest and top sections.

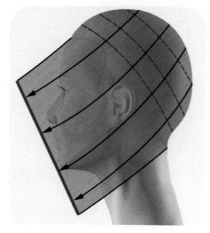

▲ **FIGURE 17-33**
Over-direction in long layered cut: design.

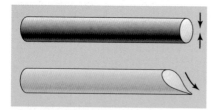

▲ **FIGURE 17-34**
Shear cut and razor cut strands.

Other Cutting Techniques

In addition to the basic haircuts, there are other techniques that can be used to create different effects in the appearance and behavior of the hair. These techniques include over-direction, razor cutting, and texturizing.

OVER-DIRECTION

Over-direction occurs when the hair is combed away from its natural fall position. This technique of shifting the hair into a different position facilitates length increase in a design and the ability to blend short and long lengths along a perimeter design line (**Figure 17-33**) or interior section.

RAZOR CUTTING

Razor cutting produces an angle at the ends of the hair that results in softer shapes with more movement and visual separation than shear-cut hair ends. Generally, haircuts that can be accomplished with shears can also be performed with a razor. Review **Figures 17-34** to **17-39** for razor applications on longer hair.

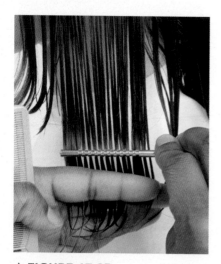

▲ **FIGURE 17-35**
Incorrect razor angle.

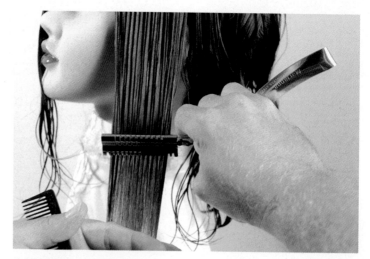

▲ **FIGURE 17-36**
Razor cutting parallel to subsection.

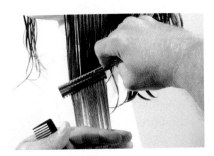

▲ FIGURE 17-37

Razor cutting at a 45-degree angle.

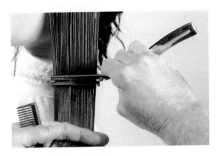

▲ FIGURE 17-38

Hand position on horizontal section.

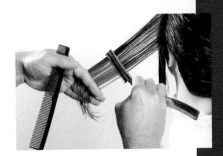

▲ FIGURE 17-39

Hand position on vertical section.

TEXTURIZING

Texturizing techniques can be used to remove excess bulk, add volume, create movement, or create wispy and spiky effects. The most commonly used texturizing techniques are point cutting, notching, slithering, slicing, and carving.

- *Point cutting* is performed at the ends of the hair using the tips of the shears at a steep shear angle in relation to the hair parting (**Figures 17-40a** and **17-40b**).

- *Notching* creates a chunkier effect than point cutting and is produced by positioning the shears at a flatter angle to the ends of the hair (**Figure 17-41**). Freehand notching is also accomplished with the tips of the shears but is usually performed within the interior sections of the haircut.

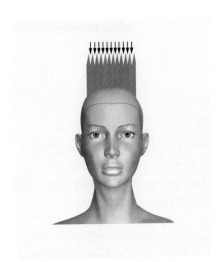

▲ FIGURE 17-40a

Point cutting with steeper shears angle.

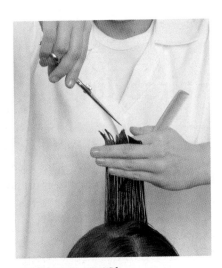

▲ FIGURE 17-40b

Point cutting.

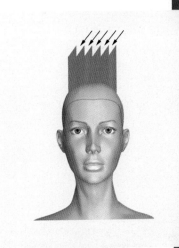

▲ FIGURE 17-41

Notching.

- *Slithering* is the process of thinning the hair to graduated lengths with the shears, which produces volume and movement. The hair is cut using a sliding shears movement with the blades kept partially opened (**Figure 17-42**).

- *Slicing* also removes bulk and adds movement in the hair. The blades are kept open, and only the portion of the blade near the pivot is used for cutting (**Figure 17-43**).

- *Carving* is a version of slicing that creates separation in the hair. The shears are moved throughout the hair with an open and closing movement that carves out sections of hair (**Figure 17-44**). Carving the ends of the hair will create texture and separation at the perimeter.

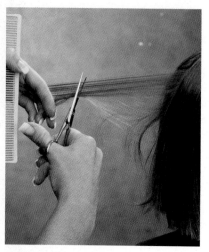

▲ **FIGURE 17-42**
Slithering.

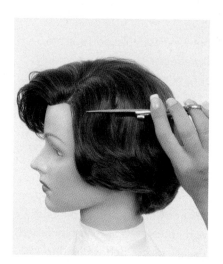

▲ **FIGURE 17-43**
Slicing.

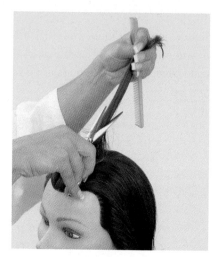

▲ **FIGURE 17-44**
Carving.

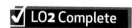

Hairstyling

As with haircutting, the first step in the hairstyling process is the client consultation. Guide the client toward the most suitable hairstyle design for her face shape, hair texture, and lifestyle. Keep styling magazines accessible for easy reference during the consultation. Hairstyling techniques include wet hairstyling, blow-dry styling, thermal styling, and natural dry styling.

TERMINOLOGY AND TECHNIQUES

This section provides a basic description of techniques and terminology used in women's hairstyling. The procedures for hair wrapping, blow-dry styling, and curling iron work are also included. For wet setting, finger waving, and pin-curling procedures, refer to *Milady's Standard Cosmetology* textbook.

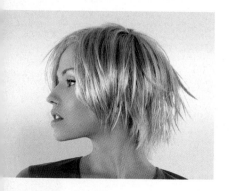

- *Wet hairstyling* is accomplished through the processes of finger waving, pin curls, hair wrapping, and roller sets. The tools needed for these processes include rollers, pin curl clips, sectioning clips, all-purpose combs, brushes, and setting lotion.

- *Finger waving* is the process of shaping and directing the hair into an S-shaped pattern through the use of the fingers, comb, and setting lotion.

- *Pin curls* serve as the basis for patterns, lines, waves, and curls, which are used in a variety of hairstyles. Pin curls are wound from the hair ends into a spiral that creates a flattened curl formation against the head, where it is secured with a hair clip.

- *Roller sets* are performed with tools called rollers. Rollers are available in a variety of materials, shapes, and sizes, which are used to set a pattern in the hair that will form the basis for a hairstyle. Plastic rollers are used for most wet roller sets. Hot rollers and Velcro rollers are used on dry hair only.

- *Hair wrapping* and *hair molding* are styling methods that use the client's head as a form or tool.

- *Blow-dry styling* is accomplished with a blow-dryer, brush, and styling products (optional) in a similar manner to that used in men's styling. Blow-dry styling also serves to prepare the hair for thermal iron curling techniques.

- *Natural dry styling* usually requires minimal manipulation of the hair. Once the hair is towel dried, it may be combed into place or arranged in a freeform style with the hands and fingers. It is then allowed to dry naturally.

- *Thermal styling* includes the procedures of thermal waving and thermal hair straightening. Heated tools are used to wave, curl, or straighten the hair.

These techniques are described and illustrated in the following sections.

HAIR WRAPPING AND HAIR MOLDING

In **hair wrapping,** the hair is wrapped around the head to create smooth, sleek styles that may or may not require finish styling with thermal irons. Hair wrapping may be used on wet or dry hair to create a temporary natural-looking curvature to the hairstyle. When the hair-wrapping technique is applied to the entire head of hair, minimal volume results at the scalp. If height or volume is desired at the crown area, two or three large rollers should be placed in this section for additional lift. **Hair molding** is the process of combing the hair straight down over the client's head form followed by drying and thermal iron finish work.

BLOW-DRY STYLING

Blow-dry styling is the technique of drying and styling damp hair in one operation. Combined with the foundation of a good haircut, blow-dry styling is a quick and relatively simple option for the client's self-styling or shop-styling procedures.

CAUTION

It is usually recommended to avoid using brushes on damp hair because some bristle styles can snag, damage, or stretch the hair during the brushing process. If the use of a brush is preferred or necessary to perform hair wrapping or molding techniques, choose a brush with wide-spaced bristles that *do not* have plastic tips attached to the ends.

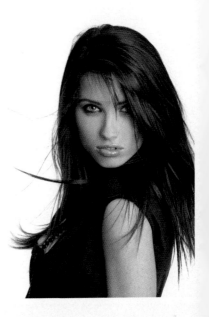

Hair Wrapping and Hair Molding

SUPPLIES

- Towels
- Shampoo cape
- Shampoo and conditioner
- Chair cloth or cape
- Neckstrip or hair-wrapping strip
- Duckbill clips
- Setting or wrapping lotion, mousse, leave-in thermal styling spray, or gel
- Tail and styling combs
- Firm-bristled brush
- Spray bottle with water
- Pressing cream, wax, or oil
- Thermal styling tools (Marcel, curling, or flat irons)

PREPARATION

1. Wash your hands.

2. Conduct the client consultation and hair analysis.

3. Drape the client and perform shampoo service. Towel blot the hair.

HAIR WRAPPING PROCEDURE

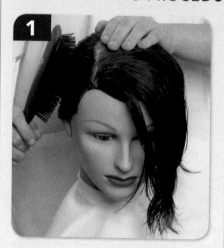

1 Apply lotion, mousse, or gel product. Comb or brush the hair clockwise around the head in the desired direction.

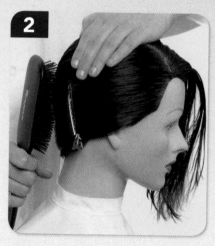

2 Use duckbill clips to keep the hair in place while wrapping.

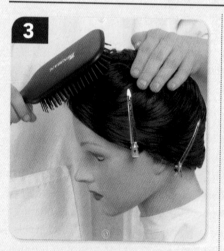

3 Continue wrapping the hair around the head. Follow the comb or brush with your hand to smooth and keep the hair tight against the head.

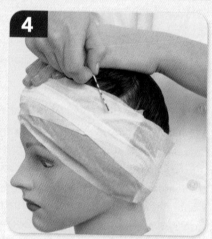

4 When the hair is wrapped, stretch a neckstrip or hair-wrapping strip around the head to keep the hair in place. Secure with a bobby pin and remove the duckbill clips.

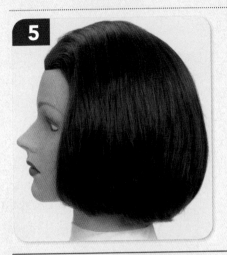

5 Place client under hood dryer. When hair is thoroughly dried, allow it to cool before combing into the finished style. Apply holding spray or oil sheen as desired.

6 Optional finish styling: Once the hair has been combed after drying, distribute pressing cream, wax, or oil through the hair. Use thermal irons to curl or further straighten the hair into the desired style. Apply holding spray or oil sheen as appropriate for the hair texture.

HAIR MOLDING PROCEDURE

1 Following the shampoo and towel-blotting process, apply mousse and leave-in thermal styling spray.

2 Comb or brush the hair straight down.

3 After the hair is smoothly molded to the head, apply a neckstrip or hair-wrapping strip around the head to keep the hair in place. Secure the strip with a bobby pin.

4 Place client under hood dryer, dry thoroughly, and allow the hair to cool before combing.

5 Distribute pressing cream, wax, or oil through the hair.

6 Use thermal irons to straighten or curl the hair as desired.

7 Comb into finished style. Apply holding spray or oil sheen as desired.

CLEAN-UP AND DISINFECTION

1. Clean and disinfect tools and implements.

2. Sanitize chair and workstation.

3. Dispose of towels and paper goods.

4. Wash your hands.

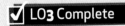
✓ **LO3** Complete

Blow-Dry Styling

SUPPLIES

- Towels
- Shampoo cape
- Shampoo and conditioner
- Chair cloth or cape
- Neckstrip or hair-wrapping strip
- Duckbill clips
- Styling lotion, mousse, or gel
- All-purpose and tail combs
- Brush of choice
- Blow-dryer with attachments
- Spray bottle with water

PREPARATION

1. Wash your hands.

2. Conduct the client consultation and hair analysis.

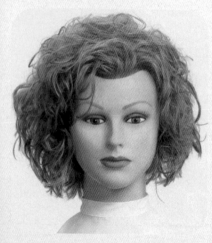

3. Drape the client and perform shampoo service. Towel blot hair.

PROCEDURE

A. ROUND BRUSH ON MEDIUM-LENGTH HAIR

1 Distribute the styling product through the hair and comb through to the ends.

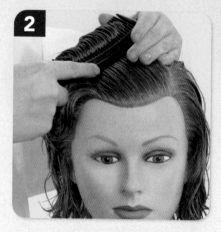

2 Use the comb to mold the hair into the desired shape.

3 Section the hair for blow-drying.

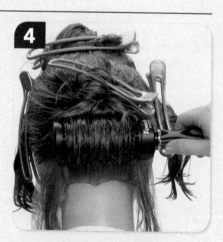

4 Beginning in the nape area, insert the brush at the base of the section. Roll the hair down to the base with medium tension at the projection appropriate for the desired volume.

5

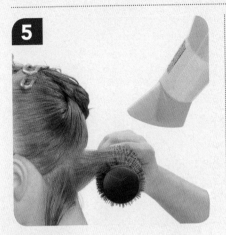

5 Direct the stream of air from the blow-dryer over the hair in a back-and-forth motion in the same direction as the hair is wound.

6 Follow the same procedure throughout the sections of the head, using the appropriate projection of hair for a given area depending on the desired style.

7

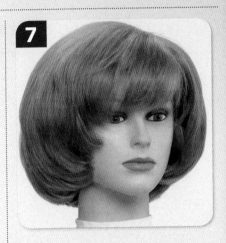

7 Make sure the hair and scalp are completely dry before combing out the style. Finish with a holding spray or other appropriate product, as client desires.

B. CURLY STYLE OPTION:

To blow-dry short, curly hair into its natural wave pattern, use a diffuser and scrunch the hair as it is being dried.

b1

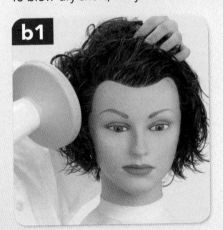

b2

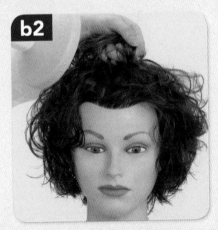

b3

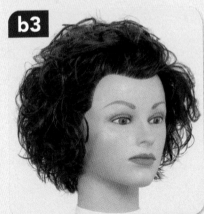

C. LONG LAYERED OPTION

Use the following as a guide to blow-dry longer hairstyles.

1 Attach the nozzle for controlled styling. Part and section the hair to facilitate working on one section at a time.

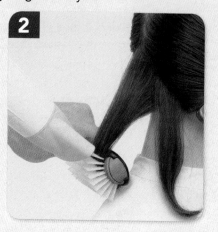

2 Begin at a nape section. Draw the brush through the hair from scalp to ends at a low elevation and follow with the dryer heat.

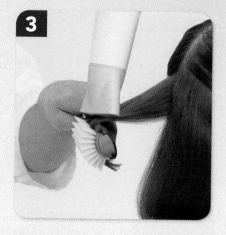

3 For increased volume, elevate the section at 45 or 90 degrees.

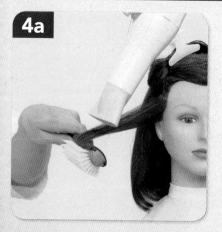

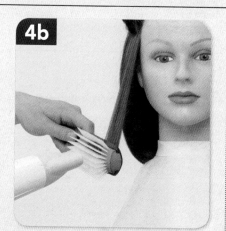

4 When reaching the ends of the hair, turn the brush under or up depending on the desired style.

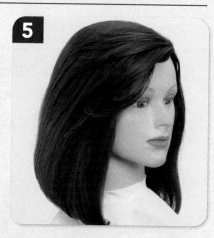

5 Continue the process until all the hair is dried. Comb or brush through the hair to finish. Apply holding spray as desired.

CLEAN-UP AND DISINFECTION

1. Clean and disinfect tools and implements.

2. Sanitize chair and workstation.

3. Dispose of towels and paper goods.

4. Wash your hands.

☑ **LO4 Complete**

THERMAL STYLING

Thermal styling uses heat to produce waving or straightening effects. Thermal waving is achieved with conventional Marcel irons or electric thermal irons. Thermal hair straightening, also known as *hair pressing*, is accomplished through the use of heated pressing combs or electric flat irons.

Thermal Waving

There are two important factors to consider when creating curls with a curling iron. The first is that the barrel size of the iron determines the size of the wave or curl; and the second is that the projection of the hair from the scalp will determine where the curl sits in relation to its base, and hence the amount of volume achieved. An understanding of the parts of a curl helps to explain the relationships between hair projection, bases, and volume.

The parts of a **curl** are the base, stem, and circle (**Figure 17-45**). The **base** is the stationary foundation of the curl on which the barrel (or roller) is placed. The **stem** is the hair between the scalp and the first arc of the circle; it gives the hair direction and mobility. The **circle** forms the curl as the hair is wrapped around the barrel or roller. The ultimate size of the curl along the length of the hair shaft depends on how it is wrapped. A hair section that is wrapped in a spiral along the curling iron barrel will have a more uniform curl formation than a hair section that is repeatedly wrapped around itself over one section of the barrel.

There are three kinds of bases used in thermal (and roller) setting. They are on-base, half off-base, and off-base.

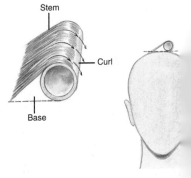

▲ **FIGURE 17-45**

Parts of a roller curl.

- **On-base** roller placement sits directly on the base and produces a full-volume curl. On-base placement is achieved by slightly over-directing the hair beyond 90 degrees in front of the base (**Figure 17-46**).

- **Half off-base,** or half-base, roller placement sits halfway on and halfway behind the base after rolling the hair parting at 90 degrees (**Figure 17-47**).

- **Off-base** roller placement produces the least amount of volume and sits completely off the base. The hair is held at 45 degrees from the base and rolled down to the scalp (**Figure 17-48**).

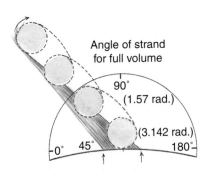

▲ **FIGURE 17-46**

On-base: full volume.

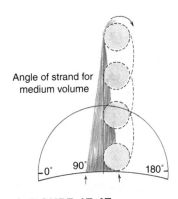

▲ **FIGURE 17-47**

Half off-base: medium volume.

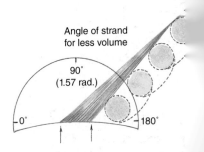

▲ **FIGURE 17-48**

Off-base: less volume.

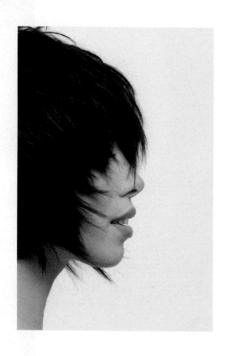

Hair Pressing

Hair pressing temporarily straightens extremely curly or hard-to-manage hair by means of a heated pressing comb or iron. Pressings generally last until the next shampoo, although high humidity and other weather conditions can cause the hair to partially revert to its natural condition. In some cases, environmental conditions may determine whether a soft, medium, or hard press is used to straighten the hair.

- A *soft press* removes 50 to 60 percent of the curl and is accomplished by applying the pressing comb once to each side of the hair section.

- The *medium press* removes 60 to 75 percent of the curl and is performed in the same manner as the soft press, but with a little more pressure.

- A *hard press* removes 100 percent of the curl formation and involves two applications of the pressing comb on each side of the hair section.

Following a shampoo and blow-dry, the hair is prepared for the pressing service with an application of a pressing cream or oil. These products make the hair softer and help to prevent the hair from burning or scorching.

Safety Precautions for Thermal Irons

- Use thermal irons only after receiving instruction on their use.

- Keep irons clean and sanitized.

- Always test the temperature of the iron before using it on a client.

- Do not overheat irons.

- Handle and remove heated irons and stoves carefully.

- Do not place heated stoves near the station mirror as the heat can cause breakage.

- Place a hard rubber comb between the client's scalp and the iron. Never use a metal comb.

- Place heated stoves and irons in a safe place to cool.

Electric Flat Irons

Electric flat irons are used to temporarily straighten curly or wavy hair. They can also be used to give direction to straighter hair texture styles while imparting a glossy, finished look to the hair. Flat irons are available in many sizes from mini-irons for short hair lengths or tight styling areas to larger irons suitable for long hair styling.

Flat irons should only be used on clean, dry hair because heat applied to hair that has oil or styling product buildup can damage the hair as well as the iron. The application of a leave-in thermal styling product is recommended before drying to protect the hair from heat damage. Excessive heat damages the hair, so care needs to be taken to monitor the temperature of the flat iron as well. Test the temperature by placing a piece of misted tissue paper between the heating plates. If the temperature is safe to apply to the hair, the moisture in the paper will evaporate without leaving any evidence of scorching.

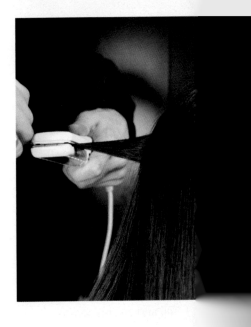

Safety Precautions for Electric Flat Irons

- Use flat irons only after receiving instruction on their use.

- Keep irons clean and sanitized.

- Choose the right size of iron for the job.

- Start with clean, conditioned, and thoroughly dried hair.

- Always test the temperature of the iron before using it on a client.

- Do not overheat irons.

- Section partings according to the density of the hair and the size of the iron.

- Handle and remove heated irons carefully.

- Place a hard rubber comb between the client's scalp and the iron when working in this area. Never use a metal comb.

- Place heated irons in a safe place to cool.

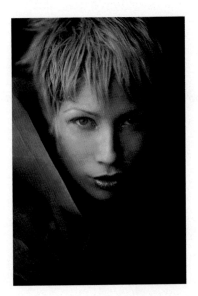

Thermal Styling with Marcel and Curling Irons

SUPPLIES

- Towels
- Shampoo cape
- Shampoo
- Chair cloth or cape
- Neckstrip
- Clips
- Leave-in thermal styling spray
- Finishing spray
- Tail and styling combs
- Brush
- Blow-dryer with attachments
- Marcel iron and stove or curling iron
- Mannequin and mannequin holder

PREPARATION

1. Wash your hands.
2. Conduct the client consultation and hair analysis.
3. Drape and perform shampoo service. Towel blot the hair.
4. Drape mannequin with chair cloth and neck strip. Heat the iron.

PROCEDURE

The manipulative techniques are basically the same for stove-heated irons and electric Marcel irons. Begin practicing by rolling the cold irons forward and then backward until comfortable with the tool.

A. PRACTICE THE FOLLOWING MANIPULATIVE MOVEMENTS BEFORE USING IRONS ON THE MANNEQUIN:

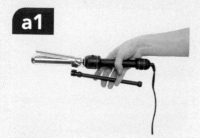
a1

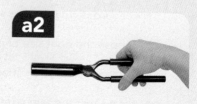
a2

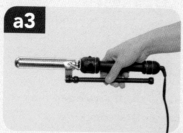
a3

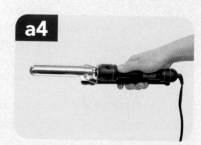
a4

- Practice turning the irons while opening and closing at regular intervals.

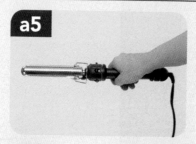
a5

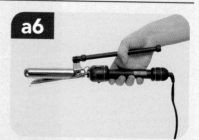
a6

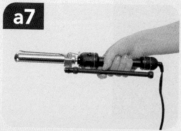
a7

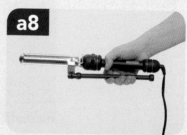
a8

- Rotate the irons downward, toward you, and upward, away from you.

- Practice releasing the hair by opening and closing the irons with a quick, clicking movement to complete a full turn.

B. PRACTICE THE FOLLOWING MANIPULATIVE MOVEMENTS ON THE MANNEQUIN:

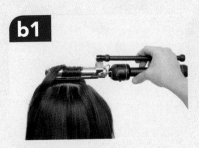

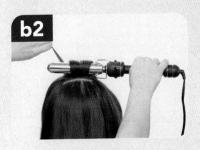

1 Section off a parting in the crown area. Open the iron and position the barrel a couple of inches from the scalp. Roll and rotate while opening and closing the iron.

2 Guide the hair section toward the center of the curl while rotating the irons.

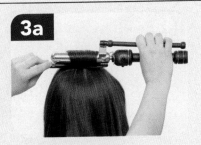

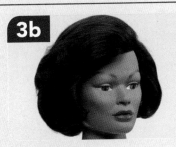

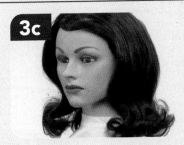

3 Position the comb to protect the scalp. Remove the curl from the iron by drawing the comb to the left and the curl to the right. Figures 3b and 3c show finished styles created with thermal irons.

CLEAN-UP AND DISINFECTION

1. Clean and disinfect tools and implements.

2. Sanitize chair and workstation.

3. Dispose of towels and paper goods.

4. Wash your hands.

Hair Pressing

SUPPLIES

- Towels
- Shampoo cape
- Shampoo
- Chair cloth
- Neckstrip
- Clips
- Pressing cream, wax, or oil
- Styling pomade
- Comb
- Brush
- Blow-dryer with attachments
- Pressing comb
- Electric heater (stove)

PREPARATION

1. Wash your hands.

2. Conduct the client consultation and hair analysis.

3. Drape client and perform shampoo service. Towel blot the hair.

4. Drape client with chair cloth and neck strip. Heat the pressing comb.

PROCEDURE

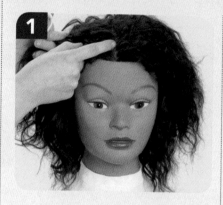

1 Blow-dry the hair. Apply pressing cream, wax, or oil.

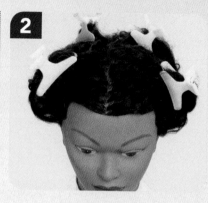

2 Comb and part off the hair into four sections.

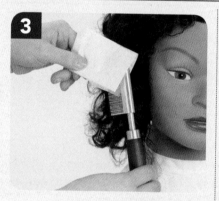

3 Divide the first section into 1" subsections. Apply additional pressing cream, wax, or oil to the subsection as needed. Test the heated pressing comb.

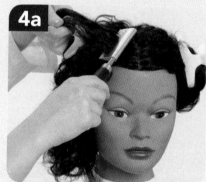

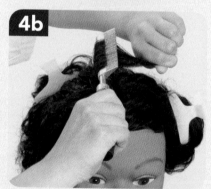

4 Hold the first subsection away from the scalp and insert the teeth of the comb into the top side of the hair section. Draw out the comb slightly, making a quick turn so that the back of the comb does the actual pressing.

5
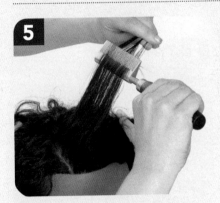

5 Press the comb slowly through the hair until the ends pass through the teeth of the comb.

6
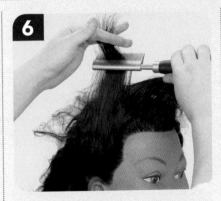

6 Reposition each completed section over to the opposite side of the head.

7 Continue this procedure until all the hair is pressed. Add pomade if desired.

8 Style and comb the hair or finish with thermal irons according to client's wishes.

8
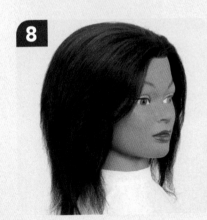

CLEAN-UP AND DISINFECTION

1. Clean and disinfect tools and implements.

2. Sanitize chair and workstation.

3. Dispose of towels and paper goods.

4. Wash your hands.

SUPPLIES

- Towels
- Shampoo cape
- Shampoo
- Styling cape
- Neckstrip
- Clips
- Leave-in thermal styling spray
- Finishing spray
- Tail comb
- Styling comb
- Brush
- Blow-dryer with attachments
- Electric flat iron

PREPARATION

1. Wash your hands.

2. Conduct the client consultation and hair analysis.

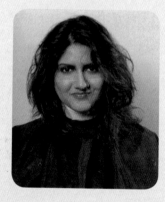

3. Drape client and perform shampoo service.

4. Towel-blot hair and apply leave-in thermal styling spray.

5. Drape client with styling cape and neck strip. Heat the flat iron.

PROCEDURE

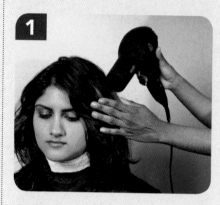

1 Blow-dry and style hair according to the cut.

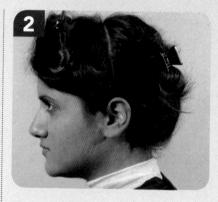

2 Comb and part off the hair into four sections.

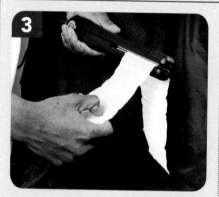

3 Divide the first section into subsections based on the density of the hair. Test the heated flat iron.

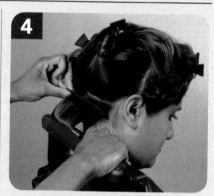

4 Hold the first subsection away from the scalp and grasp the section between the plates of the flat iron; insert the comb under the top side of the hair section to protect the scalp. Draw the iron smoothly through the subsection, re-comb, and reapply the flat iron as necessary to sufficiently straighten the hair.

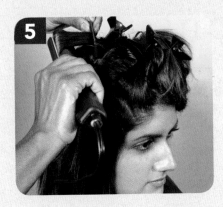

5 Repeat this process through each section until all the hair has been flat ironed. To increase lift in the top or crest sections, comb and elevate the subsection before ironing.

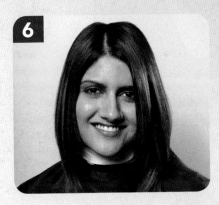

6 Comb and style the hair. Finish with styling spray or other preferred product.

CLEAN-UP AND DISINFECTION

1. Clean and disinfect tools and implements.

2. Sanitize chair and workstation.

3. Dispose of towels and paper goods.

4. Wash your hands.

✓ LO5 Complete

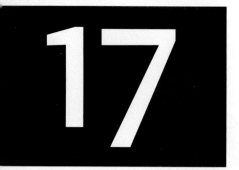

Review
Questions

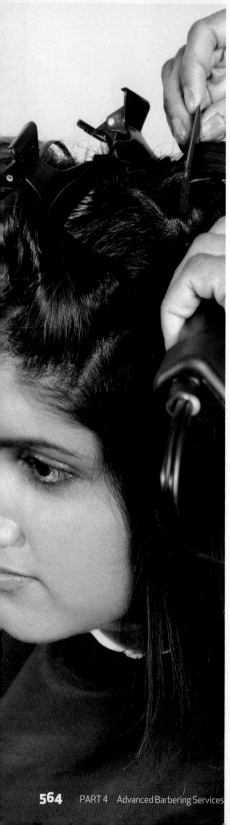

1. List the four basic cuts and the elevations or projections used to achieve them.

2. Explain over-direction.

3. List the methods used in wet hairstyling.

4. Define *on-base*, *half off-base*, and *off-base* curl placement. Explain the effects of each.

5. What is thermal hairstyling?

6. List the tools used in thermal hairstyling.

Chapter
Glossary

base the area near the scalp at which a roller or iron barrel is placed

blow-dry styling technique of drying and styling damp hair in one operation

blunt cut haircut in which all the hair comes to one hanging level at 0 elevation to form a weight line

circle also known as the curl; part of a curl that forms a complete circle

curl the hair that is wrapped around the barrel of an iron or a roller

graduated cut graduated, wedge, or stacked shape at the perimeter of a haircut; usually cut at 45 degrees

hair molding styling method that uses the head form as tool to set the hair in a straight position

hair pressing method of temporarily straightening curly or unruly hair by means of a heated pressing comb

hair wrapping method whereby the hair is wrapped around the head for drying and styling purposes

half off-base position of a curl one-half off its base; provides medium volume and movement

long layered cut hair is cut 180-degree elevation to create short layers at the top and increasingly longer layers at the perimeter

off-base position of a curl off its base; provides maximum mobility and minimum volume

on-base position of a curl directly on its base; provides maximum volume

stem the section of a curl between the base and the first arc of the circle; gives the curl direction and movement

thermal styling methods of curling or straightening on dry hair using thermal irons and pressing combs

uniform layered cut haircut in which all the hair is cut at the same length with a 90-degree elevation

18 Chemical Texture Services

☑ Learning Objectives

AFTER COMPLETING THIS CHAPTER, YOU SHOULD BE ABLE TO:

1 Explain the effects of chemical texture services on the hair.

2 Identify the similarities and differences between chemical texture services.

3 Discuss hair and scalp analysis for chemical texture services.

4 Perform a permanent wave service.

5 Perform a reformation curl service.

6 Perform a hair-relaxing service.

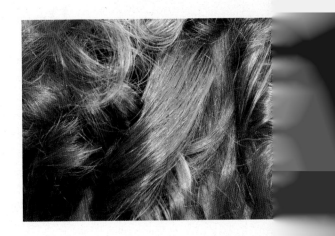

Key Terms

PAGE NUMBER INDICATES WHERE IN THE CHAPTER THE TERM IS USED.

acid-balanced waves / 584

alkaline or cold waves / 584

ammonium thioglycolate
 (ATG) / 584

base control / 582

base cream / 599

base direction / 582

base relaxers / 603

base sections / 581

basic perm wrap / 591

bookend wrap / 578

chemical blow-out / 604

chemical hair relaxing / 568

chemical texture services / 568

croquignole rodding / 583

end wraps / 578

endothermic waves / 584

exothermic waves / 585

glyceryl monothioglycolate
 (GMTG) / 584

hydroxide relaxers / 572

lanthionization / 572

lotion wrap / 583

neutralization / 589

no-base relaxers / 603

permanent waving / 568

pre-wrap solution / 586

reformation curl / 568

texturize / 604

thio relaxers / 571

true acid waves / 584

Chemical texture services such as permanent waving, reformation curls, and relaxers create chemical changes that permanently alter the natural wave pattern of the existing hair growth. These chemical services are used to curl straight hair, resize the curl in curly hair types, or straighten overly curly hair, respectively. When new hair growth occurs, retouch applications are required to maintain the altered texture and structure of the hair. Chemical texture services are practical, versatile, and lucrative services that provide clients with alternatives in haircut designs and styling.

Chemical Texture Services Defined

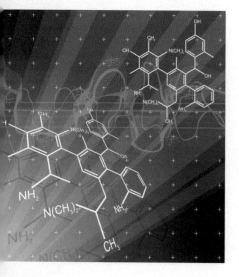

Permanent waving is a process used to chemically restructure natural hair into a different wave pattern. Most permanent waving services are performed with the objective of creating waves or curls in straighter hair types. Permanent waving requires the use of rods, end wraps, waving lotion, and a neutralizer. When performed properly, perms can increase the fullness of fine, soft hair, redirect resistant growth patterns until new growth occurs, and provide greater styling control.

A **reformation curl**, also known as a soft-curl perm, Jheri curl, or simply a curl, is a process used to restructure very curly hair into a larger curl pattern. Reformation curls require a relaxing product to partially straighten the hair, rods, end wraps, waving lotion, and a neutralizer. This makes the procedure part chemical hair-relaxer service and part permanent waving service. The reformation curl procedure offers clients with tight curl textures an additional option to the natural look or total straightening with chemical relaxing products.

Chemical hair relaxing is the process used to rearrange the basic structure of overly curly hair into a straighter hair form. The relaxing process involves the use of a relaxing cream, neutralizer or neutralizing shampoo, and conditioning product. A properly performed chemical hair-relaxing service should leave the hair in a soft, straightened form that adapts well to wet setting, wrapping, or thermal styling techniques.

Chemical services require maintenance and periodic reapplications as new growth appears. The barber who develops the ability to perform chemical texture services has yet another skill by which to establish a loyal following of satisfied clients, repeat customers, and new referrals.

The Nature of Chemical Texture Services

CHEMISTRY

Chemical texture services create permanent changes in the structure and appearance of the hair. As you learned in Chapter 11, hair is composed of three layers: cuticle, cortex, and medulla. Because the medulla is considered

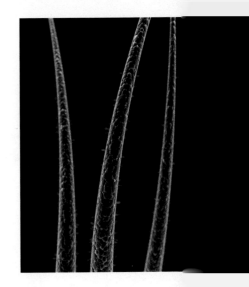

to be empty space and may be present only in medium to coarse hair types, the cuticle and cortex are the two layers most affected by chemical texture services.

The cuticle is the tough, outermost layer that protects the hair from damage. The degree to which hair is resistant to chemical changes depends on the strength of the cuticle. The alkaline solutions and substances used in chemical texture services soften and swell the cuticle, allowing for penetration into the cortex.

The cortex gives the hair its strength, flexibility, elasticity, and shape. These characteristics are derived from the millions of polypeptide chains found in the keratin that makes up the cortex of the hair. As you also learned in Chapter 11, amino acids form proteins; and, chemical reactions among proteins produce peptide linkages. The amino acids are joined end-to-end by these peptide bonds and create parallel peptide chains. The parallel chains are then held together by sulfur, hydrogen, and salt side-bonds to form a ladder-like structure. As the polypeptide chains twist together, they eventually form a fiber that becomes the cells of the cortex. As a result, the polypeptide chains in keratin are both physically and chemically bound together.

Hair develops and maintains its natural form by means of the physical and chemical cross-bonds in the cortical layer. The physical bonds are the weaker of the two types and are easily broken by the processes of shampooing and rinsing. Chemical bonds are broken or rearranged through chemical applications such as permanent waving, reformation curls, and chemical hair relaxers.

Alkaline substances used in chemical texture services create a chemical action that breaks the chemical bonds and allows for the softening and expansion of the hair. During this process, cystine (formed by disulfide or sulfur bonds) is altered slightly to become cysteine. Cysteine is an amino acid obtained by the reduction of cystine. This chemical action is important because it facilitates the chemical rearrangement of the inner structure of the hair as it assumes a new shape and form. After the hair has assumed the desired shape, it must be neutralized so that the hydrogen and sulfur cross-bonds in the cortical layer are permanently reformed. Cysteine is changed back to the cystine state during the process of oxidation and neutralization, which hardens the S bonds of the hair into the newly constructed form. Facilitated by both physical and chemical action, bonds within the cortex are rearranged and restructured when chemical texture services are performed.

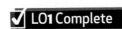
✓ LO1 Complete

PRINCIPAL ACTIONS OF CHEMICAL TEXTURE SERVICES

Chemical texture services involve two principal actions on the hair: physical and chemical. These actions are compared in **Table 18-1**.

> **TABLE 18-1** Physical and Chemical Actions of Chemical Texture Services

ACTION	PERMANENT WAVING	REFORMATION CURL	HAIR RELAXING
Physical	Shampooing and wrapping hair around rods	Smoothing or combing rearranger through the hair; wrapping hair around rods	Smoothing or combing the relaxing product; shampooing and rinsing
Chemical	Waving lotion: softens and breaks the internal hair structure	Rearranger: softens and breaks the internal hair structure	Relaxer: softens and breaks the internal hair structure
		Waving lotion (booster): softens and breaks the internal hair structure	
	Neutralizer: rehardens and rebonds the internal structure of the hair	Neutralizer: rehardens and rebonds the internal structure of the hair	Neutralizer or neutralizing shampoo: rehardens and rebonds the internal structure of the hair
			Thio relaxers may require an oxidizing neutralizer

The permanent wave process requires the *physical* actions of shampooing, rinsing, and wrapping the hair around rods. The *chemical* actions take place when a waving lotion and neutralizer produce permanent physical and chemical changes in the hair.

In permanent waving, the waving lotion (reducing agent) softens and swells the cuticle layer of the hair to allow penetration into the cortex, where the solution will break the disulfide bonds by a chemical process known as *reduction*. After processing and rinsing, the neutralizer neutralizes any remaining

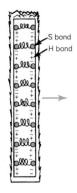

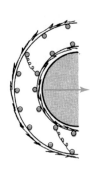

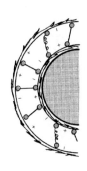

1. Straight Hair
   (Both H and S bonds
   in straight positions.)

2. Hair Wound on
   Rods and Softened
   by Shampooing and
   Cold Wave Solutions.
   (H bonds and nearly all
   S bonds broken.)

3. Hair After
   Neutralizing.
   (Some H Bonds and
   many S bonds
   reformed.)

S bond
H bond

◀ **FIGURE 18-1a**

Changes in hair cortex during permanent waving.

waving lotion in the hair and rebonds the newly arranged disulfide bonds through a process called *oxidation* (**Figures 18-1a** to **18-1c**).

The reformation curl process requires the *physical* actions of combing or smoothing a chemical rearranger through the hair for partial relaxation of the natural curl, rinsing, and wrapping the hair on rods. The *chemical* actions used to produce permanent changes in the hair are facilitated by the rearranger, waving lotion (booster), and neutralizer.

In the reformation curl process, the rearranger relaxes the natural curl by softening and swelling the cuticle, allowing for penetration into the cortex. The difference between the rearranger and the waving lotion (booster) is one of consistency. Both have the same active ingredient, ammonium thioglycolate, but the waving lotion is in lotion form and the rearranger is in a cream form. Because the rearranger will be combed through the hair, it needs to be thicker for better adhesion and control. Once the natural curl is partially relaxed and thoroughly rinsed, the waving lotion is used with rods to form a new-sized curl. The neutralization process is the same as with permanent waving.

The hair-relaxing process can be achieved with *thio relaxers* or *hydroxide relaxers*. Both product types require the *physical* actions of combing or smoothing the relaxing product through the hair, shampooing, rinsing, and conditioning. The primary *chemical* action that occurs in hair relaxing is the result of the relaxer product used to straighten the hair. Thio relaxing products, however, also require the use of a neutralizer to chemically oxidize the hair. Hydroxide relaxing products are neutralized through the physical actions of the shampooing and rinsing process because the disulfide bonds that have been broken by this type of relaxer cannot be reformed through oxidation.

When using an ammonium thioglycolate (thio) relaxer to straighten the hair, the reducing agent is of higher strength than that used in permanent waving. Most **thio relaxers** have a pH above 10 and are manufactured in cream form for better adhesion and control. The relaxer cream softens and swells the hair and breaks apart the disulfide bonds. This action permits the removal of curl from the hair as the bonds are rearranged into a straighter position through the physical

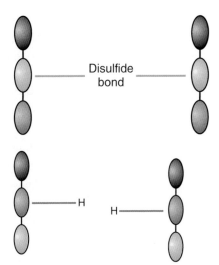

Disulfide
bond

H   H

▲ **FIGURE 18-1b**

Reduction reaction breaks disulfide bonds.

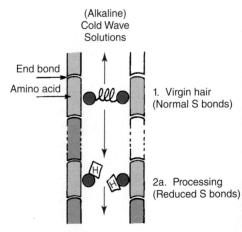

(Alkaline)
Cold Wave
Solutions

End bond
Amino acid

1. Virgin hair
   (Normal S bonds)

2a. Processing
    (Reduced S bonds)

▲ **FIGURE 18-1c**

Oxidation reaction of thio neutralizer.

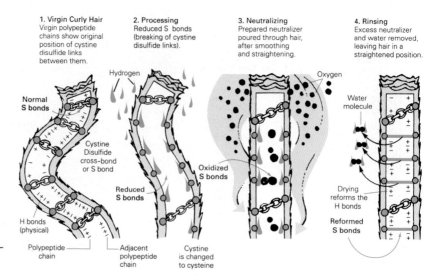

1. Virgin Curly Hair
Virgin polypeptide chains show original position of cystine disulfide links between them.

2. Processing
Reduced S bonds (breaking of cystine disulfide links).

3. Neutralizing
Prepared neutralizer poured through hair, after smoothing and straightening.

4. Rinsing
Excess neutralizer and water removed, leaving hair in a straightened position.

Normal S bonds

Hydrogen

Oxygen

Water molecule

Cystine Disulfide cross-bond or S bond

Reduced S bonds

Oxidized S bonds

Drying reforms the H bonds

Reformed S bonds

H bonds (physical)

Polypeptide chain

Adjacent polypeptide chain

Cystine is changed to cysteine

▶ **FIGURE 18-2**

Chemical hair straightening— ammonium thioglycolate.

actions of combing and smoothing the hair. The hair is then rinsed and neutralized with an oxidizing agent such as hydrogen peroxide that rebuilds the disulfide bonds broken by the relaxer **(Figure 18-2)**.

Hydroxide relaxers are strong alkalis that can swell the hair up to twice its normal diameter. Hydroxide relaxers are not compatible with thio relaxers because they use a different chemistry and can have a pH as high as 13.5. At these high concentrations, the hydroxide product permanently breaks the disulfide bonds to the point where they can never be reformed. This process is known as **lanthionization** (lan-thee-oh-ny-ZAY-shun) and occurs as the disulfide bonds are converted to lanthionine bonds when the relaxer is rinsed and the hair is still at a high pH level **(Figure 18-3)**.

1. Curly Hair
Both H and S bonds holding polypeptide chains in position.

2. Hair Being Processed
All H bonds broken, most S bonds broken. Hand and comb manipulations starting to relax wave. (Polypeptide chains shift.)

3. Neutralizing shampoo
fixes polypeptide chains in a straight position after hair has been fully relaxed.

4. Straightened Hair...
after rinsing and proper drying. Lanthionine cross-links now exist between polypeptide chains, keeping the hair in a permanently straight form. Drying reforms the physical bonds.

Neutralizer

Processing cream

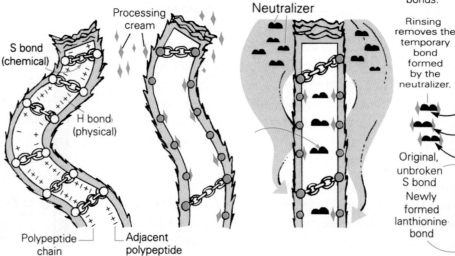

S bond (chemical)

H bond (physical)

Rinsing removes the temporary bond formed by the neutralizer.

Original, unbroken S bond

Newly formed lanthionine bond

▶ **FIGURE 18-3**

Chemical hair straightening—sodium hydroxide.

Polypeptide chain

Adjacent polypeptide chain

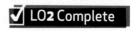

The Client Consultation

Before proceeding with any chemical service, the barber must determine the client's expectations and the degree to which those expectations can be met based on the hair type and condition. Each client has a different concept of how the chemical texture service should look. Open communication between the barber and the client helps to assure a successful chemical texture service outcome. This can be accomplished by asking open-ended questions to determine the client's desires and past experience with texture services. The barber can also use visual tools such as pictures, magazines, and stylebooks to ascertain the client's likes and dislikes. The following topics may be discussed during the client consultation.

1. *The desired hairstyle and amount of curl or straightening:* Photos or magazine pictures help to make these specifications clear to both the client and the barber.

2. *The client's lifestyle:* Does he or she have leisure time or a demanding schedule that requires a low-maintenance style?

3. *How the hairstyle relates to overall personal image:* Is the client concerned about current fashion trends?

4. *Previous experience:* Was the last chemical texture service satisfactory? If not, what were the problems?

The consultation with the client takes only a few minutes, but it is time well spent. It helps to establish your credibility as a professional, inspires the client's confidence, and makes the entire chemical texture service experience more satisfactory for both the client and barber.

Keep the information learned during the consultation in the form of a written record that includes the client's address and home and business contact information. See **Figure 18-4** for an example of an organized client record card.

In addition to determining the client's texture service desires, the barber also needs to have a clear understanding of what the finished haircut and style will look like. This information is key to a successful texture service because the desired finished look will help to determine the degree of texture or relaxation that is needed.

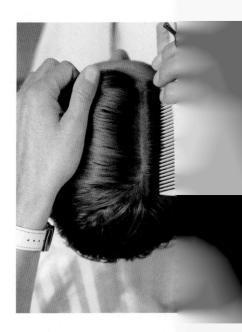

SCALP AND HAIR ANALYSIS

Before proceeding with any chemical texture service it is very important to correctly and carefully analyze the client's scalp and hair condition. The analysis should be used to determine whether the scalp and hair should receive a chemical texture service and the types of products to be used in the process.

The scalp should be examined for cuts, abrasions, or open sores. Any of these conditions can make a chemical process uncomfortable and even dangerous to a client's physical well being. Do not proceed with the service if

PERMANENT WAVE RECORD

Name .... Tel ....

Address ....

City .... State .... Zip ....

DESCRIPTION OF HAIR

Length	Texture	Type	Porosity	
□ short	□ coarse	□ normal	□ very	□ slightly
□ medium	□ medium	□ resistant	porous	porous
□ long	□ fine	□ tinted	□ moderately	□ resistant
		□ highlighted	porous	
		□ bleached	□ normal	

CONDITION

□ very good   □ good   □ fair   □ poor   □ dry   □ oily

Tinted with ....

Previouslt permed with ....

TYPE OF PERM

□ alkaline   □ acid   □ body wave   □ other ....

No. of rods .... Lotion .... Strength ....

RESULTS

□ good   □ poor   □ too tight   □ too loose

Date	Perm Used	Stylist	Date	Perm Used	Stylist
....	....	....	....	....	....
....	....	....	....	....	....
....	....	....	....	....	....
....	....	....	....	....	....
....	....	....	....	....	....

▲ FIGURE 18-4

Client record card.

abrasions or signs of scalp disease are present. Refer the client to a physician as necessary.

The hair analysis includes the hair's porosity, texture, elasticity, density, length, and direction of hair growth.

Hair Porosity

The processing time for chemical services depends more on hair porosity than on any other factor. Generally, the more porous the hair, the less time processing will take. The porosity level of the hair determines the speed with which moisture will be absorbed into the hair and is directly related to the condition of the cuticle layer. Hair porosity is classified as resistant, normal, or porous. In the case of chemical texture services, these classifications help to determine the most appropriate strength of chemical product to use on different hair types. Do not proceed with the service if the hair shows signs of breakage or over-porosity.

- *Resistant* hair has a tight, compact cuticle layer that resists penetration of chemical solutions. This hair type requires a more alkaline solution to raise the cuticle and permit uniform saturation and processing.

- *Normal* porosity means that the hair is neither resistant nor overly porous. Chemical texture services performed on this hair type will usually process as expected.

- *Porous* hair has a raised cuticle layer that easily absorbs solutions. This hair type requires a less alkaline solution that will minimize swelling and help to prevent excessive damage to the hair.

To accurately test the porosity level, use three different areas: at the front hairline, in front of the ears, and near the crown. Grasp some strands of dry hair. Hold the ends firmly with the thumb and index finger of one hand, and slide the fingers of the other hand from the ends toward the scalp. If the fingers do not slide easily, or if the hair ruffles up as your fingers slide down the strands, the hair is porous. The more ruffles that form, the more porous the hair; the fewer ruffles that form, the less porous it is. If the fingers slide easily and no ruffles are formed, the cuticle layers lie close to the hair shafts. This type of hair is the least porous and most resistant and may require a longer processing time (**Figure 18-5**).

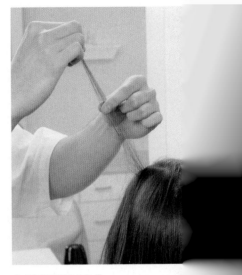

▲ **FIGURE 18-5**
Porosity test.

Hair Texture

Hair texture describes the diameter of a single strand of hair as being coarse, medium, or fine. While hair porosity is important in determining the processing time, hair texture also plays a part in the decision. For example, coarse, porous hair will usually process faster than fine, resistant hair. If the fine, resistant hair is of a wavy texture and the coarse, porous hair is very straight, however, the fine hair will probably process faster because there is already a wave formation in the hair, which usually denotes greater elasticity of the hair. Hair texture should also be considered in deciding the size of the wave pattern and when planning a hairstyle.

- *Coarse* hair usually requires more processing than medium or fine hair and may also be more resistant to chemical processes.

- *Medium* hair is the most common hair texture. It is considered normal and does not usually pose any special processing problems.

- *Fine* hair is typically more fragile, easier to process, and more susceptible to damage from chemical services. Generally, fine hair will process faster and more easily than medium or coarse hair types.

Hair Elasticity

Hair elasticity is an important factor to consider when performing chemical texture services because it is an indication of the strength of the cross-bonds in the hair. The greater the degree of elasticity, the longer the wave will remain in the hair because less relaxation of the hair occurs; thus the elasticity of the hair determines its ability to hold a curl. Hair elasticity is classified as normal or low.

- *Normal* elasticity is indicated by wet hair that can stretch up to 50 percent of its original length and then return to that length without

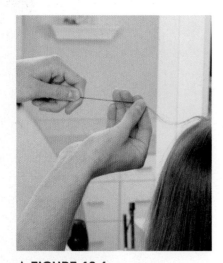

▲ FIGURE 18-6
Elasticity test.

breaking. Hair with normal elasticity usually holds the curl from wet sets and permanent waves.

- *Low* elasticity is indicated by wet hair that does not return to its original length when stretched and may not be able to hold curl patterns.

As a test of elasticity, take a few strands of damp hair and hold them between the thumb and forefinger of each hand. Slowly stretch the strands between your fingers (**Figure 18-6**). The more they can be stretched without breaking, the more elasticity the hair has. If the elasticity is good, the hair slowly contracts after stretching. Hair with poor elasticity will break quickly and easily when stretched.

Signs of poor elasticity include limpness, sponginess, and hair that tangles easily. Generally speaking, such hair will not develop a firm, strong wave. However, there are special waving solutions available that, if used in combination with smaller-diameter rods, may result in a satisfactory permanent wave or reformation curl process.

Hair Density

Hair density measures the number of hairs per square inch and indicates how thick or thin the hair is. Hair density is important to consider when performing chemical texture services because it helps to determine the number of blockings or subsections that will best facilitate the service. For example, in permanent waving, smaller blocks (subsections) and larger rods may be required for thickly growing hair. If the hair density is thin, however, smaller diameter rods are required to form a good wave pattern close to the head. Avoid large blockings on thin hair growth as the strain may cause breakage. Hair density can also indicate the amount of product that will be needed.

Hair Length

Hair length is another factor to consider when performing chemical texture services. In permanent waving and reformation curl processes, hair length may determine the rodding technique to use. For example, waving hair of average length presents no real problem. If the client's hair length is 6" or more, however, the hair may not rod closely enough to the scalp to develop a good, strong wave pattern in that area. In addition, the weight of the hair may relax or stretch the curl to the extent that the majority of the wave pattern remains mid-shaft and on the hair ends with very little lift in the scalp area.

Like hair density, the length of the hair will also help to determine the amount of product that will be needed for the texture process.

Hair Growth Pattern

The growth direction of the hair causes hair streams, whorls, and cowlicks, which influence the finished hairstyle. These characteristics must be considered when selecting the wrapping pattern and rod placement for permanent waves or reformation curls and the direction of combing and smoothing when using chemical hair relaxers.

Now that the basics that apply to chemical texture services have been explored, it is time to focus on the products, methods, and procedures associated with each individual service.

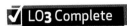

Permanent Waving

Permanent waving is a process that involves two principal actions on the hair: the physical action of wrapping the hair on perm rods and the chemical changes caused by the waving solution and neutralizer. Permanent waves are performed on hair that has been freshly shampooed and in a damp condition. A spray water bottle should be employed to maintain even moisture content throughout the hair while rodding the perm.

THE PERM WRAP

In permanent waving, the size, shape, and type of curl are determined by the type, size, and shape of the tools and the method used to wrap the hair. The tools are called *rods* and the size of the rod determines the size of the curl (**Figure 18-7**).

The proper selection of perm rods is essential for successful permanent waving. The most commonly used rods, concave and straight (**Figures 18-8** and **18-9**), are made of plastic and vary in diameter and length. The diameter of the rod controls the size of the curl. These diameters usually vary from $\frac{1}{8}$" to $\frac{3}{4}$" (**Figure 18-10**). Rods are also available in short, medium, and long lengths that typically measure from $1\frac{3}{4}$" to $3\frac{1}{2}$". An elastic band is used to secure the hair and the rod into the desired position to prevent the curl from unwinding.

Concave rods are the most commonly used perm rod. Concave rods have a smaller diameter in the center, which gradually increases to a larger diameter at both ends. This produces a tighter curl in the center and a larger curl on the sides of the hair parting (Figure 18-8). Concave rods are used when a definite wave pattern, close to the head, is desired.

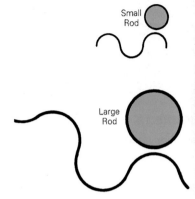

▲ **FIGURE 18-7**

The size of the rod determines the size of the curl.

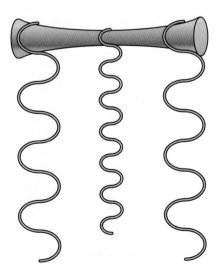

▲ **FIGURE 18-8**

Concave rod and resulting curl.

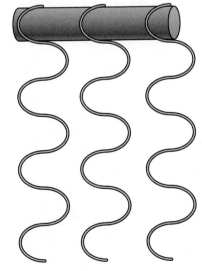

▲ **FIGURE 18-9**

Straight rod and resulting curl.

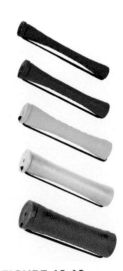

▲ **FIGURE 18-10**

Rod sizes, top to bottom: extra small, small, medium, large, extra large.

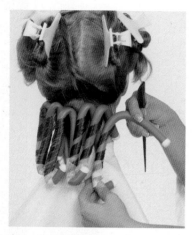

▲ FIGURE 18-11
Spiral wrapping with soft bender rods.

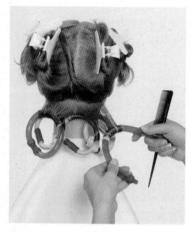

▲ FIGURE 18-12
Circle tools.

Straight rods have a uniform circumference and diameter along the rod's length. This type of rod creates a consistently sized wave from one side of the hair parting to the other (Figure 18-9). Large, straight rods are usually used for a body wave that serves as a foundation for further styling.

Other perm tools include *bender rods* and *circle tools*. Bender rods are made of stiff wires covered by soft foam that permits bending into a variety of shapes. These rods measure about 12" long and have a uniform diameter (**Figure 18-11**).

The circle tool or loop rod is a plastic-coated tool that also measures about 12" with a uniform diameter along the length of the rod. These rods are secured by fastening the ends together to form a circle (**Figure 18-12**)

End papers or **end wraps** are absorbent papers used to control the ends of the hair when wrapping and winding the hair on perm rods. End papers should extend beyond the ends of the hair to keep them smooth and straight, and to prevent "fishhooks." A fishhook is a flaw in the wrapping of the hair parting that results in the tip of the hair bending in a direction opposite to that of the rest of the curl. End papers are especially effective in helping to smooth out the wrapping of uneven hair lengths.

The most common end paper–wrapping techniques are the bookend wrap, the single flat wrap, and the double flat wrap.

- The **bookend wrap** uses one paper folded in half over the hair ends and eliminates excess paper (**Figure 18-13**). It can be used with short rods or short lengths of hair. Be careful to distribute the hair evenly over the entire length of the rod and avoid bunching the ends together toward the center of the rod. See **Figures 18-16** through **18-22** for the step-by-step procedure for a bookend wrap.

- The *single flat* or *single end wrap* uses one paper placed over the top of the hair parting being wrapped (**Figure 18-14**). See **Figures 18-23** through **18-25** for the step-by-step procedure for a single flat wrap.

- The *double flat* or *double end wrap* uses two end papers, one placed under and one over the parting of hair being wrapped. Both papers should extend beyond the hair ends (**Figure 18-15**). See **Figures 18-26** through **18-28** for the step-by-step procedure for the double flat wrap.

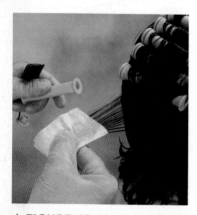

▲ FIGURE 18-13
Bookend wrap rodding a reformation curl.

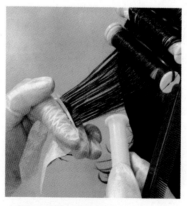

▲ FIGURE 18-14
Single flat wrap rodding a reformation curl.

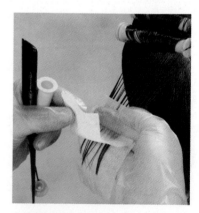

▲ FIGURE 18-15
Double end wrap rodding a reformation curl.

Bookend Wrap

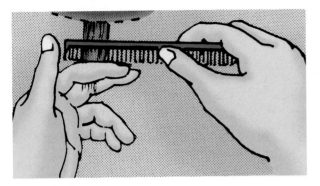

▲ **FIGURE 18-16**

Part and comb subsection up and out until all the hair is evenly directed and distributed.

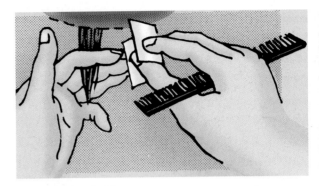

▲ **FIGURE 18-17**

Hold subsection between the index and middle fingers. Fold and place the end paper over the subsection, forming an envelope.

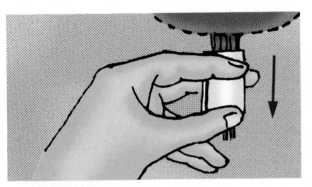

▲ **FIGURE 18-18**

Hold the subsection smoothly and evenly. Slide the paper envelope a small fraction beyond the hair ends.

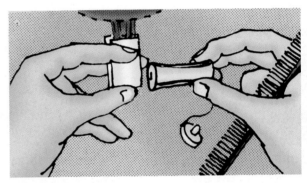

▲ **FIGURE 18-19**

With the right hand, pick up the rod.

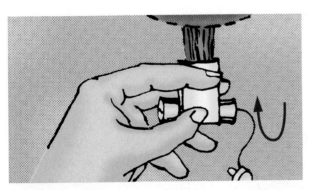

▲ **FIGURE 18-20**

Place the rod under the folded end paper, parallel to the parting. Draw end paper and rod toward hair ends until they are visible above the rod, and start winding end paper and hair under, toward the scalp.

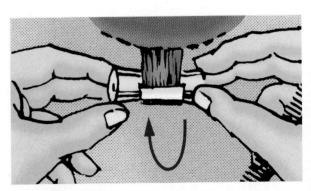

▲ **FIGURE 18-21**

Wind the hair smoothly, without tension, on the rod.

Bookend Wrap (continued)

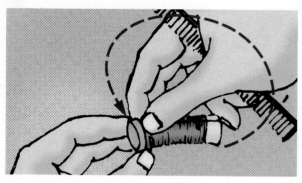

▲ FIGURE 18-22

Fasten the rod band evenly across the wound hair at the top of the rod.

Single Flat Wrap

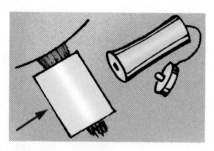

▲ FIGURE 18-23

Place the end paper on top of subsection and hold it flat to prevent bunching.

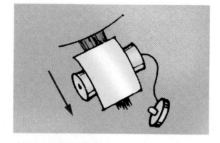

▲ FIGURE 18-24

Place rod under the subsection, holding it parallel with the parting; then draw the end paper and rod downward until hair ends are covered.

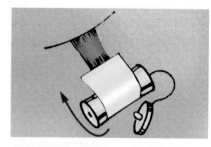

▲ FIGURE 18-25

Roll the end paper and subsection under, using the thumb of each hand to keep the strands smooth. Wind subsection on the rod to the scalp without tension. Fasten band across top of rod in the same manner as for bookend paper wrap.

Double Flat Wrap

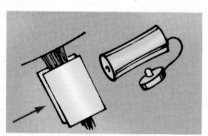

▲ FIGURE 18-26

Place one end paper beneath the hair subsection and the other on top.

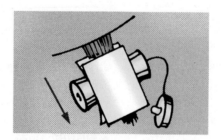

▲ FIGURE 18-27

Place rod under double end papers, parallel with the parting. Draw both papers toward hair ends.

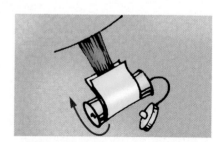

▲ FIGURE 18-28

Wind the subsection smoothly on the rod to the scalp without tension. Then fasten the band across the top of rod as for bookend paper wrap.

The preparation of the hair to receive the end wrap is the same for bookend, single, and double wrapping techniques (Refer to Figure 18-16).

Sectioning

Perm wraps begin with sectioning the hair into panels. The size, shape, and direction of these panels will vary depending on the wrapping pattern and the type of tool being used. Each panel is further divided into subsections called **base sections.** The base sections are actually partings taken from the subsection that measure *almost* the same length and width as the rod or perming tool (**Figures 18-29** and **18-30**).

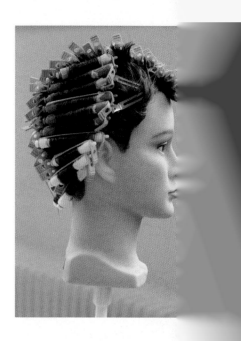

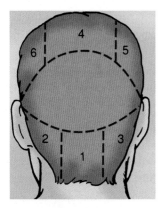

▲ FIGURE 18-29
Sectioning.

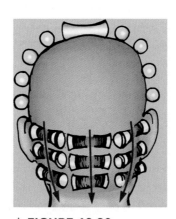

▲ FIGURE 18-30
Blocking (subsections).

The number of base sections and the rod sizes will vary with each client depending on the sectioning pattern used and the texture, density, and elasticity of the hair (**Table 18-2**). The average base section, or parting, should be slightly shorter than the length of the rod. If the rod is shorter than the length of the blocking, the hair will slip off the ends of the rod during winding and result in an uneven curl formation.

▶ TABLE **18-2** Suggested Base Sections and Rod Sizes

TEXTURE	DENSITY	ELASTICITY	BASE SECTION	DIAMETER OF ROD
Coarse	Thick	Good	Narrow	Large
Medium	Average	Normal	Smaller	Medium
Fine	Thin	Poor	Smaller	Small
Damaged	Average	Very Poor	Smaller	Large

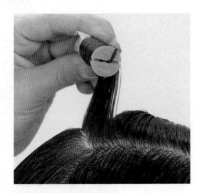

▲ **FIGURE 18-31**
On-base placement.

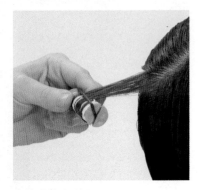

▲ **FIGURE 18-32**
Half off-base placement.

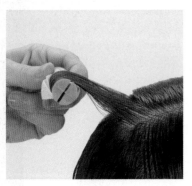

▲ **FIGURE 18-33**
Off-base placement.

The texture, elasticity, porosity, and condition of the client's hair all help to determine how the hair should be sectioned and subsectioned, which rods to use, and where the application of waving solution should begin. Be guided by your instructor.

Base Control

Base control refers to the position of the perm rod or tool in relation to its base section and is determined by the angle at which the hair is wrapped. Rods can be wound *on-base, half off-base (half-base),* or *off-base.*

In on-base placement, the hair is projected about 45 degrees beyond per-pendicular (90 degrees) to its base section and the rod is placed on the base section (**Figure 18-31**). On-base placement results in greater volume at the scalp area.

Half off-base placement results from wrapping the hair at an angle of 90 de-grees to its base section (**Figure 18-32**). At this elevation of the hair, the rod is positioned half off its base section.

Off-base placement is achieved by wrapping the hair at a 45-degree angle be-low perpendicular to its base section (**Figure 18-33**). The rod is positioned com-pletely off its base section and creates the least amount of volume in the style.

Base Direction

Base direction refers to the directional pattern in which the hair is wrapped. Although wrapping with the natural direction of hair growth causes the least amount of stress on the hair, wrapping forward, backward, or to the side can create special effects in the final hairstyle.

Base direction also refers to the horizontal, vertical, or diagonal partings and positioning of the rod on the head, as pictured in **Figure 18-34**.

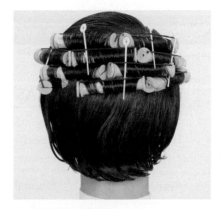

▲ **FIGURE 18-34**
Horizontal base direction.

RODDING TECHNIQUES

The two basic methods used to wrap the hair around the perm rod are the croquignole and spiral rodding techniques.

When using the **croquignole rodding** technique, the hair is wound from the ends to the scalp. This overlapping of the hair layers with each revolution of the rod increases the size of the curl as it nears the scalp area, with a tighter curl at the ends (**Figure 18-35**).

Spiral rodding can be accomplished in two ways: from the ends to the scalp, or from the scalp to the ends. In both cases, the rod or perming tool is positioned vertically as the hair parting is "rocked" or spiraled along the length of the rod. Straight rods are usually used for a spiral wrap and tend to produce a more uniform curl when the hair is spiraled properly along the rod (**Figure 18-36**).

To form a uniform wave the hair must be wrapped smoothly and neatly on each rod, without stretching. The hair should not be stretched or wrapped too tightly because that could interfere with the penetration and expansion process of the waving solution and the contraction process of the neutralizer. Tight wrapping can also result in hair breakage due to the amount of tension put on the hair.

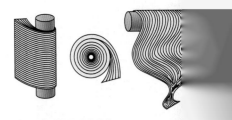

▲ **FIGURE 18-35**
Croquignole perm wrap.

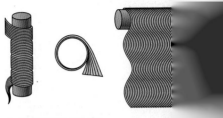

▲ **FIGURE 18-36**
Spiral perm wrap.

Wrapping Methods

There are two types of wrapping methods used in permanent waving: the water wrap and the lotion wrap. Some permanent wave solutions allow only a water wrap while others may be lotion wrapped. Always be guided by the manufacturer's directions.

- A *water wrap* is simply the action of rodding the hair in a water-damp condition. Most perms are wrapped in this manner.

- A **lotion wrap** is the application of permanent wave solution to a working panel or section of hair just prior to rodding for the purpose of pre-softening resistant hair. This technique is usually used with alkaline (cold) waves to facilitate easier rodding of resistant, straight hair types—it "jump starts" the processing action. Once the hair is rodded, the remaining solution is applied to the entire head.

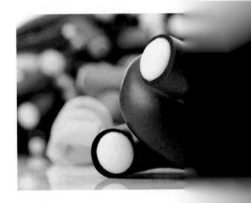

TYPES OF PERMANENT WAVES

Perm chemistry is constantly being refined and improved. Different formulas designed for a wide variety of hair types are available from today's manufacturers. Waving lotions and neutralizers for both acid-balanced and alkaline perms are available with new conditioners, proteins, and natural ingredients that help to protect and condition the hair during and after perming.

Stop-action processing is incorporated into many waving lotions to ensure optimum curl development. The curling takes place within a fixed time, without the risk of over-processing or damaging the hair. Special pre-wrapping lotions have also been developed to compensate for hair with varying degrees of porosity.

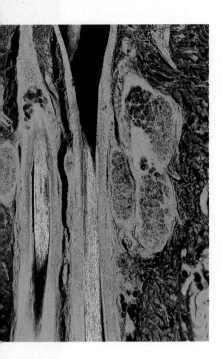

Alkaline Perms (Cold Waves)

The first **alkaline or cold waves** were developed in 1941. The main active ingredient or reducing agent in alkaline perms is **ammonium thioglycolate (ATG).** This chemical compound is made up of ammonia and thioglycolic acid. The pH of alkaline waving lotions generally falls within the range of 9.0 to 9.6, depending on the amount of ammonia. These high pH levels cause the hair shaft to swell and the cuticle layer to lift, allowing penetration into the cortex. Some alkaline perms are wrapped with waving lotion, others with water. Either type may require a plastic cap for processing. Always read the manufacturer's directions carefully before proceeding with the service.

The benefits associated with alkaline perms are strong curl patterns, fast processing time (5 to 20 minutes), and room temperature processing. Alkaline perms are generally used when perming resistant hair types, when a strong or tight curl is desired, or when the client has a history of early curl relaxation.

True Acid Waves

The first **true acid waves** were introduced in the early 1970s. These perms have a pH range between 4.5 and 7.0 and use **glyceryl monothioglycolate (GMTG)** as the primary reducing agent. This lower pH is gentler on the hair and typically produces a softer curl and less damage than alkaline cold waves. Most true acid waves require the addition of heat from a hair dryer to accelerate the processing and are considered to be *endothermic* perm products. **Endothermic waves** require the use of an outside heat source to activate chemical reactions and processing.

It should be noted that although a pH of 7.0 is neutral on the pH scale, a pH of 5.0 is neutral for hair. Since every step in the pH scale represents a tenfold change in pH, a pH of 7.0 is 100 times more alkaline than the pH of hair. Even pure water will cause the hair to swell and expand.

The benefits of true acid waves are softer curl patterns, slower but more controllable processing time (usually 15 to 25 minutes), and gentler treatment for delicate hair types. Generally, true acid perms should be used when perming delicate, fragile, or color-treated hair; when a soft, natural curl or wave pattern is desired; or when style support, rather than strong curl, is desired.

Acid-Balanced Waves

Most of today's acid waves have a pH between 7.8 and 8.2, which puts them into the category of **acid-balanced waves.** Acid-balanced waves process at room temperature and do not require the heat of a hair dryer for processing.

Although glyceryl monothioglycolate is the primary reducing agent in acid-balanced waves, these waving products usually contain some ammonium thioglycolate as well. All acid-balanced waves have three product components: permanent waving solution, activator, and neutralizer. The permanent waving solution usually contains ATG and the activator GMTG. These products must be added together immediately prior to use.

REMINDER

> Repeated exposure to GMTG has been known to cause allergic sensitivity in practitioners and clients. Watch clients closely for signs of allergy or irritation. If problems develop, suggest they see a dermatologist.

Acid-balanced waves process more quickly and produce firmer curls than true acid waves.

Exothermic Waves

Like acid-balanced perms, all **exothermic waves** have three components: permanent waving solution, activator, and neutralizer. The activator in an exothermic wave, however, contains an oxidizing agent (usually hydrogen peroxide) that causes a rapid release of heat when mixed with the waving solution. The chemical reaction that releases heat and causes the waving solution to become warm can usually be felt when holding the bottle of solution. This rise in temperature increases the rate of the chemical reaction, which in turn shortens the processing time.

Ammonia-Free Waves

Ammonia-free waves use alkanolamines (al-kan-all-AM-eenz) to replace ammonia and are gaining in popularity because of their low odor. Ammonia-free does not mean free of damage, so although these new products may not smell as strong as ammonia, they can still have a high alkaline pH. For example, an ammonia wave starts out at a pH of 9.6 and quickly drops to 8.2 during processing because ammonia evaporates quickly. This means the processing takes place at a lower pH. Alkanolamines evaporate slowly, which is why they do not give off odors, and maintain the same pH level throughout the entire processing time. This constant pH level can ultimately be more damaging to the hair than are waves containing ammonia.

Thio-Free Waves

Thio-free waves use cysteamine (SIS-tee-uh-meen) or mercaptamine (mer-KAPT-uh-meen) as the primary reducing agent. When used at high concentrations, these thio compounds with a pH range of 7.0 to 9.6 can be just as damaging as regular thio formulations.

Low-pH Waves

Sulfates, sulfites, and bisulfites offer an alternative to ATG but are weak and do not produce a firm curl. Sulfite perms are usually marketed as *body waves* and have a pH range of 6.5 to 7.0.

Strengths of Waving Solutions

Although the strength of a waving solution can be adjusted by increasing the amount of the active ingredient, today's wide range of waving products virtually eliminates the need to do so. Be cautioned that if the strength of a solution is adjusted through the addition of ammonia, the pH level should not exceed 9.6.

Most manufacturers market three or more strengths of permanent waving products:

- *Mild:* for damaged, porous, or tinted hair

- *Normal:* for normal hair with good porosity

- *Resistant:* for resistant hair with less porosity

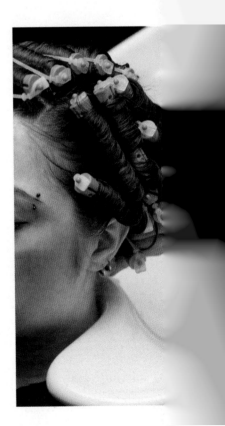

Pre-Wraps

Some permanent waving product packages contain a **pre-wrap solution** that is applied to the hair before rodding. In most cases, the pre-wrap is simply a leave-in conditioner that helps to equalize the porosity of the hair to ensure even penetration of the waving lotion and to protect the hair from unnecessary damage. Always follow the manufacturer's directions.

Perm Selection

For a successful permanent waving service, it is essential to select the proper waving product for the client's hair type and desired result. After a thorough client consultation, the barber should be able to determine which type of permanent waving product is best suited to the client's hair condition. Most resistant hair types require an alkaline wave; alkaline or acid-balanced perms can be used on most normal hair types; and acid-balanced or true acid perm formulas are the best choice for most tinted, highlighted, or delicate hair types. Use **Table 18-3** on next page as a general guide to the selection of the most common types of permanent waves.

PERMANENT WAVE PROCESSING AND WAVE FORMATION

The strength of any permanent wave is based on the concentration of its reducing agent. In turn, the amount of processing time is determined by the strength of the permanent waving solution and the porosity level of the hair. Most of the processing takes place within the first 5 to 10 minutes, so the amount of processing should be determined by the strength of the solution and not by how long the perm processes. If the hair is not sufficiently processed after 10 minutes, it may require reapplication of the solution. The next time the client receives a perm service, a stronger solution may be used. Conversely, if the client's hair has been over-processed, a weaker solution should have been used.

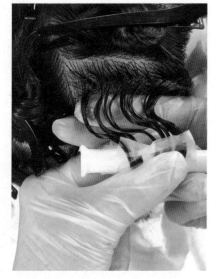

▲ **FIGURE 18-37**
S pattern.

As the hair is processing, the waves form a deep-ridged pattern. The wave has reached its peak when it forms a firm letter S shape (**Figure 18-37**). The S pattern reaches a desirable peak only once during the perm process. Shortly after the S is well formed, the hair may become frizzy unless processing is stopped. Frizziness indicates that the processing time has reached its absolute maximum. Beyond this point, the hair becomes over-processed and damaged.

Different conditions and hair textures will cause the quality of wave patterns to vary. Hair of good texture will show a firm, strong pattern, whereas hair that is weak or fine will not produce a firm pattern.

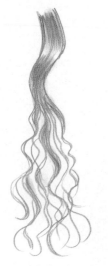

▲ **FIGURE 18-38**
Underprocessed hair.

Under-processed hair has not been sufficiently softened to permit the breaking and rearrangement of the disulfide bonds. This results in a limp or weak wave formation with undefined ridges within the S pattern. The hair retains little or no wave formation and is unable to hold the desired curl (**Figure 18-38**). Reapplication of the permanent waving solution is necessary to complete the process.

PERM TYPE	ACTIVE INGREDIENT	WRAPPING METHOD	PROCESS	RECOMMENDED HAIR TYPE	RESULTS	ADVANTAGES	DIS-ADVANTAGES
Alkaline/cold wave pH: 9.0 to 9.6	Ammonium thioglycolate (ATG)	Lotion wrap or water wrap	Room temperature	Coarse, thick, or resistant	Firm, strong curls	Processes quickly at room temperature	Unpleasant ammonia odor; may damage delicate hair
Exothermic wave pH: 9.0 to 9.6	Ammonium thioglycolate (ATG)	Water wrap	Exothermic	Coarse, thick, or resistant	Firm, strong curls	Faster processing time	Unpleasant ammonia odor; may damage delicate hair
True acid wave pH: 4.5 to 7.0	Glyceryl monothioglycolate (GMTG)	Water wrap	Endothermic	Extremely porous or very damaged	Soft, weak curls	Low pH produces minimal swelling	Requires heat from hair dryer; will not produce firm, strong curls
Acid-balanced wave pH: 7.8 to 8.2	Glyceryl monothioglycolate (GMTG)	Water wrap	Room temperature	Porous or damaged	Soft curls	Minimal swelling; processes at room temperature	Repeated exposure may cause allergic sensitivity in clients and stylists
Ammonia-free wave pH: 7.0 to 9.6	Monoethanolamine (MEA) or aminomethylpropanol (AMP)	Water wrap	Room temperature	Porous to normal	Medium to fine curls	No unpleasant ammonia odor	Overall strength varies with different manufacturers
Thio-free wave pH: 7.0 to 9.6	Mercaptamine or Cysteamine	Water wrap	Room temperature	Porous to normal	Medium to fine curls	May be gentler, depending on formula	Overall strength varies with different manufacturers
Low-pH wave pH: 6.5 to 7.0	Ammonium sulfite or ammonium bisulfite	Water wrap	Endothermic	Normal, fine, or damaged	Weak curl or body wave	Minimal swelling	Requires heat from hair dryer; produces weak curls

Over-processed hair can also appear to be too weak to hold a curl (**Figure 18-39**). Any solution that can process the hair properly can also over-process it. Solution left on the hair too long results in over-processing and, if too many disulfide bonds are broken, the hair may not have enough strength to hold the desired curl.

Signs that the hair has been over-processed include weak curl formation, a very curly appearance when wet but completely frizzy when dry, and an inability to be combed into a suitable wave pattern. In hair that has been over-processed, the elasticity of the hair has been damaged to the point where it is unable to contract into the wave formation. Over-processed hair usually feels harsh after being dried and should be given reconditioning treatments.

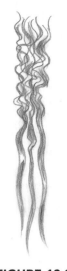

▲ **FIGURE 18-39**
Overprocessed hair.

Preliminary Test Curls

Test curls help to determine how the client's hair will react to the permanent waving process. A test curl provides information about how to obtain the best possible results out of the perm service. Test curls enable the barber to observe the following aspects of the hair:

- Speed of wave formation

- Degree of wave formation

- Exact time when peak of wave formation is reached

- Identification of resistant areas

- Appropriateness of product selection

mini PROCEDURE

PRELIMINARY TEST CURLS

Preliminary test curls are performed by rodding one parting of hair in three different areas of the head: the top, side, and nape. The procedure for performing preliminary test curls is as follows:

1 Wrap one tool in each of three different areas of the head (top, side, and nape); see **Figure 18-40**.

2 Wrap a cotton coil around each tool.

3 Apply waving lotion (**Figure 18-41**).

4 Set a timer and process according to manufacturer's directions.

5 Check each subsection frequently for proper curl development by unwinding the hair about $1\frac{1}{2}$ turns of the rod (**Figure 18-42**).

(Continued)

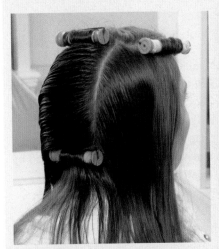

▲ **FIGURE 18-40**

Wrap rods in three areas of the head.

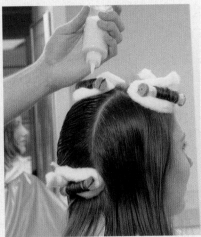

▲ **FIGURE 18-41**

Apply waving lotion to test curls.

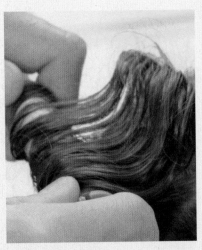

▲ **FIGURE 18-42**

Check for S formation.

6 Curl development is complete when a firm S is formed.

7 Rinse with warm water and neutralize. Do not proceed with the perm if the test curls are damaged or over-processed. If the test curls are satisfactory, proceed with the perm, but avoid re-perming the test curl partings.

NEUTRALIZATION

Permanent waving neutralizers are actually oxidizers that stop the action of permanent wave solutions and rebuild the disulfide bonds broken during processing. This process is known as **neutralization.** The most common neutralizer is hydrogen peroxide with a concentration range between 5 volume (1.5 percent) and 10 volume (3 percent). Other types of neutralizers are sodium bromate and sodium perborate.

Neutralization has two important functions:

1. Deactivate any waving solution that remains in the hair after rinsing

2. Rebuild the disulfide bonds that were broken and rearranged by the waving solution.

If the hair is not properly neutralized, the curl will relax or straighten within one to two shampoos. As with waving solutions, there may be slightly different procedures recommended for individual products. To achieve the best possible results, always read the directions carefully.

After thoroughly rinsing the permanent wave solution from the hair, it should be blotted until no excess water is absorbed into the towel. This is an important step in the neutralization process because excess water left in the hair prevents even saturation of the neutralizer and dilutes its properties.

The neutralizer should be applied to the top and bottom of each rod to assure saturation and even distribution of the product. Always give clients a towel to protect their eyes from excess or dripping neutralizer. A cotton coil should also be used for additional safety and client comfort.

Rinsing the Neutralizer

Depending on the permanent wave manufacturer's directions, neutralizers are rinsed from the hair in one of two ways: with the rods in place or after the rods have been removed from the hair.

The most commonly used method is to rinse the neutralizer from the hair with the rods in place. After a thorough rinsing with tepid water, followed by blotting, the rods are carefully removed in preparation for styling. Some directions may require a second rinse after the removal of the rods.

An alternative method is to carefully remove the rods, without stretching the hair, after neutralization has taken place. Apply the balance of the neutralizing solution and allow it to remain on the hair for an additional minute. Then rinse with tepid water and proceed with setting and/or styling the hair.

POST-PERM CARE

Most manufacturers recommend a 24- to 48-hour waiting period before shampooing freshly permed hair. Always follow the manufacture's directions and be sure to educate your clients about the most appropriate shampoos and conditioners to use after a perm service. Unless there are signs of scalp irritation, deposit-only haircolor can also be applied sooner than three days after a permanent wave.

Reconditioning treatments have a place in the after-care of a permanent wave and between permanent waves. Effective post-perm care helps to keep the hair in the best possible condition until the next chemical service. Suggest the following guidelines to permanent wave clients:

- Shampoo the hair as needed with an acid-balanced shampoo.
- Use a moisturizing hair conditioner.
- Schedule regular shop visits for trims and/or conditioning treatments to maintain the hairstyle.

PERMANENT WAVING WRAPPING PATTERNS

Once the client consultation has been completed, the barber should have a definite plan of action designed to achieve the desired results. This plan should include the selection of the permanent waving product, rod size(s), and wrapping pattern that will be used for the service.

There are five common wrapping patterns that are used in permanent waving. They are the basic, curvature, bricklay, spiral, and piggyback wraps. The parting technique most often used is a straight part. However, zigzag partings, known as the *weave technique,* can be used for an entire perm or to create smooth transitions from rodded areas to non-rodded areas within a partial perm **(Figure 18-43)**.

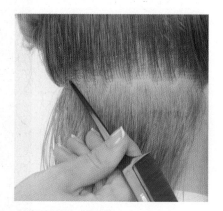

▲ **FIGURE 18-43**

Weave technique.

- *Basic perm wrap:* In this wrapping pattern, all the tools (rods) within a panel are positioned in the same direction on equal-size bases (**Figure 18-44**). All base sections are horizontal and approximately the same length and width of the rod. The base control is half off-base.

- *Curvature perm wrap:* This wrapping pattern is one of the best to use for men's styles as it produces a more natural-looking wave pattern. The movement curves within sectioned-out panels with partings and bases following the natural curvature and hair distribution of the head (**Figure 18-45**).

- *Bricklay perm wrap:* The base sections are offset from each other row by row to prevent noticeable splits in the hair (**Figure 18-46**). The bricklay pattern facilitates better blending of the hair from one area to another and may be preferred for men's styling over the basic perm wrap pattern.

- *Spiral perm wrap:* The spiral perm wrap is more a technique than a pattern. Unlike the preceding wrapping patterns, which are performed at an angle perpendicular to the rod, the spiral wrap is performed at an angle that positions the hair in a spiral pattern along the length of the rod or tool (**Figure 18-47**). This technique produces a uniform curl formation from the scalp to the ends and is especially appropriate for long hair designs.

- *Piggyback perm wrap:* The piggyback perm wrap uses two rods or tools for each parting of hair to facilitate even curl formation on long hair. The first rod is placed about midway between the scalp and hair ends. This section is rodded toward the scalp and leaves a tail of hair that extends from the mid-shaft point to the hair ends. The "tail" is then rodded from the ends to the midway point and secured and positioned across the first rod (**Figure 18-48**). In this way, the second rod is "piggybacking" the first rod.

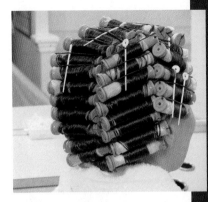

▲ **FIGURE 18-44**
Basic perm wrapping pattern.

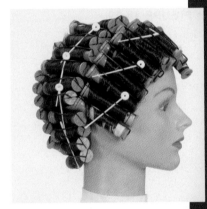

▲ **FIGURE 18-45**
Curvature perm wrapping pattern.

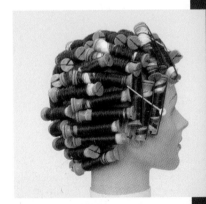

▲ **FIGURE 18-46**
Bricklay perm wrapping pattern.

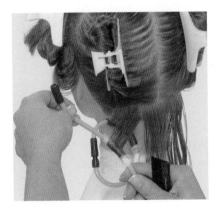

▲ **FIGURE 18-47**
Spiral perm technique.

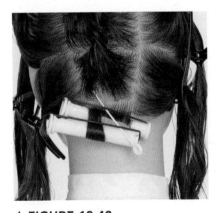

▲ **FIGURE 18-48**
Double-tool piggyback perm technique.

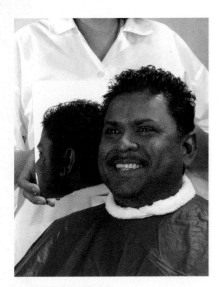

▲ FIGURE 18-49
Partial perm style.

PARTIAL PERMS

Partial perming means that only a section of the hair is permed. In men's permanent waving, this is usually hair on the top and crest area of the head **(Figure 18-49)**. Partial perms can be used to create volume and lift in these areas or to re-perm previously permed sections that have been trimmed due to normal hair growth and maintenance haircuts.

The same wrapping patterns and techniques used for a full perm can be used for a partial perm with the following considerations:

- To make a smooth transition from the rodded section to the non-rodded section, use the next larger rod size so that the curl pattern of the permed hair will blend into the non-permed hair.

- After rodding, place a coil of cotton around the wrapped rods as well as around the entire hairline.

- Before applying the waving lotion, apply a heavy, creamy conditioner to the sections that will not be permed to protect this hair from the effects of the waving lotion.

Many clients need the added texture and fullness that only a perm can give. A perm can help to temporarily overcome common hair problems by redirecting a cowlick, making limp or unmanageable hair easier to style, or making sparse hair look fuller. Although men and women's hairstyles may be different, the techniques for permanent waving are essentially the same.

SPECIAL PROBLEMS

Dry, Damaged Hair

Dry, brittle, damaged, or over-porous hair should be given reconditioning treatments prior to a permanent wave service. Avoid any treatment requiring massage or heat as this could create a sensitive scalp and irritation when the waving solution or neutralizer is applied.

Special fillers that contain protein are available for reconditioning the hair and helping to equalize its porosity. Some fillers also contain lanolin and cholesterol, which may help to protect the hair against the harshness of the permanent waving solution.

Tinted or Lightened Hair

Hair that has been tinted or lightened should be shampooed with an extra-mild shampoo before waving. It may also be advisable to use a pre-wrap or other leave-in conditioning product.

While pre-wraps and leave-in conditioners may be sufficient for stronger hair types that have been previously tinted or lightened, extremely porous hair will probably not benefit from these applications. Extremely porous hair may absorb too much conditioner, which in turn may interfere with waving solution penetration and curl formation.

Always select permanent waving solutions that are formulated for tinted and lightened hair conditions and always take the time to perform preliminary test curls.

Hair Tinted with Metallic Dye

Some over-the-counter haircoloring products still use metallic dyes in the formulations. Hair tinted with a metallic dye must first be treated with a dye remover to avoid hair discoloration or breakage. Do not wave the hair if the test curls break or discolor. This type of haircoloring product is difficult to remove so the best option is to cut the color-treated hair in a series of shop visits until all the color is removed. Then proceed with the perm service on virgin hair, followed by the application of professional haircoloring products.

Curl Reduction

Sometimes a client is displeased after a permanent wave because the hair seems too curly. If the hair is fine, do not suggest curl reduction before shampooing two or three times. This type of hair relaxes to a greater extent than does normal or coarse hair. Usually, after the second shampoo, the hair has relaxed to a satisfactory level.

If the hair has a normal or coarse texture, curl reduction may be done immediately following neutralization or after a few days.

Permanent waving solution may be used to relax the curl where required. Carefully comb it through the hair to widen and loosen the wave. When sufficiently relaxed, the hair is rinsed, towel blotted, and neutralized.

CAUTION

Do not attempt curl reduction on hair that has been over-processed, as such treatment will only further damage the hair.

Air–Conditioning and Heating Units

Because of its cooling effects, air-conditioning will usually slow the action of permanent waving solutions and additional processing time may be required. Make sure that clients are seated in an area of the shop away from drafts, vents, and fans to avoid slowing the processing time. Conversely, sitting too close to a heating vent or hood hair dryer can speed up the processing time.

Safety Precautions for Permanent Waving

- Always protect the client's clothing with the proper waterproof drape.

- Use two towels, one under the drape and one over the drape.

- Always examine the client's scalp before a perm service. Do not proceed if abrasions are present.

- Do not proceed with the perm if the client has ever experienced an allergic reaction to the products.

- Do not perm excessively damaged hair or hair that has been treated with hydroxide relaxers.

- Always apply a protective cream barrier around the client's hairline before applying the waving solution.

- Immediately replace cotton coils or towels that have become saturated with solution.

- Always protect the client's eyes when applying waving and neutralizing solutions by providing the client with a clean towel to hold over the eyes during the application. In case of accidental exposure, rinse thoroughly with cool water.

- Always follow the manufacturer's directions.

- Do not dilute or add anything to waving or neutralizing solutions unless specified in the manufacturer's directions.

- Wear gloves when applying solutions.

- Do not save opened or unused products, as the strength and effectiveness will change if not used promptly.

- Unless otherwise specified in the product instructions, apply waving and neutralizing solutions liberally to the top and underside of each rod.

- Start at the crown and progress systematically down each section. (Some barbers prefer to start at the top of the head.) Be sure that the surface area of the wound hair is wet with lotion so penetration is even.

- Follow the same application pattern for the neutralizer as used with the waving solution to avoid missing any rods.

- Sometimes it is necessary to re-saturate the rods during processing. This may be due to evaporation of the solution, dryness of the hair, hair that was poorly saturated the first time, improper selection of solution strength, or failure to follow the manufacturer's directions. Reapplying the solution will hasten processing, so watch the wave development closely as negligence may result in hair damage.

Permanent Waving

SUPPLIES

- Towels
- Waterproof drape
- Rods
- Tail comb
- End wraps
- Cotton coil
- Perm solution
- Neutralizer
- Shampoo and conditioner
- Protective cream
- Spray bottle with water
- Gloves
- Hair clips
- Timer
- Plastic cap (if required)

PREPARATION

1. Wash your hands.

2. Conduct client consultation.

3. Perform hair and scalp analysis.

4. Select and arrange required materials.

5. Drape client for a shampoo.

6. Shampoo client's hair.

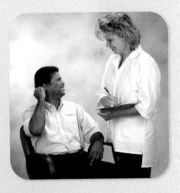

PRELIMINARY TEST CURL

1 Shampoo the hair and towel it dry.

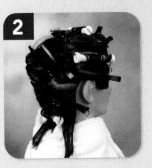

2 Following the perm directions, wrap two or three rods in the most delicate or resistant areas of the hair.

3 Wrap a coil of cotton around each rod.

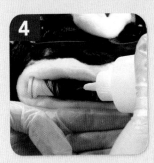

4 Wearing gloves, apply the waving lotion to the wrapped curls, being very careful not to allow the waving lotion to come in contact with unwrapped hair.

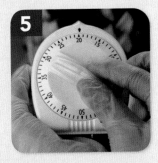

5 Set a timer and process the hair according to the perm directions.

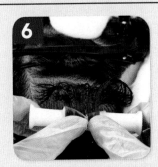

6 Check curl formation frequently.

F⊙CUS ON...

To check a test curl, unfasten the rod carefully (remember, the hair is in a softened state) and unwind the curl about 1½ turns of the rod. Do not permit the hair to become loose or completely unwound. Hold the hair firmly by placing a thumb at each end of the rod. Shift the rod gently toward the scalp so that the hair falls loosely into the wave pattern. Continue checking the rods until a firm and definite S is formed. The S reflects the size of the rod used. Be guided by the manufacturer's directions.

When the optimum curl has been formed, rinse with warm water and blot the curls thoroughly. Apply, process, and rinse the neutralizer according to the perm directions; gently dry these test curls. Evaluate the curl results. If the hair is over-processed, do not perm the rest of the hair until it is in better condition. If the test curl results are good, proceed with the perm, but do not re-perm the preliminary test curls.

PROCEDURE

1 If hair is long and a shorter cut is desired, it may be cut after the shampoo. If hair is short, cut after the permanent wave.

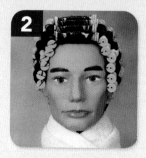

2 Section and block (subsection) the hair. Start rodding from the crown to the nape in the back to create a center panel, or from the crown forward across the top to create a front section. Use either panel of rodded hair as a guide for subsequent rod placement. Once the center back panel is rodded, rod the back side panels and then the sides. Be guided by your instructor for additional rodding patterns.

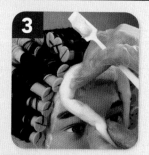

3 Apply protective cream and cotton strips around the client's hairline.

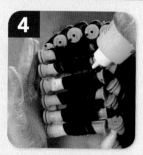

4 Apply the permanent waving solution as recommended by the manufacturer. If using a cold wave, check wave formation immediately after saturating the hair with waving solution. Take frequent test curls on different areas of the head throughout the recommended processing time.

5 Process the hair for the required time. If re-wetting the curls is necessary, apply the solution in the same order followed originally. Protect the client with fresh protective cotton strips around the hairline and neck.

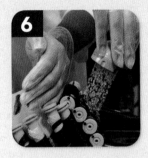

6 When the curls have processed sufficiently, rinse out the waving solution thoroughly. Use gentle water pressure and a tepid water temperature, unless the manufacturer's directions state otherwise.

CAUTION

Always rinse permanent waving lotion thoroughly from the hair before applying the neutralizer to avoid serious accidents.

7 Towel blot excess moisture from the hair wound on rods. Do not rock or roll the rods while blotting. The hair is in a softened state and any such movement may cause hair breakage. Follow towel blot with paper towel blotting to remove residual moisture.

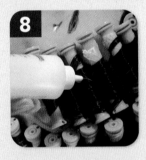

8 Apply neutralizer and process. Follow manufacturer's neutralization instructions.

9 Unwind the rods and remove them carefully (depending on manufacturer's directions).

10 Apply remaining neutralizer and work through the hair with your hands.

11 Rinse hair thoroughly.

12 Towel dry and style the hair as desired.

CLEAN-UP AND DISINFECTION

1. Clean and disinfect tools and implements, including rods.

2. Sanitize chair and workstation.

3. Dispose of towels and paper goods.

4. Sweep floor if necessary.

5. Wash your hands.

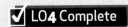

Reformation Curls

A reformation curl, also known as a *soft-curl permanent,* is a three-step process that is used to restructure very curly hair into looser and larger curls. This process uses a thio relaxer to partially relax the hair, a thio permanent wave to restructure the hair around perm rods, and a neutralizing solution to rebuild the broken disulfide bonds (see **Figure 18-2**). Styling products such as activators and moisturizing solutions are often part of the finishing process, but check with the client first.

The thio relaxer product used for the partial relaxation of the hair in a reformation curl service is most commonly known as the *rearranger.* The rearranger is an ammonium thioglycolate product in a thick cream form that is applied to dry hair in the same way as a hydroxide relaxer. The waving solution is called the *booster* and is similar in composition to alkaline permanent waving solutions or lotions. The *neutralizer* is an oxidizing solution in a clear or milky liquid form, and is part of the same product line as the rearranger and the booster. The chemical reactions of the neutralizer are the same as those created by permanent waving neutralizers.

Additional products, such as activators and moisturizers, serve as leave-in conditioners and styling products to promote curl retention, although excess application should be avoided to prevent drips and over-saturation. Depending on the texture and condition of the hair, other professional products that retain moisture and promote manageability of the hair may be preferred.

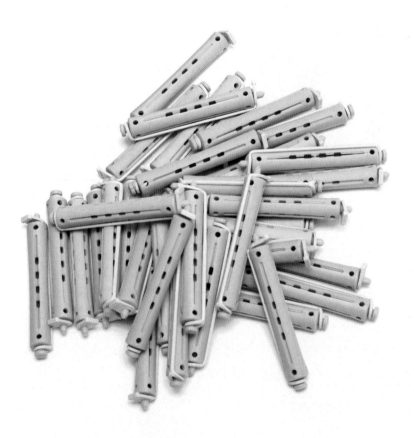

Reformation Curl

SUPPLIES

- Towels
- Waterproof drape
- Rods
- Tail comb
- End wraps
- Cotton coil
- Rearranger
- Booster
- Neutralizer
- Shampoo and conditioner
- Protective cream
- Gloves
- Hair clips
- Timer
- Plastic cap

PREPARATION

1. Wash your hands.

2. Conduct client consultation.

3. Perform hair and scalp analysis.

4. Select and arrange required materials.

5. Drape client for a chemical service.

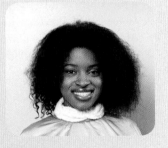

PROCEDURE

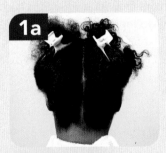

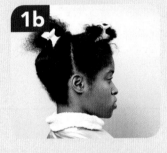

1 Part the hair into four sections from the center of the front hairline to the nape and from ear to ear. Clip hair out of the way.

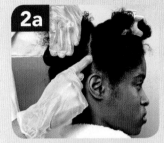

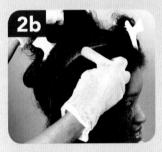

2 Apply protective **base cream** around the hairline and tops of the ears.

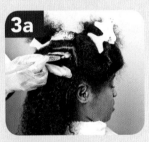

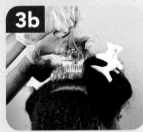

3 Wear gloves. Part off $\frac{1}{4}''$ to $\frac{1}{2}''$ partings and apply the rearranger $\frac{1}{4}''$ to $\frac{1}{2}''$ from the scalp on the top and underside of the parting. The rearranger may be applied with a brush, an applicator bottle, or the back of a comb.

4 Continue applying the rearranger until all the sections have been covered.

5

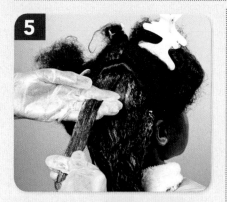

5 Use the back of the comb or the fingers to smooth and gently pull the hair partings into a more relaxed curl formation.

6 Process according to the manufacturer's directions and rinse thoroughly.

7

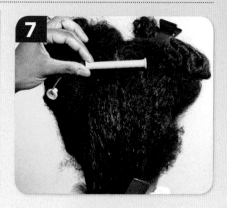

7 Part the hair into panels in preparation for rodding. Use the length of the rod to measure for the width of the panels.

8a

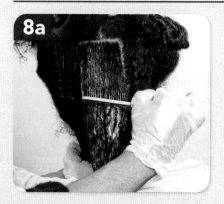

8b

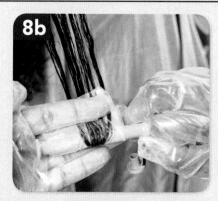

8c

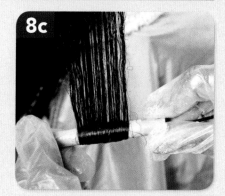

8 Apply and distribute the booster to the first panel and rod the hair.

9 Continue wrapping and rodding the remaining panels in the same manner.

10 Place a cotton coil around the hairline; apply extra booster to each curl as necessary for even saturation.

11 If a plastic cap is used, punch a few holes in it to release excess heat. Position the rim of the cap over the cotton coil so that the cap does not touch the client's skin.

12 Check cotton and towels. If saturated, replace them.

13 Process according to manufacturer's directions. Most processing takes less than 20 minutes at room temperature.

14 Check for proper curl development.

15 When processing is complete, rinse thoroughly for at least 5 minutes. Towel blot each rod to remove excess moisture.

16 Apply the neutralizer, making sure that each rod is saturated. Set the timer and neutralize according to directions.

17 Remove the rods gently and distribute the remaining neutralizer through the hair ends. Rinse thoroughly. Shampoo and condition according to manufacturer's directions.

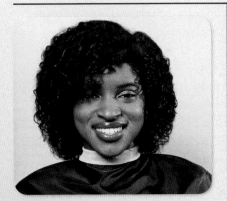

18 Style the hair as desired.

CLEAN-UP AND DISINFECTION

1. Clean and disinfect tools and implements, including rods.

2. Sanitize chair and workstation.

3. Dispose of towels and paper goods.

4. Sweep floor if necessary.

5. Wash your hands.

☑ **LO5** Complete

Chemical Hair Relaxing

Chemical hair relaxing is the process of rearranging the basic structure of extremely curly hair into a straightened form. Like the permanent waving process, chemical hair relaxers change the shape of the hair by breaking and rearranging disulfide bonds in the hair.

The basic products used in the chemical hair-relaxing process are chemical hair relaxers (straighteners), neutralizers or neutralizing shampoos, protective bases or creams, and conditioners.

TYPES OF RELAXERS

The two most common types of relaxers are thio and hydroxide relaxers. Neither type of relaxer allows pre-shampooing unless there is an excessive buildup of dirt or styling products. In rare instances when the hair requires cleansing, the shampoo service should be performed gently to avoid scalp irritation and the hair should be thoroughly dried before the relaxer is applied.

Both types of relaxers are applied in the same manner, but thio relaxers require the application of a chemical neutralizing solution whereas hydroxide relaxers are neutralized through the physical actions of rinsing and shampooing with a neutralizing shampoo product. Neutralizing shampoos or normalizing lotions are basically acid-balanced shampoos that neutralize any remaining hydroxide in the hair and help to lower the pH of the hair and scalp.

Thio (ATG) is the same reducing agent used in permanent waving, but thio relaxers usually have a pH above 10.0 and a higher concentration of ATG than permanent wave products. Thio relaxers are also thicker in consistency than permanent waving lotions for better adhesion and product control.

Hydroxide relaxers are ionic compounds formed by a metal combined with oxygen and hydrogen. Metal hydroxide relaxers include sodium hydroxide, potassium hydroxide, lithium hydroxide, and guanidine hydroxide.

Sodium hydroxide relaxers are known as lye relaxers. Sodium hydroxide is the oldest and most commonly used chemical hair relaxer. Sodium hydroxide content varies from 5 percent to 10 percent, with a pH range of 10 to over 13.5. Generally speaking, the higher the percentage of sodium hydroxide, the faster the chemical reaction on the hair. It is also true that the higher the pH factor, the greater the danger of hair damage or breakage.

Potassium and *lithium hydroxide* relaxers are often sold as "no-mix/no-lye" relaxers. Although these two relaxers are not technically lye products, their chemistry is identical and there is little difference in their performance.

Guanidine hydroxide relaxers are usually advertised as "no-lye" relaxers. These relaxers contain two products, a relaxer cream and an activator, that must be mixed immediately prior to use and are recommended for sensitive scalps.

Many *calcium hydroxide* relaxers are often mistakenly referred to as "no-lye" relaxers. Obviously, this type of marketing statement can be misleading, so care must be taken when choosing the relaxer product. Calcium hydroxide relaxers require the addition of an activator. The strength of the relaxer is determined by the amount of activator used in the mixture. Although these relaxers are considered to be mild and tend to work more slowly on the hair, there are many professionals who feel that calcium hydroxide relaxers are more damaging to the cuticle layer of the hair than other hydroxide relaxers.

Hydroxide relaxers are usually sold in *base* and *no-base* formulas. **Base relaxers** require the application of a base cream to the entire scalp prior to relaxer application. **No-base relaxers** contain a base cream that is designed to melt at body temperature and do not require the application of a separate protective base.

Most chemical relaxers are available in a variety of different strengths: mild, regular, and super. The strength of the relaxer reflects the concentration of hydroxide in its formulation. Mild strengths are recommended for fine, color-treated, or damaged hair. Regular-strength relaxers are intended for normal hair textures, and super strengths should be used for maximum straightening on extremely curly, coarse hair. Use **Table 18-4** as a guide for selecting chemical hair-relaxing products.

> TABLE **18-4** Selecting the Correct Relaxer

ACTIVE INGREDIENT	pH	MARKETED AS	ADVANTAGES	DISADVANTAGES
Sodium hydroxide	12.5 to 13.5	Lye relaxer	Very effective for extremely curly hair	May cause scalp irritation and damage the hair
Lithium hydroxide and potassium hydroxide	12.5 to 13.5	No-mix, lye relaxer	Very effective for extremely curly hair	May cause scalp irritation and damage the hair
Guanidine hydroxide	13 to 13.5	No-lye relaxer	Causes less skin irritation than other hydroxide relaxers	More drying to hair with repeated use
Ammonium thioglycolate	9.6 to 10.0	Thio relaxer, no-lye relaxer	Compatible with soft-curl permanent waves	Strong, unpleasant ammonia smell
Ammonium sulfite or ammonium bisulfite	6.5 to 8.5	Low-pH relaxer, no-lye relaxer	Less damaging to hair	Does not relax extremely curly hair sufficiently

TEXTURIZERS AND CHEMICAL BLOW-OUTS

Overly curly hair has unique characteristics that may require special styling techniques. Relaxing products can be used to **texturize** the hair, reducing it from an extremely curly state to a wave formation that makes haircutting and styling more versatile, or to perform a **chemical blow-out** service that partially straightens the hair with the intent that it will be picked out and cut. Chemical blow-outs were used for many of the semi-straightened "Afro" styles of the 1970s.

Texturizers and chemical blow-outs may be performed with either a thio or sodium hydroxide relaxer. The primary consideration with either method is to not over-relax the hair to the point where the blow-out process becomes impossible to perform.

Although thio relaxers may have a pH above 10, they are not as harsh as hydroxide relaxers. Depending on the strength of the thio relaxer, it may not straighten tightly curled hair textures completely. Since the objective of a chemical blow-out is to remove some but not all of the curl, a thio relaxer may be used for almost its entire recommended application time. Check the curl pattern every few minutes until the desired amount of curl relaxation has been achieved.

Sodium hydroxide is an extremely alkaline product and may process the hair too quickly to the point where a blow-out cannot be performed. When using sodium hydroxide, timing becomes very important. Extreme care must be taken to control the amount of processing, and the chemical should not be kept on the hair for longer than 40 percent of the recommended processing time.

The procedures for thio and sodium hydroxide relaxing have been explained thoroughly in this chapter. The important consideration to remember is to relax the hair only to the point where it has relaxed enough to facilitate the desired style.

After the relaxer has been rinsed from the hair, apply the neutralizer (stabilizer or fixative) and conditioner if using a thio relaxer, or shampoo and conditioner if using a sodium hydroxide product. In both cases, the conditioner will help to minimize possible damage or breakage and enable the hair to withstand combing, picking, and rearranging.

mini PROCEDURE

PROCEDURAL REMINDERS FOR A CHEMICAL BLOW-OUT

While the degree of curl remaining after a texturizer service should leave the hair ready for cutting and styling, the chemical blow-out requires an extra step prior to the cutting procedure. Refer to the following guidelines when performing the final steps of a chemical blow-out service after processing.

(Continued)

mini PROCEDURE

1 Use a wide-tooth comb or pick to comb the hair upward and slightly forward. The hair closest to the scalp gives direction to the hair; therefore, it must be picked upward and outward. Start at the crown and continue until all of the hair has been combed out from the scalp and distributed evenly around the head.

2 Place the client under a hood hairdryer until the hair is dried.

3 Once dried, the hair is ready for shaping. Evenness is very important at this point. Check the hair length to make sure that the shortest hair is used as the guide for the balance of the head.

4 Begin cutting at the sides. The hair is evened out around the head with clippers or shears while picking the hair outward from the scalp. Cut the hair in the direction in which it is to be combed. The object is to achieve a smooth, even cut that is properly contoured. The final cutting should be done only with shears to even out loose or ragged ends.

5 Outline the hairstyle at the sides, around the ears, and in the nape area using either shears or an outliner. After the hair is cut to the desired style, apply the finishing touches. Fluff the hair slightly with the pick where required and spray lightly to hold the shape.

STRAND TESTS FOR CHEMICAL HAIR RELAXING

Preliminary strand tests for chemical relaxer applications include the following:

- Finger test to determine the degree of hair porosity

- Pull test to determine the degree of elasticity

- Relaxer test to determine the hair's reaction to the chemical and processing time

mini PROCEDURE

RELAXER TEST PROCEDURE

1 Thread a small section of hair through a hole cut in a piece of waxed paper or paper towel. Do not use a base or cream. Apply relaxer to the hair section and smooth. Process according to manufacturer's directions.

2 Thoroughly mist the hair section with water to remove product and blot. Neutralize with neutralizer or neutralizing shampoo depending on the type of relaxing product used. Check results and note on client record card. If the hair has been satisfactorily straightened, apply conditioner or base cream to the strand, isolate it, and proceed with the relaxing treatment over the remainder of the hair.

SAFETY PRECAUTIONS FOR CHEMICAL HAIR RELAXING

- Always protect the client's clothing with the proper waterproof drape.

- Use two towels, one under the drape and one over the drape.

- Always examine the client's scalp before a relaxer service. Do not proceed if abrasions are present.

- Do not proceed if the client has ever experienced an allergic reaction to the products.

- Do not relax excessively damaged hair.

- Do not use thio relaxers on hair that has been treated with hydroxide relaxers, or hydroxide relaxers on thio-treated hair.

- Always apply a protective cream barrier around the client's hairline before applying the relaxer.

- Base the scalp with a protective cream as directed by the product manufacturer.

- Always be careful of the client's eyes when applying relaxers and neutralizing solutions. In case of accidental exposure, rinse thoroughly with cool water.

- Always follow the manufacturer's directions.

- Do not dilute or add anything to relaxer creams unless specified in the manufacturer's directions.

- Wear gloves when applying relaxers.

- Do not save mixed products, as the strength and effectiveness will change if not used promptly.

- Apply relaxer cream to the most resistant area first.

- Follow the same pattern for smoothing the relaxer as was used during the application process.

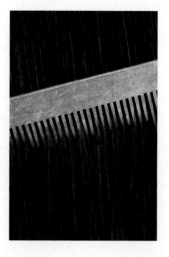

Thio and Hydroxide Relaxers

SUPPLIES

- Towels
- Waterproof drape
- Wide-toothed comb
- Tail comb
- Relaxing cream
- Neutralizing shampoo or neutralizer
- Conditioner
- Protective cream
- Gloves
- Bowl and application brush
- Hair clips
- Timer

PREPARATION

1. Wash your hands.

2. Conduct client consultation.

3. Perform hair and scalp analysis.

4. Select and arrange required materials.

5. Read product directions.

6. Drape client for a chemical service.

7. Note: Light shampooing is optional before a thio relaxer.

PROCEDURE

A. VIRGIN APPLICATION PROCEDURE

1 Part the hair into four sections from the center of the front hairline to the nape and from ear to ear. Secure hair sections with a clip.

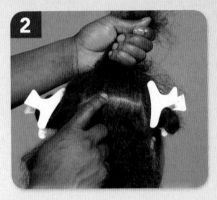

2 Apply protective base cream around the hairline and tops of the ears. Take $\frac{1}{4}$" to $\frac{1}{2}$" partings and apply base cream along each parting.

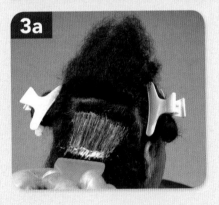
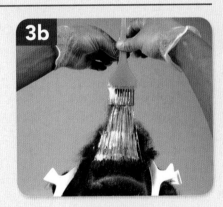

3 Wear gloves. Part off $\frac{1}{4}$" to $\frac{1}{2}$" partings and apply the relaxer $\frac{1}{4}$" to $\frac{1}{2}$" from the scalp on the top and underside of the parting. Do not apply relaxer to the scalp area or porous ends at this time. The relaxer may be applied with a brush, applicator bottle, or the back of a comb.

4 Continue applying the relaxer until all the sections have been covered.

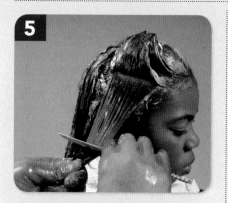

5 Use the back of the comb or fingers to smooth the hair and gently pull the hair partings into a straighter form.

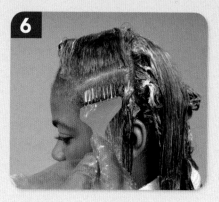

6 Process according to manufacturer's directions. During the last few minutes of processing; work the relaxer down to the scalp and through the ends of the hair. Carefully comb and smooth all sections.

7 Rinse thoroughly to remove all traces of the relaxer.

B. RETOUCH APPLICATION PROCEDURES

1 Part the hair into four sections from the center of the front hairline to the nape and from ear to ear. Clip hair out of the way.

2 Apply protective base cream around the hairline and tops of the ears. Take $\frac{1}{4}''$ to $\frac{1}{2}''$ partings and apply base cream along each parting.

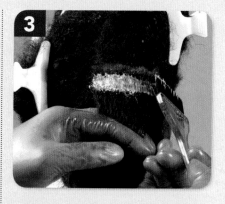

3 Wear gloves. Part off $\frac{1}{4}''$ to $\frac{1}{2}''$ partings and apply the relaxer $\frac{1}{4}''$ to $\frac{1}{2}''$ from the scalp on the top and underside of the new growth. Do not apply relaxer to the scalp area at this time. Do not overlap the relaxer onto previously relaxed hair as it may cause breakage. The relaxer may be applied with a brush, applicator bottle, or the back of a comb.

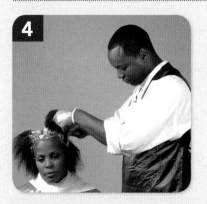

4 Continue applying the relaxer until all the sections have been covered.

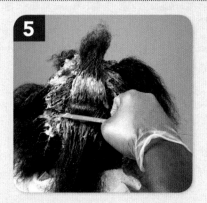

5 Use the back of the comb or fingers to smooth and straighten the new growth area.

6 Process according to manufacturer's directions. During the last few minutes of processing, work the relaxer down to the scalp.

7 Rinse thoroughly to remove all traces of the relaxer.

C. NEUTRALIZATION PROCEDURES

- Thio relaxer: Apply normalizing or neutralizing solution and comb it through to the hair ends. Process and rinse thoroughly. Follow manufacturer's directions for shampooing and conditioning.

- Hydroxide relaxer: Shampoo at least three times with neutralizing shampoo or recommended product. Rinse thoroughly and condition according to manufacturer's directions. Style as desired.

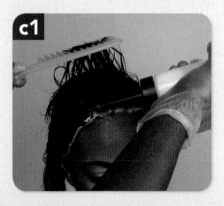

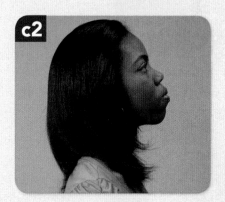

CLEAN-UP AND DISINFECTION

1. Clean and disinfect tools and implements, including rods.

2. Sanitize chair and workstation.

3. Dispose of towels and paper goods.

4. Sweep floor if necessary.

5. Wash your hands.

☑ **LO6** Complete

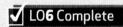

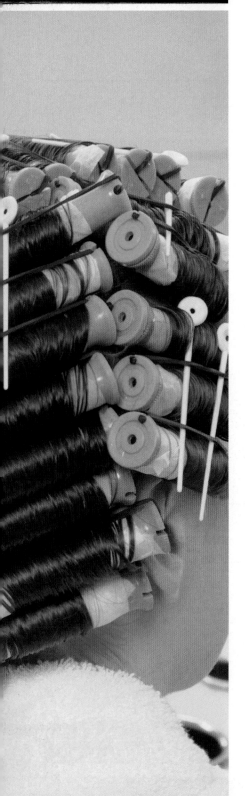

18 Review
Questions

1. Explain the physical and chemical changes that occur in the hair as a result of chemical texture services.

2. What characteristics or condition of the hair and scalp should be analyzed before performing chemical texture services?

3. List the similarities and differences between permanent wave, reformation curl, and hair-relaxing processes.

4. List the chemical products used in permanent waving.

5. List at least five permanent waving safety precautions.

6. List the chemical products used in the reformation curl service.

7. List the chemical products used with thio relaxers.

8. List the products used with hydroxide relaxers.

9. Explain the difference between base and no-base relaxers.

10. What chemical texture service requires a pre-service shampoo? Which services do not?

11. Explain the difference between a texturizer and a chemical blow-out.

12. List at least five chemical hair relaxing safety precautions.

Chapter
Glossary

acid-balanced waves perms with a 7.8 to 8.2 pH range that process at room temperature; do not require hair-dryer heat

alkaline or cold waves perms that process at room temperature without heat with a pH range between 9.0 and 9.6

ammonium thioglycolate (ATG) main active ingredient or reducing agent in alkaline waves

base control the position of the perm rod in relation to its base section

base cream protective cream used on the scalp during hair relaxing

base direction angle at which the perm rod is positioned on the head; also the directional pattern in which the hair is wrapped

base relaxers relaxers that require the use of a base or protective cream

base sections subsections of panels into which the hair is divided for rodding; one tool is normally placed on each base section

basic perm wrap rodding pattern in which all the tools within a panel are directed in the same direction

bookend wrap perm wrap in which an end paper is folded in half over the hair ends

chemical blow-out combination of a relaxer and hairstyling used to create a variety of Afro styles

chemical hair relaxing the process of rearranging the basic structure of extremely curly hair into a straightened form

chemical texture services hair services that cause a chemical change that permanently alters the natural wave pattern of the hair

croquignole rodding rodding from the hair ends to the scalp

end wraps end paper; absorbent papers used to protect and control the ends of the hair during perming services

endothermic waves perm activated by an outside heat source, usually a hood-type dryer

exothermic waves perms that create an exothermic chemical reaction that heats the solution and speeds up processing

glyceryl monothioglycolate (GMTG) main active ingredient in true acid and acid-balanced waves

hydroxide relaxers relaxers with a very high pH, sometimes over 13

lanthionization process by which hydroxide relaxers permanently straighten hair; lanthionization breaks the hair's disulfide bonds during processing and converts them to lanthionine bonds when the relaxer is rinsed from the hair

lotion wrap permanent waving wrapping technique in which the waving solution is applied to the section before rodding

neutralization process of stopping the action of a permanent wave solution and hardening the hair in its new form by the application of a chemical solution called the neutralizer

no-base relaxers relaxers that do not require application of a protective base

permanent waving a process used to chemically restructure natural hair into a different wave pattern

pre-wrap solution usually a type of leave-in conditioner that may be applied to the hair prior to permanent waving to equalize porosity

reformation curl a soft-curl permanent; combination of a thio relaxer and thio permanent, whereby the hair is wrapped on perm rods; used to make existing curl larger and looser

texturize a process used to semi-straighten extremely curly hair into a more manageable texture and wave pattern

thio relaxers relaxers that usually have a pH above 10 and a higher concentration of ammonium thioglycolate than is used in permanent waving

true acid waves perms that have a pH between 4.5 and 7.0 and require heat to speed processing; process more slowly than alkaline waves and do not usually produce as firm a curl

19 Haircoloring and Lightening

☑ Learning Objectives

AFTER COMPLETING THIS CHAPTER, YOU SHOULD BE ABLE TO:

1 Discuss the principles of color theory and their importance to haircoloring.

2 Identify the classifications of haircolor products and explain their actions on the hair.

3 Explain the action of lighteners on the hair.

4 Identify the products used in haircoloring and lightening.

5 Demonstrate the correct procedures for applying haircolor and lighteners.

6 Identify products used to color facial hair.

7 Discuss safety precautions used in haircoloring and lightening.

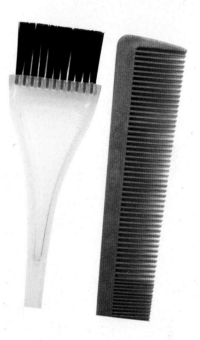

Key Terms

PAGE NUMBER INDICATES WHERE IN THE CHAPTER THE TERM IS USED.

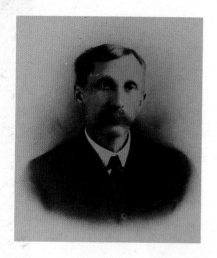

Men and women have altered their hair color for thousands of years. Early cultures considered colors to be symbols of power and mysticism. This belief led to body painting and haircoloring agents derived from vegetable and mineral dyes, as evidenced by chemicals and tools found in Egyptian tombs.

In the 1880s, American men had their beards and mustaches dyed in barbershops with coloring products that left the hair with strange iridescent tones or purple hues. These early formulations were made of silver nitrate, gold chloride, gum, and distilled water. Since the first synthetic dyes were developed in 1883, color technology and haircoloring processes have steadily improved in performance and safety.

Haircoloring is the science and art of changing the color of the hair. **Hair lightening** is the partial or total removal of natural pigment or artificial color from the hair. Haircoloring and lightening services offer the skillful barber yet another opportunity for building a loyal and lucrative clientele.

Many shop clients will express an interest in haircolor at some point or another. Clients who enjoy fashion changes, are prematurely gray, or wish to maintain a youthful appearance represent typical haircoloring service clients (**Figures 19-1a** and **19-1b**). Others may wish to change the natural color of their hair to a more attractive shade or to create decorative effects such as highlighting or streaking.

Barbers who want to provide successful haircoloring and lightening services to their clients need to understand hair structure, the laws of color, and the processes associated with color and lightening products. A skilled haircolorist is proficient in adding artificial pigment to natural, previously colored, or pre-lightened hair and understands the process of diffusing natural pigment through lightening agents.

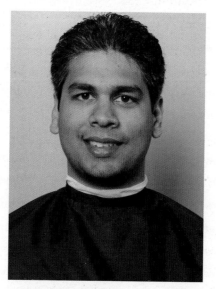

▲ **FIGURE 19-1a**
Client before haircoloring service.

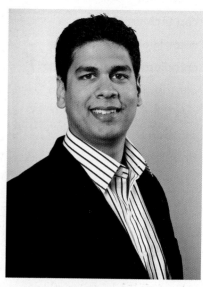

▲ **FIGURE 19-1b**
Client after haircoloring service.

Characteristics and Structure of Hair

The client's hair structure will affect the quality and ultimate success of the haircolor service. The strength of the cuticle and the amount of elasticity and natural pigment in the cortex are important considerations in determining haircoloring options and product selection. Other hair structure factors relevant to a haircoloring or lightening service are texture, density, porosity, and natural color.

- *Texture:* The diameter of the individual hair strand determines whether the hair texture is classified as fine, medium, or coarse. Melanin is distributed differently within the different textures. Melanin granules in fine hair are grouped tightly, so the hair takes color faster and may appear darker. Medium-textured hair has an average response time to haircolor products, and coarse hair may take longer to process (**Figure 19-2**).

- *Density:* To assure proper coverage, the density of the hair should be taken into account when applying haircolor or lighteners.

- *Porosity:* The porosity level of the hair influences its ability to absorb liquids. Porous hair accepts haircolor products faster and permits a darker saturation than less porous hair. Hair with a low porosity level has a tight cuticle, which makes it resistant to moisture and chemical penetration with the result that it can require a longer processing time. In hair that has an average porosity level, the cuticle is slightly raised and the hair tends to process in an average amount of time. A lifted cuticle indicates a high porosity level. This type of hair condition may take color quickly but may also fade faster than other porosity levels due to its inability to hold color pigments for the normal amount of time.

- *Natural color:* Natural hair color ranges from black to dark brown to red, and from dark blond to lightest blond. *Eumelanin* gives black and brown color to hair and *pheomelanin* is the melanin found in yellowish-blond, ginger, and red tones. The three factors that determine all natural colors, from jet black to light blond, are the thickness of the hair, the total number and size of pigment granules, and the ratio of eumelanin to pheomelanin. White hair is actually the color of keratin without the influence of melanin and therefore does not contain either type.

- **Contributing pigment** is the pigment that lies under the natural hair color. The foundation of haircoloring is based on modifying this pigment with haircoloring products to create new pigments or colors.

Gray hair is normally associated with aging, although heredity is also a contributing factor. In most cases, the loss of pigment increases as a person ages, resulting in a range of gray tones from blended to solid. The amount of gray in an individual's hair is measured in percentages, as presented in **Table 19-1**, and requires special care when formulating haircolor applications. (The challenges and solutions associated with coloring gray hair are discussed later in the chapter.)

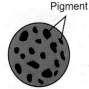

Pigment

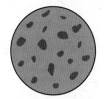

Fine-textured hair

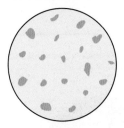

Medium-textured hair

Coarse-textured hair

▲ FIGURE 19-2

Melanin distribution according to hair texture.

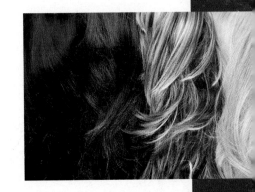

TABLE **19-1** Determining the Percentage of Gray Hair

PERCENTAGE OF GRAY HAIR	CHARACTERISTICS
30%	More pigmented than gray hair
50%	Even mixture of gray and pigmented hair
70 to 90%	More gray than pigmented; most of remaining pigment is located at the back of the head
100%	Virtually no pigmented hair; tends to look white

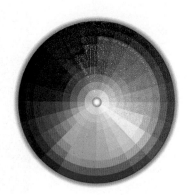

Color Theory

Color is a characteristic of visible light energy. Although the human eye sees only six basic colors, the brain is capable of visualizing the combinations of different wavelengths relevant to these three primary and three secondary colors (see Chapter 9). The light rays that are absorbed or reflected by natural hair pigment or artificial pigment added to the hair create the colors we see.

THE LAWS OF COLOR

The **laws of color** regulate the mixing of dyes and pigment to make other colors. Based in science and adapted to art, the laws of color serve as guidelines for harmonious color mixing. For example, equal parts of red and blue mixed together always make violet.

Primary Colors

Primary colors are basic or true colors that cannot be created by combining other colors. The three primary colors are yellow, red, and blue (**Figure 19-3**). All other colors are created by some combination of red, yellow, or blue. Colors with a predominance of blue are cool-toned colors and colors that are predominantly red are warm-toned colors.

- *Blue* is the darkest and the only cool primary color. Blue brings depth or darkness to any color to which it is added.

- *Red* is the medium primary color. When added to blue-based colors, red makes them appear lighter. Conversely, red added to a yellow color will cause it to become darker.

- *Yellow* is the lightest of the primary colors and will lighten and brighten other colors.

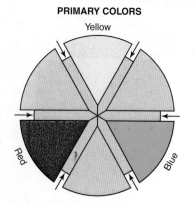

PRIMARY COLORS

Yellow

Red

Blue

▲ **FIGURE 19-3**
Primary colors.

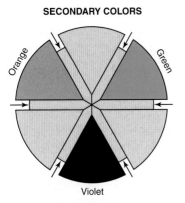

SECONDARY COLORS

Orange · Green · Violet

▲ **FIGURE 19-4**

Secondary colors.

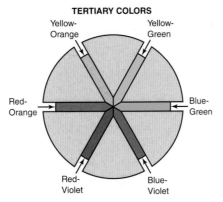

TERTIARY COLORS

Yellow-Orange · Yellow-Green · Red-Orange · Blue-Green · Red-Violet · Blue-Violet

▲ **FIGURE 19-5**

Tertiary colors.

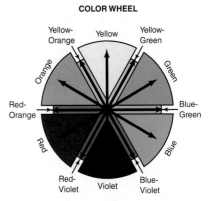

COLOR WHEEL

Yellow-Orange · Yellow · Yellow-Green · Orange · Green · Red-Orange · Blue-Green · Red · Blue · Red-Violet · Violet · Blue-Violet

▲ **FIGURE 19-6**

Complementary colors.

Secondary Colors

Secondary colors are created by mixing *equal* amounts of two primary colors. When mixed in equal parts, yellow and blue create green, blue and red create violet, and red and yellow create orange **(Figure 19-4)**. Natural hair color is made up of a combination of primary and secondary colors.

Tertiary Colors

Tertiary colors are created by mixing equal amounts of one primary color with one of its adjacent secondary colors. Presented in their order on the color wheel, tertiary colors are yellow-green, blue-green, blue-violet, red-violet, red-orange, and yellow-orange **(Figure 19-5)**.

Complementary Colors

Complementary colors are any two colors situated directly across from each other on the color wheel **(Figure 19-6)**. When mixed together their action is to neutralize each other. For example, when mixed in equal amounts, red and green neutralize each other, creating brown. Orange and blue neutralize each other, and yellow and violet neutralize each other.

Complementary colors are always composed of a primary and a secondary color, and complementary pairs always consist of all three primary colors. For example, the color wheel shows that the complement of red (a primary color) is green (a secondary color). Green is made up of blue and yellow (both primary colors). So, all three primary colors are represented to varying degrees in the complementary pair of red and green.

Hue and Tone

Hue is the basic name of a color, such as red, yellow, or violet. The color wheel is a sequential arrangement of hues that makes the relationships among colors visible. In haircoloring, **tone** describes the warmth or coolness of a color. The warm colors, also known as highlighting colors, are red, orange, and yellow. These colors produce warmer tones because they reflect more light. The cool colors, also known as ash or drab colors, are blue, green, and violet, which absorb more light and cast cool tones.

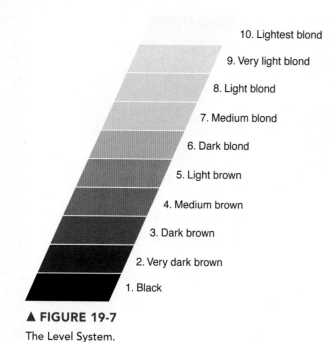

10. Lightest blond

9. Very light blond

8. Light blond

7. Medium blond

6. Dark blond

5. Light brown

4. Medium brown

3. Dark brown

2. Very dark brown

1. Black

▲ FIGURE 19-7
The Level System.

Level

The **level** is a unit of measurement used to identify the degree of lightness or darkness of a color. The level of a color reflects its saturation, density, or concentration of color. Colors lighten when mixed with white and darken when mixed with black. In haircoloring, the **level system** is used to analyze the lightness or darkness of a hair color. The colors of hair and of haircolor products are arranged on a scale of 1 to 10, with 1 being the darkest (black) and 10 the lightest (blond) **(Figure 19-7)**. Although the names for the color levels may vary among manufacturers, the level system provides a basic guide for identifying the lightness and darkness of colors, which is necessary for formulating, matching, and correcting colors.

Saturation

Saturation, or intensity, refers to the degree of concentration or amount of pigment in the color. It is the strength of a color. For example, a saturated red is very vivid. Any color can be more or less saturated. The more saturated the product, the more dramatic the change in hair color.

Base Color

Artificial haircolors are developed from primary and secondary colors to form base colors. A **base color** is the predominant tone of a color, which greatly influences the final color result. For example, a violet base color will produce cool results and help to minimize yellow tones. Blue base colors minimize orange tones, and a red-orange base creates warm, bright tones in the hair.

Identifying Natural Level and Tone

The first step in performing a haircolor service is to identify the natural level of the hair. This is accomplished by holding the manufacturer's swatches or a color ring up to the client's hair for matching. It is important to identify the natural level of the hair so that an accurate determination can be made as to what the final hair color results will look like. These results will be based on the combination of the natural hair color and the artificial color that is added to it.

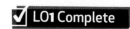

Haircoloring Products

Haircoloring products are categorized as non-oxidative and oxidative and generally fall into four classifications: temporary, semipermanent, demipermanent, and permanent **(Table 19-2)**. These classifications indicate a product's colorfastness, or its ability to remain on the hair, and are determined by the chemical composition and molecular weight of the pigments and dyes within the products **(Table 19-3)**.

TABLE **19-2** Review of Haircolor Classifications and Their Uses

CATEGORY	USES
Temporary color	Some products create fun, bold results that easily shampoo from the hair Others neutralize yellow tones or impart subtle hues
Semipermanent color	Introduces a client to haircolor services Adds subtle color results Tones pre-lightened hair
Demipermanent color	Blends gray hair Enhances natural color Tones pre-lightened hair Refreshes faded color Filler in color correction
Permanent haircolor	Changes existing haircolor Covers gray Creates bright or natural-looking haircolor changes

TABLE **19-3** Four Classifications of Color

CHARACTERISTIC	TEMPORARY	SEMI-PERMANENT	DEMI-PERMANENT	PERMANENT
Molecular weight of dye molecule	Large	Medium	Medium-small	Small
pH	Acid	Slightly alkaline	Moderately alkaline	Alkaline
Reaction or change	Physical	Chemical and physical	Chemical and physical	Chemical and physical
Color fastness	Removed with shampooing	Fades gradually	Fades slower than semipermanent color	Permanent
Color changes	Deposits	Deposits	No-lift, deposit only	Lifts and deposits

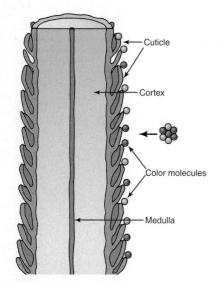

▲ FIGURE 19-8

Action of temporary haircolor.

TEMPORARY HAIRCOLOR (NON-OXIDATION COLOR)

Temporary colors utilize pigment and dye molecules of the greatest molecular weight, making these molecules the largest in the four classifications of hair color. The large size of the color molecule prevents penetration into the cuticle layer, producing only a coating action on the outside of the strand. This coating action usually results in very subtle color changes, lasting only until the next shampoo **(Figure 19-8)**.

The chemical composition of a temporary color is acidic, creating a physical change rather than a chemical change in the hair shaft. As a result, patch tests are not required when applying temporary color. Temporary rinses have a pH range of 2.0 to 4.5.

Types of Temporary Haircolor

- *Color rinses* are used to highlight the existing color or add color to the hair. These rinses contain certified colors and remain on the hair until the next shampoo. Two types of color rinses are available: instant and concentrated. Instant rinses are applied straight from the bottle and remain in the hair. Concentrated rinses are mixed with hot water before application, processed for 5 to 10 minutes, and then rinsed. Both types of rinses may leave traces of the darker shades on combs, brushes, and clothing.

- *Color-enhancing shampoos* combine the action of a color rinse with that of a shampoo. These shampoos generally contain certified colors, produce highlights, and impart slight color tones to the hair.

- *Crayons* are sticks of coloring compounded with soaps or synthetic waxes and are sometimes used to color gray or white hair between hair tint retouches. Crayons are often used by men as a temporary coloring for mustaches. They are available in several standard colors: blond; light, medium, and dark brown; black; and auburn.

- *Haircolor sprays* are applied to dry hair from aerosol containers. Color sprays are usually available in vibrant colors and are generally used for special or party effects.

- *Haircolor mousses and gels* combine slight color and styling effects in one product.

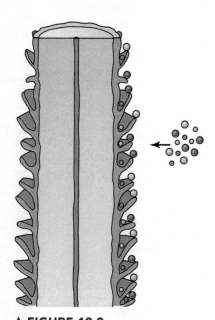

▲ FIGURE 19-9

Action of semipermanent haircolor.

SEMIPERMANENT HAIRCOLOR (NON-OXIDATION COLOR)

Traditional **semipermanent haircolor** products are sometimes known as *direct dyes* because they are not mixed with a developer. Semipermanent pigment molecules are of a lesser molecular weight than those of temporary colors. This facilitates the physical capability to partially penetrate into the cortex. While some color does enter the cortex, most of the pigment molecules stain the cuticle layer through absorption. These molecules are also small enough to diffuse out of the hair during shampooing and tend to fade with each shampoo. Most semipermanent colors will last from six to eight shampoos **(Figure 19-9)**.

The chemical composition of semipermanent color is mildly alkaline, causes the cortex to swell, and raises the cuticle to allow some penetration. This chemical composition combines small color molecules, solvents, alkaline swelling agents (mild oxidizer), and surfactants to create a type of color that is known as self-penetrating. Self-penetrating colors tend to make a mild chemical change as well as a physical change.

Most semipermanent colors do not contain ammonia and may be used right out of the bottle. Although normally gentle on the hair, semipermanent colors require a patch test prior to application to prevent the occurrence of product sensitivity or allergic reaction.

Semipermanent haircolors typically fall within the 7.0 to 9.0 pH range; however, some formulations use salt bonds to improve colorfastness and may range between 7.0 and 8.0 on the pH scale. Due to the slight alkalinity of semipermanent color, these haircolor services should be followed with a mild, acid-balanced shampoo and conditioning. This will neutralize any residual alkalinity and help to restore the hair to normal pH levels.

Semipermanent haircolor may be used to:

- cover or blend partially gray hair without affecting its natural color (most semipermanent colors are designed to cover hair that is no more than 25 percent gray).

- highlight, enhance, or deepen color tones in the hair.

- serve as a non-peroxide toner for pre-lightened hair.

DEMIPERMANENT HAIRCOLOR (OXIDATION COLOR)

Demipermanent haircolor, also known as *no-lift, deposit-only haircolor* is longer lasting than semipermanent color. These products are designed to deposit color without lifting (lightening) natural or artificial color in the hair and are considered a type of oxidation color. As such, they are not used directly out of the bottle but must be mixed with a low-volume developer or activator immediately before use. The oxidizing agent in the developer causes an oxidation reaction, which develops the color **(Figure 19-10).**

Demipermanent and other deposit-only colors darken the natural hair color when applied. They are available in gel, cream, or liquid forms and require a patch test before application.

Demipermanent haircolor may be used to:

- impart vivid color results.

- cover non-pigmented hair.

- refresh faded permanent color.

- deposit tonal changes without lift.

- reverse highlight.

- perform corrective coloring.

During the 1990s, some manufacture labeled their tube color products as semipermanent color even though mild developer wa required. Since the most manufacturer have adopted the demipermanent co classification for th products.

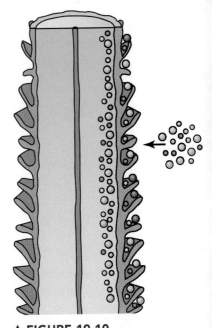

▲ **FIGURE 19-10**

Action of demipermanent color.

PERMANENT HAIRCOLOR (OXIDATION COLOR)

Permanent haircolor is mixed with a developer (hydrogen peroxide) and remains in the hair shaft. When the hair grows, a touch-up or retouch application is required to blend the color of the previously colored hair with the new hair growth. Permanent haircolor products usually contain ammonia, oxidative tints, and peroxide and require a patch test.

Permanent haircolor products can lighten and deposit color in one process. They can lighten natural hair color because they are more alkaline than demipermanent oxidation colors and are usually mixed with a higher-volume developer. The amount of lift is controlled by the pH of the color and the concentration of peroxide in the developer. As the pH of the color and concentration increase, the amount of lift increases as well. Permanent haircolor products are usually mixed with an equal amount of 20-volume peroxide and are capable of lifting one or two levels. When mixed with higher volumes of peroxide, permanent colors can lift up to four levels. Since some manufacturers recommend a 2:1 ratio of developer to haircolor, always read the manufacturer's directions.

Permanent haircolor is considered a penetrating tint because after the tint is mixed with an oxidizer it has the ability to penetrate through the cuticle into the cortex of the hair shaft. This action is facilitated by **aniline derivatives** that diffuse into the cortex and then form larger permanent tint molecules that become trapped within the cortex. In this way, the cortex undergoes permanent chemical and structural changes **(Figure 19-11)**.

Permanent tints are alkaline in reaction and generally range between 9.0 and 10.5 on the pH scale. After processing, the hair is shampooed and as it dries it begins to return to its normal pH. This causes the cortex to shrink and the cuticle to close. Both actions tend to further trap the color molecules. Except for residual color product following the haircolor application, permanent haircolor does not wash out during the shampoo process. Eventually the color will fade and may require refreshing. When new growth occurs, a **line of demarcation** will develop between the old and new growth and will require a retouch.

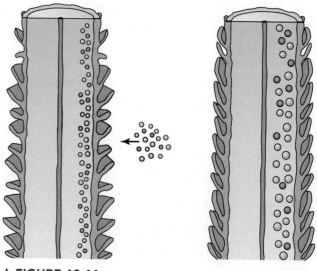

▲ **FIGURE 19-11**

Action of permanent haircolor.

Permanent haircoloring products are generally regarded as the best products for covering gray hair. This is because they simultaneously remove natural pigment through the action of lifting and add artificial color to both the gray and pigmented hair.

TYPES OF PERMANENT HAIRCOLOR

Permanent hair colors fall into four classifications: oxidation tints, vegetable tints, metallic or mineral dyes, and compound dyes.

Oxidation Tints

Oxidation tints are also known as aniline derivative tints, penetrating tints, synthetic-organic tints, and amino tints. Oxidation tints can lighten and deposit color in a single process and are available in a wide variety of colors. *Toners* also fall into the category of permanent color. **Toners** are aniline derivative products of pale, delicate shades designed for use on pre-lightened hair.

Most oxidation tints contain aniline derivatives and require a predisposition (patch) test before the service is performed. As long as the hair is of normal strength and kept in good condition, oxidation tints are compatible with other professional chemical services.

Oxidation tints are sold in bottles, canisters, and tubes, in either a semi-liquid or cream form. These products must be mixed with hydrogen peroxide, which activates the chemical reaction known as oxidation. This reaction begins as soon as the two compounds are combined, so the mixed tint must be used immediately. Any leftover tint must be discarded since it deteriorates quickly.

Timing the application of the tint depends upon the product and the volume of peroxide selected. Consult the manufacturer's directions and your instructor for assistance. A strand test should always be performed to ensure satisfactory results.

Vegetable Tints

Vegetable tints are haircoloring products made from various plants, such as herbs and flowers. In the past, indigo, chamomile, sage, Egyptian henna, and other plants were used to color the hair. Henna is still used as a professional haircoloring product, but should be used with some caution. Henna has a coating action that can build up with overuse and prevent the penetration of other chemicals. Henna also penetrates the cortex and attaches to the salt bonds. Both of these actions may leave the hair unfit for other professional treatments. Even though vegetable tints are considered permanent, they are non-oxidation color products.

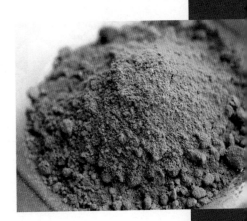

Metallic or Mineral Dyes

Metallic dyes are advertised as color restorers or **progressive colors.** The metallic ingredients, such as lead acetate or silver nitrate, react with the keratin in the hair, turning it brown. This reaction creates a colored film coating that produces a dull metallic appearance. Repeated treatments damage the hair and can react adversely with many professional chemical services. Metallic dyes are not professional coloring products.

Compound Dyes

Compound dyes are metallic or mineral dyes combined with a vegetable tint. The metallic salts are added to give the product more staying power and to create different colors. Like metallic dyes, compound dyes are not used professionally.

HYDROGEN PEROXIDE DEVELOPERS

A **developer** is an oxidizing agent that supplies oxygen gas for the development of color molecules when mixed with an oxidative haircolor product. This action creates a color change in the hair when the oxidizer combines with the melanin in the hair. Most developers range between 2.5 and 4.5 on the pH scale.

Hydrogen peroxide (H_2O_2) serves as the primary oxidizing agent used in haircoloring. As the oxygen and melanin combine, the peroxide solution begins to diffuse and lighten the melanin within the cortex. The smaller structure and spread-out distribution of the diffused melanin gives the hair a lighter appearance. This diffused melanin is called oxymelanin.

In its purest form, hydrogen peroxide has a pH level of about 7.0. When diluted with water and other substances for use in haircoloring, hydrogen peroxide has a mildly acidic pH of 3.5 to 4.0.

Strengths of Hydrogen Peroxide

Hydrogen peroxide alone produces a relatively mild lightening of the hair color and causes little damage to the hair shaft. When very pale shades are desired, however, further lightening must occur and a longer processing time or a stronger formula is required.

In the scientific world, different strengths of hydrogen peroxide are identified as percentages. In haircoloring, the term *volume* is used to denote the different strengths of hydrogen peroxide (**Table 19-4**). **Volume** is the measure of the potential oxidation of varying strengths of hydrogen peroxide. The lower the volume, the less lift is achieved; the higher the volume, the greater the lifting action.

> **TABLE 19-4** Percentages and Volumes of Hydrogen Peroxide

PERCENTAGE OF H_2O_2 IN WATER	VOLUME OF OXYGEN SET FREE
1.5%	5
3%	10
6%	20
9%	30
12%	40

Permanent haircolor products use 10-, 20-, 30-, or 40-volume hydrogen peroxide for proper color development. A 10-volume solution is recommended when less lightening is desired for color enhancement. The majority of permanent coloring products use 20-volume hydrogen peroxide for proper color development and to cover gray. A 30-volume developer is used to achieve additional lift and 40-volume developer is used with most high-lift colors to provide maximum lift in one step.

Hydrogen peroxide is distributed for use under a variety of names that include developer, oxidizer, generator, and catalyst. Regardless of the name used, hydrogen peroxide is available in three forms: dry, cream, and liquid.

- *Dry peroxide*, in either tablet or powder form, is dissolved in liquid hydrogen peroxide to boost the volume. The availability of liquid peroxide in a variety of volumes has made this product somewhat obsolete.

- *Cream peroxides* contain additives such as thickeners, drabbers, conditioners, and acids for stabilization. The thickeners help to create a product that tends to stay moist on the hair longer than liquid peroxide, is easy to control, and does not drip during the brush-and-bowl method of application.

- *Liquid hydrogen peroxide* contains a stabilizing acid that brings the pH to between 3.5 and 4.0. This form of peroxide is convenient because it can be used with most of today's bleach and tint formulas.

FYI Additives in cream peroxides may dilute the strength of the formula and make it undesirable when full strength is needed.

Hydrogen Peroxide Safety Precautions

- Use clean implements when measuring, using, and storing hydrogen peroxide. Even a small amount of dirt or impurities can cause hydrogen peroxide to deteriorate.

- Never measure the needed amount of hydrogen peroxide by pouring it into the lid of another product. The residue will cause the product in the container to oxidize as it sits on the shelf and render it unusable.

- Do not allow hydrogen peroxide formulations to come in contact with metal. Metal causes the oxidation process to occur too quickly to allow proper color development.

- Avoid breathing in vapors caused by mixing hydrogen peroxide and haircolor products.

- A hydrogen peroxide volume of 20 or more can cause skin irritations, chemical burns, and hair damage.

CAUTION

Plastic bottles of hydrogen peroxide that develop a bulge should be disposed of immediately. The bulge indicates that oxygen atoms have escaped from the hydrogen peroxide and are building up pressure within the container. Open with extreme caution!

Activators

An **activator** is an oxidizer that is added to hydrogen peroxide for the purpose of increasing its chemical action. This results in an increased lifting power, which is controlled by the number of activators that are added to the peroxide. Up to three activators can be used for on-the-scalp applications, and up to four for off-the-scalp processes.

✓ **LO2 Complete**

LIGHTENERS

Lighteners are chemical compounds that lighten hair by dispersing, dissolving, and decolorizing the natural or artificial hair pigment **(Figure 19-12)**. This is accomplished through the use of a bleach formula, hydrogen peroxide, and the chemical heat produced by the combination of these ingredients. When mixed for use, the pH of lighteners is around 10.0.

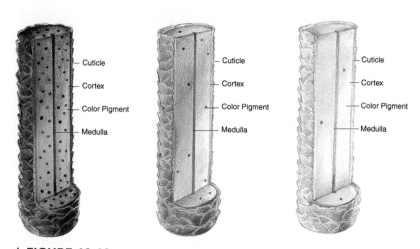

▲ **FIGURE 19-12**
Hair lighteners diffuse pigment.

The hair pigment goes through different stages of color as it lightens. The amount of change depends on how much pigment the hair has, the strength of the lightening agent, and the length of time it is processed. During the decolorization process, natural hair may go through up to 10 stages of lightening from the darkest to the lightest: natural black hair can lighten through the brown and/or red stages to orange, gold, to yellow, and finally to pale yellow **(Figure 19-13)**.

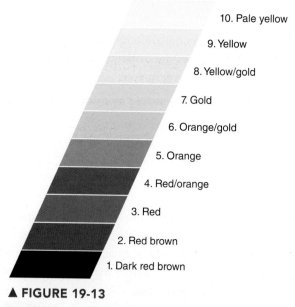

10. Pale yellow

9. Yellow

8. Yellow/gold

7. Gold

6. Orange/gold

5. Orange

4. Red/orange

3. Red

2. Red brown

1. Dark red brown

▲ **FIGURE 19-13**
Ten degrees of decolorization.

Hair lighteners are used to create blond shades that are not possible with permanent haircolor and to achieve the following effects:

- Lighten the hair to the final shade
- **Pre-lighten** the hair to prepare it for the application of a toner or tint (double-process application)
- Lighten the hair to a particular shade
- Brighten and lighten an existing shade of color

Types of Lighteners

Lighteners are available in three forms: oil, cream, and powder. Oil and cream lighteners are considered **on-the-scalp lighteners** and powder lighteners are **off-the-scalp lighteners.** Each type has unique abilities, chemical compositions, and formulation procedures.

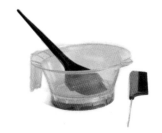

- *Oil lighteners* are usually mixtures of hydrogen peroxide with sulfonated oil. As on-the-scalp lighteners, they are the mildest form of lightener and may be used when only one or two levels of lift are desired.

- *Color oil lighteners* add temporary color and highlight the hair as they lighten. They contain certified colors, may be used without a patch test, and remove pigment while adding color tones. Color oil lighteners are classified according to their action on the hair as follows:

    ▶ *Gold:* lightens and adds golden to reddish tones depending on the base color of the hair

    ▶ *Silver:* lightens and adds silvery highlights to gray or white hair and minimizes red and gold tones in other shades

    ▶ *Red:* lightens and adds red highlights

    ▶ *Drab:* lightens and adds ash highlights. Tones down or reduces red and gold tones

- *Neutral oil lighteners* remove pigment without adding color tone. These oil lighteners may be used to pre-soften hair for a tint application.

- *Cream lighteners* are the most popular type of on-the-scalp lightener. They contain conditioning agents, bluing, and thickeners, which makes them easy to apply, and will not run, drip, or dry out. Cream lighteners provide the following benefits:

    ▶ The conditioning agents give some protection to the hair.

    ▶ The bluing agent helps to drab undesirable red and gold tones.

    ▶ The thickener provides control during application and prevents overlap.

- *Powder lighteners,* also called paste or quick lighteners, contain an oxygen-releasing booster and inert substances for quicker and stronger action. Paste lighteners will hold and not run, but do not contain conditioning agents and tend to dry out quickly.

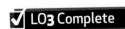

LO3 Complete

Contribution of Underlying Pigment

The natural pigment that remains in the hair after lightening contributes to the artificial color that is added. It is essential to lighten the hair to the correct stage because the pigment that remains in the hair will impact the final result of the hair lightening and coloring process.

Use **Figure 19-14** as a guide to determine the contributing pigment or undertones of color at various hair color levels.

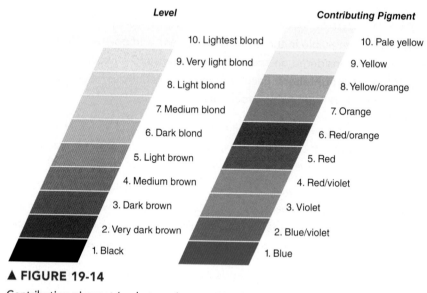

Level	Contributing Pigment
10. Lightest blond	10. Pale yellow
9. Very light blond	9. Yellow
8. Light blond	8. Yellow/orange
7. Medium blond	7. Orange
6. Dark blond	6. Red/orange
5. Light brown	5. Red
4. Medium brown	4. Red/violet
3. Dark brown	3. Violet
2. Very dark brown	2. Blue/violet
1. Black	1. Blue

▲ **FIGURE 19-14**

Contributing pigment (undertones).

TONERS

A toner is a haircoloring product that is applied to pre-lightened hair for the purpose of achieving the desired color or tones in the hair. Traditional toners are permanent aniline derivative haircoloring products that have a smaller percentage of the formula that creates delicate shades of color. Toners differ from tints only in the degree of color saturation and require a patch test.

Toners are available in pale, delicate colors. They usually have a very different color than the final shade that they produce and may appear to be purple, blue, orange, or pink in the bottle. As toner color oxidizes, it goes through several visual color changes; therefore, a strand test should be done to determine the processing time required for a desired shade.

After the hair goes through the desired stages of lightening, the color left in the hair is known as its foundation or contributing color. Achieving the correct foundation is necessary for proper toner development. This is usually the lightest degree of contributing pigment that remains after the lightening process.

Toner manufacturers provide literature that recommends the proper foundation to achieve a desired color. As a general rule, the more pale the desired color, the lighter the foundation must be. It is important to follow the guide closely. Over-lightened hair will grab the base color of the toner, while under-lightened hair will appear to have more red, yellow, or orange than the intended color.

Since toning is more of a technique than a particular product, semipermanent, demipermanent, and permanent haircolor can also be used as "toners" to achieve the desired hair color.

CAUTION: Advise clients that lightening dark hair to a pale blond tone can be very damaging to the hair.

DYE REMOVERS

The removal of haircoloring agents is sometimes desired if the client wants to change to a lighter shade, if a coloring mistake has been made, or if the hair has processed too dark due to an overly porous condition. **Dye removers** are also known as color or tint removers.

There are two basic types of products available to remove artificial pigment from the hair: oil-based products, which remove color buildup or stain from the cuticle layer of the hair shaft; and dye solvents, which diffuse and dissolve artificial pigment within the cortical layer.

- *Oil-base dye removers* lift trapped color pigments from cuticle layers and do not create structural changes in the hair shaft or pigment (natural or artificial) of the hair. These dye removers will not make drastic changes in the level of color.

- *Dye solvents* produce strong lightening effects on melanin and artificial pigment, are non-allergenic, and do not require a predisposition test. Follow the manufacturer's directions carefully.

FILLERS

Fillers are preparations designed to correct excessive porosity and/or to create a color base in the hair by penetrating the cuticle and filling in small holes in the hair. This action helps to even out porosity levels within the hair shaft that can cause uneven color deposit or lightening. The two general classifications of conditioner fillers are protein and non-protein, both of which are manufactured in gel, cream, and liquid forms. In addition to protein, color fillers may also contain conditioning agents, direct dyes, or other additives to correct high porosity and are available in clear, neutral, and a variety of color bases.

STAIN REMOVERS

Generally, soap and water will remove most tint stains from the skin. Stain removers are commercially prepared solutions that are designed for this purpose. When soap and water is not capable of removing haircolor from the skin, use one of the following methods:

- Dampen a piece of cotton with the leftover tint. Use a rotary movement to cover the stained areas and follow with a damp towel. Apply a small amount of face cream and wipe clean.

- Use a prepared stain remover.

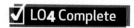

Haircoloring Procedures Terminology

Successful haircoloring usually requires a series of steps to accomplish the desired end result. Due to the wide range of haircoloring products, application methods, and procedures, it is important to have a clear understanding of the terms used in haircoloring processes. Some common procedural terms are *patch test, strand test, soap cap, tint back, record keeping,* and the *client consultation.*

PATCH TEST

An individual's reaction to aniline derivative tints can be unpredictable. Some clients may show an immediate sensitivity, while others may suddenly develop an allergy to the product after years of use. To identify a client who has a sensitivity to aniline derivatives, the U.S. Federal Food, Drug, and Cosmetic Act prescribes that a **patch test,** also known as a *predisposition test,* be given 24 to 48 hours prior to each application of an aniline derivative tint or toner.

STRAND TEST

A **strand test** is performed for color applications to determine how the hair will react to the haircolor product, how long it will take to process, and what the final outcome will look like. After the results of the patch test, the strand test is the next step in performing a haircolor service.

Patch Test

SUPPLIES

- Towels
- Waterproof drape
- Cotton-tipped applicator
- Gloves
- Haircoloring product
- Developer
- Small container for mixing color
- Client record card

PREPARATION

1. Wash your hands.
2. Conduct client consultation.
3. Perform hair and scalp analysis.
4. Select and arrange required materials.
5. Drape client for a chemical service.

PROCEDURE

1 Apply gloves. Select the test area, either behind the ear extending partly into the hairline or on the inside of the elbow.

2 Cleanse an area about the size of a quarter with mild soap and water.

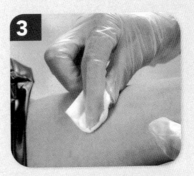

3 Dry the test area by patting with absorbent cotton or a clean towel.

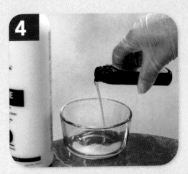

4 Prepare a small amount of the test solution according to the manufacturer's directions.

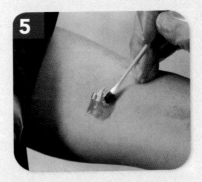

5 Apply solution to the test area with a cotton-tipped applicator.

6 Leave the test area uncovered and undisturbed for 24 hours.

7 Examine the test area for either negative or positive reactions.

8 A negative skin test will show no signs of inflammation and indicates that the color may be safely applied.

9 A positive skin test is recognized by the presence of redness, swelling, burning, itching, blisters, or eruptions. The client may also suffer from a headache and vomiting. A client showing such symptoms is allergic to aniline derivative tint, and under no circumstances should this particular kind of tint be used. The client should get immediate medical attention to avoid further complications.

10 Record the results on the client record card.

CLEAN-UP AND DISINFECTION

1. Discard disposal items.

2. Sanitize chair and workstation.

3. Dispose of towels.

4. Store products, materials, and record card.

5. Wash your hands.

Strand Test

SUPPLIES

- Towels
- Waterproof drape
- Gloves
- Tail comb
- Hair clips (plastic)
- Foil
- Haircoloring product
- Developer
- Tint bowl and brush
- Timer
- Spray water bottle
- Client record card

PREPARATION

1. Wash your hands.
2. Conduct client consultation.
3. Perform hair and scalp analysis.
4. Select and arrange required materials.
5. Drape client for a chemical service.

PROCEDURE

1 Apply gloves. Part off a $\frac{1}{2}$" square parting from the lower crown area just above the occipital. Use plastic clips to secure surrounding hair out of the way.

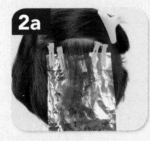 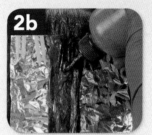

2 Place the parting of hair over a piece of foil. Formulate haircolor mixture according to manufacturer's directions and apply to the hair strand.

3 Check the development time at 5-minute intervals until the desired color is achieved. Note the time on the record card.

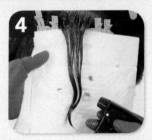

4 Once the color has developed, remove the foil and place a towel under the section. Mist thoroughly with water, add shampoo, and massage through the strand. Rinse by further misting, towel dry the strand, and observe the results.

5 Adjust the timing, product formulation, or application method as necessary and proceed with the color service.

CLEAN-UP AND DISINFECTION

1. Discard disposable items.
2. Sanitize chair and workstation.
3. Dispose of towels.
4. Store products, materials, and record card.
5. Wash your hands.

SOAP CAP

A **soap cap** is a combination of equal parts of a prepared haircolor product and shampoo that is applied like a regular shampoo. Soap caps can be used to brighten existing color, reduce unwanted yellow tones in gray hair, or blend lines of demarcation when a retouch application does not quite match the former color application.

TINT BACK

Tint back is the term used to describe the process of returning hair to its natural shade. It is important to keep in mind that previously processed hair will be more porous and, therefore, will process more quickly and possibly darker than intended. In some cases, a filler is required to even out the hair's porosity level or to achieve accurate color correction. A demipermanent haircoloring product is usually an effective choice because it is a deposit-only color formulation with minimal oxidation. Highlighting shampoos are mixtures of shampoo and hydrogen peroxide that can be used to slightly lighten hair color and are applied in the same manner.

RECORD KEEPING

Before performing a haircoloring service, a client record card should be completed for each client **(Figure 19-15).** The client record card is used to log all information pertaining to the haircoloring service. In addition to the client's contact information, the record card should be descriptive enough that it provides preservice and post-service data about the client's hair. For example, key information items should include characteristics of the hair's condition, scalp condition, haircolor history, any corrective treatments, and the results of the haircoloring process. This information can be used for future visits as a basis for other services and should be maintained from one visit to the next.

A release statement form should be used when the client's hair is in a questionable condition that may not withstand chemical processes and treatments. See **Figure 19-16** for a sample barber school release form. To some degree, the release statement is designed to protect the shop owner from responsibility for accidents and damages and is a requirement of most malpractice insurance. It should be noted, however, that a release statement is not a legally binding contract and will not fully protect the barber or the shop from liability.

HAIRCOLOR RECORD

Name _____   Tel. _____

Address _____   City _____

Patch Test: ☐ Negative ☐ Positive   Date _____

Eye Color _____   Skin Tone _____

DESCRIPTION OF HAIR

Form	Length	Texture	Density	Porosity	
☐ straight	☐ short	☐ coarse	☐ sparse	☐ very porous	☐ resistant
☐ wavy	☐ medium	☐ medium	☐ moderate	☐ porous	☐ very resistant
☐ curly	☐ long	☐ fine	☐ thick	☐ normal	☐ perm. waved

Natural hair color _____

          level   Tone   Intensity
          (1-10)   (Warm, Cool, etc.)   (Mild, Medium, Strong)

Scalp Condition
☐ normal   ☐ dry   ☐ oily   ☐ sensitive

Condition
☐ normal   ☐ dry   ☐ oily   ☐ faded   ☐ streaked (uneven)

% unpigmented _____ Distribution of unpigmented _____

Previously lightened with _____ for _____ (time)

Previously tinted with _____ for _____ (time)

☐ original hair sample enclosed   ☐ original hair sample not enclosed

Desired hair color _____

          level   Tone   Intensity
          (1-10)   (Warm, Cool, etc.)   (Mild, Medium, Strong)

CORRECTIVE TREATMENTS

Color filler used _____ Conditioning treatments with _____

HAIR TINTING PROCESS

whole head _____ retouch inches (cm) _____ shade desired _____

formula: (color/lightener) _____ application technique _____

Results: ☐ good   ☐ poor   ☐ too light   ☐ too dark   ☐ streaked

Comments: _____

_____

_____

_____

Date	Operator	Price	Date	Operator	Price

▲ **FIGURE 19-15**

Haircolor record card.

RELEASE FORM

I, the undersigned, _____
                              (name)

residing at _____
                              (street, address)

_____
                              (city, state and zip)

about to receive services in the Clinical Department of
_____

and having been advised that the services shall be performed by either students, graduate students, and/or instructors of the school, in consideration of the nominal charge for such services, hereby release the school, its students, graduate students, instructors, agents, representatives, and/or employees, from any and all claims arising out of and in any way connected with the performance of these services.

The Proprietor Is Not Responsible for Personal Property

Signed _____

Date _____

Witnessed _____

THIS RELEASE FORM MUST BE SIGNED BY THE PARENT OR GUARDIAN IF THE CLIENT BEING SERVED IS UNDER 18 YEARS OF AGE.

▲ **FIGURE 19-16**

Sample school release form.

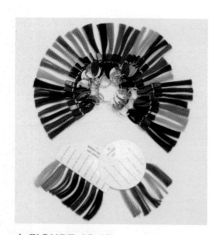

▲ **FIGURE 19-17a**

Use color swatches to determine the natural level.

CLIENT CONSULTATION

A thorough client consultation is the first step in a haircoloring service. Consultations should be held in a well-lit room that provides either a strong natural light or incandescent lighting. Fluorescent lighting is not suitable for judging existing hair colors.

Use the following as a guide to perform a haircoloring service consultation:

1. Drape the client.
2. Have the client fill out a client record card.
3. Perform a hair and scalp analysis and log the results on a record card. Use color swatches to determine client's natural level **(Figure 19-17a)**.
4. Ask the client leading questions about the desired end result to determine the preferred color, product (temporary, permanent, etc.), and method (all-over color, highlights, etc.).

5. Show examples of appropriate colors and make a determination with the client (**Figure 17b**).

6. Review the procedure, application technique, maintenance, and cost with the client.

7. Gain approval and begin the service.

8. Record end results on the client record card.

HAIRCOLOR APPLICATION TERMS

There are a variety of different haircolor application methods. Review the following to become familiar with the terms used in haircoloring procedures.

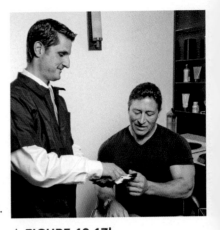

▲ **FIGURE 19-17b**
Discuss appropriate colors with client.

Virgin Application

A **virgin application** is the application of haircolor to hair that has not been previously colored. Hair that is in a "virgin" state is usually healthy hair that has not suffered any chemical damage. A virgin application also indicates that the haircoloring product will be applied to the entire hair strand versus the new growth only.

Retouch Application

When permanent haircolor or lighteners are used, new hair growth will become obvious between haircolor applications. The new growth, or re-growth, is that section of the hair shaft between the scalp and the hair that has been previously treated. This creates a line of demarcation between the natural color of the hair and the previously colored or lightened hair that requires blending by way of another color or lightener application. The term **retouch application** is used to describe this blending process.

Single-Process Haircoloring

Single-process haircoloring is a process that lightens (or lifts) and deposits color in the hair in a single application. Examples of single-process coloring are virgin tint applications and tint retouch applications. Single-process haircoloring is also known as single-application coloring, one-step coloring, one-step tinting, and single-application tinting.

Double-Process Haircoloring

Double-process hair coloring requires two separate and distinct applications to achieve the desired color. The hair is lightened before the depositing color is applied, allowing the practitioner to independently control the lightening and coloring actions. Double-process haircoloring is also known as double-application coloring, two-step coloring, two-step tinting, and double-application tinting. Double-process haircoloring may include the use of lighteners and toners, pre-softeners and tints, or fillers and color.

Pre-softening

Pre-softening is the process of treating gray or other extremely resistant hair types to facilitate better color penetration. Pre-softening swells and opens the cuticle. It can be accomplished with a mixture of 1 ounce of 20-volume peroxide and 8 drops of 28 percent ammonia water, or with an oil or cream bleach product.

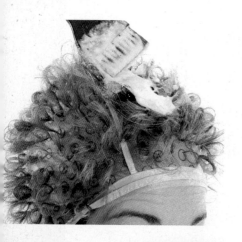

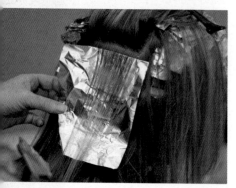

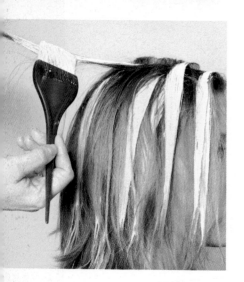

Highlighting

Highlighting is the process of coloring some of the hair strands lighter than the natural or artificial color to add the illusion of sheen and depth. Frosting, tipping, and streaking are forms of highlighting.

Lowlighting

Lowlighting or *reverse highlighting* is the process of coloring strands or sections of the hair darker than the natural or artificial color. Contrasting dark areas appear to recede and make detail less visible to the eye.

Cap Technique

The **cap technique** involves pulling strands of hair through the holes of a perforated cap with a plastic or metal hook. The number of strands pulled through the cap determines the degree of highlighting or lowlighting that is achieved.

Foil Technique

The **foil technique** involves slicing or weaving out sections of hair to be placed on a piece of foil. The color or lightening product is usually brushed onto the hair section, after which the foil is folded and sealed for processing.

Free-Form Technique

The **free-form technique**, or *balyage* (also spelled baliage), is the process of painting a lightener or color directly onto clean, styled hair. The effects can be subtle or dramatic, depending on the type of product (color or lightener) and the amount of hair that it is applied to.

Haircoloring Product Applications

Given the many choices in haircoloring formulations and applications, it is crucial that the barber provides the client with the appropriate product and follows the correct application methods. Use the following as a guide for haircoloring product selection and application.

TEMPORARY COLOR RINSES

Temporary color rinses may be used to give clients a preview of how a color change will look. They are also a satisfactory option for clients who want to highlight the color of their hair or add slight color to gray hair. These rinses wash out when shampooed and are available in a variety of color shades. Temporary rinses are easily and quickly applied at the shampoo bowl and can serve as an introduction to other, longer lasting color services.

Temporary color rinses can be used to bring out highlights, temporarily restore faded hair color to its natural shade, neutralize yellow tones in white or gray hair, or tone down over-lightened hair. Perform a preliminary strand test to determine proper color selection.

Temporary Color Rinse

SUPPLIES

- Temporary color product
- Applicator bottle (optional)
- Waterproof cape
- Towels
- Protective gloves
- Shampoo
- Color chart
- Record card
- Timer
- Comb

PREPARATION

NOTE: If the client is to receive a haircut, perform the cut prior to the color rinse application.

1. Assemble all necessary supplies.

2. Prepare the client and drape with towels and waterproof cape.

3. Examine the client's scalp and hair.

4. Select the desired shade of color rinse.

5. Perform a strand test.

PROCEDURE

1 Shampoo, rinse, and towel blot hair. Excess moisture must be removed to prevent diluting the color. Put on gloves.

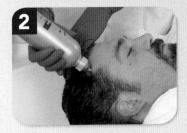

2 With the client reclined at the shampoo bowl, apply the color from the hairline through and around the entire head.

4 Do not rinse product. Towel blot excess water.

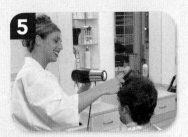

3 Use the comb to blend the color, applying more as necessary for even coverage.

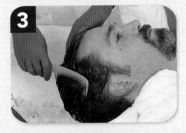

5 Proceed with styling.

CLEAN-UP AND DISINFECTION

1. Discard all disposable supplies.

2. Close and wipe off containers and store properly.

3. Sanitize implements, cape, and work area.

4. Wash hands.

5. Record results on client record card.

SEMIPERMANENT HAIRCOLOR

Semipermanent haircolor products are appropriate for the client who may want more color change than is available with a temporary rinse, but who is hesitant about a permanent color change and its related maintenance. In this way, a semipermanent tint fills the gap between temporary color rinses and permanent haircolor without replacing either of them.

Since semipermanent products are deposit-only colors, the final outcome will depend on the hair's original color and texture, the color that is applied, and the length of development time. These haircoloring products are available in liquid and cream forms in a variety of colors. Some formulations are specifically designed in blue-gray or silver-gray hues to brighten or blend gray color tones.

Characteristics of Semipermanent Tints

The basic characteristics of semipermanent haircolor that influence the decision to choose this color product over another are as follows:

- Semipermanent tints do not require the addition of hydrogen peroxide.

- The color is self-penetrating.

- The color is applied the same way each time.

- Retouching is eliminated.

- The color does not rub off, because it has penetrated the hair shaft slightly.

- Hair will usually return to its natural color after six to eight shampoos, provided a mild, non-stripping shampoo is used.

- Semipermanent tints require a 24-hour patch test.

- Some semipermanent haircolors require pre-shampooing; others do not.

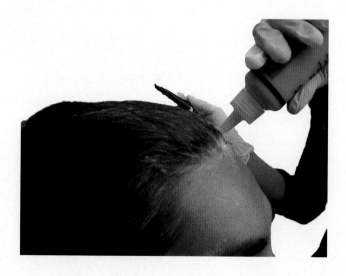

Selecting Semipermanent Color

The addition of artificial color to the natural pigment in the hair shafts creates a darker color. When using a color chart to determine the level and shade of semipermanent color to use, consider the natural color to represent half of the formula. Use the following guide to select the correct color to perform the strand test.

- On hair with no gray (solid), select a color level that is two levels lighter than the desired shade. For example: A client with a natural level of 6 desires a level 7 shade. Therefore, a level 9 shade of color should be used.

- The use of ash or cool shades will create a color that appears darker than if a warm shade is applied.

- Warm colors appear shinier due to the reflection of light.

- For clients with less than 50 percent gray, select a shade that matches the natural hair color.

- For clients with 50 percent or more gray hair, select a color one shade darker than the natural hair color.

Special Problems

Some semipermanent haircolor products have a tendency to build up on the hair shaft with repeated applications. If this should occur, apply the color to the new growth only, process until the desired color shade develops, then wet the hair with warm water and blend the color through the hair with a large-toothed comb.

DEMIPERMANENT HAIRCOLOR

Since demipermanent color is considered to be deposit-only color, the same procedures used for the application of a semipermanent haircolor product can be employed. Follow the manufacturer's guidelines for application, color selection, and processing time.

PERMANENT HAIRCOLOR

Practically all professional permanent haircoloring is done with oxidizing penetrating tints that contain aniline derivatives. These penetrating tints are considered either single-process or double-process tints and are available in liquid, cream, and gel forms.

SUPPLIES

- Semipermanent or demipermanent color product
- Color chart
- Applicator bottle or brush
- Shampoo cape
- Towels
- Protective gloves
- Shampoo
- Conditioner
- Comb
- Plastic clips (optional, depending on length of hair)
- Plastic cap (optional, depending on manufacturer's directions)
- Cotton
- Protective cream
- Record card
- Timer

PREPARATION

1. Perform a preliminary patch test 24 hours before the service. Proceed only if the test is negative.

2. Perform client consultation and record results on client record card.

3. Drape client and apply protective cream.

4. Perform a strand test and record the results.

PROCEDURE

1 Shampoo, rinse, and towel blot hair per manufacturer's directions for product type.

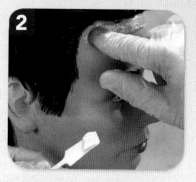

2 Part the hair into four sections. Put on gloves. Apply protective cream to hairline.

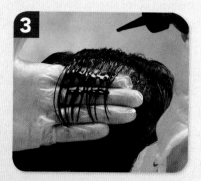

3 Working with $\frac{1}{4}$" to $\frac{1}{2}$" subsections, apply color to the entire hair shaft from scalp to ends. Use an applicator bottle or brush depending on the product's consistency. With the fingers, gently work the color through the hair until it is thoroughly saturated. Do not massage into the scalp. If the hair is long, pile it loosely on the top of the head.

4 Apply plastic cap if so instructed by the manufacturer's directions.

5 Process according to strand test results and manufacturer's directions. Check color.

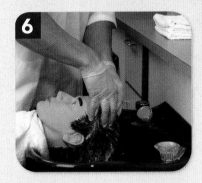

6 Following color development, wet client's hair with warm water, lather, and work through hair.

7 Rinse thoroughly, shampoo, and condition. Remove stains as necessary.

8 Rinse, towel blot, and style.

CLEAN-UP AND DISINFECTION

1. Discard all disposable supplies.

2. Close and wipe off containers and store properly.

3. Sanitize implements and tools, cape, and work area.

4. Wash hands.

5. Record results on client record card.

SINGLE-PROCESS HAIRCOLORING

Single-process tints provide a simplified method of haircoloring. In one application, the hair can be colored permanently without requiring pre-shampooing, pre-softening, or **pre-lightening**. Single-process tints usually contain a lightening agent, shampoo, aniline derivative tint, and an alkalizing agent to activate the peroxide. Most color is formulated for use with 20-volume hydrogen peroxide. When other volumes of peroxide are used, the color results change. The choice of colors varies from deepest black to lightest blond.

Characteristics of Single-Process Tints

A single-application tint is applied on dry hair. If the hair is extremely oily or dirty and a shampoo is necessary, it must be dried thoroughly before applying the tint. Some characteristics of single-process tints are that they:

- save time by eliminating pre-shampooing or pre-lightening.

- color the hair lighter or darker than the client's natural color.

- blend in gray or white hair to match the client's natural hair color.

- tone down streaks, off-shades, discoloration, and faded hair ends.

Color Selection of Single-Process Tints

The porosity of the hair is one of the most important characteristics to consider when choosing hair color tint shades. Use the following guide for choosing the level of color when tinting darker.

- *Normal porosity:* half level lighter than desired color

- *Slightly porous:* one level lighter than desired color

- *Very porous:* one to two levels lighter than desired color

General rules for single-process color selection for gray hair include:

- To match the natural color of hair and to cover gray, select the color closest to the natural shade.

- To brighten or lighten hair color and to cover gray, select a shade lighter than the natural color. The selected tint must contain enough color to produce the desired shade on gray hair.

- To darken the hair and cover gray, select a color darker than the natural hair color.

- Study the manufacturer's color chart for correct color selections.

Use the following formula for color selection when tinting lighter than the natural color.

Formulation Step Example:

1. Identify the desired level.   6
2. Identify the natural level.   − 4
3. Subtract the natural level from the desired level.   2
4. Add the level difference to the desired level.   +6
5. Total is the level of color needed.   8

Single-Process Permanent Color Applications: Virgin and Retouch

SUPPLIES

- Single-process permanent color product
- Hydrogen peroxide
- Color chart
- Applicator bottle or brush and bowl
- Shampoo cape
- Towels
- Protective gloves
- Shampoo
- Conditioner
- Comb
- Plastic clips (optional, depending on length of hair)
- Plastic cap (optional, depending on manufacturer's directions)
- Cotton
- Protective cream
- Record card
- Timer

PREPARATION

1. Perform a preliminary patch test 24 hours before the service. Proceed only if the test is negative.

2. Perform client consultation and record results on client record card.

3. Drape client and apply protective cream.

4. Perform a strand test and record the results.

VIRGIN APPLICATION PROCEDURE

1 Follow the manufacturer's directions.

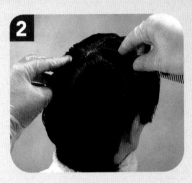

2 Put on gloves and part dry hair into four sections.

3 Prepare color formula for either bottle or brush application method.

4 Begin in the section where the hair is most resistant or where there will be the most color change.

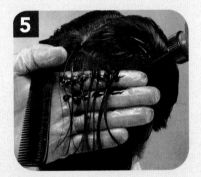

5 Part off $\frac{1}{4}''$ subsections and apply color to the mid shaft area. Stay at least $\frac{1}{2}''$ from the scalp and do not apply to the porous ends.

6 Process according to the strand test results and the manufacturer's directions.

7 Check color development. When desired color is reached, apply remaining product to hair at the scalp, then pull the color through to the hair ends.

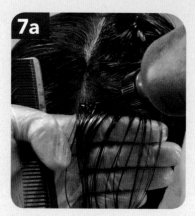

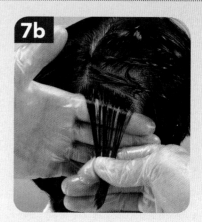

8 Lightly wet client's hair with warm water and lather. Massage lather through the hair.

9 Rinse thoroughly, shampoo, and condition. Remove stains as necessary.

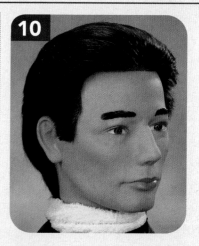

10 Rinse, towel blot, and style.

RETOUCH PROCEDURE

To retouch new hair growth, use the same preparation steps as for coloring virgin hair. Then proceed as follows:

1 Refer to the client record card for correct color selection and other data.

2 Apply the tint first to new growth at sideburns, temples, and nape area.

3 Apply the tint to new growth in $\frac{1}{4}$" partings. Do not overlap. Check frequently for color development.

4 When color has almost developed, dilute the remaining tint by adding a mild shampoo or warm water. Apply and gently work the mixture through the hair with the fingertips. Comb and blend from the scalp to the hair ends for even distribution.

5 Process for the required time. Rinse with warm water to remove excess color.

6 Use an acid-balanced shampoo and rinse thoroughly. Remove color stains, if necessary.

7 Style the hair as desired.

CLEAN-UP AND DISINFECTION

1. Discard all disposable supplies.

2. Close and wipe off containers and store properly.

3. Sanitize implements, tools, cape, and work area.

4. Wash hands.

5. Record results on client record card.

DOUBLE-PROCESS HAIRCOLORING

Double-process haircoloring begins with hair lightening, followed by a tint or toner application. This double process requires two separate steps as discussed in this section and demonstrated in Procedure 19-6.

CHARACTERISTICS OF LIGHTENERS

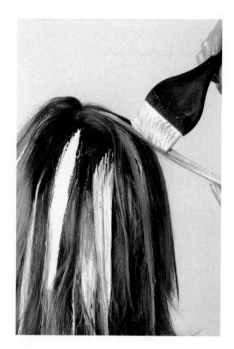

Lightening creates a desired color foundation. This new color foundation may be the finished result or it may be the first step of a double-process application. Consideration must be given to the existing hair color, processing and development time, resulting porosity, and color selection to achieve the desired shade.

Depending on the manufacturer's directions, hair lighteners can be used for the following processes.

- To lighten the entire head of hair
- To lighten the hair to a particular shade
- To brighten and lighten the existing shade
- To tip, streak, or frost certain sections of the hair
- To lighten hair that has already been tinted
- To remove undesirable casts and off-shades
- To correct dark streaks or spots in hair that has already been lightened or tinted

Selection of Lighteners

Remember to choose the appropriate lightener for the service. Cream and oil lighteners may be used on the scalp; powder lighteners are off-the-scalp products.

Together with the manufacturer's directions, be guided by the following general rules when choosing a lightening product.

- Oil lighteners are the mildest form of lightener and may be used when only one or two levels of lift are desired.
- Cream lighteners offer some protection to the hair, are controllable during application, and can be used to drab undesirable red and gold tones. For increased strength, up to three activators can be added for on-the-scalp applications and up to four activators for off-the-scalp processes.
- Powder lighteners are strong enough to produce blonding effects, but should not be used for retouch applications.

Lightener Retouch

Lightener retouch is the term commonly used when a lightener is applied only to the new hair growth to match the rest of the lightened hair. The client's record card should be consulted as a guide to the lightener used previously and the time required for the shade to develop.

Cream lightener is often used for a lightener retouch because it helps prevents the overlapping of the previously lightened hair. Black or dark brown hair usually requires more frequent retouch applications than lighter natural shades. When retouching, the lightener is applied to the new growth only. If a lighter or different level is desired overall, wait until the new growth is almost light enough or has developed fully. Then bring the remainder of the lightener through the hair shaft. One to five minutes should be ample time to create a lighter level effect.

TONERS

Other than a reduced ratio of dye load in the formula, toners have the same chemical ingredients and action as permanent haircolor products. The difference in the formulation is what allows for toners to deliver pale, delicate shades of color to pre-lightened hair.

Color Selection of Toners

Pastel colors, such as silver, ash, platinum, and beige, are popular toners for lighter blond colors. Gray hair and skin tone changes that accompany advancing years may benefit from the lighter silver tones. When extremely pale toner shades such as very light silver, platinum, or beige are desired, the hair must be pre-lightened to pale yellow or almost white.

Toner Retouch

A toner retouch must be given the same careful consideration as you would give a two-color tint retouch application. The new growth must be pre-lightened to the same degree of lightness achieved in the previous toner application. The lightener is applied to the new growth only. To avoid damage to the hair, be careful not to overlap the lightener on previously lightened hair. After the lightening process has been completed, the toner is applied to the entire length of the hair in the usual manner.

Suggestions and Reminders

- Toners are completely dependent on the proper preliminary lightening treatment, which must leave the hair light and porous enough to receive the pale toner shades.

- Semipermanent and demipermanent color can also be used with lighteners to achieve specific tones and colors.

- Strand tests are vital to correct double-process applications.

- A complete explanation of the possible outcome should be discussed with the client. It is always possible that the hair cannot be decolorized sufficiently for the color choice without resulting in serious damage to the hair. Gold or red pigments remaining in the hair after lightening indicate under-lightening; ash tones indicate over-lightening. When this happens, the shade of toner should be chosen to neutralize the unwanted tones.

Double-Process Haircoloring

STEP 1: LIGHTENING VIRGIN HAIR

SUPPLIES

- Lightener product
- Hydrogen peroxide
- Color chart
- Applicator bottle or brush and bowl
- Shampoo cape
- Towels
- Protective gloves
- Shampoo
- Conditioner
- Comb
- Plastic clips (optional, depending on length of hair)
- Cotton
- Protective cream
- Record card
- Timer

PREPARATION

1. Perform a preliminary patch test 24 hours before the service. Proceed only if the test is negative.

2. Perform client consultation and record results on client record card.

3. Drape client and apply protective cream.

4. Perform a strand test and record the results.

PROCEDURE FOR LIGHTENING VIRGIN HAIR

1 Divide dry hair into four sections.

2 Apply protective cream around hairline. Put on gloves.

3 Prepare lightening formula. Use either bottle or brush application method.

4 Begin in the section where the hair is most resistant or where there will be the most color change.

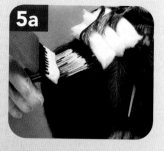 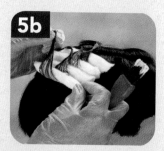

5 Part off $\frac{1}{8}$" subsections and apply lightener $\frac{1}{2}$" from the scalp up to, but not through, the porous ends. Apply to top and underside of the subsection and place a strip of cotton along the part lines to prevent seepage to the scalp area.

6 Apply lightener to other sections in the same manner. Keep lightener moist with repeated applications if necessary. Do not comb the lightener through the hair.

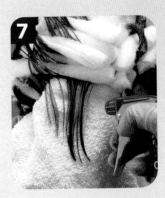

7 Process according to the strand test results and manufacturer's directions. Check lightening action by misting as for a strand test about 15 minutes before the completion of the time required. If the level is not light enough, reapply the mixture and continue testing frequently until the desired shade is almost developed.

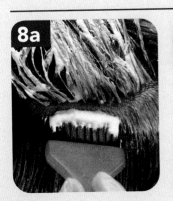 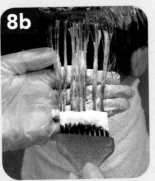

8 Remove cotton from scalp area and apply lightener near the scalp. Apply lightening product to the porous ends. Process until the entire hair shaft has reached the desired level.

9 Rinse thoroughly, shampoo, and condition. Dry the hair with a towel or under a cool dryer per the manufacturer's directions. Examine the scalp for post-service abrasions.

10 Proceed with toner application if desired.

CLEAN-UP AND DISINFECTION

1. Discard all disposable supplies.

2. Close and wipe off containers and store properly.

3. Sanitize implements and tools, cape, and work area.

4. Wash hands.

5. Record results on client record card.

STEP 2: TONER APPLICATION

SUPPLIES

- Toner product
- Hydrogen peroxide
- Color chart
- Applicator bottle or brush and bowl
- Shampoo cape
- Towels
- Protective gloves
- Shampoo
- Conditioner
- Comb
- Plastic clips (optional, depending on length of hair)
- Cotton
- Protective cream
- Record card
- Timer

PREPARATION

1. Perform a preliminary patch test 24 hours before the service. Proceed only if the test is negative.

2. Perform client consultation and record results on client record card.

3. Drape client.

4. Pre-lighten the hair to the desired level.

5. Shampoo, rinse, condition, and towel dry the hair.

6. Perform a strand test and record the results.

PROCEDURE FOR TONER APPLICATION

1 Divide dry hair into four sections.

2 Apply protective cream around hairline. Put on gloves.

3 If using an oxidative toner, mix the toner and developer. Use either bottle or brush application method.

4 Begin in the crown section and part off $\frac{1}{4}''$ subsections. Apply toner from the scalp up to, but not through, the porous ends. Apply to other sections.

5 Process according to the strand test results and the manufacturer's directions. Check toning action by misting as for a strand test. If proper color development has occurred, work the toner through the ends of the hair.

6 When the desired color has been reached, add water and massage toner into a lather.

7 Rinse thoroughly, shampoo, and condition. Remove any stains as necessary.

8 Style as desired.

CLEAN-UP AND DISINFECTION

1. Discard all disposable supplies.

2. Close and wipe off containers and store properly.

3. Sanitize implements and tools, cape, and work area.

4. Wash hands.

5. Record results on client record card.

Special-Effects Haircoloring and Lightening

Special-effects haircoloring refers to any technique that involves the partial lightening or coloring of the hair. As previously defined, highlighting is the process of lightening or coloring some of the hair strands lighter than the natural color. Frosting, tipping, and streaking are forms of highlighting application techniques. Lowlighting, or reverse highlighting, is the process of coloring strands or sections of the hair darker than the natural color. As an application process, tipping and streaking techniques can be used for lowlighting effects.

Frosting involves lightening strands of hair over various parts of the head. Either the cap technique or foils can be used for the process. The effect achieved will depend on where and how many strands of hair are treated.

Tipping is similar to frosting, except that only the ends of the hair strands are lightened or colored. Apply the product using either the cap technique or free-form technique for better placement and product control.

Streaking is also similar to frosting, but the strands of lightened or colored hair are usually thicker and more dramatic than those taken for a frosting effect. Streaking effects are best accomplished using the foil or free-form application techniques.

Special Problems and Corrective Haircolor

Each haircoloring or lightening service has the potential to create unique problems. Some problems can be avoided by performing preliminary strand tests, but others can be the result of unique properties within the client's hair structure that are unforeseen. Most haircoloring and lightening problems can be resolved with a calm approach, an accurate assessment of the problem, and the knowledge to rectify the situation.

GRAY HAIR CHALLENGES

Gray, white, or salt-and-pepper hair shades have characteristics that can present unique color challenges (**Figure 19-18**). Since both gray and white hair contain little melanin within the cortex, a large number of coloring services are performed with the intent to cover or enhance the color. Depending on the amount of gray, the hair may have a yellowish cast or process differently from one strand to another. Some gray hair also tends to be more resistant to chemical processes and may require pre-softening before a service.

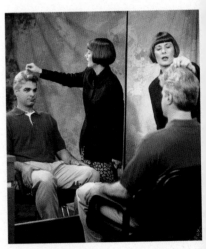

▲ **FIGURE 19-18**
Gray hair presents certain challenges.

SUPPLIES

- Lightener product
- Hydrogen peroxide
- Color chart
- Applicator bottle or brush and bowl
- Waterproof cape
- Towels
- Protective gloves
- Shampoo
- Conditioner
- Comb
- Plastic clips (optional, depending on length of hair)
- Frosting cap and hook
- Foils
- Protective cream
- Record card
- Timer

PREPARATION FOR CAP OR FOIL TECHNIQUES

1. Perform a preliminary patch test 24 hours before the service. Proceed only if the test is negative.

2. Perform client consultation and record results on client record card.

3. Drape client.

4. Perform a strand test and record the results.

PROCEDURE FOR CAP TECHNIQUE

The cap technique involves pulling strands of hair through the holes of a perforated cap with a plastic or metal hook. The number of strands pulled through the cap determines the degree of highlighting or lowlighting that is achieved throughout the hair.

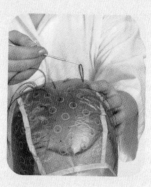

1 Shampoo the hair, if necessary, and dry.

2 Comb the hair gently.

3 Adjust a perforated cap over the head.

4 Draw the strands of hair through the holes with crochet hook. Prepare coloring or lightening product. Put on gloves.

5 Apply the color or lightener.

6 Cover loosely with a plastic cap if necessary for processing.

7 When the hair has processed, remove the plastic cap if present.

8 Rinse and shampoo the color or lightener with the perforated cap in place. Towel dry.

9 Optional: Apply toner if necessary and process accordingly.

10 Style as desired.

PROCEDURE FOR FOIL TECHNIQUE

The foil technique involves weaving out alternating strands of hair from a subsection, or slicing out $\frac{1}{8}$" partings from a straight part, to isolate the strands for coloring or lightening. The selected strands are then placed over a piece of foil wrap and the color or lightening product is applied. The foil is folded to prevent coloring or lifting any of the unwoven hair, and strands are processed to the desired shade. The foil technique facilitates strategically placed color or highlights that can accentuate a haircut or style. Frosting and streaking effects can be accomplished using the foil technique.

1 Apply to dry hair if using permanent color or lighteners. Apply to damp hair if using traditional semipermanent colors.

2 Comb the hair gently. Prepare color or lightening product. Apply gloves.

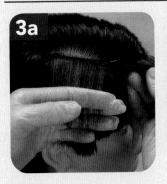

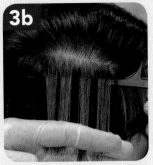

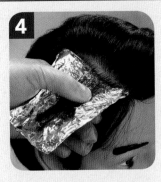

3 Slice or weave out the strands from the first parting to be processed.

4 Place the foil under the hair and grasp it firmly at the scalp between the thumb and index finger.

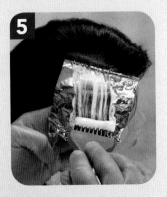

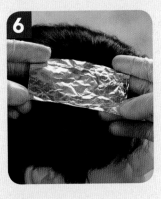

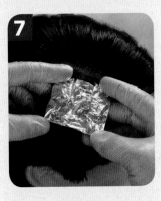

5 Brush color or lightening product onto the hair.

6 Fold the foil in half from bottom to top until the ends meet at the scalp area.

7 Fold the left and right edges of the foil halfway and crimp lightly until secure. Clip the foil upward.

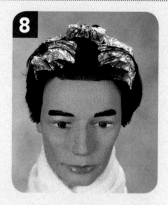

8 Continue the same process until all the areas to be foiled are completed.

9 Process according to strand test results. Check color or lightening level.

10 When processing is complete, remove foils at the shampoo bowl.

11 Rinse, shampoo, and condition according to product directions.

12 Style hair as desired.

CLEAN-UP AND DISINFECTION

1. Discard all disposable supplies.

2. Close and wipe off containers and store properly.

3. Sanitize implements and tools, cape, and work area.

4. Wash hands.

5. Record results on client record card.

F◉CUS ON...

When performing the foil technique over the entire head, the sequence of application should be lower crown, back, sides, top, and front.

✔ **LO5** Complete

Yellowed Hair

Gray, white, and salt-and-pepper hair with a yellowish cast can be treated with violet-based colors that range from highlighting shampoos and temporary rinses to lightening agents. The longevity of the product used will depend on the client's desired result and the options offered by the barber. (If lightening and coloring services are not typically offered in the barbershop, it is highly recommended that, at a minimum, highlighting shampoos or temporary rinses with violet bases be available to shop clients.)

Determining the Percentage of Gray

Since most people retain some dark hair as they turn gray, the hair must be analyzed for level, hue, and percentage of gray before the appropriate product selection can be made. Gray hair may be evenly distributed or isolated in various sections of the head, such as the temple areas. Use **Table 19-5** as a guide for determining percentages of gray and recommended formulations.

TABLE **19-5** Percentages of Gray and Recommended Formulations

PERCENTAGE OF GRAY	CHARACTERIS- TICS	SEMIPERMANENT COLOR FORMULATION	PERMANENT COLOR FORMULATION
90–100%	Virtually no pigment; white	Desired level	Desired level
70–90%	Mostly non-pigmented	Equal parts desired level and one level lighter	Two parts desired level and one part lighter level
50–70%	More gray than pigmented	One level lighter than desired level	Equal parts desired level and lighter level
30–50%	More pigmented than gray	Equal parts one level lighter and two levels lighter	Two parts lighter level and one part desired level
10–30%	Mostly pigmented	Two levels lighter than desired color	One level lighter

Formulating for Gray Hair

Gray hair will usually accept the level of the color applied. Generally, lighter shades in the level 9 range may not provide complete coverage, whereas levels 6, 7, and 8 will often cover successfully. The difference in coverage ability is due to the smaller percentage of artificial pigments found in the lighter shades of a level 9 formulation.

When a client has 80 to 100 percent gray, lighter haircolors are usually more flattering than darker shades. The client's skin tone, eye color, and personal preference will determine whether warm or cool tones are used. Reminder: when a dark level of color is applied to hair with a low percentage of gray, the

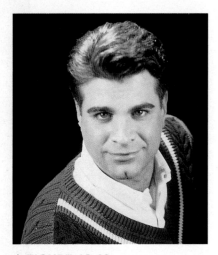

▲ FIGURE 19-19
Many haircolor options cover gray successfully.

addition of artificial pigment to the natural pigment will create a color that may be darker than the intended result. In addition, the non-pigmented strands may process lighter. To avoid these outcomes, select a color that is one level lighter than the darkest natural color (**Figure 19-19**).

Occasionally, gray hair is so resistant that pre-softening is necessary for better color penetration. Mix the product according to the manufacturer's directions and apply to the most resistant areas first. Process as directed and then perform a preliminary strand test with the desired color.

FILLERS

Color fillers are dual-purpose haircoloring products that are able to create a color base and equalize excessive porosity in one application.

Color fillers are available in clear, neutral, and a variety of colors. A clear filler is designed to correct porosity without affecting color and does not deposit a color base. Neutral fillers (a balance of all three primary colors) have minimal saturation and color correction abilities but have full power to equalize porosity. Color fillers are pre-oxidized colors that remain true during application and that will be subdued by the tint.

A color filler is recommended when there is any doubt that the finished color will develop into an even shade. The filler is applied after the hair has been pre-lightened and before the application of a toner or tint. Fillers are also used for clients who have tinted or lightened hair and desire to return it to the natural color. Color fillers have the ability to:

- deposit color to faded hair shafts and ends.
- help hair to hold color.
- help to ensure a uniform color from the scalp to the hair ends.
- prevent color streaking.
- prevent off-color results.
- prevent dullness.
- facilitate more uniform color in a tint back to the natural shade.

Fillers use certified colors as pigments and are safe to use without a predisposition test. They may be used directly from the container and applied to the hair prior to tinting, or may be added to the remainder of the tint and applied to damaged hair ends. To obtain satisfactory results, select the color filler to match the same basic shade as the toner or tint to be used.

RECONDITIONING DAMAGED HAIR

Hair that is damaged due to careless chemical applications, excessive heat, or misused styling products must be reconditioned before it can be tinted or lightened successfully.

Hair may need reconditioning for reasons other than damage resulting from the use of harmful products. Sometimes hair is naturally brittle, thin, and lifeless. Both neglect and the client's physical condition may contribute to these conditions.

Hair is considered damaged when it exhibits one or more of the following characteristics:

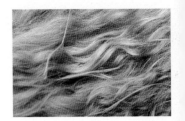

- Over-porous condition

- Brittle and dry

- Breaks easily

- Little to no elasticity

- Rough and harsh to the touch

- Spongy and mats easily when wet

- Rejects color or absorbs too much color during a tinting process

Any of these conditions may create undesirable results during a tinting or lightening treatment. Therefore, damaged hair should receive reconditioning treatments prior to and after the application of these chemical agents.

Reconditioning Treatment

To restore damaged hair to a more normal condition, commercial products containing lanolin or protein substances should be used. The reconditioning agent is applied to the hair. If heat is applied, use a heating cap, a steamer, or a heating lamp according to the manufacturer's directions. Be guided by your instructor as to the frequency and length of time for each treatment.

TINT BACK TO NATURAL COLOR

Clients who have been tinting or lightening their hair may want to return to their natural shade. Each tint back to natural color must be handled as an individual situation. The determining factors in the selection of the tint shade are the present condition and color of the hair, the final result desired, and the original color. Check the natural shade of the hair next to the scalp.

Select an appropriate shade of filler to correspond with the tint to be used; otherwise it will be difficult to obtain a uniform color from the scalp to hair ends, due to uneven porosity levels. Perform strand tests as needed to determine the expected final outcome.

COATING DYES

Many clients buy and use over-the-counter haircoloring products at home. Some such coloring agents are actually progressive dyes and must be removed prior to any other chemical service.

Hair treated with a compound, metallic, or other coating dye looks dry and dull and generally feels harsh and brittle to the touch. These colors usually fade to unnatural tones. Silver dyes have a greenish cast, lead dyes leave a purple color, and those containing copper turn red. If the barber is unsure as to whether the client has used a progressive dye, a test for metallic salts and dyes should be performed on the hair.

Test for Metallic Salts and Coating Dyes

1. In a glass container, mix 1 ounce (30 ml) of 20-volume (6 percent) peroxide and 20 drops of 28 percent ammonia water.

2. Cut a few strands of the client's hair, bind it with tape, and immerse it in the solution for 30 minutes.

REMOVING COATINGS FROM THE HAIR

The removal of metallic dyes from the hair shaft may not always be effective the first time. Performing a strand test after the treatment will indicate whether the metallic deposits have been removed. If not, the entire application must be repeated until the hair shaft is sufficiently free of metal salts to perform other chemical services.

SUPPLIES

- 70 percent alcohol

- Concentrated shampoo for oily hair

- Mineral, castor, vegetable, or commercially prepared color-removing oil

PROCEDURE

1 Apply 70 percent alcohol to dry hair.

2 Allow alcohol to stand for 5 minutes.

3 Apply the oil to the hair thoroughly.

4 Cover the hair completely with a plastic cap.

5 Place under a hot dryer for 30 minutes.

6 To remove, saturate with concentrated shampoo.

7 Work the shampoo into the oil for three minutes, then rinse with warm water.

8 Repeat the shampoo steps until the oil is removed completely.

3. Remove, towel dry, and observe the strand. Refer to the following for analysis of the hair:

- Hair dyed with lead will lighten immediately.

- Hair treated with silver will show no reaction at all. This indicates that other chemicals will not be successful because they will not be able to penetrate the coating.

- Hair treated with copper will start to boil, and will pull apart easily. This hair would be severely damaged or destroyed if other chemicals such as those found in permanent colors or perm solutions were applied to it.

- Hair treated with a coating dye either will not change color or will lighten in spots. Hair in this condition will not receive chemical services easily and the length of time necessary for penetration may result in further damage to the hair.

Coloring Mustaches and Beards

An aniline derivative tint should never be used for coloring mustaches; doing so may cause serious irritation or damage to the lips or the delicate membranes of the nostrils. Harmless commercial products are available in a variety of formulations that are appropriate for coloring mustaches and beards.

Crayons are waxy sticks that are available in several colors: blond, medium and dark brown, black, and auburn. The end of the stick is used like a pencil to apply the product by rubbing it directly on the facial hair until the desired shade is reached.

Pomades usually consist of harmless ingredients and are formulated specifically for coloring mustaches and beards. These products are available in a variety of shades including black, brown, blond, chestnut, and white (neutral). The pomade is applied to the facial hair with a small brush and is stroked from the nostrils downward until full coverage is achieved.

Liquid pomades are also available and may be preferred for use on beards. Some pomades contain heavy waxing ingredients that can be used to style mustaches with rolled or twisted ends for dramatic looks. Liquid eyebrow and eyelash tint is also available in brown and black for coloring facial hair.

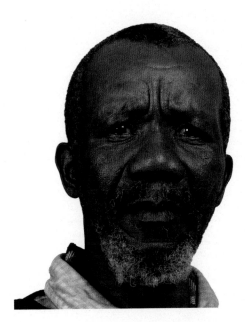

Coloring Mustaches and Beards

SUPPLIES

- Waterproof cape
- Towels
- Petroleum jelly
- Coloring solutions (No. 1 and No. 2)
- Stain remover
- Towels
- Applicator sticks

PROCEDURE

1 Seat the client in a comfortable position and drape.

2 Place a clean towel across the chest.

3 Wash the facial hair with warm, soapy water.

4 Apply petroleum jelly around the hairline of the facial hair.

5 Apply solution No. 1. Remove the cap and moisten a cotton-tipped applicator in the solution. Touch the tip of the applicator to a towel to remove excess moisture. Apply the solution to the mustache or beard, moistening it completely. Replace the cap on bottle No. 1. Discard the applicator immediately. Moisten a fresh cotton-tipped applicator with stain remover and place it on the edge of a towel for future use. Replace the cap on the stain remover bottle.

6 Apply solution No. 2 to the mustache or beard in the same manner as solution No. 1. If the skin becomes stained, use stain remover immediately. Replace the cap on bottle No. 2.

7 Wash the mustache or beard with soap and cool water.

8 Remove any stains with stain remover. Replace the bottle cap.

9 Style the mustache or beard as desired.

10 Clean-up in the usual manner.

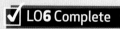 ✓ LO**6** Complete

Haircoloring and Lightening Safety Precautions

HAIRCOLORING

REMINDER

Keep up to date! Manufacturers are constantly improving and developing new haircoloring products. Be sure to attend seminars and trade shows as often as possible to stay current in your profession.

- Perform a 24-hour patch test before the application of a tint or toner.

- Examine the scalp before applying a tint.

- Do not apply tint if abrasions are present on the scalp.

- Use only sanitized swabs, brushes, applicator bottles, combs, and linens.

- Always wash your hands before and after serving a client.

- Do not brush the hair prior to a tint.

- Do not apply a tint without reading the manufacturer's directions.

- Perform a strand test for color and processing results.

- Choose a shade of tint that harmonizes with the general complexion.

- Use an applicator bottle or bowl (plastic or glass) for mixing the tint.

- Do not mix tint before ready for use; discard leftover tint.

- If required, use the correct shade of color filler.

- Make frequent strand tests until the desired shade is reached.

- Suggest a reconditioning treatment for tinted hair.

- Do not apply tint if metallic or compound dye is present.

- Do not apply tint if a patch test is positive.

- Give a strand test for the correct color shade before applying tint.

- Do not use an alkaline or harsh shampoo for tint removal.

- Do not use water that is too hot for removing tint.

- Protect the client's clothing by proper draping.

- Do not permit tint to come in contact with the client's eyes.

- Do not overlap during a tint retouch.

- Fill out a tint record card.

- Do not apply hydrogen peroxide or any material containing hydrogen peroxide directly over dyes known or believed to contain a metallic salt. Breakage or complete disintegration of the hair may result.

- Wear protective gloves.

- Analyze the condition of the hair and suggest reconditioning treatments, if required.

- When working with a cream or paste lightener, it must be the thickness of whipped cream to avoid dripping or running and resultant overlapping.

- Apply lightener to resistant areas first. Pick up $\frac{1}{8}$" sections when applying lightener. This will ensure complete coverage.

- Check strands frequently until the desired shade is reached.

- After completing the lightener application, check the skin and remove any lightener from these areas.

- Check the towel around the client's neck. Lightener on the towel that is allowed to come in contact with the skin will cause irritation.

- Lightened hair is fragile and requires special care. Use only a very mild shampoo and only cool water for rinsing.

- If a preliminary shampoo is necessary, comb the hair carefully. Avoid irritating the scalp during the shampoo or when combing the hair.

- Work as rapidly as possible when applying the lightener to produce a uniform shade without streaking.

- Never allow lightener to stand; use it immediately.

- Cap all bottles to avoid loss of strength.

- Keep a completed record card of all lightening treatments.

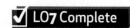

✔ LO7 Complete

sp○tlight ON

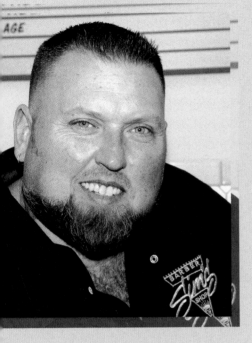

STEVE VILOT
SIM'S BARBERSHOPS
www.simsbarbershops.com

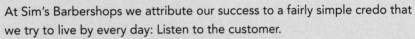

At Sim's Barbershops we attribute our success to a fairly simple credo that we try to live by every day: Listen to the customer.

I didn't come to the barbering business by the typical direct route. After graduating from college with plans of becoming a structural engineer, I worked at numerous different jobs, from technician at a gas company to bouncer at the Cask 'n' Flagon bar just outside Boston's Fenway Park. But it wasn't until I tried my hand at barbering that I found a lifelong career. I quickly discovered that the eye-hand abilities I'd picked up from drafting training at engineering school directly applied to the skills required to be a good barber, giving me a fine touch with scissors, clippers, and a straight razor. I knew that this was what I wanted to do. In 1992, I bought a small barbershop called Sim's near my home in Pittsfield, Massachusetts, and I haven't looked back since.

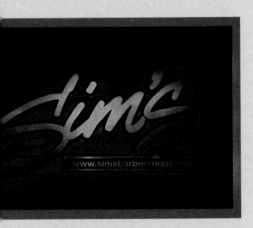

When I first took it over, Sim's was just a tiny one-chair operation. I wish I could say that at the time I had a grand master plan to expand the business and grow. But the truth is everything I've done has simply been in response to what my customers have told me. It really is that simple.

When my customers said that they didn't want to wait so long for haircuts, I added chairs and filled them with barbers by sending my friends and customers who were interested in the business to barber school. Since I've always had friends and customers of all races I developed specialties in cutting black hair and Latino hair. When my customers said that they wished I could be more accommodating to their work schedules, I decided to stay open later in the evenings during the week and I added Sunday and Monday hours.

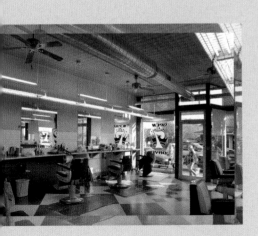

Then, when I found out that many of my customers were traveling long distances to get to Sim's, I decided to bring the barbershop to them by opening a satellite spot 20 miles south in the town of Great Barrington. And finally, when I learned that my customers wanted grooming options beyond a good haircut, I started offering premium services like professional shaves, manicures, pedicures, coloring, and waxing. We accomplished this by putting my wife Juliette's extensive spa experience to work, and in the end built a full-service barbershop for men and women.

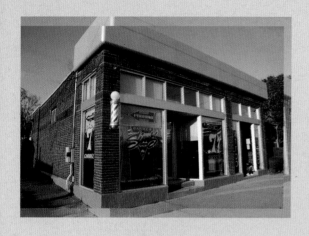

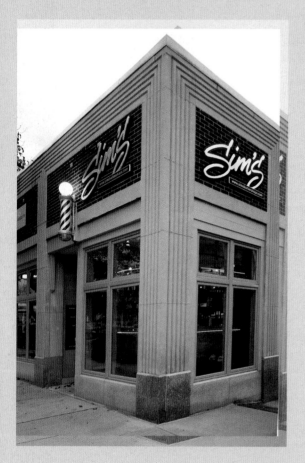

Today, what I'm hearing most from my customers and from my barber friends is a thirst for knowledge. I do a lot of professional training classes and I'm always getting questions from fledgling barbers looking for tips on the latest techniques and the hottest haircuts. That's why I established the Barber Authority as a clearinghouse for barbers to share their ideas (www.thebarberauthority.com). From my customers, I'm constantly getting questions about what new products they can use to make their hair and skin look better. Indeed, I'm finding that there are huge opportunities in men's grooming products as men are catching up to women in paying careful attention to their appearance.

In the future, I envision Sim's evolving into a full-service haberdashery. Men want to learn the best ways to shave their face, or how to style their hair a certain way, or even how to shine their shoes or tie a Windsor knot. I see Sim's as a place where a man can get a great hair cut and shave, but also gain all of this knowledge as well. Why do I see this? Because we've been listening to our customers.

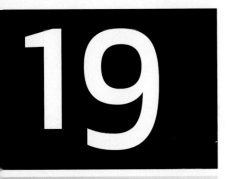

19 Review Questions

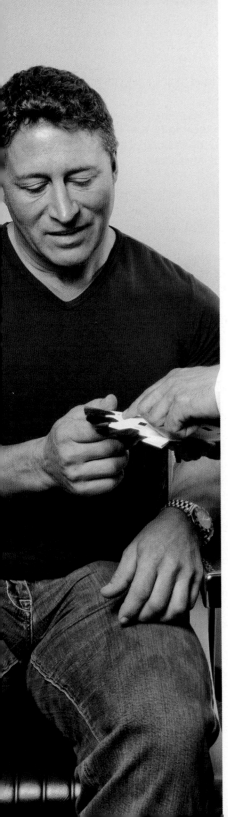

1. Define haircoloring and lightening.

2. List the colors of the color wheel. Identify primary, secondary, and complementary colors.

3. List four types of haircoloring products.

4. Identify types of non-oxidation and oxidation haircolor.

5. Explain the difference between semipermanent and demipermanent haircolor products.

6. List four types of permanent haircolor tints.

7. List the volumes of hydrogen peroxide used in haircoloring.

8. Explain how to test for sensitivities or allergies to haircolor products.

9. What is a strand test?

10. What professional products use a single-process application? Double-process application?

11. Explain the lightening process.

12. List the products used to color beards and mustaches.

Chapter
Glossary

activator an additive used to quicken the action or progress of hydrogen peroxide

aniline derivatives uncolored dye precursors that combine with hydrogen peroxide to form larger, permanent color molecules in the cortex

base color the predominant tone of an existing color

cap technique lightening technique that involves pulling strands of hair through a perforated cap with a plastic or metal hook

color fillers tinted products used to even out color processing

complementary colors a primary and secondary color positioned opposite each other on the color wheel

contributing pigment pigment that lies under the natural hair color that is exposed when the natural color is lightened

demipermanent haircolor deposit-only haircolor product similar to semipermanent but longer lasting

developer an oxidizing agent, usually hydrogen peroxide, used to develop color

double-process haircoloring a two-step combination of lightening and haircoloring

dye removers products used to strip built-up color from the hair

fillers preparations designed to equalize porosity and/or deposit a base color in one application

foil technique highlighting technique using foil

free-form technique also known as balyage; the painting of a lightener on clean, styled hair

haircoloring industry-coined term referring to artificial haircolor products and services

hair lightening the chemical process of diffusing natural or artificial pigment from the hair

highlighting coloring or lightening some strands of hair lighter than the natural color

hue the basic name of a color

laws of color a system for understanding color relationships

level unit of measurement to identify the lightness or darkness of a color

level system system used to analyze the lightness or darkness of a hair color or color product

lighteners chemical compounds that lighten hair by dispersing and diffusing natural pigment

line of demarcation a visible line separating colored hair from new growth

lowlighting coloring some strands of hair darker than the natural hair color

off-the-scalp lighteners lighteners that cannot be used directly on the scalp

on-the-scalp lighteners lighteners that can be used directly on the scalp

patch test test for identifying a possible allergy to haircolor products

permanent haircolor haircolor that is mixed with a developer and remains in the shaft

pre-lightening the first step of a double-process haircoloring; used to lighten natural pigment

pre-softening process of treating resistant hair for better color penetration

primary colors red, blue, and yellow; colors that cannot be achieved from a mixture of other colors

progressive colors haircolor products that contain compound or metallic dyes, which build up on the hair; not used professionally

retouch application application of the product to new growth only

secondary colors colors obtained by mixing equal parts of two primary colors

semipermanent haircolor deposit-only haircolor product formulated to last through several shampoos

single-process haircoloring process that lightens and colors the hair in a single application

soap cap equal parts of tint and a shampoo

strand test the application of a coloring or lightening product to determine how the hair will react to the formula and the amount of time it will take to process

temporary colors color products that last only from shampoo to shampoo

tone term used to describe the warmth or coolness of a color.

toners semipermanent, demipermanent, or permanent haircolor products used primarily on pre-lightened hair to achieve pale and delicate colors

virgin application the first time the hair is tinted

volume the measure of the potential oxidation of varying strengths of hydrogen peroxide

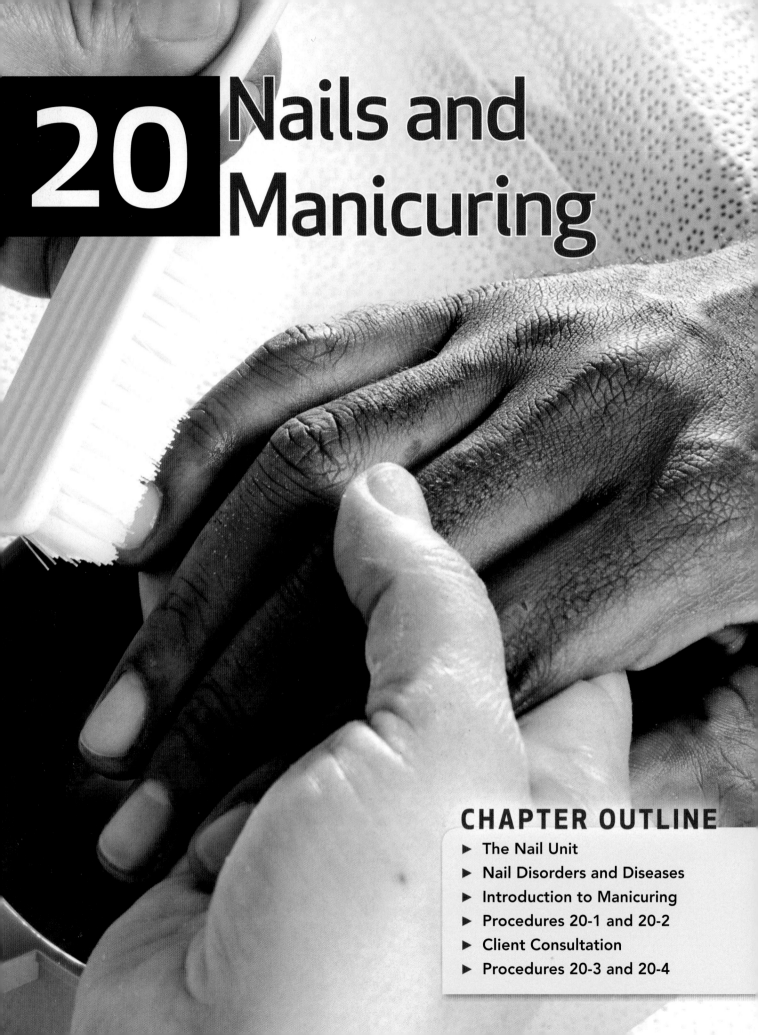

20 Nails and Manicuring

☑ Learning Objectives

AFTER COMPLETING THIS CHAPTER, YOU SHOULD BE ABLE TO:

1 Describe the composition of the nail.

2 Identify and describe nail irregularities and diseases.

3 Demonstrate the proper use of manicuring implements, equipment, and products.

4 Recognize the five general shapes of nails.

5 Demonstrate manicure and hand massage procedures.

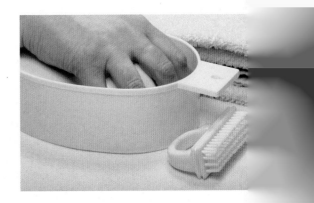

Key Terms

PAGE NUMBER INDICATES WHERE IN THE CHAPTER THE TERM IS USED.

Beau's lines / 677

bed epithelium / 673

bruised nails / 676

cuticle / 673

discolored nails / 676

eggshell nails / 676

eponychium / 673

free edge / 673

hangnails / 677

hyponychium / 673

leukonychia / 677

lunula / 673

matrix / 673

melanonychia / 677

nail / 672

nail bed / 673

nail folds / 674

nail grooves / 674

nail plate / 673

nail psoriasis / 679

nail pterygium / 678

onychia / 679

onychocryptosis / 679

onycholysis / 679

onychomadesis / 679

onychomycosis / 680

onychophagy / 677

onychorrhexis / 678

onychosis / 676

onyx / 672

paronychia / 679

pincer or trumpet nail / 678

plicatured nail / 678

pseudomonas aeruginosa / 678

pyrogenic granuloma / 680

ridges / 677

As with hair and skin services, nail care has been a part of human existence for thousands of years. This fact is evidenced through the recorded histories of Egypt and China dating back to 3000 BC. Egyptian men and women of high social rank painted their nails with henna, and by 600 BC the members of Chinese royalty were painting their nails with gold and silver paint. Later accounts of life in Rome and Babylon tell us that in addition to having their hair and beards dressed for battle, military men also colored their nails to match their lip color.

Barbershops of the first half of the 20th century routinely provided manicures as part of the traditional shave, haircut, and shoeshine service. In fact, a newspaper article of 1912 noted that in addition to shampooing, applying facial cosmetics, tinting facial hair, removing comedones, and curling hair, "the modern barbershop has a manicure girl" (Owen, 1991).

It should not be surprising that many of today's barbershops offer manicures. As a result, it is advisable that you become acquainted with the manicuring procedure and become proficient in its execution. Doing so will provide a foundation from which to offer the service or to oversee the procedure as performed by others in your employ. A basic understanding of nail composition and structure provides the first step in building this foundation of knowledge.

The Nail Unit

The **nail** is a horny, translucent plate of hard keratin that serves to protect the tips of the fingers and toes. Nails are part of the integumentary system and are considered to be appendages of the skin. The technical term for nail is **onyx** (AHN-iks).

The condition of the nail, like that of the skin, reflects the general health of the body. The normal, healthy nail is firm, flexible, and translucent with the pinkish color of the nail bed below showing through. Its surface should be smooth, curved, and unspotted, without any hollows or wavy ridges. No nerves or blood vessels are contained within the horny nail plate.

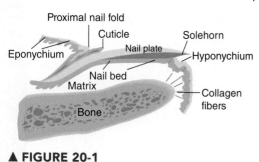

▲ FIGURE 20-1

The structure of the nail.

NAIL STRUCTURE

The nail unit consists of several basic parts (**Figures 20-1**):

- Nail bed
- Matrix
- Nail plate
- Cuticle
- Eponychium
- Hyponychium
- Specialized ligaments
- Nail folds

Nail Bed

The **nail bed** is living skin that supports the nail plate as it grows toward the free edge. It is supplied with blood vessels that provide the pinkish tone from the lunula almost to the free edge and is abundantly rich in nerves that are attached to the nail plate. The nail bed is attached to the nail plate by a thin layer of tissue called the **bed epithelium** (ep-ih-THEE-lee-um), which helps guide the nail plate along the nail bed as it grows.

Matrix

The **matrix** is embedded under the skin and is where the nail is formed. The matrix cells are nourished by nerves, lymph, and blood vessels, and produce other cells to form the nail plate. The matrix will continue to grow as long as it receives nutrition and remains healthy. The growth of nails may be affected by poor health, a nail disorder, disease, or injury to the nail matrix. The visible portion of the matrix is called the **lunula** (LOO-nuh-luh) or half-moon. It is located at the base of the nail where the matrix and the connective tissue of the nail bed join.

Nail Plate

The **nail plate** is the most visible and functional portion of the nail, and slowly slides upon the nail bed as it grows. Formed by the matrix cells, the nail plate extends to the **free edge** of the nail.

Although the nail plate seems to be made of one piece, it is actually constructed in layers. This structure can be seen in both length and thickness when a nail splits.

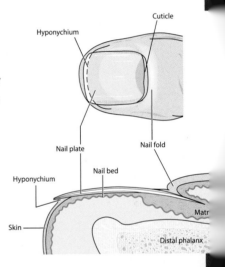

Cuticle

The **cuticle** (KYOO-tih-kul) is the crescent of dead, colorless tissue attached to the nail plate around the base of the nail. It forms a seal between the eponychium and the nail plate to prevent the entry of foreign materials or microorganisms and to help prevent injury and infection.

Eponychium

The **eponychium** (ep-oh-NIK-ee-um) is the living skin at the base of the nail plate covering the matrix area. Unlike the cuticle, which is the dead tissue on the nail plate, the eponychium is living tissue and the two should not be confused. The cuticle comes from the underside of this area where it becomes strongly attached to the new growth of the nail plate.

Hyponychium

The **hyponychium** (hy-poh-NIK-ee-um) is the slightly thickened layer of skin that lies between the fingertip and the free edge of the nail plate. It forms a protective barrier that prevents microorganisms from invading and infecting the nail bed.

Specialized Ligaments

Specialized ligaments form bands of fibrous tissue that attach the nail bed and matrix to the underlying bone. These ligaments are located at the base of the matrix and around the edges of the nail bed.

Nail Folds

The **nail folds** are folds of normal skin that surround the nail plate. These folds form the **nail grooves** on the sides of the nail that permit the nail to move as it grows.

Nail Growth

Nail growth is influenced by nutrition, health, and disease. A normal, healthy nail grows forward, starting at the matrix and extending over the fingertip. The average rate of growth in the normal adult is about $\frac{1}{10}$" (3.7 mm) per month. Typically, nails grow faster in summer than they do in winter. Children's nails grow more rapidly, whereas those of elderly persons grow more slowly. The nail of the middle finger grows the fastest and the thumbnail the most slowly. Although toenails grow more slowly than fingernails, they are thicker and harder.

Nail Malformation

If the nail is separated from the nail bed through injury, it becomes distorted or discolored. Should the nail bed be injured after the loss of a nail, a badly formed new nail will result.

Nails are not shed in the same way that hair is shed. If a nail is torn off accidentally or lost through infection or disease, it will be replaced only if the matrix remains in good condition. In some cases, the replacement nails are shaped abnormally, due to interference at the base of the nail. Replacement of the nail takes about four to six months.

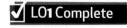
☑ LO1 Complete

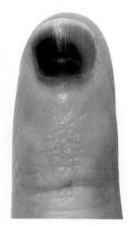

Nail Disorders and Diseases

NAIL DISORDERS

A *nail disorder* is a condition caused by injury to the nail, disease, or a chemical or nutritional imbalance. Most, if not all, clients will have had some common nail disorder, and may have one when they are scheduled for a manicure. It is important to learn to recognize the symptoms of nail disorders so that a responsible decision can be made about whether or not to perform a service on the client (**Table 20-1**). In some cases, it may be necessary to suggest the client seek a medical opinion. In others, the disorder may be improved cosmetically.

TABLE 20-1 Overview of Nail Disorders

DISORDER	SIGNS OR SYMPTOMS
Bruised nails	Dark purplish spots; usually due to injury
Ridges	Lengthwise ridges caused by uneven nail growth
Beau's lines	Depressions that run across the nail; result from illness, injury, stress, or pregnancy
Discolored nails	Nails turn a variety of colors; may indicate systemic disorder
Eggshell nails	Noticeably thin, white nail plate that is more flexible than normal; may be caused by diet, illness, or medication
Hangnail (agnail)	Cuticle splits around the nail
Infected finger	Redness, pain, swelling, or pus; refer to physician
Leukonychia (white spots)	Whitish discoloration of the nails; usually caused by injury to the base of the nail
Melanonychia	Significant darkening of the fingernails or toenails
Onychophagy	Bitten nails
Onychorrhexis	Abnormal brittleness with striation (lines) of the nail plate
Nail pterygium	Abnormal condition caused when the skin is stretched by the nail plate.
Plicatured nails	Folded nails; sharp bend in one corner of the nail plate creating increased curvature.
Pincer or trumpet nails	Edges of the nail plate curl around to form the shape of a trumpet or cone around the free edge

DISEASE	SIGNS OR SYMPTOMS
Onychia	Inflammation of the matrix with pus and shedding of the nail
Onychocryptosis	Ingrown nails
Onycholysis	Loosening of the nail without shedding
Onychomadesis	Separation and falling off of a nail from the nail bed
Onychomycosis	Fungal infection; whitish patches on nail that can be scraped off or long yellowish streaks within nail plate
Paronychia	Bacterial inflammation of the tissues around the nail; pus, thickening, and brownish discoloration of the nail plate
Pyrogenic granuloma	Severe inflammation of the nail in which a lump of red tissue grows up from the nail bed to the nail plate

In general, if the nail or skin surrounding it is infected, inflamed, or shows any sign of disease, the nail service should not be performed. Instead, the client should be referred to a physician (**Table 20-2**).

Onychosis (ahn-ih-KOH-sis) is the technical term applied to any deformity or disease of the nail, and includes the following conditions.

- **Bruised nails** occur when a blood clot forms under the nail plate. The clot is caused by injury to the nail bed. It can vary in color from maroon to black. In some cases, a bruised nail will fall off during the healing process. The application of artificial nail services to a bruised nail is not recommended.

- **Discolored nails** are a condition in which the nails turn a variety of colors such as yellow, blue, blue-gray, green, red, or purple. Discoloration can be caused by poor blood circulation, a heart condition, or topical or oral medications. It may also indicate the presence of a systemic disorder. Artificial tips or wraps, or an application of colored nail polish, can hide this condition.

- **Eggshell nails** are thin, white, and curved at the free edge (**Figure 20-2**). The condition is caused by improper diet, internal disease, medication, or nerve disorders. Be very careful when manicuring these nails. They are fragile and can break easily. Use the fine side of an emery board to file gently and do not use pressure with a metal pusher at the base of the nail.

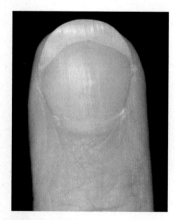

▲ **FIGURE 20-2**
Eggshell nail.

- **Ridges** are depressions that run vertically down the length of the nail. Some ridges are normal in adult nails and may increase with age **(Figure 20-3)**. If ridges are not deep and the nail is not broken, the appearance of this disorder can be corrected. Carefully buff the nails with a three-way buffer to reduce or shorten the ridges. The remaining ridges can be filled with ridge filler and covered with colored polish to give a smooth, healthy look.

- **Beau's lines** are visible depressions running across the width of the nail plate **(Figure 20-4)**. These usually result from major illness or injury that has traumatized the body, such as pneumonia, adverse drug reaction, surgery, heart failure, massive injury, or a long-lasting high fever. Beau's lines occur because the matrix slows down in producing nail cells for an extended period of time, perhaps a week or a month. This causes the nail plate to grow thinner for a period of time, but it usually returns to normal upon recovery.

- **Hangnails**, also known as *agnails* (AG-nayls), are a common condition in which the cuticle around the nail splits **(Figure 20-5)**. Hangnails are caused by dry cuticles or cuticles that have been cut too closely to the nail. The disorder can be improved by softening the cuticles with oil. Although hangnails are a simple and common disorder, they can become infected if not serviced properly.

- **Leukonychia** (loo-koh-NIK-ee-ah) is a condition in which white spots appear on the nails as a result of air bubbles, a bruise, or other injury to the nail **(Figure 20-6)**. Although the condition cannot be corrected, the nail will eventually grow out.

- **Melanonychia** (mel-uh-nuh-NIK-ee-uh) is a darkening of the nail as a result of increased and localized pigment cells within the matrix **(Figure 20-7)**. Nail polish or an artificial nail service can hide this disorder.

- **Onychophagy** (ahn-ih-koh-FAY-jee) is the medical term for nails that have been bitten enough to become deformed **(Figure 20-8)**. This condition can be improved greatly by professional manicuring techniques. Give frequent manicures, using the techniques described in this chapter.

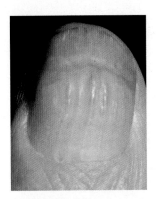

▲ **FIGURE 20-3**
Ridges.

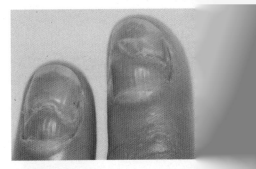

▲ **FIGURE 20-4**
Beau's lines.

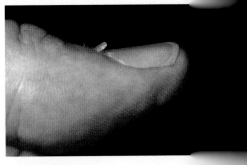

▲ **FIGURE 20-5**
Hangnail.

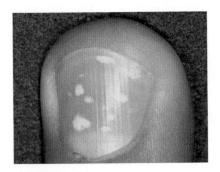

▲ **FIGURE 20-6**
Leukonychia.

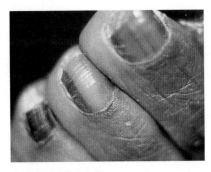

▲ **FIGURE 20-7**
Melanonychia.

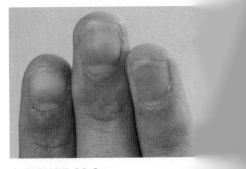

▲ **FIGURE 20-8**
Onychophagy.

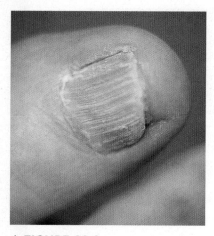

▲ FIGURE 20-9
Onychorrhexis.

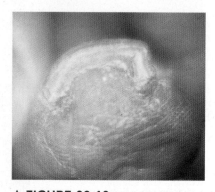

▲ FIGURE 20-10
Plicatured nail.

- **Onychorrhexis** (ahn-ih-koh-REK-sis) refers to split or brittle nails that also have a series of lengthwise ridges **(Figure 20-9)**. It can be caused by injury to the fingers, excessive use of cuticle solvents or nail polish removers, and careless, rough filing. Nail services can be performed only if the nail is not split below the free edge. This condition may be corrected by softening the nails with a reconditioning treatment, proper filing, and discontinuing the use of harsh soaps or polish removers.

- **Plicatured nail** (plik-a-CHOORD) literally means "folded nail" **(Figure 20-10)**, and is a type of highly curved nail plate often caused by injury to the matrix, but that may be inherited. This condition often leads to ingrown nails.

- A **pincer or trumpet nail** is a nail plate that has a deep or sharp curvature at the free edge caused by the curvature of the matrix. In some cases, the free edge pinches the sidewalls into a deep curve. The nail can also curl in upon itself **(Figure 20-11)** or may only be deformed only on one sidewall. In each of these cases, the natural nail plate should be carefully trimmed and filed. Extreme or unusual cases should be referred to a qualified medical doctor or podiatrist.

- **Nail pterygium** (teh-RIJ-ee-um) is an abnormal condition that occurs when skin is stretched by the nail plate as a result of damage to the eponychium or hyponychium. **(Figure 20-12)**. Do not treat nail pterygium and never push the extension of skin back with an instrument. Massaging oils or creams into the affected area may be beneficial, but irritated, painful, or infected conditions should be referred to a physician.

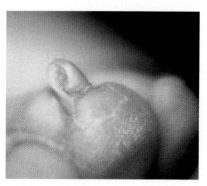

▲ FIGURE 20-11
Pincer or trumpet nail.

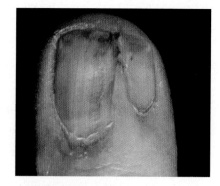

▲ FIGURE 20-12
Nail pterygium.

NAIL INFECTIONS

Discolorations of the nail plate are usually caused by a bacterial infection. Skin bacteria, such as **pseudomonas aeruginosa,** can grow out of control and cause an infection that starts with a yellow-green color and darkens to black if not properly treated. This condition should be treated by a physician **(Figure 20-13)**.

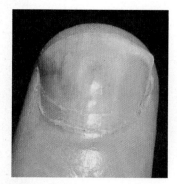

▲ FIGURE 20-13
Pseudomonas aeruginosa.

NAIL DISEASES

Any nail disease that shows signs of infection or inflammation (redness, pain, swelling, or pus) should not be diagnosed or treated in the barbershop.

- **Onychia** (uh-NIK-ee-uh) is an inflammation of the matrix with the formation of pus, redness, swelling, and shedding of the nail. Onychia is often caused by improperly sanitized implements and bacterial infection.

- **Onychocryptosis** (ahn-ih-koh-krip-TOH-sis), or ingrown nails, is a familiar condition, most commonly found in toenails, in which the nail grows into the sides of the tissue around the nail (**Figure 20-14**). Improper filing of the nail and poor-fitting shoes are causes of this disorder. If the tissue around the nail is not infected and the nail is not imbedded too deeply in the flesh, trim the corner of the nail in a curved shape to relieve the pressure on the nail groove. This condition should be treated by a physician.

- **Nail psoriasis** causes tiny pits or severe roughness on the surface of the nail plate. Sometimes these pits occur randomly, and sometimes they appear in evenly spaced rows. Nail psoriasis can also cause the surface of the plate to look as if it had been filed with a coarse abrasive, or may create a ragged free edge, or all of the above symptoms (**Figure 20-15**). Nail psoriasis is not an infectious disease, but it can affect the nail bed, causing it to develop yellowish to reddish spots underneath the nail plate.

- **Onychomadesis** (ahn-ih-koh-muh-DEE-sis) is the separation and falling off of a nail from the nail bed (**Figure 20-16**). In most cases, it can be traced to a localized infection or minor injury to the matrix bed. If there is no active infection present, a manicure may be performed.

- **Onycholysis** (ahn-ih-KAHL-ih-sis) is a condition in which the nail loosens from the nail bed, beginning usually at the free edge and continuing to the lunula, but does not come off (**Figure 20-17**). It is caused by an internal disorder, trauma, infection, or certain drugs.

- **Paronychia** (payr-uh-NIK-ee-uh) is a bacterial inflammation of the tissue around the nail (**Figure 20-18**). The symptoms are redness, swelling, and tenderness of the tissue. It can occur at the base

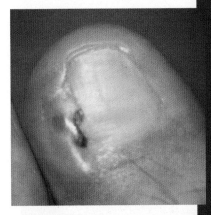

▲ **FIGURE 20-14**
Onychocryptosis.

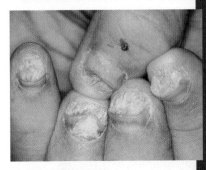

▲ **FIGURE 20-15**
Nail psoriasis.

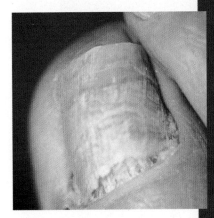

▲ **FIGURE 20-16**
Onychomadesis of a toenail.

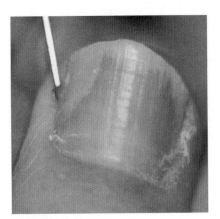

▲ **FIGURE 20-17**
Onycholysis.

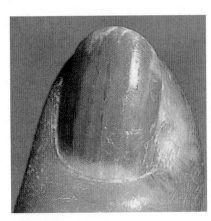

▲ **FIGURE 20-18**
Paronychia.

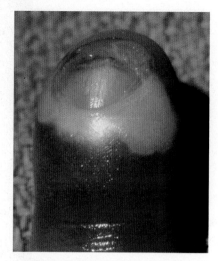

▲ FIGURE 20-19
Runaround paronychia.

of the nail, around the entire nail plate, or on the fingertip. Paronychia around the entire nail is sometimes referred to as "runaround paronychia" (**Figure 20-19**). Chronic paronychia occurs continually over a long period of time and causes damage to the nail plate (**Figure 20-20**). It can be caused by the use of unsanitary implements or by aggressive pushing or cutting of the cuticle.

- **Pyrogenic granuloma** (py-oh-JEN-ik gran-yoo-LOH-muh) is a severe inflammation of the nail in which a lump of red tissue grows up from the nail bed to the nail plate (**Figure 20-21**).

- **Onychomycosis** (ahn-ih-koh-my-KOH-sis) is a fungal infection of the nails (**Figure 20-22**). A common form is whitish patches that can be scraped off the surface. A second form is long, yellowish streaks within the nail substance. The disease invades the free edge and spreads toward the root. The infected portion is thick and discolored. In a third form, the deeper layers of the nail are invaded, causing the superficial layers to appear irregularly thin. These infected layers peel off and expose the diseased parts of the nail bed.

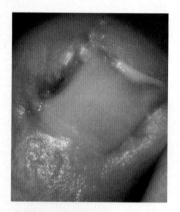

▲ FIGURE 20-20
Chronic paronychia.

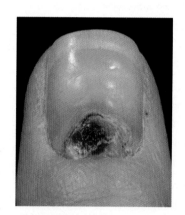

▲ FIGURE 20-21
Pyrogenic granuloma.

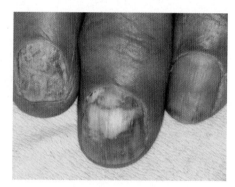

▲ FIGURE 20-22
Onychomycosis.

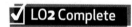
☑ **LO2 Complete**

Introduction to Manicuring

The ancients regarded long, polished, and colored fingernails as a mark of distinction between aristocrats and common laborers. Manicuring, once considered a luxury for the few, is now a service used by many men and women. The word *manicure* is derived from the Latin *manus* (hand) and *cura* (care), which means the care of the hands and nails.

To perform professional manicures, it is important to develop competence when working with nail care tools. Nail care tools consist of equipment, implements, materials, and cosmetics.

EQUIPMENT

Equipment includes the permanent tools and items used to perform nail services. These items do not require replacement until they are no longer in good repair.

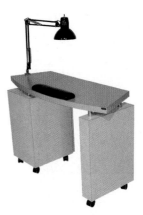

▲ **FIGURE 20-23**
Manicure table.

- *Manicure table with adjustable lamp:* Most standard manicuring tables include drawers for storage and an attached, adjustable lamp (**Figure 20-23**). The lamp should have a 40- to 60-watt bulb. The heat from a higher-wattage bulb will interfere with manicuring and sculptured nail procedures. A lower-wattage bulb will not warm a client's nails in a room that is highly air-conditioned. The warmth from the bulb will help to maintain product consistency.

- *Client's chair and nail technician's chair or stool.*

- *Finger bowl:* A plastic, china, metal or glass bowl is used for soaking the client's fingers in warm water and antibacterial soap (**Figure 20-24**).

- *Disinfection container:* This receptacle must be large enough to hold the disinfectant solution in which to immerse implements for sanitizing purposes. A cover is provided with most containers to prevent contamination of the solution when it is not in use (**Figure 20-25**).

- *Client's arm cushion:* The cushion is usually 8" to 12" long and especially made for manicuring (a towel that is folded to cushion size can also be used). The cushion or folded towel should be covered with a clean towel before each appointment.

- *Gauze and cotton container:* This container holds clean, absorbent cotton, lint-free wipes, or gauze squares.

- *Supply tray:* The tray holds cosmetics such as polishers, polish removers, and creams. It should be sturdy and easy to clean.

- *Electric nail-dryer:* A nail-dryer is an optional item used to shorten the length of time necessary for drying the client's nails.

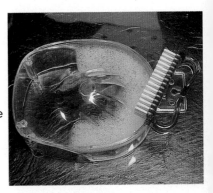

▲ **FIGURE 20-24**
Finger bath with soapy water.

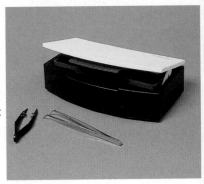

▲ **FIGURE 20-25**
Wet sanitizer.

IMPLEMENTS

Implements are tools that must be cleaned and disinfected, or discarded after use with each client. They are small enough to be sanitized in a wet sanitizer.

- *Wooden pusher:* Use a wooden pusher, also known as an orangewood stick, to loosen the cuticle around the base of a nail or clean under the free edge (**Figure 20-26**). Hold the stick similarly to a pencil. For applying cosmetics, wrap a small piece of cotton around the end.

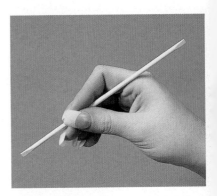

▲ **FIGURE 20-26**
Wooden pusher.

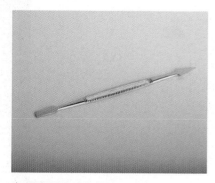

▲ FIGURE 20-27
Metal pusher.

- *Metal pusher:* The metal pusher is used to push back excess cuticle growth (**Figure 20-27**). Hold the pusher in the same way as the wooden pusher. The spoon end is used to loosen and push back the cuticle. If the pusher has rough or sharp edges, use an abrasive board to dull them. This prevents digging into the nail plate.

- *Abrasive nail file:* An abrasive nail file is used to shape the free edge of natural or sculptured nails (**Figure 20-28**). Abrasive files are available in different grits; the lower the grit number, the more aggressive its action. Most professional nail technicians use 7" or 8" nail files because some states do not allow shorter files to be used. If reusable, nail files must be sanitized after each use; if not, they should be discarded. When using a nail file, hold it with the thumb on one side of the handle and four fingers on the other side at an angle to the free edge.

  CAUTION: Always prep abrasive boards by rubbing a clean board across the sharp edges before use. Abrasive files have replaced emery boards in the salon environment but the latter are still available for the client's home use (**Figure 20-29**).

- *Nipper:* A nipper is used to trim away dead skin at the base of the nail (**Figure 20-30**). To use the nipper, hold it in the palm of the hand with the blades facing the cuticle. Place the thumb on one handle and three fingers on the other handle, with the index finger on the screw to help guide the blade around the cuticle.

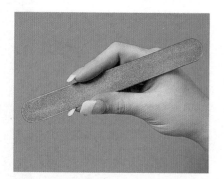

▲ FIGURE 20-28
Abrasive nail file.

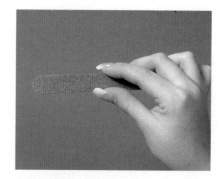

▲ FIGURE 20-29
Emery board.

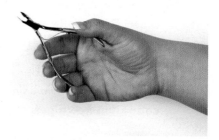

▲ FIGURE 20-30
Nipper.

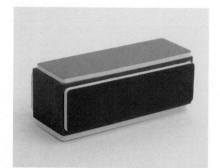

▲ FIGURE 20-31
Nail buffer.

- *Tweezers:* Tweezers can be used to lift small particles from the nail.

- *Nail brush:* A nail brush is used to clean fingernails and remove bits of cuticle with warm, soapy water. Hold the nail brush with the bristles turned down and away from you. Place the thumb on the handle side of the brush facing you and the fingers on the other side.

- *Nail buffer:* Buffers used to be made with a chamois cover, but new disposable materials have replaced them. Two- or three-way buffers are used to add shine to the nail and to smooth out corrugations or wavy ridges (**Figure 20-31**).

- *Fingernail clippers:* Fingernail clippers are used to shorten nails. For very long nails, clipping reduces filing time.

SANITATION AND DISINFECTION OF IMPLEMENTS

It is recommended that you have two complete sets of metal implements so one set is always disinfected and ready for the next client with no waiting. If there is only one set of implements available, remember that it takes 20 minutes to disinfect implements after each use.

Use the following steps to clean and disinfect implements effectively:

1 Wear gloves to prevent possible contamination of the implements by your hands and to protect your hands from the powerful chemicals in the disinfectant solution. Wash all implements thoroughly with soap and warm water and rinse off all traces of soap with plain water (**Figure 20-32**). Dry them thoroughly with a clean towel so as not to dilute the disinfectant in step 2. Brush grooved items, if necessary, and open hinged implements to scrub the area.

2 For general disinfection, metal implements must be immersed in a wet sanitizer containing an EPA-registered disinfectant (**Figure 20-33**). The required immersion time ranges from 10 to 20 minutes. Use tongs or wear gloves to remove implements from disinfectant solution. Rinse well and dry implements thoroughly with a clean towel.

3 Follow state rules and regulations for the storage of disinfected manicuring implements. Most laws stipulate storage in covered containers or a cabinet sanitizer until needed.

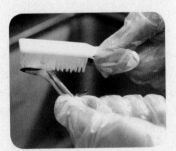

▲ **FIGURE 20-32**
Wash implements before disinfecting.

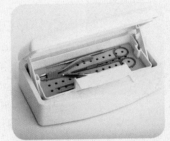

▲ **FIGURE 20-33**
Place implements in disinfectant.

MATERIALS

Materials are supplies that are used during a manicure and need to be replaced for each client.

- *Disposable towels or terrycloth towels:* A fresh, sanitized terry towel is used to cover the client's cushion before each manicure. Another fresh towel should be used to dry the client's hands after soaking in the finger bowl. Other terry or lint-free disposable towels are used to wipe spills that may occur around the finger bowl.

- *Cotton or cotton balls:* Cotton is used to remove polish, wrap the end of the wooden pusher, and apply nail cosmetics. Some nail technicians prefer to use small, fiber-free squares to remove polish because they do not leave cotton fibers on the nails that might interfere with polish application.

- *Gloves:* Use gloves when disinfecting implements and surfaces. Check with state board laws regarding required use during a manicure. Gloves are Personal Protective Equipment (PPE) worn to protect the barber from exposure to microbes during services.

- *Plastic or metal spatula:* The spatula is used to remove nail cosmetics from their containers. Never use your fingers because you will transfer bacteria into the container and contaminate the product.

- *Plastic bags:* Tape or clip a bag to the side of the manicuring table to hold materials used during a service. Line all trash cans with plastic bags. Be sure to have a generous supply of bags so that they can be changed regularly during the day.

- *Metal trash can:* The trash can should have a foot pedal and lid and be lined with a plastic bag.

- *Approved solution for jar sanitizer:* Depending on state laws, *disinfected* metal implements may be placed in a small jar containing disinfectant to maintain sanitary standards during the manicure. Always follow up with thorough washing and disinfection of the implements and jar after each use. Check your state rules and regulations for further information.

- *Antiseptic:* In the event that a nick occurs during the manicure, apply antiseptic to the injury with a sterile pledget or cotton swab.

COSMETICS

A professional nail technician needs to know how to use each nail cosmetic and what ingredients it contains. It is also important to know when to avoid using a product because of a client's allergies or sensitivities. This section identifies and describes some of the basic nail cosmetics as well as listing their basic ingredients **(Figure 20-34)**.

- *Antibacterial soap:* This soap is mixed with warm water and used in the finger bowl. It contains a detergent and an antibacterial agent that is used to sanitize the client's hands. It comes in four forms: flaked, beaded, cake, and liquid.

FYI

Gloves are available in latex, vinyl, and nitrile materials. Know that some clients are allergic to latex and that vinyl gloves do not protect the wearer from many microbes. Also, latex gloves many times shred into pieces when used to apply some lotions. For that reason, many believe nitrile gloves are the best choice for nail services. They come in boxes of 100 and are available at beauty and medical supply stores.

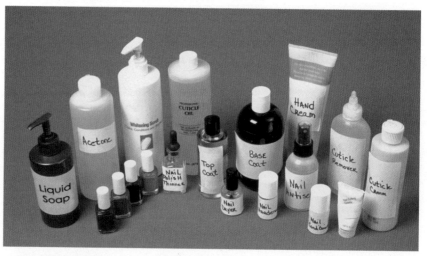

▲ **FIGURE 20-34**

Nail cosmetics.

- *Buffing powder or cream:* Buffing powder is used with a chamois buffer or three-way buffer to polish and add shine to the surface of the nail plate. The dry version may also be known as pumice powder.

- *Polish remover:* Polish remover is used to dissolve and remove nail polish. It usually contains organic solvents and acetone. Sometimes oil is added to offset the drying effect of the acetone. Use non-acetone polish remover for clients who have artificial nails, since acetone will weaken or dissolve the tips, wrap glues, and sculptured nail compound.

- *Cuticle cream:* Cuticle cream is used to lubricate and soften dry cuticles and brittle nails. It contains fats and waxes such as lanolin, cocoa butter, petroleum, and beeswax.

- *Cuticle oil:* Cuticle oil keeps the cuticle soft and helps to prevent hangnails or rough cuticles. It gives an added touch to the finish of a manicure. Cuticle oil contains ingredients such as vegetable oil, vitamin E, mineral oil, jojoba, and palm nut oil. Suggest that your clients use it at bedtime to keep their cuticles soft.

- *Cuticle solvent or cuticle remover:* Cuticle solvent makes cuticles easier to remove and minimizes clipping. It contains 2 to 5 percent sodium or potassium hydroxide and glycerin.

- *Nail bleach:* Apply nail bleach to the nail plate and under the free edge to remove yellow stains. Nail bleach contains hydrogen peroxide. If nail bleach cannot be purchased, use 20-volume (6 percent) hydrogen peroxide.

- *Nail whitener:* Nail whiteners are applied under the free edge of a nail to make the nail appear white. They contain zinc oxide or titanium oxide. Nail whiteners may be available in paste, cream, coated string, or pencil form.

- *Dry nail polish:* Dry nail polish (pumice powder) is used with the chamois buffer to add shine to the nail. Some clients prefer it to liquid clear polish. Dry nail polish contains mild abrasives that are used for smoothing or sanding, such as tin oxide, talc, silica, and kaolin, and is available in powder and cream form.

- *Nail strengthener/hardener:* Nail strengthener is applied to the nail before the base coat. It prevents splitting and peeling of the nail. There are several types of nail strengthener:

  1. Protein hardener is a combination of clear polish and protein, such as collagen.

  2. Nylon fiber is a combination of clear polish with nylon fibers. It is applied first vertically and then horizontally on the nail plate. It can be hard to cover because the fibers on the nail are visible.

  3. Hardeners do not contain formaldehyde as believed before in the industry. The ingredient is actually methylene glycol, an ingredient that creates bridges or cross-links between the keratin strands that make up the natural nail, making the plate stiffer and more resistant to bending and breaking.

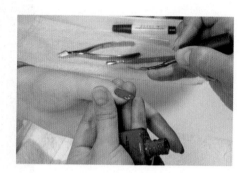

- *Base coat:* The base coat is colorless and is applied to the nail before the application of colored polish. It prevents red or dark polish from yellowing or staining the nail plate. Base coat is the first polish applied in the polish procedure, unless a nail strengthener is being used. It contains more resin than colored polish to maintain a tacky surface so the colored polish will adhere better. Base coat also contains ethyl acetate, a solvent, isopropyl alcohol, butyl acetate, nitrocellulose, resin, and sometimes formaldehyde.

- *Colored polish, liquid enamel, or lacquer:* Colored polish is used to add color and gloss to the nail. Usually it is applied in two coats. Colored polish contains a solution of nitrocellulose in a volatile solvent such as amyl acetate, and evaporates easily. Manufacturers add castor oil to prevent the polish from drying too rapidly.

- *Top coat or sealer:* The top coat, a colorless polish, is applied over colored polish to prevent chipping and to add a shine to the finished nail. It contains nitrocellulose, toluene, a solvent, isopropyl alcohol, and polyester resins.

- *Liquid nail dry:* Liquid nail dry is used to prevent smudging of the polish. It promotes rapid drying so that the polish is not tacky, and prevents the polish from dulling. It is generally available in brush-on or spray form.

- *Hand cream and hand lotion:* Hand lotion and hand cream add a finishing touch to a manicure. Since they soften and smooth the hands, they make the finished manicure as beautiful as possible. Hand cream helps the skin retain moisture. It is thicker than hand lotion and is made of emollients and humectants such as glycerin, cocoa butter, lecithin, and gums. Hand lotion has a thinner consistency than hand cream because it contains more oil. Hand cream or hand lotion can be used as the oil in a conditioning hot-oil manicure.

- *Nail conditioner:* Nail conditioner contains moisturizers. It should be applied at night, before bedtime, to help prevent brittle nails and dry cuticles.

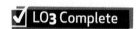

TYPES OF POLISH APPLICATION

When men choose to wear polish, it is usually a clear polish that is applied to the entire nail plate (full coverage). Other coverage options include:

- *Free edge:* The free edge of the nail is unpolished. This helps to prevent the polish from chipping.

- *Hairline tip:* The nail plate is polished and $\frac{1}{16}$" is removed from the free edge. This prevents the polish from chipping.

- *Slim-line or free walls:* Leave a $\frac{1}{16}$" margin on each side of the nail plate. This makes a wide nail appear narrower.

- *Half-moon or lunula:* The lunula at the base of the nail is left unpolished.

Colored polish is usually applied in four or five coats. The base coat is applied first, followed by two coats of color and one or two applications of topcoat. Roll the polish bottle in the palms of the hands to mix. Never shake polish. Shaking causes air bubbles to form, which can be transferred to the nail plate during application and cause marks in the finished polish. Apply all coats of polish in the following manner:

1. Remove the brush from the bottle and wipe one side on the bottle neck so that a bead of polish remains on the end of the brush. Start in the center of the nail, position the brush $\frac{1}{16}$" away from the cuticle, and brush toward the free edge.

   Using the same technique, do the left side of nail, then the right side. There should be enough polish on the brush to complete three strokes without having to dip it back into the bottle; however the amount will need to be adjusted according to the size of the nail. The more strokes used, the more lines or lumps will show on the client's nail. Small areas missed with the first color coat can be covered with the second coat.

2. Apply two coats of colored polish using the same technique used for the base coat. Complete the first color coat on both hands before starting the second coat. Polish on the cuticle should be removed with a cotton-tipped orangewood stick saturated in polish remover.

3. Apply one or two coats of top coat to prevent chipping and to give nails a glossy look. The use of an instant nail dry spray is optional, but it is effective in preventing smudging and dulling.

CHAIR-SIDE MANICURE

In some barbershops, the manicurist performs the manicure at the barber's workstation. This procedure is called a chair-side or booth manicure and requires the manicurist to either balance the supply tray on the lap or have a small table at hand. If manicures are to be performed chair-side, the styling chair should have a small, recessed hole at the end of the armrest to hold the finger bowl. The manicurist must then move around the client, depending on which hand is being manicured.

When performing a chair-side manicure, always be considerate of the barber's position during the haircutting and styling process. Try to anticipate the turn of the barber chair or a change in the client's position in order to prevent client discomfort and any interference with the barber's procedures.

A hand and arm massage is a thoroughly relaxing service that should be incorporated into manicure procedures. Use the massage techniques learned in Chapter 12 to perform the following procedures.

A. HAND MASSAGE TECHNIQUES

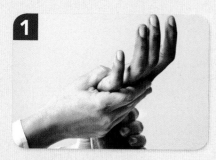

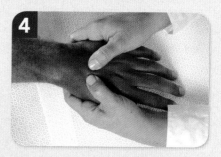

1 *Relaxation movement:* This is a form of massage known as joint movement. Apply hand lotion or cream. Place the client's elbow on a cushion. With one hand, brace the client's arm. With the other hand, hold the client's wrist and bend it back and forth slowly 5 to 10 times or until you feel the client has relaxed.

2 *Joint movement on fingers:* Lower the client's arm, bracing his right hand so you can start the massage on his little finger. Hold the finger at the base of the nail and gently rotate to form circles. Work toward the thumb, three to five times on each finger.

3 *Circular movement in palm:* Use the effleurage manipulation. Place the client's elbow on the cushion and, with your thumbs in the client's palm, rotate in a circular movement in opposite directions.

4 *Circular movement on wrist:* Hold the client's hand between your hands, placing your thumbs on top and your fingers below the client's hand. Move the thumbs in a circular motion in opposite directions, from the client's wrist to his knuckles. Move up and down three to five times. At the last rotation, wring the client's wrist by bracing your hands around the wrist and gently twisting in opposite directions.

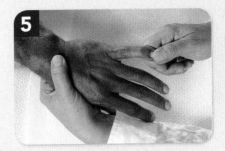

5 *Circular movement on back of the hand and fingers:* Rotate down the back of the client's hand using the thumbs. Rotate down the little finger and the client's thumb, and gently squeeze off at the tips of the client's fingers. Go back and rotate down the ring finger and index finger, gently squeezing off. Now do the middle finger and squeeze off at the tip. This tapering to the fingertips helps blood flow.

B. ARM MASSAGE TECHNIQUES

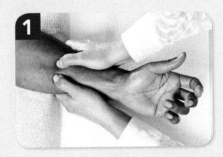

1 Warm cream or lotion in your hands, apply to the client's arm and work it in. Work from the client's wrist toward the elbow, except on the last movement, when work should be from the elbow to the wrist. Finally, squeeze off at the fingertips, as at the end of a hand massage. Apply more cream if necessary.

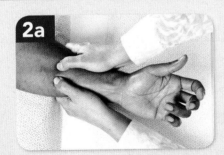
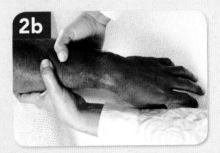

2 *Effleurage on arms:* Put the client's arm on the table, bracing the arm with your hands. Hold the client's hand palm up in your hand. Your fingers should be under the client's hand, your thumbs side by side in the client's palm. Rotate your thumbs in opposite directions, starting at the client's wrist and working toward the elbow. When you reach the elbow, slide your hand down the client's arm to the wrist and rotate back up to the elbow three to five times. Turn the arm over and repeat three to five times on the top side of arm.

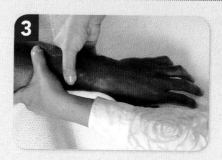

3 *Friction massage movement (wringing movement):* A friction massage involves deep rubbing of the muscles. Bend the client's elbow so the arm is horizontal in front of you, with the back of the hand facing up. Place your hands around the arm with your fingers facing in the same direction as the arm, and gently twist in opposite directions as you would wring out a washcloth, from wrist to elbow. Repeat up and down the forearm three to five times.

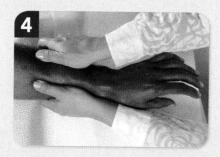

4 *Kneading movement on the arm:* Place your thumbs on the top side of the client's arm so they are horizontal. Move them in opposite directions, from wrist to elbow and back down to wrist. This squeezing motion moves the flesh over the bone and stimulates the arm tissue. Do this three to five times.

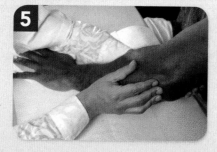

5 *Rotation of the elbow, friction massage movement:* Brace the client's arm with your left hand and apply cream to the elbow. Cup the elbow with your right hand and rotate your hand over the client's elbow. Repeat three to five times. To finish the elbow massage, move your left arm to the top of the client's forearm. Gently slide both hands down the forearm from the elbow to the fingertips as if climbing down a rope. Repeat three to five times.

Basic Table Setup

It is important that the manicure table be sanitary and properly equipped with all necessary implements, materials, and cosmetics. Anything needed during a service should be readily available. An orderly table gives the client confidence during the manicure. Since regulations regarding table setup vary from state to state, be guided by your instructor. To set up a table, you could use the following procedure.

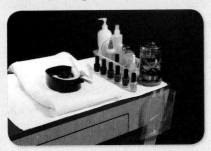

1 Apply gloves. Wipe the manicure table with an approved disinfectant.

2 Wrap the client's cushion in a clean towel. Position it in the middle of the table so the cushion is toward the client and the end of the towel is toward the operator.

3 Put cotton in the bottom of the wet sanitizer. Then fill the wet sanitizer with disinfectant 20 minutes before the first manicure of the day. Put all metal implements into the wet sanitizer. Place the wet sanitizer to the most convenient side of the table.

4 Put all cosmetics except polish on the right side of the table behind the wet sanitizer.

5 Put new emery boards and a fresh chamois buffer on the right side of the table.

6 Place a finger bowl and brush in a position convenient to the client. For a conditioning hot-oil manicure, replace the finger bowl and brush with an electric hot-oil heater.

7 Tape or clip a plastic bag to the right side of the table (if left-handed, tape to the left side). This is used for depositing used materials during the manicure.

8 Put polishes to the left.

9 The drawer can be used to keep the following items: extra cotton or cotton balls in their original container or in a fresh plastic bag; pumice stone or powder; extra chamois for buffer; instant nail dry or other supplies. Be sure to wipe the drawer with disinfectant before putting supplies in it. Never place used materials in the drawer. Only completely sanitized implements sealed in airtight containers and extra materials or cosmetics should be placed in this drawer. Always keep it clean and organized.

10 Remove gloves and wash your hands.

NOTE: Remove gloves by inverting the cuffs and pulling them off inside out and then dispose of them into the trash.

Client Consultation

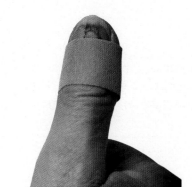

Before performing a service on a client, take time to talk with that client. During the client consultation, discuss issues of general health, the health of nails and skin, and the client's lifestyle and needs. You will use your knowledge of skin, nails, and each type of nail service to help the client select the most appropriate service. If the client has a nail or skin disorder that prevents you from performing a service, refer that client to a physician and offer to perform a service as soon as the disorder has been treated. A good client consultation can make the difference between being a professional and just doing nails.

Finish the consultation with a determination of the desired shape and polish color of the nails. Consider the shape of the hands, the length of the fingers, the shape of the cuticles, and the type of work the client does. The five standard nail shapes, illustrated in **Figure 20-35**, are described as follows:

- The *squoval nail* is a combination of a square and oval shape that is straight across the tip with the ends rounded.

- The *square, or rectangular, nail* is completely straight across with no rounding at the edges. This is a sturdy shape because the full width of the nail remains at the free edge. Clients who work with their hands usually require shorter, square nails.

- The *round nail* should be just slightly rounded at the tip of the finger.

- The *oval nail* is similar to the squoval shape with tapered, rounded corners. Clients whose hands are on display may request longer oval nail shapes.

- The *pointed nail* is suited to thin hands with narrow nail beds. The nail is tapered somewhat longer than usual to enhance the slender appearance of the hand; however, these nails can be weak and break easily.

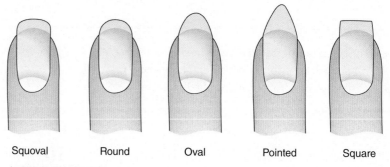

Squoval   Round   Oval   Pointed   Square

▲ **FIGURE 20-35**

Men's and women's nail shapes.

Most men prefer short nails. The square, round, or squoval shapes can be accomplished on shorter nail lengths and usually look the most appropriate on male hands. Generally, tapering the nail ends to a point or oval shape should be reserved for use on female hands and nails.

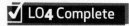
✓ **LO4 Complete**

Men's Manicure

Manicure procedures are basically the same for men and women. Table setup is the same, except that colored polish is not typically used on men. Some men like a clear liquid polish, while others prefer a dry or buffed finish. Using hand cream or lotion is optional and depends on the client's preference. The following is one method of performing a men's manicure.

SUPPLIES

- Manicure table, with lamp if needed
- Gloves (if required)
- Linen or paper towels
- Massage cream or lotion
- Finger bowl and brush
- Metal implements (fingernail clippers, nippers, file, metal pusher)
- Disposable implements (abrasive file, wooden pusher, buffers)
- Cotton or pledgets
- Hand soap or sanitizer
- Disinfection container with disinfectant solution
- Clear polish
- Buffing cream

MANICURE PRE-SERVICE

1. Apply gloves. Set up the manicuring table with implements, products, and materials.

2. Disinfect table, implements, and tools. Remove gloves.

3. Greet the client.

4. Wash your hands. Have the client wash his hands or apply a hand sanitizer. Thoroughly dry hands and nails with a sanitized towel. Apply new gloves if required.

5. Perform a client consultation. Check for nail disorders and decide if it is safe and appropriate to perform the manicure. If the client should not receive the service, explain the reasons and suggest that he seek a medical consultation. If it is safe to proceed, discuss the service options with the client.

6. Begin working with the left hand so you can work from right to left.

PROCEDURE

NOTE: This procedure is written for the right-handed client

1 If the client has clear polish from a previous manicure, it must be removed. Begin with the little finger of the left hand, using cotton saturated with polish remover. Repeat on the right hand.

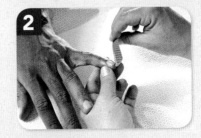

2 Shape the nails. Most men keep their nails fairly short. If the nails are long, shorten them with fingernail clippers before filing. File from the corners to center in one direction; do not saw back and forth.

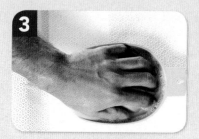

3 Soften the cuticles. After filing the nails of the left hand, soak them in a soap bath while filing the second hand.

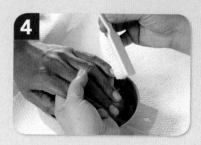

4 Clean the nails. Use a nail brush to clean fingertips and nails and to remove surface debris from nails. Remove the left hand from the soap bath while placing the right hand into the bath, and brush the fingers with downward strokes, starting at the first knuckle and brushing in one direction toward the free edge.

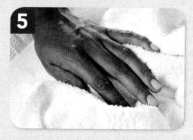

5 Dry the hand. Use the end of a clean towel, making sure to dry between the fingers. As you dry, gently push back the eponychium with the towel.

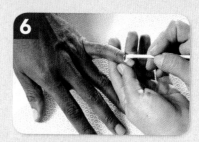

6 Apply cuticle remover. Use a cotton-tipped wooden pusher to apply cuticle remover to each nail on the left hand. Put left hand back into the bath while repeating cleansing steps on the right hand. Apply cuticle remover to right hand, remove left hand from bath, and replace with right hand.

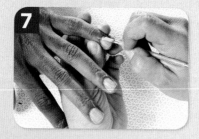

7 Loosen the cuticles. Men generally have more cuticle than women; therefore, more work may need to be done on them than in a women's manicure. Use the spoon end of the pusher or a wooden pusher to gently push back and lift the cuticle off the nails of the left hand. Repeat on right hand.

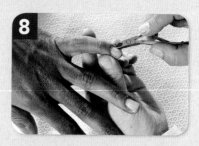

8 Use sharp nippers to remove any loosely hanging tags of dead skin (hangnails). Never rip or tear the cuticle tags or the living skin, since this may lead to infection. State regulations do not permit nail technicians to cut or nip living skin.

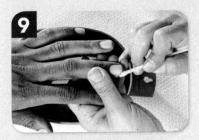

9 Clean under the free edge with a cotton-tipped wooden pusher while holding the left hand over the soap bath, and brush a last time to remove bits of cuticle and nail debris that remain on the nail. Rest the left hand on a clean towel and repeat this procedure on the right hand.

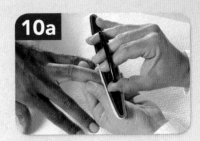

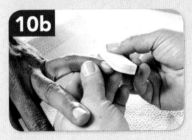

10 Apply buffing powder or cream and buff.

11 Apply cuticle oil. Use a cotton-tipped wooden pusher, a cotton swab, or an eyedropper to apply, and massage oil into the nail plate and surrounding skin using a circular motion.

12 Bevel nails if necessary.

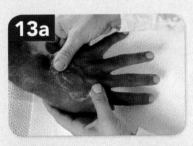

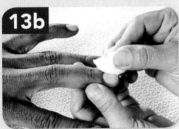

13 Apply hand lotion and massage the hands and wrists; wipe excess lotion off nails.

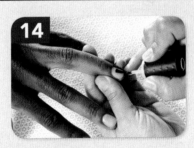

14 Polish the nails with a clear matte polish if desired or buff gently.

15 Complete manicure post-service procedure.

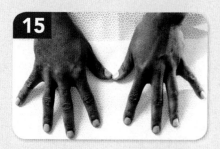

CLEANUP AND DISINFECTION

1. Schedule another appointment with the client to maintain the manicure or to perform another service; complete client's record card.

2. Clean up work area. Disinfect table, tools, and implements. Take the time to restore the basic table setup.

3. Place all used materials in the plastic bag at the end of the table and discard into a closed trashcan.

4. Wash your hands.

Women's Plain Manicure

The following procedure is just one of several correct ways to perform a plain manicure. Be guided by your instructor for alternative methods.

SUPPLIES

- Manicure table, with lamp if needed
- Gloves (if required)
- Linen or paper towels
- Massage cream or lotion
- Finger bowl and brush
- Metal implements (fingernail clippers, nippers, file, metal pusher)
- Disposable implements (abrasive file, wooden pusher, buffers)
- Cotton or pledgets
- Hand soap or sanitizer
- Disinfection container with disinfectant solution
- Polish selection

MANICURE PRESERVICE

1. Set up the manicuring table with implements and materials.

2. Sanitize table, implements, and tools.

3. Greet the client.

4. Wash your hands. Have the client wash her hands. Thoroughly dry hands and nails with a clean towel.

5. Perform a client consultation. Refer to the client record card for responses and observations during the client consultation. Check for nail disorders and decide if it is safe and appropriate to perform a service on the client. If the client should not receive service, explain the reasons and make a medical referral, if necessary. If it is safe to proceed, discuss the service desired by the client.

6. Begin working with the hand that is not the client's favored hand. The favored hand will need to soak longer, because it is used more often.

PROCEDURE

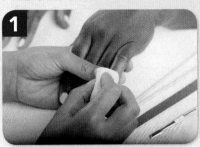

1 *Remove polish:* Begin with the little finger. Saturate cotton with polish remover. If the client is wearing artificial nails, use non-acetone remover to avoid damaging them. Hold saturated cotton on the nail for approximately 10 seconds. Wipe the old polish off the nail with a stroking motion toward the free edge. If all the polish is not removed, repeat this step until all traces of polish are gone. It may be necessary to put cotton around the tip of an wooden pusher and use it to clean polish away from the cuticle area. Repeat this procedure on each finger.

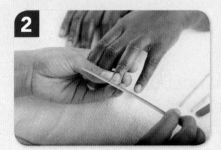

2 *Shape the nails:* Using an emery board or nail file, shape the nails. Start with the little finger, holding it between the thumb and index finger. Use the coarse side of an emery board to shape the nail. File from the right side to the center of the free edge and from the left side to the center of the free edge. Do not file into the corners of the nails. File each hand from the little finger to the thumb.

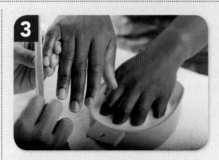

3 *Soften the cuticles:* After filing the first hand, put it in a soap bath while filing the second hand, to soak and soften the cuticles.

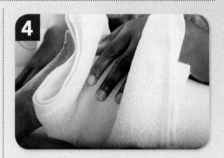

4 *Clean the nails:* Brushing the nails and hands with a nail brush cleans the fingers and pieces of cuticle from the nails. Remove the first hand from the soap bath and brush the fingers with a nail brush. Use downward strokes, starting at the first knuckle and brushing toward the free edge. Dry the hand with a fresh towel. Make sure to dry between the fingers.

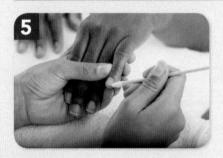

5 Apply cuticle remover using a cotton-tipped wooden pusher. Saturate cotton with cuticle remover and spread the remover generously around the cuticles and under the free edge of each finger. Put the second hand into the soap bath to soak.

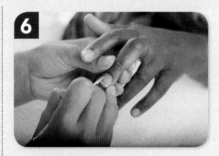

6 *Loosen the cuticles:* Use a wooden pusher and/or the spoon end of a steel pusher to push back gently and lift the cuticle off of the nails. Use a circular movement to help lift cuticles that cling to the nail plate. The cuticle remover will probably remove enough cuticle so that clipping will be unnecessary.

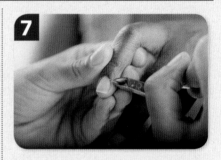

7 Carefully nip the cuticles if allowed by your state board. Use a cuticle nipper to remove any loosely hanging tags of dead skin (hangnails). Try to remove the cuticle in one piece. Wipe away excess cuticle remover if necessary to see the cuticle clearly. Brush gently to clean.

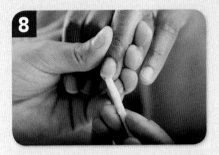

8 Clean under the free edge using a cotton-tipped wooden pusher. Remove the second hand from the soap bath. Hold the first hand over the soap bath and brush a last time to remove any bits of cuticle and traces of solvent. Then let the client's first hand rest on the clean towel.

9 Repeat steps 4 through 8 on the second hand.

10 *Bleach nails:* Bleaching the nails is an option if the client's nails are yellowed. Use a prepared nail bleach or 20-volume (6 percent) hydrogen peroxide. Apply the bleaching agent to the yellowed nail with a cotton-tipped wooden pusher. Be careful not to brush bleach on the client's skin or cuticle as it will cause irritation. Apply the bleach several times if the nails are extremely yellow. Certain clients' nails will need to be bleached every time as part of each manicure for a period of time, since all the yellow may not fade after one service.

11 *Buff nails:* Buffing with a disposable chamois or other buffer is optional. To buff nails, apply dry polish to the nail with a wooden pusher. Buff on a diagonal, from the base of the nail to its free edge. Buff in one direction, from left to right with a downward stroke and then from right to left with a downward stroke, forming an X pattern. While buffing, lift the back of the buffer off the nail to prevent friction, which will cause a burning sensation. After buffing, the client's hands should be washed to remove any traces of abrasive or dry polish. The buffer also can be used to smooth out wavy ridges or corrugated nails.

12 Using a cotton-tipped wooden pusher, apply cuticle oil to each nail. Start with the little finger of the left hand and rub oil into each cuticle in a circular motion. Repeat on the right hand.

13 *Bevel nails option:* To bevel the underside of the free edge, hold an emery board at a 45-degree angle and file with an upward stroke. This removes any rough edges or cuticle particles.

14 Apply hand lotion and massage hands and arms. A hand massage is a pleasant touch before applying polish. Apply lotion or cream to the hand and arm with a clean spatula.

15 Remove traces of oil so that the polish will adhere to the nail. Use a small piece of cotton saturated with alcohol or polish remover.

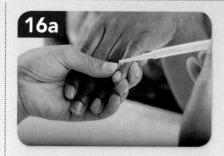

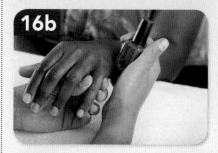

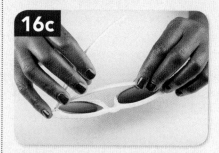

16 Apply base coat. Apply polish and remove excess. Apply top coat.

CLEAN-UP AND DISINFECTION

1. Schedule another appointment with the client to maintain the manicure or to perform another service. Complete client's record card.

2. Clean up work area. Disinfect table, tools, and implements. Take the time to restore the basic table setup.

3. Place all used materials in the plastic bag at the end of the table. If the bag is full or contains used materials from artificial nail services, discard it in a closed pail.

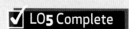

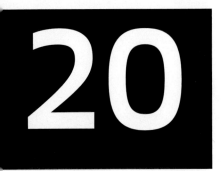

Review Questions

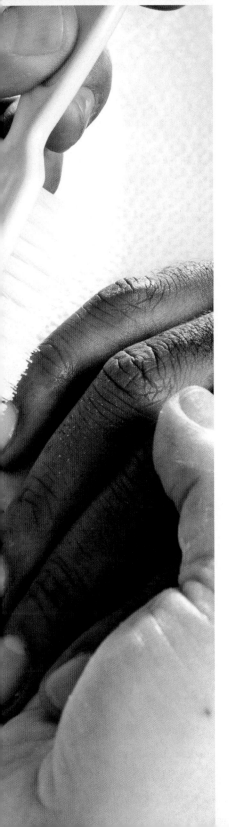

1. Explain the location of the following: (a) nail bed, (b) matrix, (c) nail plate, (d) free edge, and (e) cuticle.

2. What is the average growth rate of a nail?

3. What are five nail disorders that may be serviced by a manicurist?

4. List five nail disorders that should not be serviced by a manicurist.

5. List the basic materials needed to perform a men's manicure.

6. What are the five basic nail shapes?

7. Identify nail shapes that look appropriate on a man's hand.

8. Name five hand massage techniques and four arm massage techniques.

9. Briefly list the steps of a basic manicure procedure.

10. Explain the manner in which a chair-side manicure is performed.

Chapter
Glossary

Beau's lines lengthwise ridges caused by uneven nail growth

bed epithelium thin layer of tissue between the nail plate and the nail bed

bruised nails blood clots that form under the nail plate; appear as dark purplish spots

cuticle dead, colorless tissue attached to the nail plate around the base of the nail

discolored nails a condition in which the nails turn a variety of colors such as yellow, blue, blue-gray, green, red, or purple; can be caused by poor blood circulation, a heart condition, topical or oral medications, or a systemic disorder

eggshell nails have noticeably thin, white nail plates that are more flexible than normal

eponychium living skin at the base of the nail plate and covering the matrix area

free edge part of the nail plate that extends over the tip of the finger

hangnails condition in which the cuticle splits around the nail

hyponychium slightly thickened layer of skin between the fingertip and free edge of the nail plate

leukonychia condition of white spots on the nails due to air bubbles, bruising, or injury to the nail

lunula half-moon shape at the base of the nail

matrix area where the nail is formed; produces cells that create the nail plate

melanonychia darkening of the nail due to increased and localized pigment in the matrix

nail an appendage of the skin; horny protective plate at the end of the finger or toe

nail bed portion of the skin on which the nail plate rests

nail folds folds of normal skin around the nail plate

nail grooves slits or furrows on the sides of the nail

nail plate horny plate resting on and attached to the nail bed

nail psoriasis tiny pits or roughness on the surface of the nail plate

nail pterygium abnormal condition occurring when skin is stretched by the nail plate

onychia inflammation of the matrix with pus, redness, swelling, and shedding of the nail

onychocryptosis ingrown nails

onycholysis loosening of the nail without shedding

onychomadesis the separation and falling off of the nail from the nail bed

onychomycosis fungal infection; whitish patches on nail that can be scraped off or long yellowish streaks within nail plate

onychophagy bitten nails

onychorrhexis abnormal brittleness of the nail plate

onychosis technical term for any deformity or disease of the nail

onyx technical term for nail

paronychia bacterial infection of the tissues surrounding the nail

pincer or trumpet nail edge of nail plate curls around to form a trumpet or cone shape at the free edge

plicatured nail "folded nail"; highly curved nail plate often caused by injury

Pseudomonas aeruginosa skin bacteria that can cause an infection of the nail

pyrogenic granuloma severe inflammation of the nail in which a lump of red tissue grows up from the nail bed to the nail plate

ridges depressions running vertically down the length of the nail

PART 5

THE BUSINESS OF BARBERING

21 State Board
PREPARATION AND LICENSING LAWS

☑ Learning Objectives

AFTER COMPLETION OF THIS CHAPTER, YOU SHOULD BE ABLE TO:

1 Discuss how to prepare for written state board examinations.

2 Discuss barber board laws, rules, and regulations in your state.

3 Discuss how to prepare for practical state board examinations.

4 Explain what information may be found in candidate information booklets/materials.

5 Identify the primary objectives of state barber board rules and regulations.

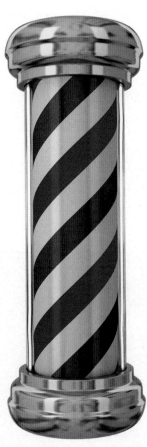

Key Terms

PAGE NUMBER INDICATES WHERE IN THE CHAPTER THE TERM IS USED.

candidate information
booklet / 713

practical exams / 710

written exam / 706

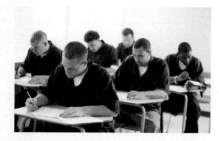

▲ FIGURE 21-1
Candidates preparing for the licensing examination.

By the time you have reached this chapter in the textbook, you should be well on your way to taking your state board examinations (**Figure 21-1**). This is a crucial milestone that marks the beginning of your professional career as you put all that you have learned and mastered into practice.

As with the basic education that is behind you, and the successes that lie ahead, the preparation for your state board examinations is under *your* control. Many factors will influence how well you perform on these tests, including your mastery of course content, physical health and psychological attitude, time management skills, and study skills.

Preparing for State Board Exams

Most states require written theory and practical hands-on examinations. Others may employ written test instruments for both theory and practical testing. In either case, you may be experiencing some test anxiety. This is a perfectly natural feeling no matter how well you perform behind the chair or in the classroom. Let's face it, thinking and working under the pressure of career-changing events can be challenging! Sometimes self-doubt creeps in and you might find yourself asking questions such as, "Can I pass the written test? Will I pass the practical? What if my model doesn't show up? What if I nick my model during the shave? What if the questions are taken from a different textbook? What if, what if, what if . . . ?" Sound familiar? Probably, but there are steps you can take to reduce stress so that you can perform to your optimum level.

WRITTEN EXAMS

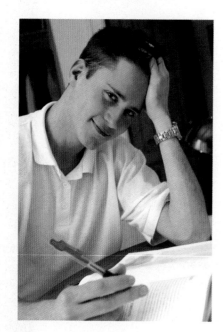

First of all, you must know the basics. Last-minute cramming is not going to help you answer a situational question about repairing a reddish cast on chemically relaxed hair unless you know the laws of color theory and how chemicals affect the hair. Use the study skills learned in Chapter 1 and organize your review strategy; then use every resource that is available to review the basics for the **written exam,** including:

- Textbooks and workbooks

- Past quizzes and tests

- State barber board rules and regulations

- Examination candidate information booklet or materials

- Instructors

If you feel particularly weak in a certain subject or confused about a procedure, ask your instructor to help you review. *Always* study your state barber board rules and regulations to prepare for related questions on the written exams.

Test Formats

Most written barber exams consist of multiple-choice questions, although some may include true–false or situational questions as well. Refer to the barber law or candidate information materials of your state for this information.

Tests typically begin with oral and/or written directions that tell you how the questions should be answered and what the time limits are. *Listen* and/or *read* carefully before you begin!

Although the most important strategy of test taking is to know your material, there are some general guidelines that might help you answer different types of questions:

- *True/False:* Absolute qualifiers such as *all, none, always,* and *never* are generally not true, and for a statement to be true, each part of the entire statement must be true.

- *Multiple Choice:* Read the directions carefully to see if the questions require more than one answer. For example, there is a big difference between "Select the best *answer* to each question" and "Select the best *answers* to each question."

- Read the entire question and try to answer it in your head first, then read through the possible answers (**Figure 21-2**). First impressions are often correct so don't second-guess yourself. Select the answer closest to your own or eliminate answers you *know* are incorrect, then look for the best answer among the remaining choices.

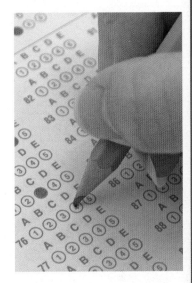

FINAL EXAM

1. The study of the hair is called:
   a) hairology
   b) dermatology
   c) trichology
   d) biology

2. Hair is not found on the palms of the hands, soles of the feet, lips, and:
   a) neck
   b) eyelids
   c) ankles
   d) wrists

3. The technical term for eyelash hair is:
   a) cilia
   b) barba
   c) capilli
   d) supercilia

4. Hair is composed chiefly of:
   a) oxygen
   b) keratin
   c) melanin
   d) sulfur

5. The two main divisions of the hair are the hair root and:
   a) hair shaft
   b) follicle
   c) papilla
   d) bulb

6. The hair root is located:
   a) above the skin surface
   b) below the skin surface
   c) under the cuticle
   d) within the cortex

7. The hair root is encased by a tubelike depression in the skin known as the:
   a) bulb
   b) arrector pili
   c) papilla
   d) follicle

8. The club-shaped structure that forms the lower part of the hair root is the:
   a) arrector pili
   b) bulb
   c) papilla
   d) hair shaft

▲ **FIGURE 21-2**

Sample of a multiple-choice test.

When two possible answers are similar, one of them is probably correct. For example:

1. A comb that is dropped on the floor must be:
   a. cleansed and rinsed before used on a client
   b. cleansed and disinfected before used on a client
   c. cleansed and dried before used on a client
   d. disinfected before used on a client

Although answers b and d are similar, the important word *cleansed* is missing in d, so the answer is b.

When two or more possible answers mean the same thing, they must both be wrong. For example:

2. The epidermis is also known as the:
   a. scarf skin
   b. derma
   c. true skin
   d. corium

The answer is a because *derma, true skin,* and *corium* refer to the dermis.

Answers that include "all of the above" are often—but not always—the correct response. Sometimes test questions are confusing when words like *not, except,* or *but* are used. Pay attention to these words and reread the question if it does not seem clear.

- *Matching:* Read all the items in each list before beginning and then check off the items from the response list to eliminate choices.

- *Essays:* Organize your answer according to the cue words in the question and develop an outline before you begin writing. Make sure to write in a complete, accurate, clear, and well-organized manner.

- *Situational:* Situational test items usually provide a scenario and several different questions are asked that relate to the scenario. The sample scenario that follows provides an example of this type of test item.

Scenario: Henry's new client, Angie, likes to wear her hair in a short bob with a tapered nape area and was not happy with the last haircut she received at a different shop. Angie had asked to have the back tapered, but the stylist created a bi-level instead.

Question 1: What do you think the stylist did to create the bi-level effect?
a. Cut the hair too close in the nape area
b. Cut the hair all the same length in the nape area
c. Did not cut the hair to gradually increase in length from the hairline to the occipital area
d. Any of the above

Answer: d, because the results of a, b, or c could all create a bi-level effect.

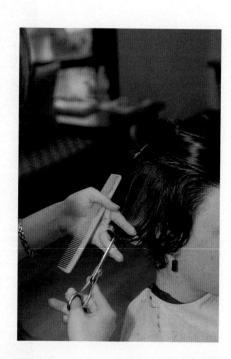

Question 2: How can Henry avoid the same mistake?

a. Use a shear-over-comb technique to taper the hair in the nape area.

b. Use a clipper-over-comb technique to taper the hair in the nape area.

c. Use a fingers-and-shear technique to taper the hair in the nape area.

d. Any of the above.

Answer: Again, the answer is d because any one of these methods could be used to accomplish a tapered nape to occipital area.

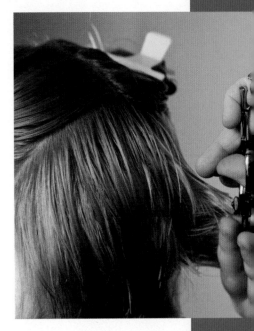

Question 3: At what elevation or projection should Henry cut Angie's hair at the occipital area to create the "bobbed" effect?

a. 0 elevation

b. 45 degrees

c. 90 degrees

d. 180 degrees

Answer: b, because projecting the hair at 45 degrees will create a stacked or "bobbed" effect.

Question 4: What should the hair from the nape to the occipital area look like from a side view when projected at 90 degrees from a vertical parting?

a. Longer at the nape; shorter at the occipital

b. A 45-degree angle from nape to occipital; shorter at the nape, longer at the occipital

c. Uniform layers

d. Increased layers

Answer: b, because the hair will be shorter at the hairline and gradually increase in length to the occipital area; this creates a 45-degree angle when held at 90 degrees.

If a scenario question confuses you, go back to the original scene or break the question down for clarity. For example, if you were unsure about the answer to Question 4, refer back to what you already know—namely, that Angie had a bi-level cut but wanted a tapered cut. In Questions 1–3, choices were provided that could accomplish the taper. Question 4 simply asks what the taper will look like when held at a specific projection (90 degrees) from a specific type of parting (vertical). Visualize the scenario—you know the taper is shorter at the hairline and there is length at the occipital. You know how to hold vertical partings. What would your finger placement look like if you were cutting the hair from the nape to the occipital? That's right—a 45-degree angle!

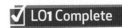

✓ LO1 Complete

Barber Law

In addition to testing basic theory concepts, the written exam will contain questions about your state's barber laws and rules. The overview of state barber board rules and regulations at the end of this chapter provides some general information that is applicable to all the boards; however, you will probably have

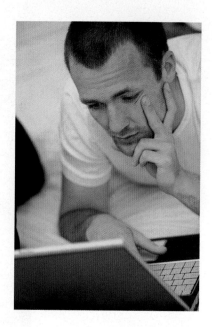

to learn about the specific laws or rules of your state. For example, there may be a test question that asks, "How many members of the barber board must be licensed barbers?" The answer to this question varies from state to state, so you will need to know what the configuration of the barber board is in your state. Other questions relating to barber laws and regulations that may vary from state to state include, but are not limited to, the following:

- Chapter or administrative code number

- Number of board members

- Configuration of the board (barbers, public members, etc.)

- Terms of office

- Definitions

- Exemptions and exceptions

- Examination prerequisites (school hours, age, service requirements, etc.)

- Re-examination requirements

- Types of licenses

- License display

- License renewal dates

- Fees and penalties

- Minimum square footage for a barbershop

- Continuing education requirements

- Prohibited acts

- Qualifications for endorsement

Obtain copies of the barber board rules and regulations and candidate information literature for your state. Review these documents thoroughly and be guided by your instructor when preparing for written exams.

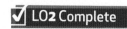

LO2 Complete

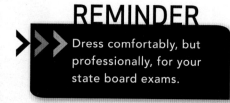

REMINDER

Dress comfortably, but professionally, for your state board exams.

PRACTICAL EXAMS

After completing the barber school curriculum, examination candidates should be competent in their technical skills and ready for state board **practical exams.** Although performance criteria for practical examinations vary from state to state, the basic skills or procedures that are usually evaluated are haircutting, shaving, shampooing, sanitation, and possibly blow-drying or a chemical service. A fairly standard testing protocol requires candidates to demonstrate competence with the comb, shears, razor, and clippers. Safety precautions, proper draping procedures, and the safe handling of tools are also important performance standards. Review barber board rules and candidate information literature for details about what you will be tested on at the practical exam.

Practical exams require a different approach than written exams because you have to perform the procedures. After all, performing services is what barbering is all about and practical exams are the best way to evaluate a person's competency in barbering techniques.

Basic preparation for practical exams should always include practice on the model that you will be taking to the examination. To feel confident about your performance, you must be familiar with the model's hair texture and the haircut that you will be performing. Many states require a taper hair cut (Figure 21-3) and knowing the characteristics of your model's hair and the

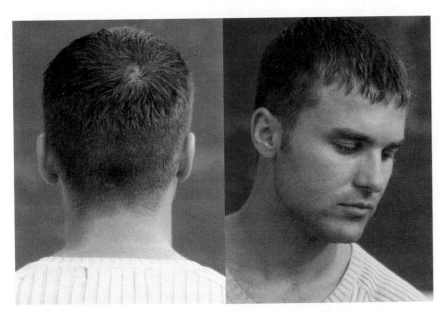

▲ **FIGURE 21-3**
One variation of a taper cut.

best techniques for cutting it will help to eliminate some nervousness and stress during the practical exam. When practicing for practical exams, make sure to:

- set up your station as if you were at the state board examinations.

- ensure that all tools and implements have been disinfected and are in good working order.

- practice all sanitation and disinfection procedures, including hand washing.

- time yourself.

- request feedback from instructors and the model.

- be clear about what examiners will check and look for in the performance of procedures.

- read your state board rules and regulations to find specific exam information.

- review the candidate information booklet for specifics about practical testing.

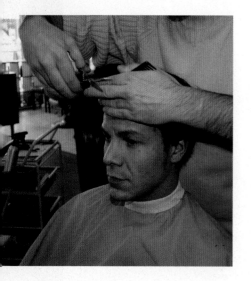

If the correct procedures for performing the services of your state's practical exam are not already second nature to you, it is time for some honest reflection and self-assessment.

Begin by envisioning yourself at the test site. Your model is in place and the lead examiner has given the signal to begin. What do you do first? Next? Think through all the steps of all the procedures and then write each step down on a piece of paper (Figure 21-4). During the next haircut or other practice exam procedure that you perform, use the list for reference. Pretend that you are at the exam and follow as many of the procedures as the situation allows, for example, washing your hands, practicing proper draping, disinfecting tools, or deciding at what section of the head you will begin the haircut. Refer to your list and make notes as necessary. Revise the list as you notice steps that were left out or overlooked.

Practical Exam–Haircut Procedure Plan

After given the signal to begin, I will:

Set up tools and linens
Sanitize tools
Wash hands
Drape model for shampoo
Perform shampoo and towel dry the hair
Store soiled linen
Remove shampoo cape and store
Drape model for haircut
Wash hands
Rinse sanitized comb
Start haircut at the top
Proceed with haircut
Shake off cape and remove neckstrip
Drape for outline shave
Perform outline shave
Store soiled linen
Comb model's hair
Wash tools and return to disinfectant
Wash hands and indicate completion of test

▲ FIGURE 21-4

Sample procedure plan.

Preliminary Planning for Practical Exams

- *Model*: In addition to studying and practicing for state board examinations, most barbering test candidates will have to arrange to bring a model for their practical exams. This is not an arrangement that can be left to the last minute and, ideally, you should have been practicing on this model for several months. Several weeks before the test date, confirm the date, time, and travel arrangements with your model. Turn the trip to the examinations into a shared adventure and schedule time to have a celebration breakfast, lunch, or dinner. Plan to see some local attractions after the exams. Reward yourself. You've earned it!

- *Travel*: Arrange any travel plans that need to be made if you are testing in a city other than your own. If you have to travel out of town, consider arriving the day before your exams and staying overnight. This will give you the opportunity to find the test site and reduce the risk of arriving late or getting lost. It should also allow you to get a good night's sleep since you will not have a great distance to travel the day of your exams.

- *Packing*: Create a checklist of tools, implements, and equipment that you will need for the practical exams. Have your instructor review the list to make sure it is complete or compare it to the candidate information that most states send out when application for examination is made. Make sure that all tools are thoroughly cleaned and disinfected. Make sure there are no identifying names on your kit bag. If the written exams are paper tests, bring several sharpened pencils.

- *Attire*: Wear comfortable, professional-looking attire to the exams. A barber's jacket is appropriate but do not wear clothing with your name or the name of the school inscribed. Do not wear sandals, clogs, Crocs, or other open footwear that is unsafe in the work environment. Do wear comfortable closed-toed, closed-heel shoes with support and non-skid soles. Avoid excess jewelry or accessories.

- *Health*: Make a conscious effort to eat well and get sufficient rest for several days before and up to the examination date. Vitamin supplements can help to give you a nutritional edge when you are nervous or under stress. Relax. Trust in yourself and do your best.

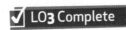

REMINDER

>> Be sure to label the contents of generic containers like spray bottles (water, alcohol, etc.)

CANDIDATE INFORMATION BOOKLETS

The extent of information made available to exam candidates varies from state to state. Some states may produce a 12-page booklet, while others provide only a few pages of information. Regardless, most states now have their candidate information online for easy access so be sure to review these valuable test-taking tools.

In most cases, **candidate information booklets** or materials will contain the following:

- Introduction to written and practical exams

- Examination rules

- Location and contact information for exams

- Manner of testing (computer-based, paper and pencil, etc.)

- Requirements, procedures, and reservation information for computer-based testing, if applicable.

- Content overview—written (number of questions, subject areas, sample questions, etc.)

- Content overview—practical (specific procedures to be tested, possible points, etc.)

- Model requirements (practical)

- Tool and equipment requirements (practical)

- What to bring and what not to bring (written and practical)

- References used to write or develop the examinations

- Grading and scoring policies (re-examination information, notification of results, etc.)

- Administrative polices (late arrivals, cancellations, exam review process, etc.)

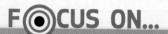

F⊙CUS ON...

Arrive 15 to 30 minutes early for your state board exams.

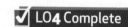

State Barber Board Rules and Regulations

Although state barber board rules and regulations may vary from state to state, the basic concept and functions of state barber boards remain the same: to protect the health, safety, and welfare of the public as it relates to the practice of barbering (See Appendix for State Barber Board contact information). Be guided by your instructor and the specific rules and regulations of your state. The following statements are designed to review these general concepts and functions.

- The governing body that is responsible for the efficient and orderly administration of barbering rules and regulations is the state barber board or other board that governs the profession.

- The authority to conduct disciplinary hearings rests with the state barber board.

- Additional authority given to the state barber board for the purposes of properly administering barber license law is the power to issue rules and regulations.

- The primary objective of the barber license law is to protect the health, safety, and welfare of the public as it relates to the practice of barbering.

- The governor of the state appoints barber board members.

- The state senate confirms the appointment of barber board members.

- The state barber board regulates educational requirements, testing, licensing, inspections, investigations, and disciplinary action.

- The objective of barber license examinations is to evaluate a license applicant's competency.

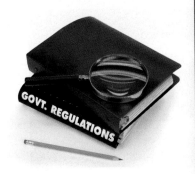

- State barber board rules and regulations may not be used to limit the number of licenses or licensees.

- An important personal requirement for a barber license applicant is to be of good moral character.

- Barbers may be forbidden to perform services on clients when the barber is suffering from a communicable disease.

- State barber boards may discipline a barber by revocation or suspension of the barber's license.

- Licensed barbers are protected by the laws of the state against unlawful action by the state barber board.

- Licensed barbers must be granted a hearing before the state barber board can take action to revoke or suspend a license.

- A licensee who violates the provisions of the barber license law can be cited and subject to disciplinary action.

- Persons who act as a barber without obtaining a license are guilty of practicing unlawfully.

- A barber who has his or her license suspended or revoked has the right to appeal to the courts.

- A person convicted of violating any of the provisions of the license law is guilty of a misdemeanor.

- The purpose of periodic inspections of barbershops is to ascertain compliance with sanitation regulations and licensure compliance.

- A licensee who willfully fails to display a license or certificate is guilty of a violation of the barber law.

- Barber law requires that suspended or revoked licenses must be surrendered to the state barber board.

- The state barber board may suspend or revoke the license of a licensee who is guilty of gross malpractice.

- The barbershop owner is responsible for posting sanitation rules, barber law, and/or the state board rules and regulations in the barbershop.

- The state barber board may suspend or revoke the license of a licensee who is guilty of immoral behavior.

- An apprentice practices barbering under the constant and direct supervision of a licensed barber.

- Generally speaking, persons who are legally exempt from barber law provisions while working within the provisions of their own professions include medical personnel, military personnel, and cosmetologists.

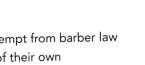

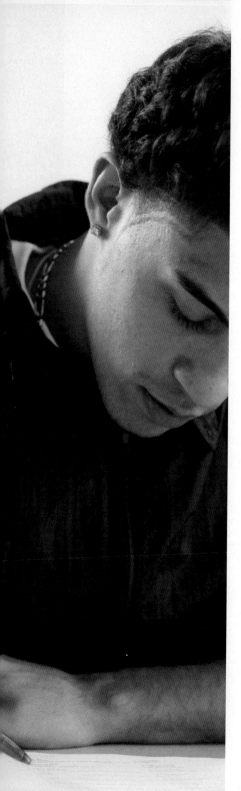

21 Review Questions

1. List the ways in which a student can prepare for written-theory state board exams.

2. List at least five strategies that may assist candidates to prepare for practical examinations.

3. List the practical exam procedures you will have to perform in your state.

4. What document provides exam candidates with important test-taking information?

5. Explain the primary purpose of barber laws, rules, and regulations.

6. Identify the full name of the barber board in your state.

Chapter
Glossary

candidate information booklet literature provided to examination candidates by the barber board

practical exams hands-on test on a live model

written exam paper-and-pencil or computer-based testing covering theoretical concepts related to barbering and barber law specific to the state

22 The Job Search

Job Application

Personal Information

NAME (LAST NAME FIRST)

CITY

ADDRESS

PHONE NO.

☑ Learning Objectives

AFTER COMPLETING THIS CHAPTER, YOU SHOULD BE ABLE TO:

1 Discuss industry positions available for barbering students.

2 Explain the guidelines of goal setting.

3 List and discuss personal characteristics important for employment.

4 Discuss employment classifications and wage structures.

5 Write a résumé and perform a job search.

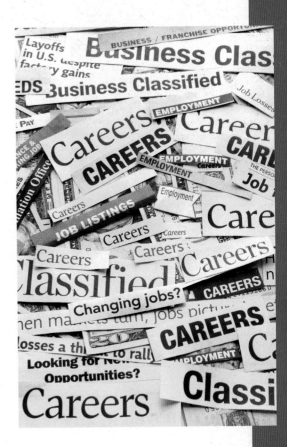

Key Terms

PAGE NUMBER INDICATES WHERE IN THE CHAPTER THE TERM IS USED.

booth rental / 725

commission / 726

cover letter / 729

employee / 724

independent
  contractor / 725

model release form / 730

portfolio / 729

résumé / 728

This chapter has been provided to assist you in your search for employment in the barbering field. Unlike many other job markets, which may have more applicants than positions available, the need for barbers and barbershops has been on a steady increase since the 1970s. While there may be some who would argue with this statement, a short historical perspective may change their minds and provide you with a context from which to view your own future in barbering.

Industry Trends: Then and Now

Prior to the Vietnam War, the Beatles, and the hippie generation of the 1960s, most average-sized towns had at least one, if not two or three, barbershops. Many of these shops were what might be thought of as a traditional barbershop, with 4 to 10 chairs, leather strops hanging at their sides, and hair tonics situated in front of the mirror. Some shops did not have shampoo bowls or even offer the service, and the majority of haircuts were performed on dry hair. Phrases such as "just a trim" or "a little off the top" were commonly heard instructions from customers.

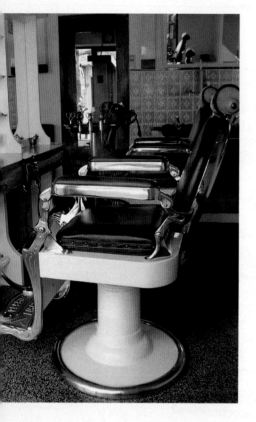

While there were certainly exceptions to the stereotypical barbershops just described, the majority of high-end barbershops or barbering salons were usually located in cities. It should be understood that 40 or more years ago, today's thriving suburbs, which abut each other and link cities to rural areas in many parts of the country, started out as little more than isolated villages and towns with populations of about 20,000 people. Independently owned businesses, from drugstores and bakeries to banks, butcher shops, and beauty parlors, were the norm. Chain and franchise salons were virtually nonexistent.

Most of the larger corporations and businesses were located in the cities, which had the population to support the higher-end barbershops and salons. Busy executives and professional people were more apt to indulge in shampoo, manicure, facial, or chemical services on a regular basis, in addition to their cuts, shaves, or beard trims. As the suburbs grew, more of these shops could be found in the outlying areas, but they were still few and far between in terms of distance and the inclination to offer a full range of services.

The impact of the long-hair trend generated by musicians and social groups of the 1960s and early 1970s was felt in the traditional barbershops. Some barbers chose not to adapt their skills to the long-hair look and lost customers as a result. While it is true that many young people allowed their hair to grow long without any form or design, there were others who preferred a longer but more controlled look. This look necessitated a different method of cutting and styling, which included preliminary shampoos, more precision cutting of the interior sections of the hair, and blow-drying. At about the same time, unisex salons were introduced and began to capitalize on the longer-hair market. The barbershops' clientele began to dwindle and fewer young people were studying to be barbers. This was also about the time that certain social and industry factions generated the notion that barbers and barbering were a thing of the past, regardless of whether it was true or not.

Eventually, with fewer young barbers to take their place, some veteran barbers retired and simply closed the doors to their shops. Conversely, younger barbers who enhanced their skills to include new techniques that would satisfy the haircutting needs of their clients are still in business today. As this group now prepares for retirement, new barbers are needed to replace them.

From the 1970s through the 1990s, unisex salons garnered much of the male market; this has resulted in entire generations of males who are more familiar with unisex and beauty salons than with barbershops. Fortunately for the next generation of barbers, of which you are a part, the cycle has gone full circle and men are again seeking out barbershops for their personal grooming services.

The male baby boomer, which is now in his 50s or 60s, craves a return to the shops he knew while growing up. He does not want to be surrounded by the smell of acrylics or chemicals. He wants to feel comfortable and secure in a male domain when he has a haircut or manicure. Young men are wearing shorter styles such as fades, military cuts, and shaved heads. These styles require the expertise of a barber and the industry knows it. Barbers are in demand in barbershops, unisex salons, and even in some beauty shops. Check the classifieds from any average-size newspaper and it is likely that you will see a help-wanted ad for a barber or barber-stylist.

The preceding historical perspective should help to explain why it is accurate to say that the need for barbers and barbershops has actually been on a steady increase since the 1970s. At that time, the profession needed barbers who could adapt to new trends. The profession needed barbers to maintain and offer an alternative to unisex and beauty salons for men's hair care. The profession now needs barbershops that have been designed to meet the expectations and service requirements of a variety of male preferences, from traditional shops and high-end salons to those with upbeat and trendy motifs. The profession needs barbers who will pass along their skills and the standards of the profession to others as teachers, state board members, and association leaders. The profession needs skilled artisans who challenge the skill of others in friendly competition at hair and trade shows. The profession needs lobbyists to protect the barbering profession and its future. The profession has needed new and young barbers to replace retiring practitioners all along.

The need is there. How you choose to fill that need will decide your future.

Preparing for Employment

At this stage in your barbering education you probably have some ideas as to where you would like to work upon graduation and licensure. Depending on the barber board regulations in your state, some students in the class may already be working in a barbershop or salon as a receptionist, assistant, or manicurist. When students take advantage of opportunities to work in

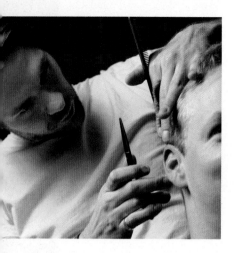

a barbershop while still in school, they are engaging in valuable learning experiences that will prove beneficial when entering the profession full time. Participation in the actual day-to-day operations of a shop or salon benefits students by providing the following:

- Exposure to the overall duties, responsibilities, and services of the shop

- Understanding of individual tasks and responsibilities of shop personnel

- Experience in communicating with clients and coworkers

- Experience in perfecting customer service skills

- Observation of advanced services, techniques, and skills

- Familiarity with shop procedures and standards

- Opportunity to lay the foundation for future employment

- Financial gain

If you are not quite sure where you will be working in the near future, think about what you really want out of your career, the services you prefer to perform, and the work environment in which you see yourself as most comfortable. Visit area shops and salons with the intention of finding the right atmosphere and environment for your personality and skills. This journey should not be considered solely as a job hunt, but rather as an exploration of available options. At this stage you should simply explore those options and decide which are the most suitable for you.

Preparing for employment also includes other practical issues such as goal setting, participation in professional activities, gaining an understanding of worker classifications and wage structures, résumé writing, and the development of a portfolio.

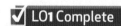

GOAL SETTING

The topic of goal setting was discussed in Chapter 3. Now that you are on your way to employment in the field, it may be time to either revise those initial plans or put them into motion to achieve your professional goals. Review the following guidelines in preparation for this exciting journey.

- *Be realistic.* Too often expectations are set so high that, regardless of the outcome, the reality is a disappointment. For example, it is unrealistic to expect that a newly licensed barber will be booked solid during his or her first week of employment. Be realistic when planning goals.

- *"Look before you leap."* Apply this old but useful principle whenever a major decision has to be made. Be cautious in business dealings and always seek legal counsel when contracts are involved.

- *Keep an open mind.* Doing so can create more opportunities and probable successes. Personal and professional growth can be the result of keeping an open mind in a field that is technically and professionally advancing each year. There are always new things to learn, new interests to develop, and new roads to explore.

- *Be flexible.* Timing can be extremely important and being flexible will help you to adjust to the circumstances of life. Flexibility and timing, combined with realistic goals and expectations, may produce a very workable plan that allows you to realize your full potential in a steady progression of insight, experience, and skill.

- *Believe in yourself.* Realize that with a realistic approach, flexibility, and an open mind, goals can be achieved.

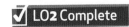 ✓ **LO2 Complete**

PARTICIPATION

There will be many opportunities while you are still in school to attend special events relating to barbering that can help prepare you for employment. Attendance at trade shows and educational seminars can enhance your product knowledge, technical skill, and overall understanding of the industry. In addition, trade shows are fun, stimulating, and a good way to get a feel for the profession. Seminars are offered on a myriad of subjects and topics, and platform demonstrations educate in the hands-on arena.

Becoming a member of an industry association or organization on a student level is one of the best ways of getting involved. Trade organizations are usually involved in all aspects of the profession, including the hosting of trade shows and the representation of the industry in legislative circles. Membership in such groups may include benefits such as discounted trade show and educational tickets, student competitions, leadership training or other educational opportunities.

Student competitions offer yet another opportunity to experience a thrilling aspect of the profession. Competitions may be sponsored by barber schools, vocational or professional organizations; distributors, manufacturers, suppliers; or other educational groups. Participation in competition hones the student's professional image, skills, and sense of self-esteem while laying the foundation for future professional performance.

Your school also may offer other opportunities for self-growth and industry awareness. Many instructors use students as teachers' aides. The duties vary and may include office or classroom assistance, either of which will be noted and appreciated by the instructor and create a learning experience for the student. If your school does not have such a program, consider approaching your instructor with the idea.

Participation in any of the preceding or similar activities is of value to a potential employer. It indicates a student's initiative and interest in the profession. Such activities also may indicate a student's willingness to be a team player, the ability to be a leader, or the drive of an achiever. Keep a record of the dates and descriptions of all your participation activities for inclusion in your résumé.

PERSONAL CHARACTERISTICS

There are several key personal characteristics that will help you get the job you want and keep it. Review the following characteristics and make a mental note of your personal strengths and those that may need enhancement.

- *Motivation* is the drive necessary to take action to achieve a goal. Externally motivated activities may produce results, but internally driven motivation is the most fulfilling and long-lasting.

- *Integrity* is a strong commitment to a code of morals and values. It is the compass that guides you in everything you say and do.

- *Technical and communication skills* must be developed to reach the level of desired success. About 80 percent of your success will depend on communication and people skills; the remaining 20 percent will be based on technical skills.

- *Strong work ethics* are demonstrated by a belief that work is good and by a commitment to delivering quality service for the value received from your employer.

- *Enthusiasm* demonstrates your passion for what you are doing and is contagious in a very positive way.

- *Your attitude* is one of the strongest marketing tools you possess. The other is your personality. Your attitude affects other people and the way in which you view life in general. A positive attitude generates a positive response in those you meet and is easily seen by potential employers (**Figure 22-1**).

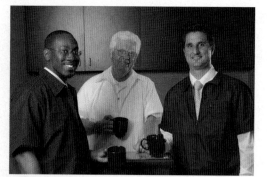

▲ **FIGURE 22-1**
A positive attitude is contagious.

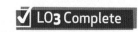

EMPLOYMENT CLASSIFICATIONS

The way you will be paid for services performed in the barbershop will depend primarily on your employment status as an employee, independent contractor, or booth renter. Most barbers work as independent contractors or booth renters, although employee positions are available in some shops and salons. The U.S. Internal Revenue Service (IRS) categorizes independent contractors and booth renters as self-employed workers; these worker categories have certain required criteria and restrictions that are used to separate them from designation as an employee for tax liability purposes.

Employee Status

As an **employee,** you might work on a salary, commission, or salary-plus-commission basis. You can expect to be told when and where to work in the form of required work hours, how to perform the job, and whether or not a uniform is required. Your clients will more than likely be booked for you and you probably will not handle any money for services other than your tips. Training may be offered or required, depending on the needs of the business, and some establishments may provide insurance or vacation benefits.

As an employee, your employer is responsible for withholding income and Medicare taxes, paying a portion of your social security tax, paying unemployment taxes, and providing you with a Form W-2, *Wage and Tax Statement*. Your responsibilities as an employee include reporting all wages, tips of $20.00 or more per month, commissions for product sales, and filing your personal income tax statement.

Independent Contractor Status

As an **independent contractor,** you may rent a chair or work for a percentage of the proceeds of services you perform, but you must apply for a tax identification number and provide your own business insurance coverage. You are also responsible for your own income and self-employment taxes and should receive a Form 1099-MISC from the shop owner when you earn over $600.00 a year. Although business expenses may be deducted, all income and tips are to be reported and estimated quarterly tax payments may be required. In order to prove that you are working as an independent contractor for tax purposes, there must be a written agreement or contract between you and the shop owner. This agreement must include how you will be compensated, your responsibilities, what is included in the chair rental, and an end date for your work. When set up properly, independent contractor agreements may be renewable. Refer to the list of stipulations provided in Chapter 23 and be guided by an accountant to ensure the agreement conforms to current federal tax laws.

Booth Renter Status

In a **booth rental** arrangement, you are actually setting up a small business. This requires a contract with the shop owner, appropriate business licenses, insurance, a tax ID number, and tax designation as a booth renter or independent businessperson. As a booth renter, you lease space from the shop owner and are solely responsible for your own clientele, supplies, record keeping, workstation maintenance, and accounting. You handle all money transactions and are responsible for booking your own appointments. Usually, the only obligation to the shop owner is the weekly or monthly rent. You should be given a key to the establishment and be able to set your own hours and schedule.

One of the main advantages of booth rental is that you can become self-employed for a relatively small investment. The initial expenses are fairly low and usually limited to the costs incurred for rent, supplies, products, and personal promotion or advertising. For some booth renters, a very low overhead may balance equitably with the income generated as a beginning barber with a small clientele. However, a good rule to follow is to make sure your clientele is large enough to cover all overhead costs *and* pay you a salary.

REMINDER

>>> The IRS has stipulated that, "The penalty for failure to pay or file taxes can be as high as 75% of the tax due if willfully negligent or fraudulent. The penalty for not reporting tips to an employer is equal to 50% of the social security and Medicare taxes due on those tips."

Chair or booth rental may also be ideal for those individuals who are interested in part-time employment, want to supplement another income, or prefer to take a stepping-stone approach to shop ownership. Regardless of the motivation, a booth rental arrangement provides the means for an individual to retain most of the control and decision making as it applies to work schedules and professional goals.

Position availability, personal choice, convenience, and the level of responsibility you care to assume will influence the capacity in which you work. Be sure to familiarize yourself with applicable state and federal tax laws. Working as an independent contractor or booth renter are forms of self-employment, which means that paid holidays or vacation benefits are nonexistent. Instead, you will have to plan ahead and set aside savings for times when you are not working or an emergency arises.

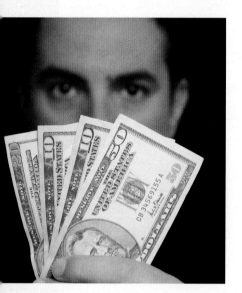

WAGE STRUCTURES

As discussed previously, booth rental involves paying the shop owner a fixed amount of rent for the space. All the fees brought in from the performance of services are basically yours after paying for the rent and supplies. For the employee or independent contractor, however, compensation may be structured in one of several different ways.

Straight or hourly salaries are most often seen in chain or franchise salons, but can provide you with a chance to earn a fixed income while building a clientele. With experience in the field and increased clientele, the fixed salary arrangement may evolve into a commission-based form of compensation.

In a **commission** compensation structure, the employer pays you a percentage of the gross service sales you generate. Commission percentages for barbers can vary greatly, anywhere from 40 to 70 percent, and depend on a variety of factors that may include your level of experience or the number of clients the shop services on a regular basis.

A *salary-plus-commission* (sometimes called a guarantee) compensation arrangement usually guarantees a minimum base salary with a percentage of the amount over the base added to it for a total wage. As with salaried compensation, salary-plus-commission may also evolve into a commission-only wage status.

Commission wages are usually paid as a straight percentage of the total fees taken in for services; however, sometimes a fee is taken "off the top" for the shop, and the commission percentage is based on the remainder. Both employees and independent contractors may be paid on a commission basis. Using Table 22-1, compare the differences between the various wage structures based on total service sales of $500.

TABLE 22-1 Wage Structure Comparison

	EMPLOYEE		INDEPENDENT CONTRACTOR		BOOTH RENTER	
	Salary @ $10 per hour	Salary plus 70% commission	70% commission only	70% commission less off the top fee	Chair rental	Booth rental
Service Sales	$500.00	$500.00	$500.00	$500.00	$500.00	$500.00
Salary	400.00	−125.00				
Fees				−75.00		
		= $375.00		= 425.00		
		×70%	×70%	×70%		
Commission		= 262.50	= 350.00	= 297.50		
		+125.00				
		= 387.50				
Rent					150.00	150.00
Supplies					25.00	50.00
Wage before taxes	$400.00	$387.50	$350.00	$297.50	$325.00	$300.00

NOTE: Employees may also be compensated on a commission-only basis

NOTE: Although commission percentages vary from shop to shop, the 70-percent commission rate that was once a union barber's standard commission may still be available in some barbershops.

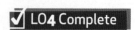

THE RÉSUMÉ

A **résumé** is a written summary of your education, work experience, and achievements. While there are many different types of résumé formats that can be customized to suit your needs **(Figure 22-2)**, some basic guidelines are as follows:

- Include your name, address, phone number, and e-mail address on both the résumé and the cover letter.

- List work experience and education information in chronological order from the most recent activities to the earliest.

- State your objective. Make sure it is relevant to the job.

- Limit the résumé to one page whenever possible and print on high-quality paper.

- Always use correct grammar, punctuation, and indentation.

- Include the names of educational institutions from which you have graduated.

Name
Address
Phone Number E-Mail

Objective:

Experience:

Accomplishments:

Special Projects:

Honors & Awards:

Education:

► **FIGURE 22-2**

Sample résumé format.

- List your abilities and accomplishments.

- Focus on information that is relevant to the position you are seeking.

- Add numbers and percentages when appropriate to expand on your accomplishments.

- List awards, special commendations, and honors.

- Use action verbs such as *achieved, designed, developed*, etc. to begin accomplishment statements.

- Make your résumé easy to read by using clear, concise sentences.

- Emphasize transferable skills mastered at other jobs that can be used in a new position.

- E-mail addresses and personal identification labels should be professional and appropriate for business use.

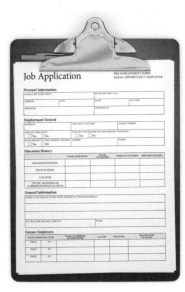

A **cover letter** should be used to introduce yourself to the employer and to reference the position you are seeking. It also provides an opportunity to expand on specific accomplishments that were only briefly mentioned in the résumé.

THE PORTFOLIO

A **portfolio** is a collection of photographs depicting your ability to provide hair care services. The concept of creating a portfolio for the purpose of marketing a skill or talent is not new to individuals in the fields of art, photography, and modeling. Until recently, however, its application to the barber's job search has been almost nonexistent.

The presentation of a portfolio is a graphic way to demonstrate your full range of talent, creativity, and skill to a prospective employer. Therefore, it should contain before-and-after photos of your work **(Figure 22-3)**.

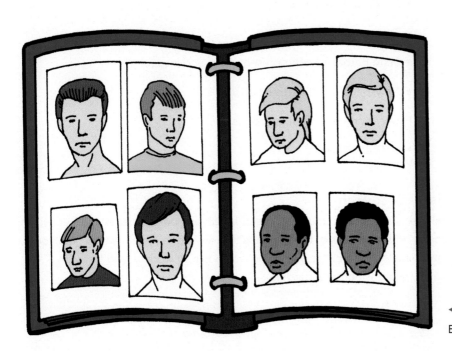

◀ **FIGURE 22-3**
Before-and-after photos in a portfolio.

As a marketing tool, a portfolio should represent a barber's best work. Consider keeping an inexpensive camera or extra memory cards for your cell phone in your kit. After obtaining the client's permission, take before-and-after photographs of your work. Keep a log of the dates, names, and services performed so the pictures can be labeled. To avoid the possibility of any future complaints or conflicts, ask the client to sign a **model release form** or waiver (**Figure 22-4**).

MODEL RELEASE FORM

I, _____ , hereby grant permission to _____ , student

barber, to photograph the hair services rendered to me on _____ for the

purpose of creating a portfolio of his/her work.

▲ **FIGURE 22-4**
Sample model release form.

WHERE TO LOOK

Your school is one of the best places to begin a job search. Most barber schools maintain contact with shops and salons and post openings at a central location in the school.

Use all the resources available to locate shops and salons in your area, including:

- Fellow students and instructors

- Suppliers who visit the school

- Distributor seminars and classes

- Trade shows

- State barber board representatives and inspectors

- Newspaper classified section

- Telephone book (yellow pages)

- Online job banks

Field Research

Field research should actually be used for several purposes: first, to become familiar with the types of barbershops that are in the area; next, to help you determine the type of shop that you would like to work in; and lastly, to search for a position as a barber.

Once you have targeted several shops to visit, contact the owners or managers by telephone. Introduce yourself and explain that you are preparing to graduate from barber school and that you would appreciate being allowed to visit the shop. Any mutual contacts you have can also be mentioned at this time. For example, if your uncle Charlie is one of the shop's customers, explain that he suggested you visit the shop because he always gets a good haircut there. This puts networking on a very personal level and you will probably end up with an open invitation to visit.

Field research can also lead to a job that you might not have known was available. Many times there will be a simple "Barber Wanted" sign in the window that would have been missed if you had relied solely on printed ads in the newspaper.

The Employment Interview

ARRANGING THE INTERVIEW

After you have passed your state board examinations, you will be ready to pursue a position in the barbershops located in your field research. The next step is to contact the establishments you are interested in by sending them a résumé with a cover letter that requests an interview. Make sure that you offer to bring a model so the owner can observe your technical skills.

In the event that you do not get a response from sending out a résumé, you may have to make some cold-call visits to barbershops. Although this may not seem to be the most desirable way to seek a position, it can work. Remember to have your résumé and barber's license with you, just in case.

INTERVIEW PREPARATION

Job hunting and interviewing is a familiar exercise for most people. The unfamiliar element is that you are seeking a position as a barber. A review of the material on professional image in Chapter 3 should serve as a reminder of the qualities that a shop owner or manager is looking for in an employee. Many employers require job applicants to perform a haircut or other services on a live model. This is a standard practice so do not feel intimidated by it.

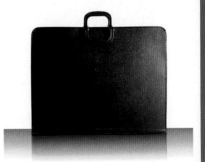

Another way in which you can prepare for the interview is to have all your support materials in one place. This includes your identification, licensing information, résumé, portfolio, and the employment application if available (**Figures 22-5** and **22-6**). Be prepared to answer questions about your skills and abilities, including how you might handle a difficult client or provide excellent customer service. Think about the questions you would like answered before making the decision to work there.

EMPLOYMENT APPLICATION

Applicants are considered for all positions, and employees are treated during employment without regard to race, color, religion, sex, national origin, age, marital or veteran status, medical condition, or handicap.

PERSONAL INFORMATION

SS#__________ Phone __________ Date __________

Last name__________ First __________ Middle __________

Present street address City State Zip

Permanent street address City State Zip

If related to anyone employed here, state name: __________

Referred to barbershop by: __________

EMPLOYMENT DESIRED

Position __________

Date you can start __________ Salary Desired__________

Current Employer __________

May we contact? __________

Ever applied with this company before? __________ Where? __________ When? __________

EDUCATION

Name/location of School	Years Completed	Subjects Studied

Subject of special study or research work:

What foreign languages do you speak fluently?

Read fluently: __________

Write fluently: __________

US Military Service Rank Present Membership

In Nat'l Guard/Reserve

▲ FIGURE 22-5

Employment application form.

Activities (other than religious) Civic, Athletic, Fraternal, etc. (Exclude organizations for which the name or character might indicate race, creed, color or national origin of its members.)

FORMER EMPLOYMENT

List below last four employers, beginning with the most recent one first.

DATE: Month/Year	Name, Address of Employer	Salary	Position	Reason For Leaving
From:				
To:				
From:				
To:				
From:				
To:				
From:				
To:				

REFERENCES

Give below the names of three persons not related to you whom you have known at least one year.

Name	Address	Business	Years Known

PHYSICAL RECORD

Please list any defects in hearing, vision, or speech that might affect your job performance.

In case of emergency, please notify:

Name   Address   Telephone

I authorize investigation of all statements contained in this application. I understand that misrepresentation or omission of facts called for is cause for dismissal if hired.

Signature _____ Date _____

▲ **FIGURE 22-6**

Employment application form.

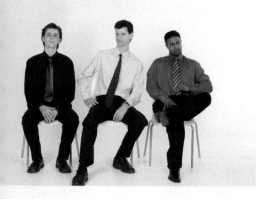

THE INTERVIEW

On the day of the interview, dress for success and make sure that your attire is clean, pressed, and appropriate for an interview. Be aware that there are certain behaviors that should be demonstrated during the interview itself:

- Be prompt.

- Carry yourself with good posture.

- Be courteous, be polite, and smile.

- Speak clearly.

- Answer questions honestly.

- Do not bring food or drinks to the interview.

- Never criticize former employers.

- Remember to say *thank you* at the end of the interview.

When you are invited to ask questions of the interviewer, consider the following:

- Does the shop advertise regularly?

- How will I be compensated?

- What is the procedure for walk-in customers?

- Is there customer overflow and will they be directed to my chair?

- Shall I call you or will you contact me with your decision?

Other factors that an applicant needs to consider are as follows:

- Wage percentage scale

- Pay schedule

- Percentage scale for retail sales

- Benefits (health, life, and dental insurance)

- Sick leave and vacation policies

- Dress code

- Equipment and supplies provided by the shop

- Hours of operation

- New-client policies

Legal Aspects of the Interview

Questions that *may not* be included in an employment application or interview include those involving:

- Race, religion, or national origin

- Citizenship status

- Disabilities or physical traits

- Marital status

- Height and weight

- Arrest record

- Sexual orientation

Questions that *may* be asked include those related to drug use, convictions for a crime, or smoking. Age is usually avoided in an interview unless it is needed to verify that the candidate meets the minimum age requirement for the job. Employers are permitted to ask whether an applicant is over the age of 18 and, if not, whether they can provide work papers. To find out more information, check with your state and federal employment law offices or the Equal Employment Opportunity Commission (EEOC).

Hopefully this chapter has provided you with some innovative ideas and useful suggestions for your job search in the field of barbering. Good luck and happy job hunting!

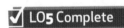

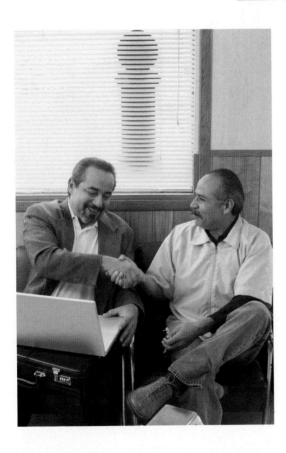

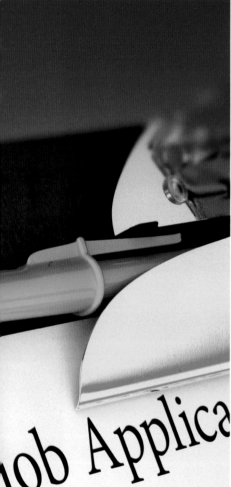

22 Review
Questions

1. List this textbook's guidelines for setting personal and professional goals.

2. List potential shop or salon positions available to student barbers.

3. List three common employment classifications for barbers.

4. Identify two marketing tools that require preparation.

5. What does a résumé summarize?

6. What is the purpose of a cover letter?

7. What important form must be signed before a photo is used in a portfolio?

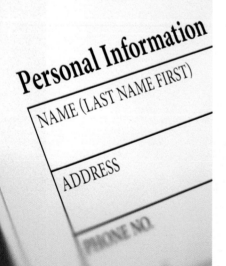

Chapter
Glossary

booth rental a form of self-employment, business ownership, and tax designation with certain responsibilities for bookkeeping, taxes, insurances, etc.

commission a certain percentage of the fees charged for services that become the employee's wages

cover letter a letter attached to a résumé that introduces the applicant to the employer and references the position being sought

employee employment classification in which the employer withholds certain taxes and has a high level of control

independent contractor a form of self-employment and tax designation with specific responsibilities for bookkeeping, taxes, insurances, etc.

model release form form used to permit the use of a model's pictures for print or exposure

portfolio collection of photographs depicting the barber's work

résumé written summary of a person's education and work experience

23 Barbershop Management

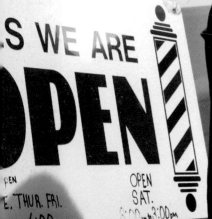

☑ Learning Objectives

AFTER COMPLETING THIS CHAPTER, YOU SHOULD BE ABLE TO:

1 Discuss self-employment and barbershop ownership.

2 Understand responsibilities associated with business development and ownership.

3 Discuss types of business ownership.

4 Explain the differences among employment classifications.

5 Discuss the features of a business plan.

6 Design a floor plan.

7 Discuss different types of advertising.

8 Identify the types of records that barbershop owners must maintain.

9 Demonstrate services and retail product sales techniques.

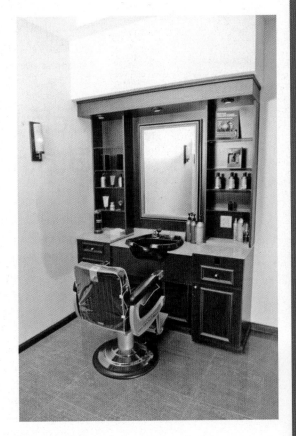

Key Terms

PAGE NUMBER INDICATES WHERE IN THE CHAPTER THE TERM IS USED.

booth rental / 748	**employee** / 745	**S-Corp** / 744
business plan / 754	**franchise** / 744	**target market** / 753
capital / 754	**independent contractor** / 747	
corporation / 742	**partnership** / 742	
demographics / 753	**sole proprietorship** / 741	

Many opportunities exist for a successful career as the owner or manager of a barbershop. Starting one's own business is an enormous responsibility that requires thorough and careful research followed by a detail-oriented implementation plan. Business ownership requires the knowledge and application of business principles, regulatory and business law, financial management, salesmanship, human relations skills, and operational management expertise. It also requires the type of personality that has the ability to see the "big picture" while multi-tasking all the many factors that help to create a viable and successful enterprise.

Barbershop ownership and daily management involve the direct control and coordination of all operational activities. This chapter introduces some basic business and management principles as an overview to self-employment in the barbering industry. It is intended for use as a general guide from which to springboard into performing the detailed research and implementation that business ownership entails.

Self-Employment and Business Ownership

One of the best aspects of barber licensure is the range of employment options it facilitates for working within the industry. You may choose a position as a part-time or full-time employee, independent contractor, or booth renter—or, after a few years in the business with an established clientele, you may decide to open your own barbershop.

STEPS TO BARBERSHOP OWNERSHIP

Business ownership is a serious step that requires commitment and follow-through. The aspiring barbershop owner should be prepared to research the business idea thoroughly before making any final decisions or signing any contractual documents.

Business *ownership* involves planning; decision making; financial obligations; contractual agreements; policy making; compliance with local, state, and federal laws; insurance; hiring and firing; purchasing; and all other details of business operations. *Management* is associated with production and involves an understanding of the daily operations involved in the business and of the people working within the establishment. In most barbershops, the owner is the manager as well as one of the practicing barbers.

There are many tasks that need to be performed once the decision to open a barbershop has been reached. The following list provides some of the steps required to achieve this goal.

1. Determine the type of ownership: sole proprietorship, partnership, corporation, limited liability company, subchapter s-corporation, or franchise. Decide whether you want to buy an existing business, start one from the ground up, or invest in a franchise business.

2. Review current tax law to plan the best worker classification(s) for the business.

3. Retain a lawyer and an accountant.

4. Determine the services to be offered and the market to be reached.

5. Determine the type of shop environment desired, including theme, mood, and décor of the premises. These decisions, along with the intended market, will help to determine the best location for the business.

6. Find a suitable location, research costs, and design a floor plan.

7. Create a business plan including financial projections, budgets, sales estimates, start-up costs, and so forth.

8. Arrange for financing or capital investment.

9. Plan and research equipment, fixtures, and furnishings purchases.

10. Establish a record-keeping system.

11. Establish shop policies, procedures, and protocols.

12. Arrange for advertising and publicity.

13. Recruit barbers; hire and train employees as applicable.

14. Design a plan to establish good public relations within the community.

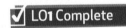 **LO1 Complete**

TYPES OF BUSINESS OWNERSHIP

There are several types of business organizational structures that may be considered for a barbershop: sole proprietor, partnership, corporation, limited liability company, subchapter s-corporation, and franchise. Thorough research should be done before deciding which type of organizational structure is the most desirable for your individual circumstances. A CPA (Certified Public Accountant) should be able to provide all the information necessary to make this decision. In some cases, the type of business chosen will depend on the amount of available capital; in others, personal preference will dictate the choice. The way in which your workers are classified for federal tax purposes may also influence the organizational structure you select. Some of the characteristics of each business structure are described in the following sections.

Sole Proprietor

If an individual has enough money to finance the cost of setting up and operating the barbershop, individual ownership or **sole proprietorship** should be considered.

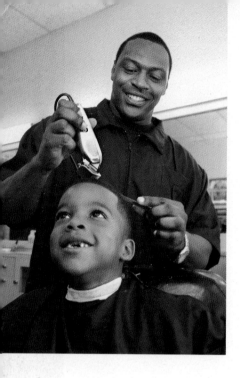

A sole proprietorship has certain advantages over a partnership or corporation:

- The owner is the boss and manager.

- The owner determines policies and makes all decisions.

- The owner receives all profits.

Sole proprietorship has the following disadvantages:

- The owner's working capital is limited by the amount of personally available funds.

- The owner is personally liable for all business debts and bears all losses.

- The owner is personally responsible for all business operations.

Partnership

When two or more individuals share ownership they form a **partnership**, although not necessarily equally. One reason for forming a partnership arrangement is to generate more capital for investment in the business. This can be facilitated through a "silent partner" arrangement in which an investing partner looks for a financial return on an investment but does not actively take part in the daily operations of the business. Other partnerships are based on the partners working together within the business with similar goals and responsibilities.

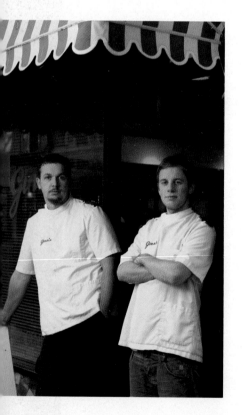

The advantages that a partnership has over individual ownership are:

- More capital is made available to equip and operate the business.

- Work, responsibilities, and losses are shared.

- Combined abilities and experience assist in the solution of business problems.

The chief disadvantages of a partnership are:

- Each partner is responsible for the business actions of the other.

- Disputes and misunderstandings may arise between partners and become irresolvable.

- Each partner is personally liable for all debts of the business.

There should always be a written agreement defining the duties, responsibilities, and percentage of ownership of each member. Shop policies, procedures, and protocols should be drawn up together and a consensus reached before implementation.

Corporation

When three or more individuals intend to operate a barbershop, a **corporation** may be a good alternative to a partnership. A corporation has the advantage over a partnership in that its stockholders are not legally responsible in case of loss or bankruptcy. Other factors associated with a corporate organizational structure include:

- The division of profits is proportionate to the number of stocks owned by each individual.

- A charter is required by the state and identifies each individual in the corporation.

- A board of directors governs the management, policies, and decision-making in accordance with the corporation's charter.

- The stockholders cannot lose more than their original investment in the corporation.

- The corporation is subject to taxation and regulation by the state. Federal tax laws allow some types of small corporations to be taxed on a partnership basis. This option should be explored since most barbershops would fall into a small-corporation category. An accountant and lawyer should be consulted on all matters.

Limited Liability Company

The formation of a limited liability company (LLC) is yet another alternative business structure for barbershop owners. Formed at the state level, a LLC can provide owners with protection from acts or debts associated with the company. There is also flexibility in how a LLC is taxed; owners can choose from a sole proprietorship tax structure or a corporate tax structure. The LLC business structure has become very popular with small businesses because it combines the best aspects of partnerships and corporations to create an advantageous structure for a single individual or a group of owners.

Benefits of a limited liability company include, but are not limited to:

- Management guidelines are flexible, similar to those of a partnership.

- Tax advantages derive from profits and losses factored at the individual level.

- There is no taxation on the company itself.

- Members bear limited personal liability for business debts, as in a corporation.

- There is no limit on the number of owners.

- Owner salaries and business expenses are deductible as in a corporation.

- LLCs allow flexibility to elect taxation as a sole proprietorship, partnership, S-Corp, or corporation.

Some disadvantages of a limited liability company are:

- The majority of LLC owners (members) will have to pay self-employment taxes.

- There is a lack of uniform statutory regulations from state to state.

- Some states tax LLCs.

- Two members are required in order to meet criteria for classification as a partnership for federal tax purposes.

Subchapter S-Corporation (S-Corp)

Similar in structure to a regular corporation, an **S-Corp** also has some features of a LLC in that double taxation of the company's earnings is offset by reporting income on the owners' income tax returns. An S-Corp must also meet specific criteria that include a limit to the number of shareholders and the U.S. citizen or resident alien status of those shareholders. In addition, an S-Corp must adhere to an organizational structure similar to that of a corporation and maintain the same type of formal record keeping, including meeting minutes, annual reports, and the like. One of the advantages an S-Corp has over a LLC is that employment tax is paid only on employee-owners' salaries, which would impact only part of the total earnings, whereas a LLC member is subject to taxation on the total income or earnings.

Franchise

To be successful in today's business market requires a competitive edge. Building name recognition (branding) and developing business savvy costs money, time, and hard work. A **franchise** is a form of a chain organization with a regional or national name, a consistent image, and a proven business formula that is used throughout the business locations. Franchisees are individuals who have met the criteria established by the franchisors as likely to be successful in operating the business. Depending on the company, the initial financial investment for a new franchisee may be expensive; however, franchisors typically provide expert business support and training in addition to a business plan and broad-scale marketing campaigns. Decisions such as location, size, décor, and pricing are usually determined by the parent company and employees may receive the same benefits as in corporately owned shops and salons. Franchise ownership may work to your advantage because the necessary systems, knowledge, and expertise are already in place.

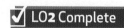 LO2 Complete

EMPLOYMENT CLASSIFICATIONS

An important consideration in business planning for barbershop ownership is determining the capacity in which other barbers will be working in the shop. Will your fellow barbers work as employees, independent contractors, or booth renters? This may be a tough decision to make because the entrepreneurial spirit that drives a person to implement their own vision in their own way may be impacted by the criteria or restraints assigned by the U.S. Internal Revenue Service (IRS), such as worker classifications associated with the barbering industry.

Worker classifications are used to determine the party or entity that has the responsibility to pay federal taxes. The current designations were developed from research about the way the barbering industry does business, followed by a court decision that based worker classifications on facts associated with the level of behavioral control, the level of financial control, and the relationship of the parties. It should be understood that no single fact is a determining factor and that each case may be reviewed independently by filing a *Form SS-8: Determination of Worker Status for Purposes of Federal Employment Taxes and Income Tax Withholding*. This should be done prior to deciding the extent of ownership control you wish to retain or the capacity in which your barbers will be paid.

The employment status descriptions that follow provide a basic look at various factors that impact the extent of legal and tax responsibilities, control over shop workers, and financial obligations for a shop owner. As such, they may also help you to determine the best business structure for your barbershop (Table 23-1).

Employer–Employee Classification

As an employer, you can opt to pay your **employee** barbers on a *salary, commission, or salary-plus-commission* basis. Straight or hourly salaries are most often seen in chain or franchise salons and provide new hires with a chance to earn a fixed income while building their clientele. While this arrangement may be advantageous to a newly licensed barber, it generates additional financial responsibility on the employer to earn and then cover any lost wage costs. At some point, the employer may choose to evolve the fixed salary arrangement into a commission-based form of remuneration or compensation.

In a *commission* compensation structure, the employer pays the barber a percentage of the gross service sales generated by that barber. Considerations for determining the commission percentage depend on a variety of factors that include, but are not limited to:

- The polices and practices of the shop.

- The costs associated with running the shop.

- The amount taken "off the top" for operating expenses.

- The employee barber's level of experience.

- The ability of the employee barber to bring new business to the shop.

- The amount of "overflow" clientele the shop generates on a regular basis.

A *salary-plus-commission* compensation arrangement may offer the best of both previous structures for new barbers because it guarantees a minimum salary while providing compensation for increased production. The potential upside for the employer in this arrangement may be a more secure worker who is motivated to increase production. As with salaried compensation, salary-plus-commission may also evolve into a commission-only wage status.

TABLE 23-1 Employment Classification Overview

EMPLOYEE	INDEPENDENT CONTRACTOR	BOOTH RENTER
Work instructions are provided	No instruction, training, or evaluation is provided	No instruction, training, or evaluation is provided
Training may be provided or required	May require personal investment in advanced training	Requires personal investment in advanced training
Operating hours are set or scheduled	Sets own hours and schedule with agreement	Sets own hours and work schedule
Appointments are scheduled by business	May schedule own appointments	Schedules own appointments
Job performance is evaluated	Services revenue may be collected at front desk	Services revenue is collected by booth renter
Equipment and facilities are provided	May pay for certain equipment or arrange an agreement; Opportunity for profit and loss exists	Certain equipment included in lease; Opportunity for profit and loss
Benefits may be provided	No benefits are provided	No benefits are provided
No rental agreement exists	Independent contractor agreement required. Requires agreement with an end date, wage payment information, responsibilities, etc.	Booth rental agreement is required. Requires lease with dates, fee, booth renter responsibilities, etc.
Expenses may be reimbursed	Expenses are not usually reimbursed	Expenses are not reimbursed
May be paid on hourly, salaried, commission, or salary-plus-commission basis	May work on percentage, commission or flat fee; and agreements may be renewed. May work in more than one location	Responsible for collecting all service revenues
Uniforms may be required	Attire may be discussed in agreement	Generally the renter's decision
Income tax, portion of social security tax, Medicare tax, and unemployment tax are paid by employer	Is responsible for all taxes, licenses, and insurance	Is responsible for all taxes, licenses, insurance, and advertising
Amount of tips are recorded by employer	Responsible for own tips and taxes	Responsible for own tips and taxes
Employer is required to provide *Form W-2, Wage and Tax Statement*	May work within confines of shop hours Owner is required to provide 1099 form	Requires submitting 1099 form to owner for rent paid

As an employer, you should provide work guidelines for employees that include scheduled work hours, where to do the work, appointment scheduling, tools or equipment to be used, how work is to be performed, uniform requirements, and required on-the-job training. You are also required to withhold income, Medicare, unemployment, and your share of employees' social security taxes and provide *Form W-2: Wage and Tax Statement* forms for all employees. You may or may not offer insurance or training benefits to employees.

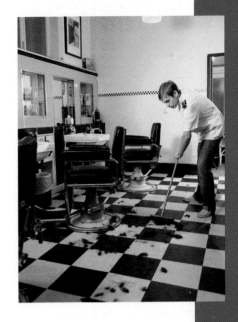

Also as an employer, you retain all control of the monies coming into and being disbursed from the shop. This includes general bookkeeping and the maintenance of records that document the accrual of your employees' monthly tips over $20.00 and commissions paid for product sales.

Independent Contractor Classification

Although the term **independent contractor** has been used for decades to describe the worker status of most barbers, under current tax law many may have been working as employees without any of the benefits of that classification. The factors that distinguish an independent contractor from an employee or a booth renter include a number of variables that may seem overlapping or vague given the nature of the business and how most barbershops are run. Again, filing a *Determination of Worker Status for Purposes of Federal Employment Taxes and Income Tax Withholding* form should resolve any questions.

As a general guideline, independent contractors may rent a chair or work for an agreed percentage of barbering service sales, but must have their own business insurance coverage and tax identification number. They are responsible for their own income and self-employment taxes and should receive a *Form 1099-MISC* from the business owner when they earn over $600.00 a year.

Additionally, the business arrangements between the shop owner and contractor need to be established in a written contract that clearly stipulates the following:

- How (tickets, receipts, etc.) and where (front desk, cash register, etc.) service revenues will be collected

- Length of time contractor will be employed; may be renewed

- Business hours of operation

- Commission percentage or flat fee amount for services performed

- Responsibility of the contractor for income and quarterly taxes, tips, licenses, and insurances

- Responsibility of the shop owner to provide contractor with a 1099-MISC form annually.

- Percentage or flat fee amount for chair rental and due date

- Inclusions in rent (e.g., utilities, signage)

- Supplies, materials, and equipment maintenance responsibility of contractor

- Provision of phone line by contractor

Did **You** Know...

The commission percentage a shop owner can offer an employee or independent contractor is usually guided by the basic operating costs of the business; the percentage the owner keeps is normally used to offset these operating costs.

Because an independent contractor is self-employed, the shop owner has no jurisdiction over the contractor's ability to work at other barbershops as well. For example, if Joe Barber has a contractual agreement with Barbershop A to work Mondays through Wednesdays and a second agreement with Barbershop B to work Thursdays through Saturdays, neither shop owner can tell Joe not to do so. In this way, the independent contractor classification actually helps to protect the worker so that someone else cannot limit his or her work potential.

Booth Renter Classification

In a **booth rental** arrangement, the shop owner provides space to be leased and the barber actually operates a small business within the confines of the shop. The booth renter needs to set up the business accordingly to include a lease contract with the shop owner, all the appropriate business licenses and insurances, tax identification number, and IRS tax designation as a booth renter or independent *businessperson*, not *contractor*. Booth renters are solely responsible for their own clientele, supplies, record keeping, tools and equipment, workstation maintenance, accounting, and so forth. Usually, the only obligation to the shop owner is the weekly or monthly rent. As the shop owner, you will need to provide booth renter(s) with a key to the establishment so they are able to set their own hours and schedule.

FYI

In some states the term *Booth Renter/Rental* has been renamed *Area Renter/Rental* on licensure applications.

The current laws and definitions used to assign tax liability to the appropriate individuals may require some practicing owners and renters to revise their contracts of just a few years ago. For example, if a booth rental contract stipulates the time or hours of operation, dress code, or other forms of behavioral or financial control, the booth renter may actually be designated as an employee by tax law. At the minimum, a booth rental agreement should clearly state the following:

- Amount and due date of rent to be collected by the shop owner

- Possession of a key to the establishment

- Responsibility of renter for their own operating expenses, taxes, tips, insurances, etc.

- Responsibility of renter for collecting all income for services performed

- Responsibility of renter to provide owner with a 1099-MISC form at the end of the tax year for rent paid

ALERT!

The IRS has stipulated that "the penalty for failure to pay or file taxes can be as high as 75% of the tax due if willfully negligent or fraudulent. The penalty for not reporting tips to an employer is equal to 50% of the social security and Medicare taxes due on those tips."

It is highly recommended that legal counsel and a tax accountant be retained before creating or signing any employment, independent contractor, or booth rental agreement.

> TABLE **23-2** Sample IRS Tip Reporting Form

DATE TIPS RECEIVED	DATE OF ENTRY	A. TIPS RECEIVED DIRECTLY FROM CUSTOMERS AND OTHER EMPLOYEES	B. CREDIT CARD TIPS RECEIVED	C. TIPS PAID OUT TO OTHER EMPLOYEES	D. NAMES OF EMPLOYEES TO WHOM YOU PAID TIPS
1		Off			
2					
3					
4					
5					
Subtotals					blank
Week 2 ▼					
Week 3 ▼					
Week 4 ▼					
Subtotals from pgs. 1, 2, and 3					blank
Totals	blank	$	$	$	blank

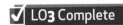

✓ LO3 Complete

PURCHASING AN ESTABLISHED BARBERSHOP

An *established barbershop* is one that is in operation at the time that it is put on the market for sale and that has a solid, repeat clientele. Empty storefronts that formerly housed a barbershop, or barbershops that have been in existence for less than a few years, do not qualify as "established." Each purchase opportunity needs to be well researched and looked at closely before any financial investment is made or contracts signed.

The purchase of an existing barbershop could be a golden opportunity, especially if the owner is retiring. In this type of situation, many of the established customers will probably continue to patronize the shop if they receive equal or better service. There may also be the option of offering the former owner the opportunity to work part-time, even one or two days a week. This can be a win-win situation for both the former owner and the new owner. The former owner adds financially to his or her retirement years with less responsibility and time being required by the business, while the new owner reaps the benefit of a business that maintains some continuity and goodwill for the customers.

While a retiring-owner scenario may provide the best options and opportunities for an aspiring barbershop owner, it is a scenario that may not come along very often. In many cases, the shop space is rental property and what is actually for sale is not much more than fixtures, furnishings, and possibly some equipment. In this type of situation, you would not be buying a business per se, but rather simply taking advantage of the fact that the space was previously set up as the same type of business. It might be worth considering since the plumbing or equipment might already be in place, or because the local populace is familiar with seeing a barbershop in that location. If the location is a good one, and depending on the reasons for the business closure by the former owner, pursuing the purchase of the equipment and signing the lease might prove to be a good opportunity for business ownership.

A third scenario that may present itself is the purchase of an existing barbershop that is operating as a viable enterprise with established employees and their clientele. This case would call for disclosure by the owner of the business assets, income, expenses, and profit and loss statements. In any of these scenarios, it is essential to seek the professional assistance of an accountant and a lawyer (Figure 23-1).

Before any sale agreements are signed, an investigation should be made to answer the following questions:

- Is the mortgage, bill of sale, or lease transferable without any liens against it?

- Are there any defaults in the payment of debts?

- Are all the state and federal taxes, including property, Social Security, etc., paid and current?

- Are there lease or current tenant obligations that have to be addressed?

Once the business has been cleared of any financial or ownership obligations, a purchase agreement to buy the barbershop should be drawn up and include the following:

- A written purchase and sale agreement with the names and contact information of both parties

- A complete, signed statement of inventory, from fixtures to supplies, indicating the value of each item

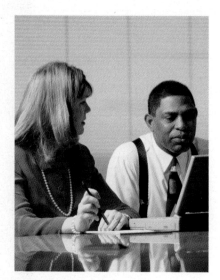

▲ FIGURE 23-1
Seek professional accounting and legal advice.

- Use of the shop's name and reputation for a definite amount of time (if desired)

- Disclosure of the business's accounts, tax information, and profit-and-loss statements

- Disclosure of any and all information regarding the shop's clientele and purchasing and service habits

- A statement that prohibits the seller from competing with the new owner within a specified distance from the present location

ESTABLISHING A BARBERSHOP

Services and Markets

Welcome to the conceptualization stage of establishing a barbershop (Figure 23-2). When you envision yourself working behind the chair in *your* barbershop, what do you see? What does the environment look like? Who is sitting in your chair: a man, woman, teenager, or child? What types of services are you performing: haircuts, shaves, chemical services? Do you think that your barbershop concept has the potential for success based on what you envision?

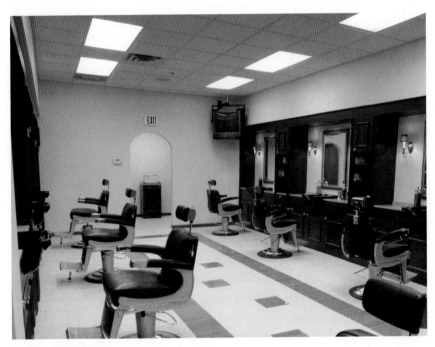

▲ **FIGURE 23-2**

Envision your barbershop.

When it has been decided which services are to be marketed to a specific group or groups, a vital starting point has been established from which to develop the barbershop. These decisions will initially serve as a guide when choosing the shop location and design. Next, they will help you to organize your thoughts concerning the equipment, products, and supplies required to service the clientele you hope to attract. This information will then be used to develop the business plan, estimate start-up costs, design a marketing strategy, and secure the necessary capital.

The decisions made about services and targeted markets guide important aspects of establishing the barbershop and help to determine the barbershop's potential for success. For example, consider a scenario in which male teenagers have been chosen as the targeted market. Explore the following questions that might be asked to help determine the feasibility and potential success of a barbershop that is targeted exclusively to a teenage male clientele:

- Where is the most ideal shop location to capitalize on this market?

- What is the concentration of male teenagers at the proposed location?

- Is the concentration at the proposed location (near schools, parks, sports fields, etc.) seasonal in nature?

- Is there any direct competition in the area?

- What is the average income or expendable funds of the targeted age group?

- How many haircuts would have to be performed to cover overhead expenses? What is the estimated frequency of shop visits per person?

- What should the shop look like to appeal to male teenagers?

- In what ways could the shop be promoted to this particular group?

- What hours of operation would best optimize teenagers' accessibility to the shop?

- Why is targeting this group the best plan for the shop—or is it?

The results you arrive at after exploring, developing, and researching the concept for the barbershop will guide you in making modifications or changes to the general plan. These changes are to be expected and should be handled with a positive problem-solving approach. If your idea does not appear to be viable or realistic after getting all the facts, work through a variation of it or develop a different concept. Take the time to work through ideas and plans before committing to actual contracts and expenditures. If the plan does not work on paper, there is little likelihood that it will work in reality.

The Shop Environment

At this stage, you have a well-thought-out plan, the research to support it has been done, and you are ready to move ahead with creating your barbershop. When you envisioned yourself behind the chair, you may have caught a glimpse of the way your shop would look. Now it is time to take a closer look at that image. What do you see? How big is the space? How many barber chairs do you see? Does every station have a shampoo bowl? What is the color scheme? Is there a reception or retail display area? What style of furniture or cabinetry do you see? Is there music playing, and if so, what kind?

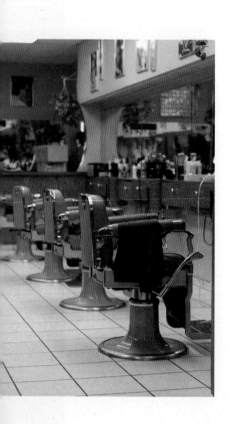

The answers to these questions, among others too numerous to mention, will help you make specific decisions about the business environment that you want to create for yourself, your clients, and your employees. Creating your own barbershop provides a golden opportunity to project your personality, style, and standards into an environment in which you will spend a good portion of your time. Therefore, it should be clean, comfortable, functional, and appealing to yourself and others.

Location

Location, location, location is a mantra sung by many small-business owners, especially those in service industries such as barbering. Visibility, parking, signage, competition, even public transportation access, are just some of the features associated with a good location.

The barbershop must be located in a population area large enough to support it. It should be near other active businesses such as supermarkets, restaurants, or banks that attract walk-by and drive-by traffic. Signage is crucial and should be visible from the roadway.

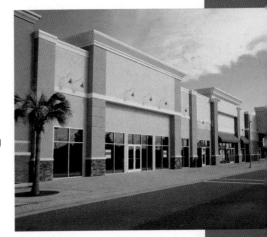

In general, the shop location should reflect your **target market**, the group that has been identified as the desired clientele and to which marketing and advertising efforts will be directed. Check the local **demographics** concerning the size of the area, population, and average income. Consult with local merchants, banks, and real estate agents to get a feel for the area. This information will assist you in developing shop policies and prices.

When judging the merits of a particular site, consider signage, the entrance, the inside area of the space, window placement, water supply, interior and exterior lighting, air-conditioning and heating units, toilet facilities, and parking facilities. Make a list of any structural or plumbing and electrical changes the space will require to facilitate its use as a barbershop and discuss it with the landlord. Although you may be able to negotiate with the landlord, the costs incurred by these changes are usually the tenant's responsibility and should be factored into the startup costs.

The Lease

In many cases, owning your own business does not mean that you own the building that houses the business. Most of the better business locations, such as strip malls or downtown commercial buildings, are owned by investment property corporations that only lease storefronts and offices.

After the site has been selected, and before signing a lease, check the local zoning ordinances to make certain that the area is zoned to permit the operation of a barbershop.

After all the facts have been checked and any drawbacks or obstacles addressed, a lease should be negotiated for the premises. A lease protects the barbershop owner against unexpected increases in rent, protects the right of continued occupancy, and clearly sets forth the rights and obligations of both the landlord and the barbershop owner.

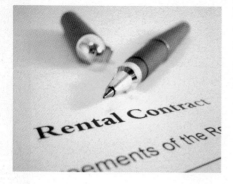

Before signing a lease, it should be read carefully and clearly understood by the parties involved. Be sure to have an attorney review the lease to ensure that it contains all the provisions and agreements made between the landlord and you, the tenant. These agreements may include, but are not limited to, the following:

- An exemption that allows for the removal during renovation of certain fixtures or structures unnecessary to the barbershop, without violation of the lease

- All agreements concerning renovations, repairs, plumbing, painting, fixtures, and electrical installations

- An option that makes provision for you to assign the lease to another person in case a partnership develops or a new owner takes over the business

The Business Plan

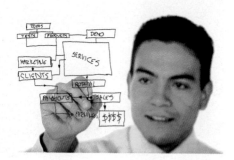

A **business plan** is a written description of the proposed business as it appears now and as it will appear in the future. It is a necessary tool to obtain financing and to provide a blueprint for future growth. The business plan should be developed from the information gathered during the preliminary research and should include the following:

- A general description of the business and the services it will provide

- The number of personnel to be hired, their anticipated salaries or rental contributions, and other benefits

- An operations plan including the price structure of services offered and monthly expenses such as rent, supplies, repairs, laundry, advertising, taxes, and insurance

- A financial plan that includes a profit-and-loss statement

- A detailed listing of start-up costs including construction, fixtures, furnishings, and equipment

Seek professional guidance if you have any questions about how to develop and write a business plan.

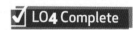
✓ LO**4** Complete

Finances

One of the results of a good business plan is that it provides an accurate estimate and assessment of the financial investment necessary to start up and sustain the business for a given length of time. The investment, or working **capital**, should be sufficient to cover the rent, wages, and monthly expenditures for a minimum of one year. The number one reason businesses fail is under-capitalization! It will take time to build a clientele in a new location, even when an established clientele follows you there, so you must be prepared financially to weather those early lean months.

The shop owner usually has all the financial responsibility, and a certain percentage of the fees taken in for services will have to be allocated to cover overhead costs. Many times, whatever is left becomes the owner's salary. Obviously, this is not the best way to do business but it happens quite often nevertheless. The best way to avoid this situation is to have enough money set aside to make it through the clientele-building process.

How much money is enough money? The answer can be determined in part by considering some individual circumstances that may include:

- The clientele and its willingness to move from the previous location

- The availability of other barbers with a following who will work in the shop

- The owner's personal status and financial situation, that is, single, married, single with dependents, previous debt, etc.

- The availability and type of financing, and its source

As a general rule, no less than one year's worth of operating expenses should be available. If there is no existing clientele, two years of operating capital is not an unrealistic requirement.

Legal Responsibilities

When conducting a business and employing other individuals, it is necessary to comply with local, state, and federal regulations and laws.

- *Local regulations* may include local building codes, zoning laws, and occupational or business licenses.

- *State laws* cover sales taxes, professional and business licenses, and workers' compensation.

- *State and federal* governments administer income tax laws.

- *Federal law* governs income tax, Social Security, unemployment insurance, cosmetics and luxury tax payments, and OSHA safety and health standards.

Insurance for business establishments include malpractice, premises liability, fire, burglary and theft, and business interruption coverage.

Barbershop Layout

When the location of the shop has been decided and the lease signed, it is time to formalize the layout or floor plan of the barbershop. The shop should be designed to achieve maximum efficiency and economy of space to ensure a smooth operation and traffic pattern (**Figures 23-3** and **23-4**).

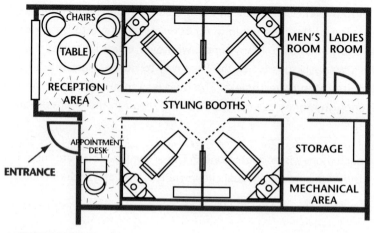

▲ **FIGURE 23-3**
Sample floor plans.

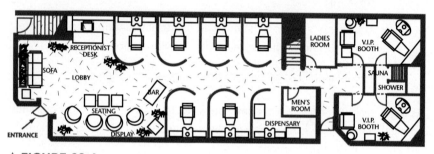

▲ **FIGURE 23-4**
Sample floor plans.

In addition, the shop design should be planned to provide:

- Adequate aisle space

- Adequate space for each piece of equipment

- Quality mirrors

- Fixtures, furniture, and equipment chosen on the basis of cost, durability, utility, and appearance. (Avoid closeout or odd-sized fixtures or equipment that may be a problem to maintain or replace. The purchase of standard equipment, either new or renovated, is a better investment because it is usually easier to replace or match standard parts and fixtures.)

- Premises that are painted and decorated in colors that are restful and pleasing to the eye

- Adequate restrooms for clients and employees

- Handicap-access facilities and doors

- Good plumbing and sufficient lighting for services

- Proper ventilation, air-conditioning, and heating

- Sufficient electrical outlets and current to adequately service all equipment

- Adequate storage areas

- Sufficient display areas

- An attractive reception or waiting area adequately furnished and comfortable, can be one of the barbershop's best promotional features.

REMINDER

>>> Always refer to your state's barber board rules and regulations before purchasing or opening a barbershop.

Cleanliness and comfort are two of the most important requisites for a professional-looking barbershop. The equipment should be easily accessible, arranged in an orderly manner, and maintained in good working order. Sanitation and disinfection procedures must be strictly enforced at all times. *Always consult state barber board regulations in your state when designing the barbershop.*

✓ **LO5 Complete**

Advertising

Advertising includes all activities that attract attention to the barbershop. The personalities and abilities of the owner, manager, and staff; the quality of the work performed; and the attractiveness of the shop are all natural advertising assets.

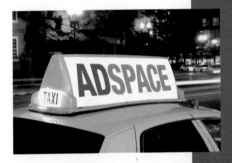

The right kind of publicity is important because it acquaints the public with the various services offered. To be effective, advertising must attract and hold the attention of those individuals to whom it is directed. It must create a desire for the services or merchandise offered.

The choice of an advertising medium is based on the form that will accomplish the desired objective most effectively. For advertising to be effective, it must be repeated. One-time ads or radio spots will produce little return on the investment; conversely, frequent and timely ad placement can make advertising dollars work for the business. Some advertising venues that may be considered for implementation are:

- Newspaper advertising

- Circulars and flyers

- Direct mail

- Classified advertising in yellow pages

- Promotional giveaways

- Radio advertising

- TV advertising

- Window displays

- Exterior banners

- Client referrals

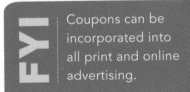

FYI Coupons can be incorporated into all print and online advertising.

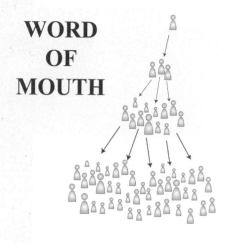

WORD OF MOUTH

- Contacting clients

- Telemarketing

- Community outreach and networking

- Websites and blogs

- E-mails

Once clients are attracted to the barbershop, courteous and efficient service will encourage their return and recommendation of the shop to others. Remember that, regardless of where advertising dollars are spent, word-of-mouth referrals from pleased and satisfied clients are the best form of advertising.

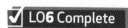
✓ LO6 Complete

Protection Against Fire, Theft, and Lawsuits

- Keep the premises securely locked.

- Follow safety precautions to prevent fire, injury, and lawsuits.

- Purchase liability, malpractice, fire, and burglary insurance.

- Never violate the medical practice law of your state by attempting to diagnose, treat, or cure disease. Refer the client to a physician.

- Become thoroughly familiar with the barbering laws and sanitation codes of your state.

- Keep accurate records of the number of workers and their salaries, length of employment, and Social Security numbers for various state and federal laws affecting the social welfare of employees.

- Maintain client record cards, especially for chemical services.

- Maintain a Material Safety Data Sheet notebook.

Business Operation

Successful business operation requires an owner or manager who possesses good business sense, leadership abilities, an understanding of sound business principles, good judgment, and diplomacy. These are all skills that develop over time with experience and application. To jump-start that development, seek out educational opportunities in the form of business seminars or mentoring programs that will help to hone personal management skills that need enhancement. If you are interested in purchasing a franchised shop or salon, utilize all the business operation data the franchisors offer.

In addition to efficient and effective management, the success of a business depends on the following factors:

- Sufficient investment capital

- Cooperation between management and employees

- Professional business procedures

- Trained and experienced personnel

- Competitive pricing of services

- Quality customer service

Business problems can be numerous, especially when a new business is just getting started. The first year is the most crucial, and every effort should be made by the owner or manager to ensure the shop's success. Some contributing causes to business failure include:

- Inexperience in dealing with the public and employees

- Insufficient capital to sustain the business until established (under-capitalization)

- Poor location

- High cost of operation

- Lack of proper basic training

- Neglect of the business

- Lack of qualified personnel

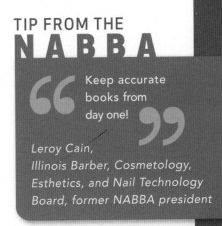

TIP FROM THE
NABBA

"Keep accurate books from day one!"

*Leroy Cain,
Illinois Barber, Cosmetology,
Esthetics, and Nail Technology
Board, former NABBA president*

Record Keeping

Good business operation requires a simple and efficient record system. Records are of value only if they are correct, concise, and complete. *Bookkeeping* means keeping an accurate record of all income and expenses. *Income* is usually defined as the money generated from services and retail sales. *Expenses* include rent, utilities, salaries and commissions, advertising, supplies, equipment, and repairs. Retain all check stubs, canceled checks, receipts, and invoices. The services of a professional accountant are recommended to help keep records accurate and processed in a timely manner.

Proper business records are necessary to meet the requirements of local, state, and federal laws regarding taxes and employees. All business transactions must be recorded in order to maintain proper records and are required for:

- Efficient operation of the barbershop.

- Determining income, expenses, profit, and loss.

- Assessing the value of the business for prospective buyers.

- Arranging a bank loan.

- Providing data on income tax, Social Security, unemployment and disability insurance, wage and hour law, accident compensation, and percentage payments of gross income required in some leases.

One cause for business failure is the lack of complete and systematic records. Business transactions must be recorded in order to judge the condition of the business on an ongoing basis; simple bookkeeping is usually sufficient for most barbershops. One easy method is to maintain a daily account of the income and expenses of the shop. Daily income receipts can be totaled from the cash register and daily expenditures tracked by keeping receipts, invoices, and canceled checks. It should always be known how much money is coming in and where it is being spent.

Additionally, changes in the tax laws for shops and salons now require barbers and stylists to keep monthly tip logs. Employees need to provide employers with their tip information; independent contractors might be required to provide the shop owner with tip information depending on the structure of their agreement; and booth renters need to maintain their own tip records for tax purposes.

The difference between the total income and the total expense is the *net profit*. A profit occurs when the income is greater than the expenses. When the expenses are greater than the income, a loss occurs. An operating budget helps to keep expenditures on track and maximizes the probability of having sufficient income to cover expenses.

Expenses common to operating a barbershop include salaries, insurance, rent, repairs, advertising, utilities, telephone, depreciation, laundry, cleaning, products and supplies, and miscellaneous items.

When transferred to a weekly or monthly summary sheet, daily records enable the owner or manager to evaluate the progress of the business. A summary sheet helps the business owner to:

- Make comparisons with other years.

- Detect any changes in demand for different services.

- Order necessary supplies.

- Check on the use of materials according to the type of service rendered.

- Control expenses and waste.

Each expense item affects the total gross income. Accurate records show the cost of operation in relation to income. Keep daily sales slips, appointment books, and petty cash books for at least one year. Payroll records, canceled checks, and monthly and yearly records are usually held for seven years. Be guided by your accountant as to how long these documents should be kept.

Purchase and inventory records also are important to keep. An organized inventory system can be used to maintain a perpetual inventory, which prevents overstocking or shortage of supplies. These records also help to establish net worth at the end of the year.

Service Records

Always keep service records or client cards that describe the treatments given and merchandise sold to each client. A card file system or computer-based program kept in a central location can be used for these records. All service records should include the name and address of the client, date of each purchase or service, amount charged, product used, and results obtained. Note the client's preferences and tastes for future reference.

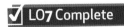

Operating a Successful Barbershop

While there are many factors that contribute to the success of the business, the key to a prosperous barbershop is to take care of the customer. Excellent service, courteous attitudes, and a professional environment promote referrals and repeat business. In order to achieve these standards, the owner or manager must guide employees and the daily operations that contribute to the overall success of the shop.

Personnel

The number of employees will be determined in part by the barbershop's size and type. For example, a four-chair shop offering basic services such as haircuts and shaves may employ three to four barbers and be very successful. The daily maintenance and sanitation duties are usually shared, as are booking appointments and ringing up monetary transactions. Conversely, a larger full-service shop will probably require a full-time receptionist, a manicurist, or other staff to keep the operation running smoothly.

Since the success of the business depends largely on the quality of the work produced by the staff, consider the following when interviewing prospective employees:

- Personality and attitude

- Image and personal grooming as it relates to the barbershop environment

- Communication skills

- Level of skill

- The clients they bring with them

Making good hiring decisions is crucial and undoing bad ones is painful to all involved. Develop a system or checklist for hiring that grades the job applicant in those categories that are important to the success of the shop. Design objective statements that can be evaluated with *yes* or *no* answers and/or that measure statements in terms of *satisfactory, needs improvement,* or *unsatisfactory*. These distinctions become a tool that can be used in the hiring process because they focus on those areas that need discussion or attention prior to and/or after employment. For example, a job applicant scores satisfactorily in personality, image, and communication, but is rated as needing improvement during a haircut demonstration. The employer now has a better indication of the applicant's strengths and weaknesses and can make the decision to hire with realistic expectations.

The decision to hire should include weighing the positive aspects of the applicant against those that may need improvement. In the preceding example, the employer may decide that since the applicant has the human relations skills so important to the business, coaching the applicant's technical skills would be time well spent for the benefit of the shop. Conversely, if the employer has just lost an employee or has more clients than his or her existing staff can effectively service, he or she may not have the time to mentor the applicant.

The sample Interview Evaluation Inventory in **Figure 23-5** should be customized for your own use, but it is recommended that job applicants always perform a practical service that demonstrates their barbering skills as part of the interview process.

Managing Employees

Managing employees effectively can be a challenging experience for many new barbershop owners. As with most other aspects of business ownership, managing people is a skill that can be enhanced with knowledge and experience. Some general guidelines for effective personnel management are as follows:

- *Be honest with employees.* Make clear your expectations for employee behavior and attitudes. Let employees know how and when they will be evaluated. Do not wait to give an employee feedback, whether it is positive or negative. Make sure you are both in a private area of the shop and tell him or her what you are thinking or what you have observed.

- *Expect the best.* Always give employees the benefit of the doubt and expect the best intentions from them. Never assume or immediately jump to negative conclusions. Most often, employees are simply trying to be helpful but may not know how to go about accomplishing it.

- *Be a mentor.* As the shop owner you will be viewed as an experienced veteran. Along with this comes the responsibility to help and guide whenever possible. Teach employees what you know and be willing to learn new things from them as well.

- *Share information.* Whenever possible and appropriate, share information regarding shop decisions with employees so that they become part of the process. Share your goals for the shop so that employees can help you attain them.

- *Follow the rules.* If you expect an employee to follow the rules, you must set the example and follow them as well. There should be no evidence or demonstration of double standards in the barbershop.

Name:			Phone:		Date:	
Address:				Zip Code:		
Background Information	Yes	No	Comments	Satisfactory	Needs Improvement	Unsatisfactory
Recent graduate						
Valid Barber License						
Experienced			# of years:			
Personality/Attitude						
Projected self-confidence						
Positive & professional						
Image						
Hair appropriately styled						
Appropriate attire						
Clothing neat/clean						
Shoes neat/clean						
Nails clean/manicured						
Communication Skills						
Maintained eye contact						
Good voice pitch/tone						
Engaged in conversation						
Answered questions						
Asked relevant questions						
Level of Skill						
Performed haircut						
Performed neck shave						
Performed facial shave						
Performs chemical services:						
Permanent waves						
Reformation curls						
Chemical relaxers						
Haircoloring						
Performs women's styling						
Performs other						
Clientele						
Established						
Within range to follow						
Client contact cards viewed						
Totals						

▲ **FIGURE 23-5**

Sample Interview Evaluation Inventory.

Benefits

The best business environment is one in which everyone feels appreciated, enjoys working hard, and strives to provide excellent service to the customers. Acknowledge and welcome staff members each day. Show a genuine interest in their well-being. One way to maintain this type of positive work environment is to share the barbershop's success whenever it is financially feasible to do so. Another way is to provide benefit opportunities through thoughtful and careful shop management.

The concept of sharing the shop's success can manifest itself in ways that range from small tokens of appreciation to professional development opportunities. Supply employees with tickets to trade shows and educational events or schedule group activities. You might sponsor a local team, provide membership to a local gym, or make sure everyone is pictured in the promotional ad. Any method that demonstrates to employees that they are valued and appreciated will enhance the work environment and atmosphere of the barbershop. And don't forget those more simple forms of appreciation such as "Thank you," "Good job," or "I'm glad you're part of our team."

Employee benefits, such as health insurance or paid vacations, may or may not be financially feasible for some barbershop owners. If the owner's financial situation does not allow for covering the costs of benefits, there are small-group plans employees may purchase on their own as an alternative to paying for individual coverage.

OTHER BUSINESS OPERATIONS

Pricing of Services

The cost of services is generally based on operational costs, the location of the shop, and the type of clientele it serves. The price list should be posted in a place where it will be easily seen, usually near the reception or checkout desk. Be sure to monitor what the competition is charging for comparable services to remain competitive with pricing.

The Reception Area

First impressions count, and since the reception area is the first thing clients see, it should be attractive, appealing, and comfortable. The receptionist, phone system, and retail merchandise may be located in this area. There should be a supply of business cards with the address and phone number of the shop on the reception desk. This is also the place where the client's financial transactions are often handled (Figure 23-6). Be sure to allocate space for a cash register, credit card machine, and/or computer system when designing the shop layout.

Booking Appointments

Booking appointments must be done with care as services are sold in terms of time on the appointment page. Appointments should be scheduled to make the most efficient use of everyone's time. Under ideal conditions, a

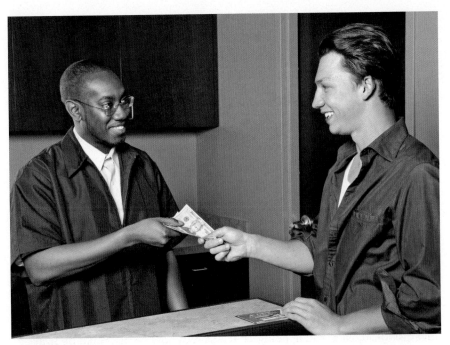

▲ FIGURE 23-6

Financial transactions are often handled at the reception desk.

client should not have to wait past his appointment time for a service and a barber should not have to wait for the next client. Appointment books are available in traditional heavy stock paper or computer software versions (Figure 23-7).

The size and style of the barbershop usually determines who books the appointments. Large shops often have a receptionist who books the appointments; barbers in smaller shops may book their own appointments, depending on the owner's preferences.

Occasionally it becomes necessary to provide services to a client who cannot travel to the barbershop due to injury or illness. When this type of situation arises, the barber may be allowed to go to the client, but the appointment information and location must be written in the appointment book. Check your barber board's rules and regulations to see if a provision has been made for such circumstances in your state.

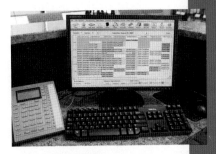

▲ FIGURE 23-7

A computerized appointment book.

Telephone Techniques

The majority of barbershop business is handled over the telephone. Good telephone habits and techniques make it possible for shop owners and barbers to increase business. With each call to the shop, there is opportunity to build on the shop's reputation and clientele base.

During a typical workday in the barbershop, the telephone is used to:

- Make or change appointments.

- Seek new business.

- Remind clients of their appointments.

- Answer questions and render friendly service.

- Handle complaints to the client's satisfaction.

- Receive messages.

- Order equipment and supplies.

- Give directions to clients (post a small map near phones).

- Provide shop hours.

- Determine who is on staff that day.

The phone is usually located at the reception desk or near the cash register. The appointment book should be readily accessible, along with the usual desk supplies. Keep an up-to-date list of frequently called numbers and a recent telephone directory.

The shop's telephone number should be prominently displayed on stationery, advertising circulars, and in newspaper ads. Business cards should be available in the waiting area and at each station.

Good telephone etiquette requires the application of a few basic principles that add up to common sense and common courtesy. When using the shop or cell phone, follow these basic rules.

- Answer all calls as quickly as possible, preferably by the second ring.

- Express an interested and helpful attitude. Your voice, what you say, and how you say it all make a definite impression on others.

- Identify yourself and the shop when making or receiving a call. If the requested information is not readily available, ask the client to please hold while you get it.

- If there are multiple phone lines, ask permission to place the current call on hold to answer the incoming call.

- Be tactful. Avoid saying or doing anything that may offend or irritate the caller.

  ▶ Inquire who is calling by saying, "Who is calling, please?"

  ▶ Address people by their titles and last names, as in "Mr. Jones."

  ▶ Use polite expressions such as *thank you, I'm sorry,* or *I beg your pardon.*

  ▶ Avoid making side remarks or speaking to others during a call.

  ▶ Let the caller end the conversation.

  ▶ Do not hang up loudly at the end of a call.

- All greetings and automated messages should be business appropriate, with no offensive music, language, or slang.

As a general rule, the most effective speech is that which is correct and at the same time natural. A cheerful, alert, and enthusiastic voice most often comes from a person who has these same personal qualities. A good telephone personality includes clear speech, correct speech patterns, and a pleasing tone of voice.

To make a good impression over the phone, assume a good posture, relax, and then draw in a deep breath before answering the phone. Pronounce words distinctly, use a low-pitched, natural voice, and speak at a moderate pace. Clear voices carry better than loud voices over the phone.

If your listeners sometimes break in with such remarks as "What was that?" or "I'm sorry, I didn't get that," it usually means that your voice is not doing its job well. Try to find out what is wrong and correct it. Some common conditions that cause problems for the person at the other end of the line include the following:

- Speaking too loudly or too softly
- Speaking too closely or too far away from the mouthpiece
- Speaking in very low or very high pitches
- Using incorrect pronunciation

While there may be one main phone line to the barbershop, almost everyone has a cell phone today, and if you are a booth renter, the calls will come directly to you. The practices of telephone etiquette include turning off the phone and allowing calls to go to voice mail while working on clients. Return calls in-between clients or whenever you take a break to avoid annoying a client in the chair or losing the focus of your work.

Booking Appointments by Phone

When booking appointments, take down the client's name, phone number, and the desired service. You should be familiar with all the services and products available in the shop and their costs. Be fair when making appointment assignments. Do not schedule six appointments for one barber and two for another unless the client requests a particular individual. When a client requests an appointment with a specific barber, every effort should be made to accommodate the request. If the barber is not available, there are several ways to handle the situation:

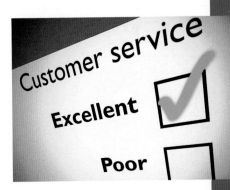

- Suggest other times the barber is available.
- If the client cannot come in at any of those times, suggest another barber.
- If the client is unwilling to try another barber, offer to call the client if there is a cancellation at the desired time.

Handling Complaints by Telephone

Handling complaints, particularly over the phone, is a difficult task. The caller is probably upset and short-tempered. Respond with self-control, tact, and courtesy, no matter how trying the circumstances may be. This will reassure the client that they are being treated fairly.

Your tone of voice must be sympathetic and reassuring. Your manner of speaking should convince the caller that you are really concerned about the complaint. Do not interrupt the caller. Listen to the entire problem. After hearing the complaint in full, try to resolve the situation quickly and effectively. The following are suggestions for dealing with some problems. If other problems arise, follow the policy of the shop or check with the owner or manager for advice.

- Tell the unhappy client that you are sorry for what happened and explain the reason for the difficulty. Tell the client that the problem will not happen again.

- Sympathize with the client by saying that you understand and that you regret the inconvenience suffered. Express thanks that the person called this matter to your attention.

- Ask the client how the shop can remedy the situation. If the request is fair and reasonable, check with the owner or manager for approval.

- If the client is dissatisfied with the results of a service, suggest a visit to the shop to see what can be done to remedy the problem.

- If a client is dissatisfied with the behavior of a particular barber, call the owner or manager to the phone.

The Business Venture Checklist in **Figure 23-8** serves as a basic guideline for aspiring barbershop owners. It is not meant to be inclusive of all the tasks or items that need attention in the start-up of a business, but it should point you in the right direction. The checklist may also serve as a self-assessment instrument that can be used to determine specific areas that require further study before committing to the responsibilities of business ownership.

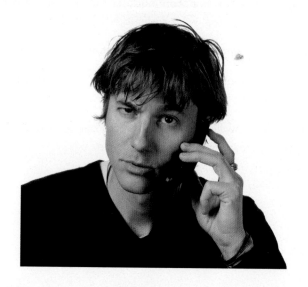

CHECKLIST	ACTION	RESULTS	✔
Capital			
Amount available			
Amount required			
Organization			
Individual			
Partnership			
Corporation			
Banking			
Bank Accounts			
Business Plan			
Checks			
Monthly Statements			
Notes and Drafts			
Location			
Area Businesses			
Parking			
Population			
Public Transportation			
Quality of Area			
Signage			
Space Required			
Traffic (drive/walk)			
Zoning			
Layout/Renovation			
Cabinetry			
Design Plan			
Electrical Outlets			
Entrance/Exits			
Exterior Painting			
Floor Covering			
Interior Painting			
Laundry Area (optional)			
Lighting			
Mirrors			
Plumbing			
Reception Area			
Retail Area			
Shampoo Area (optional)			
Shampoo Bowls/Sinks			
Square Footage			
Storage Area			
Telephone Installation			
Toilet Facilities			
Window Placement			
Window Signage			
Workstations			
Equipment/Furnishings			
Barber Chairs			
Coat Rack			
Computer			
Electric Sanitizers			
Fire Extinguisher			
Reception Desk/Counter			
Reception Furniture			
Retail Display			
Trash Receptacles			
Products/Supplies			
Back-bar Products			
Business Cards			
Cleaning Products			

▲ **FIGURE 23-8**

Business Venture Checklist.

CHECKLIST	ACTION	RESULTS	✔
Cleaning Tools			
Disinfectants			
Office Supplies			
Paper Goods			
Retail Products			
Services Products			
Record-Keeping System			
Appointment Books			
Computer Software			
Disbursements			
Inventory			
Invoices			
Petty Cash			
Profit and Loss			
Receipts			
Advertising			
Marketing Strategy			
Selection of Media			
Track Coupon Strategies			
Legal			
Business License			
Claims and Liens			
Contracts (other)			
Labor Law Compliance			
Lease/Purchase Contract			
Operational License			
State Board Compliance			
Tax Compliance			
Unemployment			
Wages/Compensation			
Insurance			
Fire, Theft, & Burglary			
Health/Disability			
Liability			
Malpractice			
Management			
Business Reputation			
Community Outreach			
Daily Operations			
Disputes/Complaints			
Employee Hire/Fire			
Ethics/Standards			
Promotions (marketing)			
Monthly Budget			
Advertising			
Depreciation			
Rent/Mortgage			
Repairs			
Services (laundry, etc.)			
Supplies/Products			
Taxes			
Wages			
Methods of Payment			
C.O.D.			
In Advance			
On Account			
Time Payments			

▲ **FIGURE 23-8**

(Continued).

Selling in the Barbershop

The success of any barbershop is based on the professional skill and selling ability of its personnel. Revenue is derived from both the performance of the services offered and the sale of grooming aids. The ability of the professional barber to sell additional services and grooming supplies can greatly influence earnings and profits and it also helps clients to maintain the look you worked hard to achieve (Figure 23-9)!

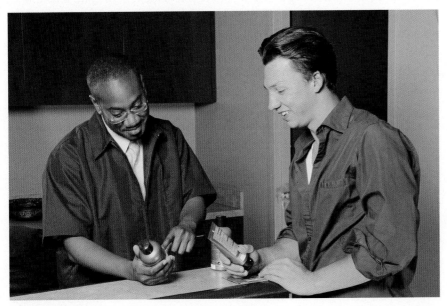

▲ **FIGURE 23-9**
Selling retail products benefits everyone and affects profits.

THE PSYCHOLOGY OF SELLING

Successful selling requires a clear and definite understanding of the client's needs and desires. It does not matter how good a service or a grooming aid may be—unless the client feels a need for it, there will be no sale. To close a sale, the client must perceive the service or product as necessary. Usually this simply requires an explanation of the benefits for clarification and understanding. A hard-sell approach should never be used.

Some motivational factors for purchasing services or products are based on a desire to:

- Improve appearance.

- Improve social relationships.

- Retain one's appearance.

- Get the most value for the money.

- Feel good.

Clients usually resent high-pressure selling tactics and care must be taken to avoid creating antagonism instead of confidence. The approach should be subtle, friendly, honest, and sincere to encourage the client's confidence in the barber's judgment. Remember, barbering services may be obtained in many places, but the personality behind the service is what brings the client back.

SELLING SERVICES

The barber's professional image can influence and arouse a client's interest in other styling and grooming services. The barber should be a living example of the services and products available in the shop. For example, if the barber wears a hair replacement system, his client may feel more confident about trying one as well. If the barber uses a particular shampoo or tonic on the back bar, the client will be more inclined to purchase a bottle from the retail display on his or her way out.

To sell additional services to clients, the barber must be aware of each service, know how to perform it, and be able to explain the benefits to be derived from it.

The client usually considers the barber to be an expert in good grooming and looks to him or her for suggestions and advice. It is the responsibility of the barber to be well informed on all grooming matters so that when advice is asked for, it is correct and appropriate.

Tips on Selling Services

- *New cuts and styles:* Tactfully suggest changes that will keep your clients current with modern trends. Have pictures and posters available for easy reference.

- *Facials:* As you cut your client's hair, notice the condition of his or her skin and tactfully suggest one of the following facials: plain facial, dry skin, oily skin, or acne.

- *Mustache and beard trims:* If the client wears a mustache and/or beard, the best policy is to ask if he would like a trim. Some clients prefer to trim their own facial hair while others expect the barber to offer the service. This policy should be followed in regards to trimming ear and nose hair as well.

- *Shampoo service:* Today, many barbershops include a shampoo as part of the haircutting service. Promote the relaxing effects of the massage that is part of a shampoo service along with the cutting and styling benefits of working with freshly shampooed hair. Clean hair facilitates greater precision in cutting and styling and helps to maintain sanitation standards in the shop.

- *Scalp treatments:* A scalp and hair analysis should be performed before every haircut. Treatments for normal maintenance and for dry, oily, dandruff, and alopecia conditions should be available in the barbershop. Explain the benefits of the recommended treatment to the client.

- *Hair treatments:* Suggest deep conditioning, bluing, temporary color, or dandruff rinses whenever it is appropriate for the condition of the client's hair.

- *Chemical texture services:* Permanent waves, reformation curls, texturizers, and chemical hair relaxers can provide clients with minimal to drastic hair texture changes. Educate clients about the advantages, disadvantages, and maintenance requirements of these "permanent" services. Remember, chemical changes to the hair cannot be shampooed out. When discussing the option of a permanent wave with a client, offer to "set" the hair on perm rods to help the client envision the finished look. Offer the potential relaxer client a hair-pressing service to envision straight hair or a texturizing process that will gradually ease him or her through the transition of changing from curly to straight hair.

- *Haircoloring:* Clients with gray hair may welcome the suggestion of a color rinse that matches or brightens their client's natural shade and that can be rinsed out if not satisfactory. Explain the differences between coloring products in terms of how long they last, the degree of color change or enhancement, maintenance, and cost.

- *Hair replacement systems:* Many of the hair replacement products available today are so natural looking that, from a distance, even barbers may have a hard time distinguishing a hair solution from a natural head of hair.

For barbers who wear hair replacements, specializing in this type of sale is a perfect spin-off of their professional skills and experience with artificial hair. Barbers who do not wear hairpieces, but would like to provide them for their customers nonetheless, can utilize subtle marketing techniques such as displaying a hair replacement on a mannequin head or advertising posters from the replacement supplier.

SELLING GROOMING SUPPLIES

The sale of grooming aids and supplies should go hand in hand with the sale of services. The purchase of such items as shaving creams, powders, lotions, and styling aids is a natural extension of the barbershop as the center of and source for good grooming.

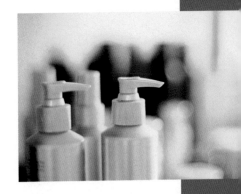

Shops should maintain an assortment of quality grooming aids to meet the demands and tastes of their clients. When clean, tasteful display cabinets are placed in strategic areas in the shop, little additional effort is required to call a client's attention to the variety of grooming supplies available.

The barber should be able to explain the qualities and benefits of the retail products sold in the shop. Some clients want to know every detail about a product and others just want to know if it works. In either case, barbers need to understand the purpose and contents of the products and their effects on the hair or skin. When barbers provide accurate purchasing advice to clients, the sale of one item almost inevitably leads to the sale of others on a regular basis.

Display cabinets should always be maintained and well dusted. Update with new items and periodically create more client interest by changing the displays to reflect holidays, sports seasons, or new styling trends.

A well-equipped barbershop with an interest in promoting retail sales should have a variety of grooming supplies available for its clients, such as shaving supplies, lotions and tonics, shampoos, conditioners, styling aids, mustache and beard supplies, hairpiece supplies, and hair supplies.

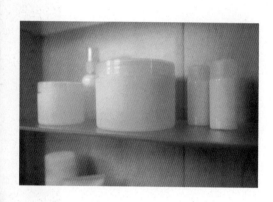

- *Shaving supplies:* razors, blades, shaving creams, lather brushes and mugs, pre-shave lotion, and aftershave lotion

- *Lotions and tonics:* facial cleansers, moisturizing lotion, toners, Bay Rum, hair tonics, astringents, and sunscreens

- *Powders and styptics:* aftershave powder, body talc, and styptic powder or liquid

- *Shampoos:* acid-balanced, regular, dry hair, oily hair, and dandruff formulas

- *Conditioners:* regular, moisturizing, deep-conditioning, protein, and dandruff formulas

- *Styling products:* styling lotions, gels, mousses, tonics, hairsprays, pomades, and butch wax

- *Mustache and beard supplies:* mustache wax, mustache combs and scissors, and electric trimmers

- *Hair replacement accessories:* adhesives, cleaners, solvents, and double-sided tape

- *Hair grooming supplies:* combs, brushes, and blow-dryers and attachments

- *Mustache and/or nose trimmers*

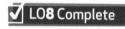
✓ LO8 Complete

GREG ZORIAN, III

The Zorian family has been in the barber business for more than 70 years, ever since Greg Zorian, Sr. opened the first Gregory's Barbershop in 1934 in Troy, New York. The second Gregory's Barbershop was started in 1968 in Westmere, New York, by Greg Zorian, Jr.

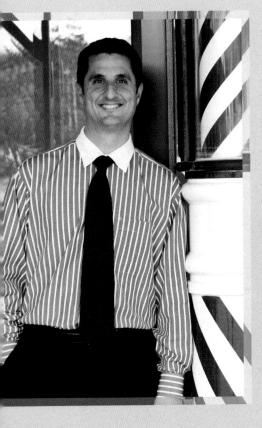

The third Gregory's Barbershop was started as a partnership between my father and I in 1996 in Delmar, New York. My sister, Nicole, also works there and is a third-generation barber like myself and also served a two-year apprenticeship under my father, who along with being a barber for 40 years has also been heavily involved in education for various companies. After receiving my master barber's license I worked with the Oster Clipper company for five years, traveling throughout the east coast and Canada teaching men's clipper cutting.

Since the opening of our first shop we opened another barbershop in Clifton Park, New York. Our barbershops service 800 to 1000 loyal customers per week and employ up to 20 barbers at a time, with an average retention rate of 6 years. Gregory's barbershops have received numerous accolades including "Top Five in the World" by Four Seasons magazine, "Best Men's Barbershop" from Hudson Valley Magazine, and "Best Barbershop in the Capital District" four years in a row in the *Times Union* and *Metroland* magazine.

The key to our barbershops' continued success is keeping up with the latest trends while still offering the traditional services such as scalp massages, manicures, and hot towel shaves. My father's famous saying is, "We're what I call old school and new school." Half of our work is classic; the other half is still classic, but with a modern twist.

Gregory's Barbershops offer full-service men's grooming, from hair and beard coloring to shaves and facials. The mainstay, however, is providing the comfortable and friendly atmosphere and professionalism of a family barbershop, with a men's club feel. We also carry an array of high-quality men's grooming products.

I feel very fortunate for the success I have had in my first 18 years in the barber business and look forward to sharing my knowledge and experience with current and future students. I am also in the process of assisting some of our local schools teaching men's haircutting and developing continuing education programs. Along with partnering with the schools, I will be starting my own education company to coach and mentor licensed barbers and cosmetologists in the technical and customer-service skills that have made our business a success.

Currently Gregory's Barbershop is embarking on using a variety of marketing programs to enhance and expand our business. Data-based marketing and Web-based programs are currently in development stages along with Facebook and other social networking tools to keep our customers informed of all of our special events and charity community events. We are also using video e-mail, which gives a more personal touch and keeps us on the cutting edge of technology. I look forward to meeting and working with as many of you as possible and wish you much success.

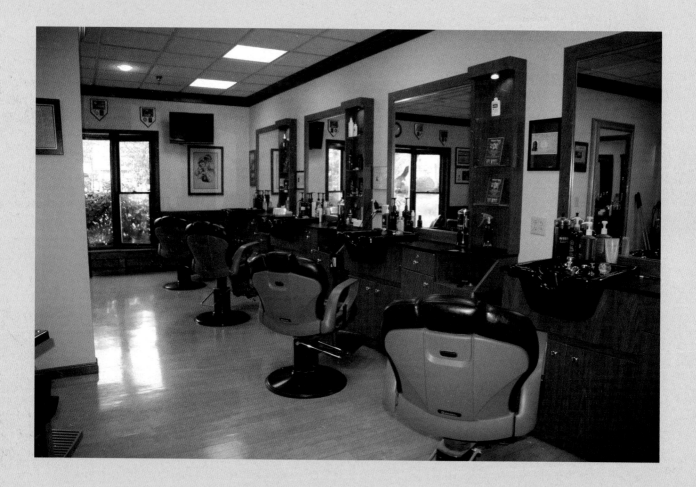

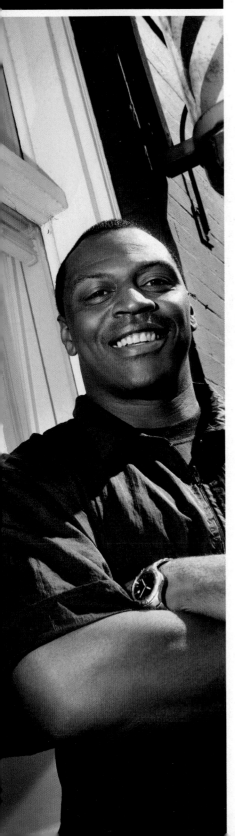

23 Review
Questions

1. Identify two ways a barber may be self-employed in the barbershop.

2. Define *booth rental*.

3. List and define six types of ownership under which a business may operate.

4. List 14 tasks that should be performed before opening a barbershop.

5. Define *established barbershop business*.

6. Describe the best location for a barbershop.

7. What is the best form of advertising?

8. Explain the value of summary sheets.

9. Identify two ways in which revenue is generated in the barbershop.

10. Explain why product knowledge is important to successful retail sales.

Chapter
Glossary

booth rental a form of self-employment, business ownership, and tax designation with certain responsibilities for bookkeeping, taxes, insurances, and so forth

business plan a written plan for a business as it is seen in the present and envisioned in the future

capital the money needed to start a business

corporation business ownership shared by three or more people, called stockholders

demographics information about the size, population, average income, and so forth of a given area

employee employment classification in which the employer withholds certain taxes and has a high level of control

franchise business ownership in which there is brand name recognition, support, group purchasing, and ongoing training for self and staff

independent contractor a form of self-employment and tax designation with specific responsibilities for bookkeeping, taxes, insurances, and so forth

partnership business structure in which two or more people share ownership, although not necessarily equally

S-Corp business entity with features similar to a corporate structure that allows company income to be reported through the owners' personal income tax returns like a limited liability company

sole proprietorship business structure with a single owner and manager of a business

target market the group that has been identified as the desired clientele and to which marketing and advertising efforts will be directed

Appendix

State Barber Boards

ALABAMA (334) 242-1918 Fax (334) 242-1926	**NO BARBER BOARD—NO BARBER LAW (Cosmetology licensing only)** RSA Union Building, 100 North Union Street, Suite 300 Montgomery, Alabama 36130 Email: bob.mckee@aboc.Alabama.gov Web: http://www.aboc.state.al.us
ALASKA (907) 465-2547 Fax (907) 465-2974	ALASKA STATE BOARD OF BARBERS & HAIRDRESSERS 333 Willoghby, 9th Floor State Office Bldg., Occupational Licensing, Juneau, AK Mailing Address: PO Box 110806, Juneau, AK 99811-0806 Colleen Wilson, Licensing Examiner Email: colleen.wilson@alaska.gov Web: http://www.commerce.state.ak.us/occ/pbah.htm
ARIZONA (602) 542-4498 Fax (602) 542-3093	ARIZONA BOARD OF BARBERS 1400 West Washington, Rm. 220, Phoenix, AZ 85007 Sam Barcelona, Assistant Director E-mail: sam.barcelona@azbarberboard.us Web: http://www.boardofbarbers.az.gov
ARKANSAS (501) 682-2806 Fax (501) 682-5073	ARKANSAS STATE BOARD OF BARBERS EXAMINERS 501 Woodlane Avenue, Room 212 North, Little Rock, AR 72201-1025 Charles Kirkpatrick, Executive Secretary E-mail: charles.kirkpatrick@arkansas.gov Web: http://www.arbarber.com
CALIFORNIA (916) 574-7570 Fax (916) 575-7281	CALIFORNIA BUREAU BOARD OF BARBERING & COSMETOLOGY 2420 Del Paso Road #100, Sacramento, CA 95834 Kristy Underwood, Executive Director E-mail: barbercosmo@dca.ca.gov Web: http://barbercosmo.ca.gov
COLORADO (303) 894-7772 Fax (303) 894-7693	COLORADO BOARD OF BARBERS & COSMETOLOGISTS 1560 Broadway, Suite 1340, Denver, CO 80202 Ofelia Duran, Program Director E-mail: Barber-Cosmetology@dora.state.co.us Web: http://www.dora.state.co.us/barbers_cosmetologists

(Continued)

CONNECTICUT (860) 509-7603 Fax (860) 509-8457	**CONNECTICUT EXAMINING BOARD FOR BAR-BERS, HAIRDRESSERS & COSMETOLOGISTS** Dept. of Health & Public, 410 Capitol Ave. M.S. #12 APP PO Box 340308, Hartford, CT 06134 Frank Manna, License & Applications Analyst E-mail: oplc.dph@ct.gov Web: http://ct.gov/dph/site/default.asp
DELAWARE (302)-744-4518 (302)-744-4500 Fax (302) 739-2711	**DELAWARE BOARD OF COSMETOLOGY & BARBERING** 861 Silver Lake Blvd. Suite 203, Dover, DE 19904 Judy Letterman E-mail: judy.letterman@state.de.us Web: http://www.dpr.delaware.gov
DISTRICT OF COLUMBIA (202) 442-4472 Fax (202) 698-4329	**DISTRICT OF COLUMBIA BOARD OF BARBERING AND COSMETOLOGY** 941 North Capitol Street N.E. Suite 7200, Washington, DC 20002 Sheldon J. Brown, Board Administrator E-mail: SheldonJ.Brown@dc.gov
FLORIDA (850) 487-1395 Fax (850) 921-2321	**FLORIDA BARBER BOARD** 1940 N. Monroe St., Tallahassee, FL 32399-0790 Robyn Barineau, Executive Director E-mail: Robyn.barineau@dbpr.state.fl.us Web: http://www.myflorida.com/dbpr/pro/cosmo/cos_index.shtml
GEORGIA (478) 207-2440 Fax (866) 888-1176	**THE GEORGIA BOARD OF BARBERS** 237 Coliseum Drive, Macon, Georgia 31217 Lisa Durden, Executive Director Web: http://sos.Georgia.gov/plb/barber/default.htm
HAWAII (808) 586-2696 Fax (808) 586-2874	**HAWAII BOARD OF BARBERING AND COSMETOLOGY** 335 Merchant St., Room 329, Honolulu, HI 96813 Mailing Address: P.O. Box 3469, Honolulu, HI 96801 Laureen M. Kai, Executive Officer E-mail: Barber_cosm@dcca.Hawaii.gov Web: http://hawaii.gov/dcca/pvl/boards/barber/
IDAHO (208) 334-3233 Fax (208) 334-3945	**IDAHO BOARD OF BARBER EXAMINERS** Owyhee Plaza, 1109 Main St., Suite 220, Boise, ID 83702 Tana Cory, Bureau Chief E-mail: bar@ibol.Idaho.gov Web: http://www.ibol.idaho.gov/BAR/General/BAR_BOARD.htm

ILLINOIS (217) 785-0800 Fax (217) 782-7645	**ILLINOIS BARBER, COSMETOLOGY, ESTHETICS, AND NAIL TECHNOLOGY** Dept. of Professional Regulation, 320 W. Washington St., 3rd Floor, Springfield, IL 62786 E-mail: http://www.idfpr.com/dpr/e_mail/prfgrp01.asp Web: http://www.idfpr.com/dpr/WHO/brbr.asp
INDIANA (317)234-3031 Fax (317) 233-4236	**INDIANA STATE BOARD OF BARBER EXAMINERS** 402 West Washington, Room W072, Indianapolis, IN 46204 Tracy Hicks, Director E-mail: pla12@pla.in.gov Web: http://www.in.gov/pla/barber.htm
IOWA (515) 281-6959 Fax (515) 281-3121	**IOWA BOARD OF BARBERING** Iowa Dept. of Public Health, 321 E 12th St., Des Moines, IA 50319-0075 Ella Mae Baird, Board Executive E-mail: ebaird@idph.state.ia.us Web: http://www.idph.state.ia.us/licensure
KANSAS (785) 296-2211 Fax (785) 368-7071	**KANSAS STATE BARBER BOARD** Jayhawk Tower, 700 S.W. Jackson St., Suite 1002 Topeka, KS 66603-3758 H.R. (Rocky) Vacek, Administrator E-mail: barberboard@yahoo.com
KENTUCKY (502) 429-7148 Fax (502) 429-7149	**KENTUCKY BOARD OF BARBERING** Leesgate Rd., Suite 6, Louisville, KY 40222-5055 Karen Greenwell, Administrator E-mail: karen.greenwell@ky.gov Web: http://barbering.ky.gov
LOUISIANA (225) 933-5923 (225) 925-1703	**LOUISIANA STATE BOARD OF BARBER EXAMINERS** 4626 Jamestown Avenue, Suite 1, PO Box 14029, Baton Rouge, LA 70898-4029 Sharon Cobb, Executive Director E-mail: LJangelnickcole@cs.com
MAINE (207) 624-8603 Fax (207) 624-8637	**MAINE BOARD OF BARBERING AND COSMETOLOGISTS** Dept. of Professional & Financial Regulation, 122 Northern Ave., Gardiner, ME 04345 Mailing Address: 35 State House Station Augusta, ME 04333 Debra Thompson E-mail: barbercosm.lic@maine.gov Web: http://www.maine.gov/professionallicensing

(Continued)

MARYLAND (410) 230-6194 Fax (410) 333-6314	**MARYLAND STATE BOARD OF BARBERS** 500 N. Calvert, Room 307, Baltimore, MD 21202-3651 Brian Logan, Administrator E-mail: Blogan@dllr.state.md.us Web: http://www.dllr.state.md.us
MASSACHUSETTS (617) 727-9970 Fax (617) 727-5339	**MASSCHUSETTS DIVISION PROFESSIONAL LICENSURE—BARBER BOARD** 1000 Washington Street, 7th Floor Boston, MA 02118-6100 Ms. Zane Skerry, Executive Director E-mail: zane.b.skerry@state.ma.us Web: http://www.mass.gov/dpl/boards.htm (NOTE: Office relocated April 2010)
MICHIGAN (517) 241-8720 Fax (517) 373-1044	**MICHIGAN STATE BOARD OF BARBER EXAMINERS** 2501 Woodlake Circle, Okemos, MI 48864 Mailing Address: PO Box 30018, Lansing, MI 48909 E-mail: bcslic@michigan.gov Web: http://www.michigan.gov/barbers
MINNESOTA (651) 201-2820 Fax (651) 617-2248	**MINNESOTA BOARD OF BARBER EXAMINERS** 2829 University Ave. S.E., Suite 310, Minneapolis, MN 55414 Thora Fisko, Executive Secretary E-mail: bbe.board@state.mn.us Web: http://www.barbers.state.mn.us/board.asp
MISSISSIPPI (601) 359-1015 Fax (601) 359-1050	**MISSISSIPPI STATE BOARD OF BARBER EXAMINERS** 510 George St., Room 240, Jackson, MS 39205 Mailing Address: P.O. Box 603, Jackson, MS 39205-0603 Sondra Clark, Administrator E-mail: MSBBE@bellsouth.net
MISSOURI (573) 751-0805 Fax (573) 751-8167	**MISSOURI STATE BOARD OF COSMETOLOGY AND BARBER EXAMINERS** 3605 Missouri Blvd., P.O. Box 1062 Jefferson City, MO 65102 Darla Fox, Executive Director E-mail: darla.fox@pr.mo.gov Web: http://www.pr.mo.gov/cosbar.asp
MONTANA (406) 841-2335 Fax (406) 841-2309	**MONTANA BOARD OF BARBERS AND COSMETOLOGISTS** P.O. Box 200513, 301 South Park, 4th Floor Helena, MT 59620-0513 E-mail: dlibsdcos@mt.gov Web: http://www.cosmetology.mt.gov

NEBRASKA (402) 471-2051 Fax (402) 471-2052	**NEBRASKA BOARD OF BARBER EXAMINERS** State Office Bldg., 301 Centennial Mall South, 6th Floor, Lincoln, NE 68509 Mailing Address: P.O. Box 94723, Lincoln, NE 68509 Ronald Pella, Director E-mail: barbers.board@nebraska.gov Web: http://www.barbers.state.ne.us
NEVADA (702) 456-4769 Fax (702) 456-1948	**NEVADA STATE BARBERS HEALTH & SANITATION BOARD** 4710 East Flamingo Rd., Las Vegas, NV 89121 Eloy Maestas, Secretary E-mail: N/A Web: http://www.barber.state.nv.us
NEW HAMPSHIRE (603) 271-3608 Fax (603) 271-8889	**NEW HAMPSHIRE BOARD OF BARBERING & COSMETOLOGY & ESTHETIC** 2 Industrial Park Drive, Concord, NH 03301 Lynda Elliott, Director E-mail: Lelliott@NHSA.state.nh.us Web: http://www.nh.gov/cosmet
NEW JERSEY (973) 504-6419 Fax (973) 648-3536	**NEW JERSEY BOARD OF COSMETOLOGY & HAIRSTYLING** 124 Halsey Street, P.O. Box 45003, Newark, New Jersey 07101 Jay A. Malanga, Executive Director E-mail: malangaj@dca.lps.state.nj.us Web: http://www.njconsumeraffairs.gov/cosmetology/
NEW MEXICO (505) 476-4690 Fax (505) 476-4665	**NEW MEXICO BOARD OF BARBERS & COSMETOLOGISTS** 2550 Cerrilos RD., 2nd Floor, Santa Fe, NM 87504 Mailing Address: P.O. Box 25101, Santa Fe, NM 87504 Monica Garcia, Administrator E-mail: N/A Web: http://www.rld.state.nm.us/BarbersCosmetologists/index.html
NEW YORK (518) 474-4429 Fax (518) 473-2730	**NEW YORK STATE BARBER BOARD—DEPT. OF STATE** Alfred E. Smith Office Bldg, 80 South Swan St, 10th Floor Mailing Address: P.O. Box 22001, Albany, NY 12201 Kathleen McCoy, Assistant Director, Division of Licensing Service, Dept. of State E-mail: licensing@dos.state.ny.us Web: www.dos.state.ny.us/lcns/professions/barber/barber.html
NORTH CAROLINA (919) 981-5210 Fax (919) 981-5068	**NORTH CAROLINA STATE BOARD OF BARBER EXAMINERS** 5809-102 Departure Dr., Raleigh NC 27616 Kelly Braam, Director E-mail: kbraam@ncbarbers.com Web: http://www.ncbarbers.com

(Continued)

NORTH DAKOTA (701) 838-4459 Fax: N/A	**NORTH DAKOTA STATE BOARD OF BARBER EXAMINERS** 2030 California Drive NW, Minot, ND 58703 Tona Stevenson, President E-mail: tona@min.midco.net Web: http://governor.state.nd.us/boards/boards-query.asp?Board_ID=17
OHIO (614) 466-5003 Fax (614) 387-1694	**OHIO STATE BARBER BOARD** 77 S. High St., 16th Floor, Columbus, OH 43215-6108 Howard L. Warner, Executive Director E-mail: howard.warner@brb.state.oh.us Web: http://www.barber.ohio.gov
OKLAHOMA (405) 271-5779 Fax (405) 271-5286	**OKLAHOMA STATE BARBER BOARD** 1000 Northeast 10th Street Oklahoma City, OK 73117-1299 Dhuann Robertson, Administrative Assistant E-mail: dhuannr@health.ok.gov Web: http://old.health.ok.gov
OREGON (503) 378-8667 Fax (503) 585-9114	**OREGON HEALTH LICENSING AGENCY, BOARD OF COSMETOLOGY** 700 Summer St. NE, Suite 320, Salem, OR 97301-1287 E-mail: ohla.info@state.or.us Web: http://www.oregon.gov/OHLA/COS
PENNSYLVANIA (717) 783-3402 Fax (717) 705-5540	**PENNSYLVANIA STATE BOARD OF BARBER EXAMINERS** 2601 North Third St, Harrisburg, PA 17110 Mailing Address: P.O. Box 2649, Harrisburg, PA 17105-2649 Kelly Diller, Board Administrator E-mail: ra-barber@state.pa.us Web: http://www.dos.state.pa.us/barber
RHODE ISLAND (401) 222-2828 Fax (401) 222-1272	**RHODE ISLAND BOARD OF HAIRDRESSING AND BARBERING BOARD** 3 Capitol Hill, Room 104, Providence, RI 02908-5097 Gail Giuliano, Administrator E-mail: Gail.giuliano@health.ri.gov Web: http://www.health.ri.gov/hsr/professions/hair_barb_app.php
SOUTH CAROLINA (803) 896-4540 Fax (803) 896-4484	**SOUTH CAROLINA STATE BOARD OF BARBER EXAMINERS** Synergy Business Park—Kingstree Building 110 Centerview Dr. Ste. 201 Columbia, SC 29210 Eddie L. Jones, Administrator E-mail: jonese@llr.sc.gov Web: http://www.llr.state.sc.us/pol/barber

SOUTH DAKOTA (605) 642-1600 Fax (605) 722-1006	SOUTH DAKOTA BOARD OF BARBER EXAMINERS 810 N. Main #298, Spearfish, SD 57783 Paula Spargur, Executive Assistant E-mail: PROFLIC@rushmore.com Web: http://dol.sd.gov/bdcomm/barber/bbboard.aspx
TENNESSEE (615) 741-2294 Fax (615) 741-1310	TENNESSEE STATE BOARD OF BARBER EXAMINERS 500 James Roberston Pkwy, Nashville, TN 37243-1148 Beverly Waller, Executive Director E-mail: Beverly.waller@state.tn.us_ Web: http://tennessee.gov/commerce/boards/barber/
TEXAS (512) 463-6599 Fax (512) 463-2951	TEXAS DEPARTMENT OF LICENSING AND REGULATION 920 Colorado Street, P.O. Box 12157, Austin, TX 78711 William Kuntz, Executive Director E-mail: Margie.weaver@license.state.tx.us Web: http://www.license.state.tx.us
UTAH (801) 530-6179 Fax (801) 530-6511	UTAH COSMETOLOGY AND BARBER BOARD 160 E. 300 South, P.O. Box 146741 Salt Lake City, UT 84114-6741 Sally A. Stewart E-mail: Sstewart@utah.gov Web: http://www.dopl.utah.gov/licensing/ cosmetology_barbering.html
VERMONT (802) 828-1134 Fax (802) 828-2465	VERMONT BOARD OF BARBERS AND COSMETOLOGISTS Office of Professional Regulation, National Life Bldg, North Floor 2, Montpelier, VT 05620-3402 Christopher Winters, Director; Kara Shangraw, Administrative Assistant E-mail: kshangraw@sec.state.vt.us Web: http://www.vtprofessionals.org/opr1/cosmetologists/
VIRGINIA (804) 367-8509 Fax (804) 527-4295	VIRGINIA BOARD FOR BARBERS & COSMETOLOGY Perimeter Center, Suite 400, 9960 Mayland Drive Richmond, VA 23233-1463 Zelda D. Williams, Board Administrator E-mail: barbercosmo@dpor.virginia.gov Web: http://dpor.virginia.gov/dporweb/bnc_main.cfm
WASHINGTON (360) 664-6626 Fax (360) 664-2550	WASHINGTON COSMETOLOGY, MANICURIST, BARBER & ESTHETICIAN ADVISORY BOARD 405 Black Lake Blvd. SW, Olympia, WA 98502 Mailing Address: P.O. Box 9026, Olympia, WA 98507-9026 Trudie Touchette E-mail: plssunit@dol.wa.gov Web: http://www.dol.wa.gov/business/cosmetology/

WEST VIRGINIA (304) 558-2924 Fax (304) 558-3450	**WEST VIRGINIA STATE BOARD OF BARBERS & COSMETOLOGISTS** PO BOX 6768, Charleston, WV 25362 Adam L. Higginbotham, Director E-mail: mindi.d.stewart@wv.gov Web: http://www.wvbbc.org
WISCONSIN (608) 261-4486 Fax (608) 267-3816	**WISCONSIN BARBERING & COSMETOLOGY EXAMINING BOARD** 1400 E. Washington, Bureau of Business & Design Professions Mailing Address: P.O. Box 8935, Madison, WI 53708-8935 Yolanda McGowan, Bureau Director E-mail: web@drl.state.wi.us Web: http://drl.wi.gov
WYOMING (307) 777-8572 Fax (307) 777-3681	**WYOMING STATE BOARD OF BARBER EXAMINERS** 2515 Warren Ave. Suite 302, Cheyenne, WY 82002 Betty Abernethy, Executive Secretary Email: babern@state.wy.us Web: http://www.cosmetology.wy.gov

Glossary / Index

Angle, the space between two lines or surfaces that intersect at a given point; in haircutting, the hair is held away from the head to create an angle of elevation, 398–399

Angular artery, artery that supplies blood to the sides of the nose, 160

Anhidrosis, deficiency or lack of perspiration, 235

Aniline derivatives, uncolored dye precursors that combine with hydrogen peroxide to form larger, permanent color molecules in the cortex, 622

Anionics, 188–189

Anode, positive electrode, 209–210, 319

Anterior auricular artery, artery that supplies blood to the front part of the ear, 160

Anthrax, inflammatory skin disease characterized by the presence of a small, red papule, followed by the formation of a pustule, vesicle, and hard swelling, 232

Antiseptics, chemical agents that may kill, retard, or prevent the growth of bacteria; not classified as disinfectants, 81–82

Aorta, largest artery in the body, 158

Aponeurosis, tendon that connects the occipitalis and the frontalis, 149, 302

Appointment booking, 764–765, 767

Arching technique, method used to cut around the ears and down the sides of the neck, 410–411

Arm bones, 146

Arm massage, 689–690

Arrector pili, involuntary muscle fiber attached to the follicle, 244

Arteries, muscular, flexible tubes that carry oxygenated blood from the heart to the capillaries throughout the body, 158, 160–161, 302

affected by facial massage, 306–307

Aseptic, free of disease germs, 60, 66

Associated Master Barbers and Beauticians of America (AMBBA), 23–24

Asteatosis, condition of dry, scaly skin due to lack of sebum, 234

Astringent, tonic lotions with an alcohol content of up to 35%; used to remove oil accumulation on oily and acne-prone skin, 192, 194, 320, 327

Atom, smallest particles of an element that still retains the properties of that element, 175

Atrium, one of the two upper chambers of the heart through which blood is pumped to the ventricles, 157

Attire, safety precautions with, 97

Attitude, a manner of acting, posturing, feeling, or thinking that shows a person's mood, disposition, mindset, or opinion, 36–37

Auricularis anterior, muscle in front of the ear that draws the ear forward, 149, 151, 303

Auricularis posterior, muscle behind the ear that draws the ear backward, 149, 151, 303

Auricularis superior, muscle above the ear that draws the ear upward, 149, 151, 303

Auriculotemporal nerve, nerve that affects the external ear and skin above the temple, up to the top of the skull, 155, 305

Autonomic nervous system, the part of the nervous system that controls the involuntary muscles; regulates the action of the smooth muscles, glands, blood vessels, and heart, 153

Axons, 153

B

Bacilli, rod-shaped bacteria that produce diseases such as tetanus, typhoid fever, tuberculosis, and diphtheria, 57–58

Back, bones of, 146

Backhand position/stroke, razor position and stroke used in 4 of the 14 basic shaving areas: **Numbers 2, 6, 7, and 9,** 351, 354–355, 363, 365, 367

Bacterial infections, 59–60. *See also* Infectious diseases

Bacteria, one-celled microorganisms also known as germs or microbes, 56–60

Bacteriology, 56–60

bloodborne pathogens, 60, 75

immunity, 68

parasites, 67–68

Balancing shampoos, designed for hair and scalp conditions, 190

Barba, Latin, for beard, 16

Barber(s)

modern, 22–24

training of, 24

Barber boards, 25–26, 714–715

Barber Code of Ethics, 24

Barbering

history of, 16–20, 26–28

modern, 22–24

tools used in. *See* Tools

Barber pole, most often a red, white, and blue striped pole that is the iconic symbol of the barbering profession, 22, 31

Barber's Company of London, 21

Barbershop

environment, 752–753

establishing of, 751–761

layout, 755–757

location, 753

management of, 740–745

operation of, 761–770

ownership, 741–755

purchasing established, 749–751

reception area, 764

selling in, 772–774

Barber-surgeons, early practitioners who cut hair, shaved, and performed bloodletting and dentistry, 20–22

Barbicide, 85

Basal cell carcinoma, most common and least severe type of skin cancer, 235

Base, the area near the scalp at which a roller or iron barrel is placed, 555

Base color, the predominant tone of an existing color, 618

Base control, the position of the perm rod in elation to its base section, 582

Base cream, protective cream used on the scalp during hair relaxing, 603

Base direction, angle at which the perm rod is positioned on the head; also the directional pattern in which the hair is wrapped, 582

Base relaxers, relaxers that require the use of a base or protective cream, 603

Bases, also known as alkalis, 178–179, 181

Base sections, subsections of panels into which the hair is divided for rodding; one tool is normally placed on each base section, 581

Basic perm wrap, rodding pattern in which all the tools within a panel are directed in the same direction, 591

Beaded hair, 265

Beards
  clipper-cut, 387
  coloring, 661–662
  designing, 379–387
  traditions concerning, 19–20

Beau's lines, lengthwise ridges caused by uneven nail growth, 675, 677

Beauty soaps, 186

Belgian hones, 121

Beliefs, specific attitudes that occur as a result of our values, 35

Belly of a muscle, middle part of a muscle, 148

Bi-level styles, 420

Binary fission, 58

Blackhead, an open comedone; consists of an accumulation of excess oil (sebum) that has been oxidized to a dark color, 234, 338

Blades, the cutting parts of the clippers, usually manufactured from high-quality carbon steel and available in a variety of styles and sizes, 113–114. *See also* Razor(s)
  changing razor, 117

Bloodborne pathogens, disease-causing bacteria or viruses that are carried through the body in the blood or body fluids, 60, 75

Bloodletting, 20–21

Blood, nutritive fluid circulating through the circulatory system that supplies oxygen and nutrients to cells and tissues and removes carbon dioxide and waste from them, 158–159

Blood-spill disinfection, the procedures to follow when the barber or client sustains an injury that results in bleeding, 91–92

Blood vascular system, group of structures (heart, veins, arteries, and capillaries) that distribute blood throughout the body, 156

Blood vessels, 157–158

Blow-dryers, 129–130

Blow-dry styling, the drying and styling of the hair with a blow-dryer and implements or fingers; technique of drying and styling damp hair in one operation, 471–475, 549, 552–554

Blue light, 213–214, 322

Bluing rinses, temporary colors or shampoo products with a blue base used to offset yellow and gray tones in hair, 193

Blunt cut, haircut in which all the hair comes to one hanging level at 0 elevation to form a weight line, 523–527, 540

Bobs, 540

Body systems, 142–164
  circulatory system, 142, 156–161
  digestive system, 142, 162
  endocrine system, 142, 162
  excretory system, 142, 162
  integumentary system, 142, 164
  lymphatic (immune) system, 142, 161
  muscular system, 142, 147–151
  nervous system, 142, 152–156
  reproductive system, 142
  respiratory system, 142, 163–164
  skeletal system, 142–146

Bones, 143–146

Bookend wrap, perm wrap in which an end paper is folded in half over the hair ends, 578–580

Booth rental, a form of self-employment, business ownership, and tax designation with certain responsibilities for bookkeeping, taxes, insurances, etc., 725–727, 746, 748

Boric acid, 197

Braids, 476–477

Brain, largest and most complex nerve tissue; part of the central nervous system contained within the cranium, 141, 153

Breathing, 163–164

Bricklay perm wrap, 591

Brittle hair, 265

Bromhidrosis, foul-smelling perspiration, 235

Bruised nails, blood clots that form under the nail plate; appear as dark purplish spots, 675–676

Brush machine, 313–314

Buccal nerve, 156, 305

Buccinator, thin, flat muscle of the cheek between the upper and lower jaws, 149–150, 302

Bulla, large blister containing a watery fluid, 229

Business issues
  advertising, 757–758
  appointment booking, 764–765, 767
  barbershop ownership, 741–755
  booth rentals, 725–727, 746, 748
  business plan, 754
  finances, 754–755
  leases, 753–754
  legal responsibilities, 755
  personnel issues, 761–764
  pricing, 764
  record keeping, 759–760
  self-employment, 740–744
  service records, 761

Business operation, 758

Business ownership, 741–744

Business plan, a written plan for a business as it is seen in the present and envisioned in the future, 754

Business Venture Checklist, 768–770

C

Cake makeup, 194

Calcium hydroxide, 603

Candidate information booklet, literature provided to examination candidates by the barber board, 713–714

Canities, technical term for gray hair, 265

Canvas strops, 122–123

Capes, 89, 273–275

Capillaries, thin-walled vessels that connect the smaller arteries to the veins
  blood, 158
  lymph, 161

Capital, the money needed to start a business, 754

Cap technique, lightening technique that involves pulling strands of hair through a perforated cap with a plastic or metal hook, 638, 654

Carbuncle, the result of an acute, deep-seated bacterial infection in the subcutaneous tissue, 264

Cardiac muscles, 147

Cardiovascular system, 156–161

Carpus, the bones of the wrist, 146

Carving, 548

Catabolism, the phase of metabolism that breaks down complex compounds within the cells; releases energy to perform functions, 140

Catagen phase, transition phase of the hair growth cycle, 251–252

Cataphoresis, process of forcing acidic substances into tissues using galvanic current from the positive toward the negative pole, 211, 319–320

Cathode, negative electrode, 210, 319

Cationics, 189

CDC. *See* Center for Disease Control and Prevention

Cell, basic unit of all living things, 140–141
  blood, 159
  nerve, 153–156

Cell growth, 140

Cell membrane, part of the cell that encloses the protoplasm; permits soluble substances to enter and leave the cell, 140

Cell metabolism, 140–141

Cell reproduction, 140

Center for Disease Control and Prevention (CDC), 90

Central nervous system, cerebrospinal nervous system consisting of the brain, spinal cord, spinal nerves, and cranial nerves, 152

Cervical cutaneous nerve, nerve located at the side of the neck; affecting the front and sides of the neck to the breastbone, 156

Cervical nerves, nerves that originate at the spinal cord, affecting the scalp and back of the head and neck, 156, 305–306

Cervical vertebrae, seven bones that form the top part of the spinal column in the neck region, 145

Chairs, hydraulic, 133

Changeable-blade straight razor, a type of straight razor that uses changeable, disposable blades, 116–117

Chemical blow-out, combination of a relaxer and hairstyling used to create a variety of Afro styles, 604–605

Chemical change, change in the chemical composition of a substance by which new substances are formed, 177

Chemical compounds, 178–179

Chemical disinfectants, 80–85

Chemical hair relaxing, the process of rearranging the basic structure of extremely curly hair into a straightened form, 568, 570–571, 598, 602–609

Chemical properties, characteristics that can only be determined with a chemical reaction, 177

Chemicals, safety precautions with, 98–99

Chemical texture services, hair services that cause a chemical change that permanently alters the natural wave pattern of the hair
  chemistry of, 568–569
  client consultation for, 573–577
  defined, 568
  hair relaxing, 568, 570–571, 598, 602–609
  permanent waving, 568, 570–571, 577–597
  principal actions of, 570–572
  reformation curls, 568, 570–571, 598–601
  scalp and hair analysis for, 573–577

Chemistry, the science that deals with the composition, structures, and properties of matter, 174–179
  chemical texture services, 568–569
  cosmetic, 183–186
  hair, 245–249
  inorganic, 174
  organic, 174
  shampoo, 272–273, 276–283
  United States Pharmacopeia (U.S.P.), 197–198
  of water, 179–183

Chest bones, 146

Children, safety precautions with, 97

Chinese culture, 18

Chloasma, non-elevated spots due to increased pigmentation in the skin, 231

Chronic disease, 66, 227

Cicatrix, technical term for scar, 230

Circle, also known as curl; part of a curl that forms a complete circle, 555

Circuit breaker, switch that automatically interrupts or shuts off an electric circuit at the first sign of overload, 206

Circulatory system, system that controls the steady circulation of blood through the body by means of the heart and blood vessels, 142, 156–161

Clarifying shampoos, shampoos containing an acidic ingredient that cuts through product buildup, 190

Clay masks, 327

Clean (Cleaning), to remove all visible dirt and debris from tools, implements, and equipment by washing with soap and water, 73, 80

Cleansers, 326

Cleansing creams, 194

Cleansing lotions, 194

Client consultation
  for haircoloring, 636–637
  for haircutting/styling, 392–393
  for manicures, 692
  for texture services, 573–577

Client consultation cards, 325–326

Client record card, 493, 574

Clients, dealing with, 41–45

Clipper blades, 113–114

Clippercide, 85

Clipper cut styles, 418–419

Clipper cutting, 412–419, 446–452, 544–546

Clipper guards, 113–114

Clipper-over-comb, cutting over a comb with the clippers, 412, 446–452

Clippers, electric haircutting tools with a single adjustable blade or detachable blade system; used in freehand or clipper-over-comb cutting to shape, blend, or taper the hair, 112–115, 135
  beard trimming uses of, 387
  care of, 115
  cordless, 113
  disinfecting of, 88–89
  holding, 114
  magnetic, 112, 115
  pivot motor, 112
  rotary motor, 112, 115

Cutis, another name for the dermis, 221

Cuts, 91–92

Cutting above the fingers, method of holding the hair section between the fingers so that cutting can be performed on the outside of the fingers; used with horizontal and vertical projections of hair, 403–405

Cutting below the fingers, method of holding the hair section between the fingers so that cutting can be performed on the inside of the fingers; used in 0- and 45-degree elevation cutting, 403, 405

Cutting line, the position of the fingers when cutting a section of hair, 400

Cutting stroke, the correct angle of cutting the beard with a straight razor, 351

Cyst, closed, abnormally developed sac containing fluid or morbid matter, above or below the skin, 229

Cysteine, 569

Cytoplasm, all of the protoplasm of a cell except that in the nucleus, 140

D

Damaged hair
perming, 592
reconditioning, 658–659
Dandruff, 259–261, 292
DC. *See* Direct current
Decontamination, the removal of pathogens from tools, equipment, and surfaces, 89, 92
Deep-conditioning treatments, chemical mixtures of concentrated protein and moisturizers, 192
Dehydration, 236
Demipermanent color, deposit-only haircolor product similar to semipermanent but longer lasting, 619, 621, 641–643
Demographics, information about the size, population, average income, and sodium forth of a given area, 753
Dendrites, 153
Deodorant soaps, 186
Depilatories, 195
Depression, 38
Depressor labii inferioris, muscle surrounding the lower lip, 149–150, 302

Derma, technical name for skin; also another name for the dermis, 221

Dermal papilla, small, cone-shaped elevation located at the base of the hair follicle that fits into the hair bulb, 243

Dermatitis, an inflammatory condition of the skin, 232

Dermatitis venenata, an eruptive skin condition due to contact with irritating substances such as tints or chemicals, 232

Dermatology, medical science that deals with the study of the skin, 220
skin disorders, 226–236
skin histology, 220–226

Dermis, second or inner layer of the skin; also known as the derma, corium, cutis, or true skin, 221

Design line, usually the perimeter line of the haircut, 401

Desincrustation, process used to soften and emulsify oil and blackheads in the hair follicles, 211, 318–319

Developer, an oxidizing agent, usually hydrogen peroxide, used to develop color, 624–625

Diagnosis, 66, 227

Diagonal, lines positioned between horizontal and vertical lines, 398

Diaphragm, muscular wall that separates the thorax from the abdominal region and helps control breathing, 163–164

Diet, 244

Diffused drying, 473, 475

Digestive system, the mouth, stomach, intestines, and salivary and gastric glands that change food into nutrients and wastes, 142, 162

Dihydrotestosterone (DHT), 256

Dilute solution, 184

Diphtheria, 68

Diplococci, round-shaped bacteria that cause diseases such as pneumonia, 57

Diplomacy, the art of being tactful, 36

Direct current, constant current that travels in one direction only and produces a chemical reaction, 205, 207

Direct surface application, high-frequency current

performed with the mushroom- or rake-shaped electrodes for its calming and germicidal effect on the skin, 316–317

Disclosure, 95

Discolored nails, a condition in which the nails turn a variety of colors such as yellow, blue, blue-gray, green, red, or purple; can be caused by poor blood circulation, a heart condition, topical or oral medications, or a systemic disorder, 675–676

Disease, 66, 227

Disinfectants, chemical agents used to destroy most bacteria and some viruses and to disinfect tools, implements, and surfaces, 80–85

Disinfection, the second-highest level of decontamination; used on hard, non-porous materials, 80
blood-spill, 91–92
rules for, 92
Universal Precautions for, 90
Displaying of products, 343
Disposable towels, 89
Disulfide bonds, also known as sulfur bonds; a type of chemical cross bond found in the hair cortex, 248
Double end wrap, 578, 580
Double flat wrap, 578, 580
Double-process haircoloring, a two-step combination of lightening and haircoloring, 637, 648, 650–652
Drafting, putting thoughts and information into cohesive sentences and paragraphs, 7, 13
Draping, covering the client's clothing with a cape or drape for sanitation and protection, 273–276
Dreadlocks, 477–478
Drugs, 244
Dry (cabinet) sanitizer, an airtight cabinet containing an active fumigant used to store sanitized tools and implements, 86, 103
Dry hair, perming, 592
Dry or powder shampoos, shampoos that cleanse the hair without water, 190, 283
Dry skin, 324
facial for, 335

Dye removers, products used to strip built-up color from the hair, 629

E

Ear hair trimming, 470

Ear muscles, 149–150

Eczema, inflammatory skin condition characterized by painful itching; dry or moist lesion forms, 232–233

Edgers. *See* Trimmers

Editing, the task of proofreading and correcting a paper in terms of punctuation, spelling, grammar, and so forth, 7, 13

Ed Jeffers Barber Museum, 29

Efferent nerves, 154

Efficacy, the effectiveness of a disinfectant solution in killing germs when used according to the label, 83, 103

Effleurage, light, continuous stroking movement applied with the fingers (digital) or the palms (palmar) in a slow, rhythmic manner, 309

Eggshell nails, have noticeably thin, white nail plates that are more flexible than normal, 675–676

Egyptian culture, 16–17

Elastin, protein base similar to collagen that forms elastic tissue, 224

Electrical equipment. *See also specific types*
  safety precautions with, 322–323

Electrical measurements, 205–206

Electric charge, 207

Electric circuit, 207

Electric clippers. *See* Clippers

Electric current, the flow of electricity along a conductor, 204–205

Electric facial machines
  galvanic machines, 132, 318–320, 336–337
  high-frequency machines, 132, 315–318, 337
  infrared-ray lamps, 321, 336
  microdermabrasion, 320–321
  ultraviolet-ray lamps, 321

Electric field, 207

Electric hair vacuum, 129

Electricity, 204–209
  basics, 207–208
  electrical terms, 204–205

modalities, 209–212

polarities, 209–210

safety devices, 206–207

safety precautions with, 96, 208–209

Electric latherizers, 128

Electric massager, massaging unit that attaches to a barber's hand to impart vibrating massage movements to the skin surface, 133, 285, 313, 329, 332

Electric wire, 204

Electrode, an applicator used to direct electric current from a machine to the skin, 207, 209

Electromagnetic spectrum, 212

Electromagnetism, 207

Electron, 207

Electrotherapy, electronic scalp and facial treatments, 209. *See also* Electric facial machines

Elemental molecules, 175, 178

Element, the simplest form of matter, 175

Elevation, angle or degree at which a subsection of hair is held, or elevated, from the head when cutting; also referred to as projection, 399

Eleventh cranial nerve, spinal nerve branch that affects the muscles of the neck and back, 156

Emotional disturbances, 244

Emotional stability, 36

Emotions, 38

Employee benefits, 764

Employee, employment classification in which the employer withholds certain taxes and has a high level of control, 724, 727, 745–747, 761–764

Employment, preparing for, 722–731

Employment applications, 732–733

Employment interviews, 731–735

Emulsions, mixtures of two or more immiscible substances united with the aid of a binder or emulsifier, 185

End bonds, also known as peptide bonds; chemical bonds that join amino acids end to end, 246

Endocrine glands, 244

Endocrine system, group of specialized glands that affect growth, development, sexual function, and general health, 142, 162

Endothermic waves, perm activated by an outside heat source, usually a hood-type dryer, 584

End wraps, end paper; absorbent papers used to protect and control the ends of the hair during perming services, 578

Environmental Protection Agency, also referred to as EPA; develops and enforces the regulations of environmental law in an effort to protect human health and the environment, 74, 103

Envisioning, the process of visualizing a procedure or finished haircut style, 393

EPA-registered disinfectant, a product that has been approved by the Environmental Protection Agency as an effective disinfectant against certain disease-producing organisms, 83

Epicranius, broad muscle that covers the top of the skull; also known as occipito-frontalis, 148–149, 302

Epidemic, 66, 228

Epidermis, outermost layer of the skin; also called the cuticle or scarf skin, 220–221

Epilators, 195

Eponychium, living skin at the base of the nail plate and covering the matrix area, 673

Equipment
  brush machines, 313–314
  electric facial machines, 320–321
  electric massagers, 133, 285, 313, 329, 332
  galvanic machines, 132, 318–320, 336–337
  high-frequency machines, 132, 315–318, 337
  hot-towel cabinet, 132, 314
  hydraulic chairs, 133
  manicuring, 681
  massage, 313–323
  safety precautions with, 96
  steamers, 314–315
  therapeutic lamps, 213

Ergonomics, the study of human characteristics related to the specific work environment, 40–41

Implements (Continued)
shears, 108–111
tweezers, 133
Inactive stage (spore-forming), the stage in which bacteria do not grow or reproduce, 58–59
Income, 759
Independent contractor, a form of self-employment and tax designation with specific responsibilities for bookkeeping, taxes, insurances, etc., 727, 746–748
Indirect application, high-frequency current administered with the client holding the wire glass electrode between both hands, 317–318
Indirect division, the method by which a mature cell reproduces in the body, 140
Industry trends, 720–721
Infected finger, 675
Infection control
chemical disinfectants, 80–85
physical agents for, 81
prevention and control, 80–85
public sanitation, 81, 93–94
for shaving, 348–350
solution strengths, 85–86
Infection, the result when the body is unable to cope with the invasion of bacteria and their harmful toxins, 59, 70
Infectious diseases, 59–60, 66, 228. *See also* Sanitary measures
parasitic, 262–263
public sanitation and, 93–94
staphylococci infections, 263–264
Universal Precautions for, 90
Inferior labial artery, artery that supplies blood to the lower lip, 160
Inflammation, 66, 228
Infraorbital artery, artery that supplies blood to the eye muscles, 160
Infraorbital nerve, nerve that affects the skin of the lower eyelid, side of the nose, upper lip, and mouth, 155, 305
Infrared-ray lamps, 321, 336
Infrared rays, invisible rays with long wavelengths and deep penetration; produce the most heat of any therapeutic light, 215
Infratrochlear nerve, nerve that affects the membrane and skin of the nose, 155, 305

Innovative learners, 8
Inorganic chemistry, chemistry dealing with compounds lacking carbon, 174
Insertion of a muscle, the more moveable attachment of a muscle, 147
Instant conditioners, conditioners that typically remain on the hair from one to five minutes and are rinsed out, 191
Insulator, substance that does not easily transfer electricity, 204, 208
Integumentary system, the skin at its appendages, 142, 164
Interactive learners, 8–9
Internal carotid artery, artery that supplies blood to the brain, eyes, eyelids, forehead, nose, and ear, 159
Internal jugular vein, vein located at the side of the neck; collects blood from the brain and parts of the face and neck, 161
Interview Evaluation Inventory, 763
Interviews, 731–735
Intestines, 141
Intuitive learners, 9
Ionization, the separating of a substance into ions, 180
Ions, an atom or molecule that carries an electric charge, 180, 208
Iontophoresis, process of introducing water-soluble products into the skin through the use of electric current, 211, 318, 320
Ivy dermatitis, a skin inflammation caused by exposure to the poison ivy, poison oak, or poison sumac, 233

J
Jheri curls. *See* Reformation curls
Job search
employment interviews, 731–735
field research, 730–731
preparing for, 722–731
Journeymen barber groups, barber employee unions, 22
Journeymen Barbers' International Union, 22–23

K
Keloid, thick scar resulting from excessive tissue growth, 231
Keratinization, 246

Keratin, the protein of which hair is formed, 242
Keratoma, technical name for a callus, caused by pressure or friction, 231
Kidneys, 141
Kilowatt-hour, 208
Knotted hair, 265
Knotting, 488

L
Labeling, 78
Lace-front, popular hair solution style used for off-the-face styles, 488, 501–502
Lacrimal bones, small bones located in the wall of the eye sockets, 144
Lanthionization, process by which hydroxide relaxers permanently straighten hair; lanthionization breaks the hair's disulfide bonds during processing and converts them to lanthionine bonds when the relaxer is rinsed from the hair, 572
Lanugo, vellus hair, 250
Latex allergies, 479
Lather brushes, 128
Lathering, 360
Lather mugs, 128
Lather receptacles, 128–129
Laws of color, a system for understanding color relationships, 616–618
Lawsuits, 758
Layers, graduated effect achieved by cutting the hair with elevation or over-direction; the hair is cut at higher elevations, usually 90 degrees or above, which removes weight, 400–401
Learning styles, classifications that are used to identify the different ways in which people learn, 8–10
Leases, 753–754
Leave-in conditioners, conditioners and thermal protectors that can be left in the hair without rinsing, 192
Legal responsibilities, 755
Lentigines, technical name for freckles, 231
Lesion, a structural change in the tissues caused by injury or disease, 229–231

Melanin, coloring matter or pigment of the skin; found in the stratum germinativum of the epidermis and in the papillary layers of the dermis, 224

Melanocytes, 224

Melanonychia, darkening of the nail due to increased and localized pigment in the matrix bed, 675, 677

Melanosomes, 224

Memory, improving, 4–5

Men

    facial massage for, 300–307

    facial treatments for, 323–340

    skin care for, 300, 328–329, 341–343

Mentalis, muscle that elevates the lower lip and raises and wrinkles the skin of the chin, 149–150, 302

Mental nerve, nerve that affects the skin of the lower lip and chin, 155, 305

Merchandising of products, 343

Meryma'at, Egyptian barber commemorated with a statue, 17

Metabolism, a complex chemical process whereby cells are nourished and supplied with the energy needed to carry out their activities, 140–141

Metacarpus, contains the metacarpal bones in the palm of the hand, 146

Metallic dyes, 593, 623, 659–660

Methicillin-resistant *Staphylococcus aureus,* 59, 70

Microbes. *See* Bacteria

Microbiology, 56

Microdermabrasion, 320–321

Middle Ages, 20

Middle temporal artery, artery that supplies blood to the temples, 160

Miliaria rubra, technical name for prickly heat, 235

Milia, technical name for milk spots; small, benign, whitish bumps that occur when dead skin is trapped in the surface of the skin, commonly seen in infants, 234

Milliampere, 206

Milliampere meter, 208

Mind-mapping, a graphic representation of an idea or problem that helps to organize one's thoughts, 5–6

Mineral dyes, 623

Minoxidil, topical medication used to promote hair growth or reduce hair loss, 259, 515

Miscible, 184

Mitosis, cells dividing into two new cells (daughter cells), 58, 70, 140

Mixed-hair products, 487

Mixed nerves, nerves that contain both sensory and motor nerve fibers; can send and receive messages, 154

Mnemonics, any memorization device that helps a person to recall information, 5

Modalities, currents used in electric facial and scalp treatments, 209–210

Model Release Form, form used to permit the use of a model's pictures for print or exposure, 730

Moisturizers, 327

Moisturizing conditioners, contain humectants to absorb and promote the retention of moisture in the hair, 192

Moisturizing creams, 196

Moisturizing or conditioning shampoos, products formulated to add moisture to dry hair, 191

Molecules, two or more atoms joined chemically, 175–176

Moler, A. B., he wrote the first barbering textbook; opened the first barber school in Chicago in 1893, 23

Mole, small brownish spot on the skin, 231

Monilethrix, 265

Moses, 17

Motivation, a desire for change, 47

Motor nerve fibers, nerve fibers distributed to the arrector pili muscles, which are attached to the hair follicles, 223

Motor nerves, nerves that carry impulses from the brain to the muscles, 154

Motor points, a point on the skin, over a muscle, where pressure or stimulation will cause contraction of that muscle, 308–309

Mouth muscles, 149–151

MRSA, acronym for methicillin-resistant *Staphylococcus aureus;* a type of staph infection resistant to certain antibiotics, 59, 70, 101

MSDS. *See* Material Safety Data Sheet

Muscles, system that covers, shapes, and supports the skeleton; contracts and moves various parts of the body, 300

    ear, 149, 151

    eyebrow, 150

    face, 148–151

    hand, 151

    mastication, 148–149, 151

    mouth, 149–151

    neck, 149, 151

    nose, 149–150

    scalp, 148–149

    stimulation of, 148, 303

    structure of, 147–148

Muscular system, body system that covers, shapes, and supports the skeletal tissue, 142, 147–151

Mustaches

    coloring of, 661–662

    designing of, 377

    trimming of, 378, 384, 386

Myology, study of the structure, function, and diseases of the muscles, 147

N

Nail bed, portion of the skin on which the nail plate rests, 673

Nail brush, 682

Nail buffer, 682

Nail cosmetics, 684–686

Nail folds, folds of normal skin around the nail plate, 674

Nail fungus, 67

Nail grooves, slits or furrows on the sides of the nail, 674

Nail plate, horny plate resting on and attached to the nail bed, 673

Nail psoriasis, tiny pits or roughness on the surface of the nail plate, 679

Nail pterygium, abnormal condition occurring when skin is stretched by the nail plate, 675, 677

Nails, an appendage of the skin; horny protective plate at

the end of the finger or toe, 672–674. *See also* Manicuring
disorders and diseases, 674–680
growth of, 674
malformations, 674
structure of, 672–674
Nasal bones, **bones that form the bridge of the nose,** 144
Nasal nerve, **nerve that affects the point and lower sides of the nose,** 155, 305
National Association of Barber Boards of America, **the association of the state barber boards,** 24–25
National Association of Barber Schools, 24
National Association of State Board of Barber Examiners, 24
National Educational Council, 24
Natural drying, 470–471
Natural dry styling, 549
Natural hones, 121
Natural immunity, **natural resistance to disease that is partially inherited and partially developed,** 68
Neck bones, 145
Neck dusters, 129
Neck lengths, 396
Neck muscles, 149, 151
Neck shave, **shaving the areas behind the ears, down the sides of the neck, and at the back neckline,** 373–375, 429
Neck strip, 276
Negative thoughts, 46
Nerves (neurons), 153–156, 300, 303–306
skin, 223
stimulation of, 303
Nervous system, 142, 152–156
Net profit, 760
Neurology, 152
Neurons. *See* Nerves
Neutralization, **process of stopping the action of a permanent wave solution and hardening the hair in its new form by the application of a chemical solution called the neutralizer,** 589–590
Neutralizer, 598
Neutron, 208
Nevus, **technical name for a birthmark,** 232
No-base relaxers, **relaxers that do not require application of a protective base,** 603

Nonionics, 189
Nonpathogenic bacteria, **beneficial or harmless bacteria that perform many useful functions,** 57
Nonstriated muscles, 147
Normal skin, 324
Nose muscles, 149–150
Nose shapes, 395
Nostril hair trimming, 470
Notching, 428, 547
Note-taking, 6
Nucleus, **dense, active protoplasm found in the center of a cell; important to reproduction and metabolism,** 140
Nutrition, 38

O

Objective symptoms, **symptoms that can be seen by anyone,** 60, 66, 228
Occipital artery, **artery that supplies the scalp and back of the head up to the crown,** 161, 307
Occipital bone, **hindmost bone of the skull; located below the parietal bones,** 143
Occipitalis, **back of the epicranius; muscle that draws the scalp backward,** 149, 302
Occupational disease, 66, 228
Occupational Safety and Health Act, **an act that led to the creation of OSH Act,** 75
Occupational Safety and Health Administration (OSHA), **also referred to as OSHA, whose primary purpose is to assure, regulate, and enforce safe and healthful working conditions in the workplace,** 75
Oculomotor nerve, 304
Off-base, **position of a curl off its base; provides maximum mobility and minimum volume,** 555, 582
Off-the-scalp lighteners, **lighteners that cannot be used directly on the scalp,** 627
Ohm (O), **the unit of electrical resistance in an electrical current,** 206, 208
Oil glands, 225
Oily skin, 324
facial for, 338
Ointments, 186
Olfactory nerve, 304

On-base, **position of a curl directly on its base; provides maximum volume,** 555, 582
Once-over shave, **single-lather shave in which the shaving strokes are made across the grain of the hair,** 371
One-length cut, 523–527
On-the-scalp lighteners, **lighteners that can be used directly on the scalp,** 627
Onychia, **inflammation of the matrix with pus, redness, swelling, and shedding of the nail,** 676, 679
Onychocryptosis, **ingrown nails,** 676, 679
Onycholysis, **loosening of the nail without shedding,** 676, 679
Onychomadesis, **the separation and falling off of the nail from the nail bed,** 676, 679
Onychomycosis, **fungal infection; whitish patches on nail that can be scraped off or long yellowish streaks within nail plate,** 676, 680
Onychophagy, **bitten nails,** 675, 677
Onychorrhexis, **abnormal brittleness of the nail plate,** 675, 677
Onychosis, **technical term for any deformity or disease of the nail,** 676
Onyx, **technical term for nail,** 672. *See also* Nails
Opponent muscles, **muscles in the palm that bring the thumb toward the fingers,** 151
Optic nerve, 304
Orbicularis oculi, **ring muscle of the eye socket,** 149–150, 302
Orbicularis oris, **flat band around the upper and lower lips,** 149–150, 302
Organic chemistry, **study of substances that contain carbon,** 174
Organic shampoos, **formulated from natural organic ingredients,** 191
Organization, **a method used to store new information for short-term and long-term memory,** 4–5
Organs, **structures composed of specialized tissues performing specific functions,** 141

of a substance, 180–182, 187, 273

pH scale, a measure of the concentration of hydrogen ions in acidic and alkaline solutions, 180–181

Physical appearance, 37–41

Physical change, change in the form of a substance without the formation of a new substance, 177

Physical mixtures, combination of two or more substance united physically, 178–179

Physical properties, characteristics of matter that can be determined without a chemical reaction, 176

Physiology, study of the functions or activities performed by the body's structures, 139

Pick combs, 106

Piggyback perm wrap, 591

Pincer or trumpet nail, edge of nail plate curls around to form a trumpet or cone shape at the free edge, 675, 678

Pin curls, 549

Pityriasis capitis simplex, dry dandruff type, 260

Pityriasis steatoides, waxy or greasy dandruff type, 260

Pityrosporum, 260

Pivot motor clippers, 112

Planning, any action taken prior to the draft writing process when preparing a report or presentation, 7, 13

Plasma, fluid part of blood and lymph, 159

Plastic mold form, 494–497

Platelets, blood cells that aid in forming clots, 159

Platysma, muscle that extends from the chest and shoulder to the side of the chin; depresses lower jaw and lip, 149, 151, 303

Plicatured nail, "folded nail"; highly curved nail plate often caused by injury, 675, 678

Plug, 208

Point cutting, 547

Polarity changer, 208

Polarity, negative or positive pole of an electric current, 209–210

Polish application, 686–687

Polymer, 192

Polypeptide chain, long chain of amino acids linked by peptide bonds, 247

Portfolio, collection of photographs depicting the barber's work, 729–730

Port wine stain, 232

Posterior auricular artery, artery that supplies blood to the scalp, behind and above the ear, 161, 307

Posterior auricular nerve, nerve that affects the muscles behind the ear at the base of the skull, 156, 305

Postperm care, 590

Posture, 38–40

Potassium hydroxide, 198, 602–603

Potential hydrogen. *See* pH

Powders, 183

Practical exam, hands-on test on a live model, 710–713

Pre-lightening, the first step of a double-process haircoloring, used to lighten natural pigment, 627, 644

Preservative treatments, 323

Pre-softening, process of treating resistant hair for better color penetration, 637

Press-button can latherizers, 128

Pressing combs, 131

Pre-wrap solution, usually a type of leave-in conditioner that may be applied to the hair prior to permanent waving to equalize porosity, 586–587

Prewriting, 7

Pricing, 764

Primary colors, red, blue, and yellow; colors that cannot be achieved from a mixture of other colors, 616

Primary lesions, 229–230

Primary terminal hair, short, thick hairs that grow on the eyebrows and lashes, 250

Procerus, muscle that covers the bridge of the nose, depresses the eyebrows, and wrinkles the nose, 149–150, 302

Product labeling, 78

Professional ethics, 44–45

Professional image, the impression projected by a person in any profession, consisting of outward appearance and

conduct exhibited in the workplace, 34–41

Professional responsibilities, 99

Profiles, 395

Prognosis, 67, 228

Progressive colors, haircolor products that contain compound or metallic dyes, which build up on the hair; not used professionally, 623

Projection, angle or elevation that hair is held from head for cutting, 399–400

Protein conditioners, products designed to slightly increase hair diameter with a coating action and to replace lost proteins in hair, 192

Proteins, 246–247

Proton, 208

Pseudofolliculitis barbae, a chronic inflammatory form of folliculitis known associated with "razor bumps," resembling folliculitis papules and pustules; generally accepted to be caused by ingrown hair, 263–264

Pseudomonas aeruginosa, skin bacteria that can cause an infection of the nail, 678

Psoriasis, skin disease characterized by red patches and silvery-white scales, 233

Public sanitation, the application of measures used to promote public health and prevent the spread of infectious diseases, 81, 93–94

Pure substance, matter that has a fixed chemical composition, definite proportions, and distinct properties, 177–178

Pus, a fluid that contains white blood cells, dead and living bacteria, waste matter, tissue elements, and body cells; a sign of infection, 59

Pustule, inflamed pimple, containing pus, 230

Pyrogenic granuloma, severe inflammation of the nail in which a lump of red tissue grows up from the nail bed to the nail plate, 676, 680

Witch hazel, 198
Women
    haircutting for, 522–563
    hairstyling for, 548–563
Word associations, 5
Worshipful Company of Barbers
    guild, 21
Wrinkles, 324–325
Wrinkle treatment creams, 196
**Written exam, paper and pencil
    or computer-based testing**
covering theoretical concepts
related to barbering and bar-
bering law specific to the state,
706–710

Z

Zero elevation, 399
Zinc oxide, 198
**Zygomatic bones, bones that
    form the prominence of the
    cheeks,** 144

Zygomatic nerve, nerve that
    affects the skin of the temple,
    side of the forehead, and upper
    cheek, 155–156, 305
Zygomaticus major, 149–150
Zygomaticus minor, 149–150
Zygomaticus, muscle extend-
    ing from the zygomatic bone
    to the angle of the mouth;
    elevates the lip as in laughing,
    149–150, 303